RADIATION PROTECTION
IN MEDICAL
RADIOGRAPHY

RADIATION PROTECTION
IN MEDICAL
RADIOGRAPHY

Mary Alice Statkiewicz Sherer, AS, RT(R), FASRT
Paula J. Visconti, PhD, DABR
E. Russell Ritenour, PhD, DABR, FAAPM, FACR
Kelli Welch Haynes, MSRS, RT(R)

8TH EDITION

ELSEVIER

ELSEVIER

3251 Riverport Lane
St. Louis, Missouri 63043

RADIATION PROTECTION IN MEDICAL RADIOGRAPHY, EIGHTH EDITION ISBN: 978-0-323-44666-2

Notices

Knowledge and best practice in this field are constantly changing. As new research and experience broaden our understanding, changes in research methods, professional practices, or medical treatment may become necessary.

Practitioners and researchers must always rely on their own experience and knowledge in evaluating and using any information, methods, compounds, or experiments described herein. In using such information or methods they should be mindful of their own safety and the safety of others, including parties for whom they have a professional responsibility.

With respect to any drug or pharmaceutical products identified, readers are advised to check the most current information provided (i) on procedures featured or (ii) by the manufacturer of each product to be administered, to verify the recommended dose or formula, the method and duration of administration, and contraindications. It is the responsibility of practitioners, relying on their own experience and knowledge of their patients, to make diagnoses, to determine dosages and the best treatment for each individual patient, and to take all appropriate safety precautions.

To the fullest extent of the law, neither the Publisher nor the authors, contributors, or editors, assume any liability for any injury and/or damage to persons or property as a matter of products liability, negligence or otherwise, or from any use or operation of any methods, products, instructions, or ideas contained in the material herein.

Library of Congress Cataloging-in-Publication Data

Names: Statkiewicz-Sherer, Mary Alice, 1945- author. | Visconti, Paula J., author. | Ritenour, E. Russell, 1953- author. | Haynes, Kelli (Kelli Welch), author.
Title: Radiation protection in medical radiography / Mary Alice Statkiewicz Sherer, Paula J. Visconti, E. Russell Ritenour, Kelli Welch Haynes.
Description: Eighth edition. | St. Louis, Missouri: Elsevier, [2018] | Includes bibliographical references and index.
Identifiers: LCCN 2017039022 (print) | LCCN 2017039993 (ebook) | ISBN 9780323566780 (ebook) | ISBN 9780323446662 (pbk. : alk. paper)
Subjects: | MESH: Radiation Protection–methods | Radiography–adverse effects | Radiation Monitoring–methods
Classification: LCC RC78.3 (ebook) | LCC RC78.3 (print) | NLM WN 650 | DDC 616.07/570289–dc23
LC record available at https://lccn.loc.gov/2017039022

Executive Content Strategist: Sonya Seigafuse
Content Development Manager: Lisa Newton
Senior Content Development Specialist: Laura Selkirk
Publishing Services Manager: Deepthi Unni
Project Manager: Manchu Mohan
Design Direction: Amy Buxton

Printed in Canada

Last digit is the print number: 9 8 7 6 5 4 3 2 1

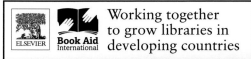

Working together to grow libraries in developing countries

www.elsevier.com • www.bookaid.org

In memory of my parents, Felix J. and Elizabeth M. Krohn,
To my sons, Joseph F. Statkiewicz, Christopher R. Statkiewicz, and Terry R. Sherer, Jr., with love,
And
To all with whom I may share my knowledge.

REVIEWERS

James Adams, MHA, RT(R) (CT) (MR) (QM) (BD) (ARRT)
Radiography Academic Program Director
Jefferson Community College & Technical College
Department of Allied Health & Nursing
Louisville, Kentucky

Janet E. Akers, MET, RT(R) (M)
Program Director
Jefferson College Radiologic Technology Program
Department of Health Occupations
Hillsboro, Missouri

Deanna Butcher, MA, RT(R)
Program Director
St. Cloud Hospital School of Diagnostic Imaging
St. Cloud, Minnesota

Mary Ellen Carpenter, MA, RT(R) (CV) (CT)
Radiography Program Faculty
Essex County College
Newark, New Jersey

Doyle B. Decker, MA, RT(R) (CT)
Radiography Program Coordinator
Somerset Community College
Somerset, Kentucky

Mary C. Doucette, MS, RRA RT(R) (M) (MR) (QM) (CT)
Program Director
Great Basin College
Elko, Nevada

Ursula A. Dyer, MS, BS, RT(R) (CT)
Program Director
Radiologic Science
Kilgore College
Kilgore, Texas

Gail J. Faig, BS, RT(R) (CV) (CT)
Program Director
Shore Medical Center
School of Radiologic Technology
Somers Point, New Jersey

Lisa Fanning, MEd, RT (R) (CT)
Chair, School of Medical Imaging & Therapeutics
MCPHS University
Boston, Massachusetts

Joe A. Garza, MS, BS, RT(R)
Professor/Clinical Coordinator
Lone Star College Montgomery
Conroe, Texas

Steven Iacono, MBA, BE, RT(R)
Director, Radiography Program
Northampton Community College
Bethlehem, Pennsylvania

Barbara A. Kissel, MBA, RT(R), CRT, F
Assistant Professor, Program Director
Radiologic Technology
Pasadena City College
Pasadena, California

Kristi Klein, MS, Ed, RT(R) (M) (CT)
Program Director
Madison Area Technical College
Radiography Program
Madison, Wisconsin

Carol R. Kocher, MS, RT(R) (M)
Program Director
Olney Central College
Olney, Illinois

Cynthia A. Meyers, MS, RT(R)
Program Coordinator
Niagara County Community College
Sanborn, New York

Elizabeth Price, EdD, RT(R) (M) (CT)
Associate Dean, STEM
Rowan College at Burlington County
Mt. Laurel, New Jersey

Amy C. VonKadich, MEd, RT(T)
Department Chair, Diagnostic Medical Imaging
NHTI: Concord's Community College
Department of Diagnostic Medical Imaging
Concord, New Hampshire

Patricia Weber, MHA, RT(R) (CT)
Assistant Professor
Radiologic Technology and Medical imaging
Clarkson College
Omaha, Nebraska

Diana S. Werderman, MS, Ed, RT(R)
Assistant Professor
Trinity College of Nursing & Health Sciences
Rock Island, Illinois

The books on the shelves in my office are positioned by subject: medical physics, health physics, radiobiology, radiography/fluoroscopy, mammography, computed tomography, magnetic resonance imaging, and diagnostic ultrasound. My copy of Sherer et al's *Radiation Protection in Medical Radiography (RPMR)* rests with a dozen other books whose principal effort is health physics, or as most of us think of it, "radiation protection."

But RPMR is much more than radiation protection because it deals with most areas of medical imaging to a sufficient depth that it could rest among my medical physics volumes. What I like best about the textbook is its breadth yet its brevity. It is not a thick, heavy textbook to be avoided, but rather a complete coverage of radiation protection in medical imaging while at the same time providing substantial medical physics text to satisfy that subject for most students and educators.

I particularly like the layout of this text, which greatly improves its readability. RPMR is well organized with properly highlighted and richly illustrated tables, figures, and photographs to aid in quick comprehension.

This eighth edition of RPMR is totally up to date on its principal mission: radiation protection. Recent years have seen the expression of increasing concern regarding patient radiation dose and potential population responses.

The authors cover this admirably with discussions of Image Gently, Image Wisely, and several new documents from NAS/BEIR (National Academy of Sciences Committee on the Biological Effects of Ionizing Radiation) and NCRP (National Council on Radiation Protection and Measurements).

The publisher has done its part, too. The early editions were published by the C. V. Mosby Company, which was bought by Elsevier, and Elsevier has done a super job with very helpful supplementary material for all. Some of this assistance is described in the highly complete and complementary appendices. The user is encouraged to visit the appendices early in the use of this textbook. The user will also find lots of help at the publisher's website, Evolve.

The training and experience of the authors are apparent. They are scientists, clinical practicing radiologic technologists, and educators. This shows in their practical writing skill.

Stewart Carlyle Bushong, ScD, FAAPM, FACR
Professor of Radiologic Science
Baylor College of Medicine
Houston, Texas

PREFACE

CONTENT

Extensively revised and expanded, the eighth edition of *Radiation Protection in Medical Radiography* continues to offer radiation science professionals on multiple levels essential and timely information on the elements of radiation safety. This includes extended discussions on radiation protection, radiobiology, and relevant radiation physics, all designed to fully educate professionals in the safe use of x-rays in diagnostic imaging.

Information in this edition begins with an introduction to radiation protection followed by reviews of various types and sources of radiation and radiation doses received. Other subject matter includes topics such as the interactions of x-radiation with matter, radiation quantities and units, and radiation monitoring. A chapter covering an overview of cell biology prepares the reader for the discussion of molecular and cellular radiation biology that follows.

Readers become aware of recent changes in concepts and terminology in the two chapters entitled "Early Tissue Reactions and Their Effects on Organ Systems" and "Stochastic Effects and Late Tissue Reactions of Radiation in Organ Systems." This updated information is also addressed in later chapters.

Priority is also given to the topic of dose limits for exposure to ionizing radiation. Because x-ray and ancillary equipment constantly undergoes change, equipment design for radiation protection is also covered. Great emphasis is placed on management of patient radiation dose during diagnostic procedures, and special considerations on safety in computed tomography and mammography are also addressed. Because management of imaging personnel radiation dose during x-ray procedures is extremely important, it, too, is discussed in detail.

To create awareness of opportunity for advancement in other imaging modalities and the special safety considerations needed in procedures in those disciplines, the final chapter covers radioisotopes and their associated radiation protection. This chapter also contains relevant information on radiation emergencies, such as the use of radiation as a terrorist weapon and the appropriate handling and procedures to follow in such situations.

Another invaluable feature of this textbook is an appendix that presents a wealth of additional material in 12 separate appendices. These address topics that complement and expand information in the various chapters.

The format of each chapter remains the same as in previous editions. Bullets continue to be used to enhance readability by calling attention to specific information, and key terms as before, are identified in bold print. The authors have endeavored to present material in this textbook in a succinct but reasonably complete fashion to meet the ongoing needs of the various members of the health care sector. With each edition, the authors have sought to expand the scope of the subject matter covered in the text to provide the reader with a broader base of knowledge.

New to This Edition

Many extra figures and improved illustrations are presented throughout the textbook. These and other artwork enhance the visual impact of the text, thereby promoting visual learning and aiding the reader's understanding of various material.

The number of chapters in the textbook has increased from 14 to 15 to accommodate the inclusion of specific new information. In addition, the order of selective materials in some chapters has been rearranged to facilitate more effective and efficient delivery of all subject matter covered. This edition also contains an updated and much-expanded glossary of relevant terms associated with radiation protection, radiobiology, and relevant radiation physics. The authors believe that this glossary can serve as a very useful overall quick-review tool.

Chapter Contents

Information covered in **Chapter 1** includes a discussion of the use of ionizing radiation in the healing arts, beginning with the discovery of x-rays in 1895, the fundamental properties of x-rays, team concept in the medical field, and the control of radiant energy. Goals and concepts of radiation protection have now been moved to this chapter. In addition, a simplified introduction to the three main radiation quantities and their units of measure is presented to acquaint students with these concepts earlier in their education. Sections on the justification and responsibility for imaging procedures, and the *as low as reasonably achievable* (ALARA) principle remain but have been updated.

Other revised topics include patient protection and patient education, which bring into consideration the risk of imaging procedures versus the potential benefit of such procedures. Ongoing discussion of the use of background equivalent radiation time (BERT) to inform patients of the amount of radiation they will receive during a specific x-ray procedure continues to be an important component of this chapter. Segments on the increased radiation sensitivity in children, the Alliance for Radiation Safety in Pediatric Radiology, the Image Gently, and the Image Wisely Campaigns have been moved forward to this first chapter to foster awareness of the magnitude of these topics to the learner. Other new sections in Chapter 1 are monitoring and reporting radiation dose, the NEXT Program, and reference values and protocols for dose alert.

Chapter 2 presents information on radiation types, sources, and doses received. Current discussions on the electromagnetic spectrum, ionizing and nonionizing radiation, and particulate radiation are also included. A section on the *concept of radiation dose* has been added to give an appreciation of radiation doses that humans can receive and have received. Updated information on biologic damage potential and various sources of this, both natural and manmade, are included in this section to expand the reader's knowledge of radiation and its ability to cause injury in living tissue. Follow-up data regarding nuclear power plant accidents are covered under the section on manmade radiation.

Relevant radiation physics, such as the interactions of x-radiation with matter, are covered in **Chapter 3**. This information has been both revised and expanded in order to offer the reader a clearer, yet more detailed, discussion of these topics. The purpose of this is to make learning easier by providing essential background knowledge and the comprehension of those concepts of radiation protection and the subject matter of radiobiology, which are presented in later chapters.

Whereas the first two chapters provided a brief introduction to the topic of radiation quantities and units of measure, **Chapter 4** offers a much more detailed discussion of this subject. Beginning with their historical evolution, the chapter progresses with updated information on radiation quantities and units of measure and focuses on what is now currently in use. Thus great emphasis is placed on the utilization of the metric system to increase the learner's comprehension of the Systems International (SI) units of measure. A strong effort has also been made to more clearly define all terms involving radiation dose.

Radiation monitoring for personnel and information on types of radiation survey instruments and their usage are covered in **Chapter 5**. Discussion on the newest type of personnel monitor, the personnel digital ionization dosimeter, is now included in this chapter, and information on other types of personnel monitors currently in use has been updated. The section on radiation survey instruments for area monitoring has also been updated.

A detailed overview of cell biology is presented in **Chapter 6**. This basic chapter covers cell chemical composition, cell structure, and cell division. Where appropriate, material has been updated. New information also has been added in some sections (e.g., the human genome, various cell components and functions, more expanded definitions of terms and processes, and added figures), all of which are intended to lend much greater learning value to this chapter. Information contained in this chapter serves as a prerequisite for the material covered in the next chapter.

Chapter 7 covers molecular and cellular radiation biology. Main topics included in this section are the molecular effects of irradiation and radiation energy transfer determinants, such as the oxygen effect and the consequences of exposure to different types of radiation. Also covered in detail are cell radiosensitivity and survival curves for mammalian cells. Discussions of subject matter under these categories have been updated and enhanced.

With changes in both concept and terminology, **Chapter 8** is dedicated to covering material on the somatic effects of radiation, which are effects of radiation upon the body that was irradiated. These specific outcomes examined occur within minutes, hours, days, or weeks of irradiation and as a result of this are named *early tissue reactions*. Added material relating to this new terminology is presented.

Stochastic effects and *late tissue reactions* of radiation in organ systems are considered in **Chapter 9**. Effects that occur months or years after exposure to radiation are the focus of this chapter. These late effects can be either delayed tissue reactions, such as the formation of cataracts, or stochastic effects, such as the induction of cancer or genetic alterations. Extra material has been added to clarify the use of the new terminology. In addition, chapter contents include detailed coverage of epidemiology, radiation dose–response relationship, late somatic effects, and genetic effects. The contents of many subtopics in this chapter have also been updated.

Chapter 10 addresses the subject of current dose limits for exposure to ionizing radiation. The basis of the effective dose limiting system is also discussed, along with the identification and function of the various current radiation protection organizations. Existing US regulatory agencies are identified, and their tasks are earmarked. Other topics include requirements for a radiation safety program and information about the necessity for and duties of the radiation safety committee. The responsibilities, needed training, and authority of the radiation safety officer (RSO) is also described at length in this chapter. Although the ALARA concept has been covered earlier in the text, it is now discussed in greater detail. The position of the US Food and Drug Administration (FDA) as it relates to patient radiation dose is identified in a self-published document called the "White Paper." This information is given within the chapter. The value and importance of the Consumer-Patient Radiation Health and Safety Act of 1981 are also explained. Radiation-induced responses of concern in radiation protection are identified by category, and new terminology recently introduced is fully described. Risk associated with radiation exposure in medical imaging is also covered. Use of tissue weighting factors and the concept underlying radiation protection are presented. Current National Council on Radiation Protection and Measurements recommendations are reviewed, and action limits for emergency situations are identified. Subject matter on radiation hormesis has been expanded and updated. Finally, occupational and nonoccupational dose limits are discussed.

Equipment design for radiation protection is dealt with in **Chapter 11**. The latest advances in imaging equipment that pertain to safety as well as other devices and accessories that may be used to provide radiation protection for the patient and for the equipment operator are reviewed.

Chapter 12 concentrates on management of patient radiation dose during diagnostic x-ray procedures. Many topics in this chapter have been revised with the latest available information. Material covered includes discussion of the need for effective communication, immobilization methods used to minimize or prevent patient motion during a radiographic exposure, and the need for protective shielding for the patient's gonadal area or another specific area. Selection of appropriate technical exposure factors obtained from standardized technique charts is stressed, as is the use of higher kVp with lower mAs exposure technique factors to reduce dose to the patient. Other topics considered are the need for correct radiographic image postprocessing and the importance of a having a quality control program. Use of a high kVp air gap technique to reduce scattered radiation is also reviewed. Emphasis is placed on the topic of *repeat images,* and consequences of such repeats are identified. The value of having a repeat analysis program is demonstrated. Again, the topic of *benefit* versus *risk* as it pertains to x-ray examinations is discussed. Nonessential radiologic examinations are specified, and concern about risk of exposure from diagnostic imaging procedures is addressed. This includes a discussion of the importance of eliminating the unethical practice of *fluoroscopically guided positioning.* Considerable space is allotted to the topic of protecting pregnant or potentially pregnant patients. Several subtopics in this section have been updated. Finally, the chapter reviews pediatric considerations during radiographic imaging. The Image Gently Campaign for reducing radiation dose for children and the Image Wisely Campaign for reducing dose for adults are also detailed in this chapter.

Special considerations on safety in computed tomography (CT) and mammography are now covered in **Chapter 13**. This is a newly created chapter designed to inform about the various methods employed for radiation protection in these selective procedures. Many of the topics and subtopics covered contain relatively new information. The section on patient dose in CT includes the following subtopics: radiation exposure, skin dose and dose distribution, direct patient shielding, and characteristics of spiral, or helical, CT. Under the topic of methods for reduction of patient dose in CT, the following items are addressed: tube current modulation, iterative reconstruction, optimization of tube voltage, and patient centering. There are also sections on dose parameters, effective CT dose, and the goal of CT imaging from a radiation protection point of view. The section on patient dose in mammography includes the following subtopics: mammography screening, digital mammography, filtration for mammography equipment, and a brief explanation of a new imaging method: digital tomosynthesis.

Management of imaging personnel radiation dose during general diagnostic x-ray procedures is the prime focus in **Chapter 14**. Information contained within this chapter has been updated to reflect the most current radiation safety practices. Annual limits for occupationally exposed personnel are identified. The ALARA concept as it pertains to protection of personnel in the clinical setting is discussed. Various methods to lower occupational dose are identified and described. Special attention is given to protection for pregnant personnel. The cardinal, or basic, principles of radiation protection for personnel exposure reduction is addressed, and methods of protection during general fluoroscopic procedures are examined. The use of protective garments and where a radiographer should stand while performing a mobile radiographic examination are reviewed. Protection for the operator during C-arm fluoroscopy and during high-level-control interventional procedures is also given much attention. In addition, an overview of diagnostic x-ray suite protection design, which includes the following subtopics: requirement for radiation-absorbed barriers, reasons for overshielding, calculating barrier shielding requirements, and new approaches to shielding, is presented. Finally, there is a discussion about radiation warning signs.

Chapter 15, the last chapter in the text, covers the topics of radioisotopes and their associated radiation protection. This chapter, which has been updated, provides an excellent resource for qualified individuals wanting to advance into other disciplines beyond diagnostic imaging such as nuclear medicine or radiation therapy. Under the main heading of medical usage, the following subtopics are included: radiation therapy, handling and disposal of radioactive materials, nuclear medicine, positron emission tomography combined with computed tomography, and radiation protection. The second half of the chapter discusses radiation emergencies and the use of radiation as a terrorist weapon. Subtopics include contamination, cleanup of a contaminated urban area, and medical management of persons experiencing radiation bioeffects.

As previously mentioned in the preface, this latest edition of the text contains a considerable number of new and revised figures and illustrations. These include photographs, diagrams, information boxes, and tables. They have been added or updated throughout the book as required to increase the reader's comprehension of various subject matter, thereby promoting visual learning.

LEARNING ENHANCEMENTS

Each chapter begins with a list of learning objectives to master, followed by a chapter outline, and a list of key terms that will appear in bold print in each chapter. Following the list of key terms, an introductory paragraph provides an overview of the material to be covered. Bullets are used throughout the text to facilitate readability and to call attention to specific information.

Chapter content is followed by a bulleted summary that highlights the most important information in each chapter. A list of references follows the chapter summary. A list of general discussion questions comes after the list of references. These general discussion questions are then followed by a series of multiple-choice review questions that the reader can use to assess knowledge acquired from completing each chapter. Instructors may also use the general discussion questions or the multiple-choice review questions to stimulate discussion of selected topics of interest. Bold print has been used to focus the attention of the reader on the key terms in each chapter. These key terms may also be found in the enhanced glossary now located in the back matter of the textbook. Throughout the text, information boxes are present to direct the reader to important information. The back matter of the book also contains a series of well-developed appendices that provide supporting material for subject matter contained within the chapters of the text and offer additional relevant information. Answers to the multiple-choice review questions may be found on the publisher's website, Evolve.

Information has been presented in this textbook as clearly and concisely as possible in a style that builds from basic to more complex concepts. Radiographic images, photographs, tables, information boxes, and graphs reinforce and enhance learning and facilitate retention of material. Throughout the textbook useful examples are included after discussion of concepts that may be difficult to comprehend.

Ancillaries
Workbook

A workbook to accompany this textbook is also available in written form. It contains a variety of exercises for each of the 15 chapters in the book. Exercises included in the workbook are matching of terms or phrases with their definitions, multiple-choice questions, true or false statements, fill-in-the-blank statements, labeling of diagrams or missing information in boxes or charts, short-answer questions, general discussion or opinion questions, and a chapter posttest. Use of the workbook in conjunction with the textbook will provide a challenging experience for the learner. It will reinforce learning and help students remember important concepts and material covered in each chapter of the book. The answers for all exercises are located in the back of the workbook. Using both the textbook and workbook simultaneously will be of significant value in helping the radiography student prepare for credentialing examinations such as the American Registry of Radiologic Technologists (ARRT) certification examination for full-scope radiographers. Limited-scope x-ray students preparing for credentialing examinations administered through individual state licensing boards can also use the textbook in conjunction with the workbook to prepare for their state licensing examinations.

INSTRUCTOR'S ANCILLARIES

Instructor's ancillaries are also available with this eighth edition to assist radiologic technology educators. Ancillaries include a test bank containing multiple-choice questions for each chapter, a collection of images from the textbook, and a PowerPoint lecture presentation. These additional materials are available on the publisher's website, Evolve. The web address is: http://evolve.elsevier.com/Sherer/radiationprotection.

USING THE BOOK

In general, the presentation of the eighth edition presumes that the reader has some background in elementary physics, human anatomy, and medical and imaging terminology. Basic knowledge of units of measure (metric and English), atomic structure, the physical concepts of energy, electric charge, subdivision of matter, electromagnetic radiation, x-ray production (both quality and quantity), and the process of ionization is useful but not mandatory. The reader will be able to substantially build on their existing knowledge level by assimilating information presented in this textbook.

To facilitate a working comprehension of the principles of radiation protection, radiobiology, and physics related to radiation protection, study materials presented in the eighth edition remain sophisticated enough to be true to the complexity of the subject matter, yet simple and concise enough to permit comprehension by all readers. For student radiographers and radiology residents, this text is best used in conjunction with formal instruction from a qualified instructor. Practicing radiographers, new medical physicists, newly appointed radiation safety committee chairs, and radiologists may make use of this book as a self-teaching instrument to broaden and reinforce their existing knowledge of the subject matter and as a means to acquaint themselves with changing concepts and new material. The textbook can serve as a resource for continuing education because it provides an extensive range of information that has been expanded and updated with each new edition.

By mastering the material covered in this radiation protection textbook and its ancillaries and by applying this knowledge in the performance of radiologic procedures in the clinical setting, the reader will help to ensure the safety of patients, all diagnostic imaging personnel, and the general public.

Mary Alice Statkiewicz Sherer, AS, RT(R), FASRT

ABOUT THE AUTHORS

Mary Alice Statkiewicz Sherer, AS, RT(R), FASRT, Radiologic Technology Educator/Instructor/Technologist Emeritus, is the primary author of this textbook and the accompanying workbook and ancillary materials. Ms. Sherer continues to be available as a private radiography education, radiation safety, and medical publishing consultant. In the past, she was employed for 6 years as an instructor for the Limited Scope X-Ray Program at High-Tech Institute, Inc. (Anthem College), a career college that was located in Nashville, Tennessee. Before assuming that position in January 2004, Ms. Sherer worked at Summit Medical Center in Hermitage, Tennessee, for 13 years, where she performed diagnostic imaging procedures and served as that department's Compliance/ Education Coordinator. Prior to that position, Ms. Sherer was employed at Memorial Hospital of Burlington County (now Virtua Health System Memorial Hospital) in Mount Holly, New Jersey, where she served for more than 16 years as radiography program director and then as educational administrative assistant for the Department of Radiology.

After earning an ARRT certification in 1965, Ms. Sherer filled several technical and teaching positions in the New Jersey area and in 1980 graduated with an associate degree in science from the College of Allied Health Professions, Hahnemann Medical College and Hospital of Philadelphia (Hahnemann University). She has been an active and leading member of several professional organizations, having served on committees and task forces of the American Society of Radiologic Technologists, as president of the 28th Mid-Eastern Conference of Radiologic Technologists, and as president and chairman of the Board of Directors of the New Jersey Society of Radiologic Technologists. Services to the ASRT include functioning as chairman of the Radiologic Technology editorial review board for the membership year 1989–1991 and participating as a member of the Committee on Memorial Lectures for the membership years 1989–1991 and 1991–1993. For her services and contributions to the profession of radiologic technology, in June 1990, Ms. Sherer was elevated to the status of Fellow of the American Society of Radiologic Technologists. She continues to hold this professional honor.

In addition to being the primary author of the first edition of *Radiation Protection for Student Radiographers* and the second, third, fourth, fifth, sixth, and seventh editions of *Radiation Protection in Medical Radiography*, as well of this edition, Ms. Sherer is the author of *Q & A: Preparation for Credentialing in Radiography*, published in 1993 by W.B. Saunders Company. In 1984 she served as co-author for the textbook, *Radiation Protection for Dental Radiography*, which was published by Multi-Media Publishing, Denver. Articles written by Ms. Sherer have been published in *Radiologic Technology, The Journal of the American Society of Radiologic Technologists,* and *ADVANCE for Imaging and Radiation Therapy Professionals,* a national biweekly newspaper published by Merion Publications. She has also served as a consultant to ADVANCE.

In 1999 Mosby produced Radiobiology and Radiation Protection, the fourth program in Mosby's Radiographic Instructional Series, a CD-ROM (and slide series) presentation consisting of eight modules, approximately 1 hour each in duration. A Study Guide and an Instructor's Manual accompanied the audiovisual materials. Ms. Sherer served as chief consultant for the development of the program and as a technical reviewer.

More recently, Ms. Sherer served as a member of the advisory board for the second, third, fourth, and fifth editions of *Radiography Essentials for Limited Practice,* a Saunders/Elsevier publication.

Paula J. Visconti, PhD, DABR, was the chief of medical physics and radiation safety officer at Virtua Health System Memorial Hospital in Mount Holly, New Jersey, for over 30 years. She had also served for a period as the radiation safety officer for the entire Virtua Health System in southern New Jersey, which comprises four hospitals.

Dr. Visconti received her PhD in experimental atomic physics from the City University of New York in 1971. She was a full-time instructor in the Physics Department at the City College of New York for several years thereafter. Dr. Visconti began her career in medical physics at

Montefiore Hospital and Medical Center in New York City, where she remained for 5 years as an associate physicist. During that time, she lectured extensively in radiologic physics to both therapeutic radiology residents and student radiographers.

Dr. Visconti is a member of the Society of the Sigma Xi, the American Association of Physicists in Medicine, and the American College of Radiology and is certified in therapeutic radiologic physics by the American Board of Radiology.

E. Russell Ritenour, PhD, DABR, FAAPM, FACR, is currently professor and chief medical physicist of the Department of Radiology and Radiological Science at Medical University of South Carolina. Previously, he served as professor and chief of the physics section, Department of Radiology, University of Minnesota Medical School and was director of graduate studies in biophysical sciences and medical physics, University of Minnesota Graduate School. Dr. Ritenour received his PhD in physics from the University of Virginia and completed a postdoctoral fellowship sponsored by the National Institutes of Health in medical physics at the University of Colorado Health Sciences Center. He stayed on the faculty at the University of Colorado for 10 years, serving as director of the graduate medical physics training program, until moving to the University of Minnesota in 1989.

Dr. Ritenour has served as radiation safety officer for several hospitals and research facilities. He has also served as a consultant to the US Army for resident training programs and has written a number of audiovisual training programs and educational websites for radiologic technologists, radiology residents, and medical physicists. In addition, he is a co-author of four books, two of which have gone into subsequent editions.

Dr. Ritenour is past president of the Rocky Mountain Chapter of the Health Physics Society and a frequent contributor to that society's website's feature, "Ask the Expert." He has chaired education and training committees of the American College of Radiology and the American Association of Physicists in Medicine and has served as board examiner and written examination committee chair for the American Board of Radiology. Dr. Ritenour is a Fellow and Past President of the American Association of Physicists in Medicine and a Fellow of the American College of Radiology.

Kelli Welch Haynes, MSRS, RT (R), is a tenured associate professor and Program Director for the Bachelor of Science program at Northwestern State University in Shreveport, Louisiana. She is also a graduate faculty member. Mrs. Haynes graduated from Northwestern State with her Bachelor of Science degree in 1995, and she graduated summa cum laude from Midwestern State University in Wichita Falls, Texas, in 2000 with her Master of Science in Radiologic Sciences with a concentration in Administration. Before becoming an educator in August 2000, Mrs. Haynes was the Director of Radiology at Lagniappe Hospital (now Promise Hospital) in Shreveport, Louisiana, for 5 years, where she performed diagnostic radiography exams and computed tomography.

She has been an active member of several professional organizations, having served on the boards, committees, and task forces of the American Society of Radiologic Technologists, chapter director of the Louisiana Alpha chapter of Lambda Nu, the national honor society for the radiologic and imaging sciences, and currently serves as the President for the Association of Educators in Imaging and Radiologic Sciences and as site visitor for the Joint Review Committee on Education in Radiologic Technology. She is also a member of the Association of Collegiate Educators in Radiologic Sciences.

She has created six online continuing education modules for the American Society of Radiologic Technologists. Mrs. Haynes has served as a reviewer for many radiologic sciences textbooks. In radiography, she has developed the *Mosby's Radiographic Online (MRO) for Radiation Protection in Medical Radiography*, 7th edition, *Bontrager's Textbook of Radiographic Positioning and Related Anatomy*, and *Sectional Anatomy for Imaging Professionals*. Mrs. Haynes has presented over 75 presentations at the state, regional, national, and international levels. She has also published articles in *Radiologic Technology, The Journal of the American Society of Radiologic Technologists, Radiologic Science and Education*, and *ADVANCE for Imaging and Radiation Therapy Professionals*.

ACKNOWLEDGMENTS

The ongoing encouragement and support of my family, collaborating authors, professional colleagues, friends, and the competent staff of Elsevier, Inc., have made the development and production of the eighth edition of *Radiation Protection in Medical Radiography* and all its ancillaries possible.

To my family—sons, Joseph, Christopher, and Terry—a very special acknowledgement and sincerest thanks are given. The consistent love, support, and encouragement you provide give me the strength and determination to accomplish my goals in life. You are my greatest blessing. Also included with my family are two little shih-tzus, Dexter and Roxie, who were always by my side during the writing of this edition.

The technical integrity of this edition is attributed to the collaborative efforts of two brilliant and exceptional medical physicists, Paula J. Visconti, PhD, DABR, and E. Russell Ritenour, PhD, DABR, FAAPM, FACR, and an extremely competent radiologic technologist educator, Kelli Welch Haynes, MSRS, RT (R), who has enhanced our team with her professional expertise. Each of these individuals has made valuable contributions in terms of technical information, numerous recommendations, reviewing, editing, and development of new materials and illustrations for this new edition, thereby increasing the overall technical accuracy, timeliness, and value of the textbook. I am deeply indebted to both Dr. Visconti and Dr. Ritenour, not only for their technical contributions and recommendations, but also for the many hours each has spent in reviewing, writing, and assisting with editing of materials for this new edition and previous editions. Paula and Russ, thank you for everything that you have done to help make this textbook the best it can be. Special thanks is given to Kelli Haynes for conducting a photo shoot to obtain new photographs for our book. Thanks is also given to Kelli's students: Chassity Thomas, Taylor Atkins, Christine Mettenbrink, Christina Thiels, Garon Gaspard, and Lashayla Ester for their participation in the photo shoot. You have greatly helped to modernize and increase the visual appeal of this publication. Sincere appreciation is also given to Kelli Haynes for development of the PowerPoint slide presentation, which is available on Evolve to accompany the textbook.

A very special thank you is given to Stewart Carlyle Bushong, ScD, FAAPM, FACR, Professor of Radiologic Science, Baylor College of Medicine, Houston, Texas, and renowned author, for writing the foreword for our eighth edition. We appreciate your professional comments and endorsement of our textbook.

Thanks are given to the anonymous reviewers selected by Elsevier, Inc., to review the manuscript for the eighth edition. We are most appreciative of your commitment to quality education in the radiation science field and your patience for taking the necessary time to review our manuscript and make very helpful and thoughtful recommendations and suggestions to improve both the technical aspects and grammatical clarity of the manuscript. Your constructive feedback is very much appreciated.

Our sincerest thanks are given to Dr. Uwe Busch, Director, Deutsches Roentgen Museum, Remscheid, Germany, for verification of historical information that validates specific points of data.

Over the years many contributions to our editions have been made by many individuals, companies, and organizations in the form of materials borrowed, such as selective technical information, photographs, and other illustrations from various sources. These materials have helped to enhance the technical value and visual appeal of this and previous editions. We are very grateful for permission for use of these materials and acknowledge their use in the book through the process of citation, where applicable.

We acknowledge the ongoing use of some photographs that were taken for previous editions of the book and continue to be used in this edition. Thanks are given to those persons who participated in earlier photo shoots. The original photos obtained continue to complement various sections of the text and have enhanced the visual appeal of the book.

Sincere gratitude for effective communication, hard work, and ongoing support of our project is given to the highly competent and wonderful staff of Elsevier, Inc. Special acknowledgement and thanks are given to Executive Content Strategist Sonya Seigafuse, Senior Content Development Specialist Laura Selkirk, and Project Manager Manchu Mohan. We applaud your efforts to bring the eighth edition of this textbook to publication. We couldn't have accomplished this task without you! Thank you all.

Those who seek to learn the art and science of medical imaging are the future of the profession. To the radiography students and radiology residents who will use this textbook, it is my hope that the material contained within this edition will greatly contribute to providing you with a foundation in radiation protection and radiation biology and the means to enhance your knowledge in this subject matter. Education is an ongoing process; each person who enters into the radiation sciences assumes a responsibility to continue learning to enhance their skills and overall knowledge. This growth will enable imaging professionals to better serve patients entrusted to their care.

Finally, as I have stated in preceding editions, a very special remembrance is given to my parents, the late Felix and Elizabeth (Markovitch) Krohn, for all they did for me. Their many words of wisdom and lifelong encouragement remain with me. The education in my chosen profession they made possible helped me gain the knowledge necessary to prepare this new and previous editions. My personal accomplishments in the field of medical imaging serve as a tribute to them.

Mary Alice Statkiewicz Sherer, AS, RT(R), FASRT

CONTENTS

Introduction to Radiation Protection

OBJECTIVES

After completing this chapter, the reader will be able to perform the following:

- Define all key terms.
- Identify the consequences of ionization in human cells.
- List the properties, or characteristics, of x-rays.
- Describe the concept of teamwork in the medical field, and state the potential benefit that such an organized collaborative approach can have on radiation safety.
- Give examples of how radiologic technologists and radiologists can exercise control of radiant energy while performing imaging procedures.
- State the goals and discuss the concept of radiation protection.
- List the three main types of radiation quantities, and identify the unit(s) of measure in which each quantity is specified.
- Explain the justification and responsibility for imaging procedures.
- Explain how diagnostic efficacy of an imaging procedure can be maximized.
- Explain how imaging professionals can help ensure that both occupational and nonoccupational doses remain well below maximum allowable levels.
- State the ALARA principle, and discuss its significance in diagnostic imaging.
- List the three basic principles of radiation protection.
- List employer requirements for implementing and maintaining an effective radiation safety program in a facility that provides imaging services, and identify the responsibilities that radiation workers must fulfill.
- Describe the importance of patient education as it relates to medical imaging.
- Explain how radiographers should answer patients' questions about the risk of radiation exposure from an imaging procedure, and give some examples.
- Compare radiation sensitivity of children with radiosensitivity of adults.
- Explain the difference between the Image Gently Campaign and the Image Wisely Campaign.
- Discuss the reasons for monitoring and reporting radiation dose.

CHAPTER OUTLINE

KEY TERMS

absorbed dose
ALARA
alert levels
Alliance for Radiation Safety in
    Pediatric Imaging
background equivalent radiation
    time (BERT)
biologic effects
coulomb per kilogram (C/kg)
diagnostic efficacy

effective dose
exposure
gray (Gy)
Image Gently Campaign
Image Wisely Campaign
ionizing radiation
milligray (mGy)
milliroentgens (mR)
millisievert (mSv)

occupational and
    nonoccupational doses
optimization for radiation
    protection (ORP)
radiation
radiation protection
reference values
risk
sievert (Sv)

The transfer of kinetic energy, or energy of motion, from one location to another that is called **radiation** has been present on our planet in all of its various manifestations since the beginning of time. The use of radiation within the healing arts did not occur until after the discovery of an energetic form of radiation called *x-rays* in 1895. Since the early 1900s, both their beneficial and destructive potentials have been known. When passing through normal matter, x-rays were observed to produce electrically charged particles along their path. The altered atoms or molecules comprising these charged particles were called *ions*. Because of this effect the x-rays were classified as **ionizing radiation**. The production of these ions, as well as the electrons ejected in the process, is the event that may cause injury in normal biologic tissue. Consequences of ionization in human cells are listed in Box 1.1.

In the years following their discovery, most of the fundamental properties of x-rays were discovered by experiment. Briefly, they can be described as follows:
- X-rays are invisible.
- X-rays can have varying degrees of penetration in normal tissue, ranging from very superficial (skin surface) to much deeper (5 cm or greater) depending on their energy.
- X-rays are not deflected from their paths by either electric or magnetic fields and so are classified as electrically neutral.
- Although visible light may be focused with a lens, x-rays cannot be.

> **BOX 1.1   Consequences of Ionization in Human Cells***
>
> - Creation of unstable atoms
> - Production of free electrons
> - Production of low-energy x-ray photons
> - Creation of highly reactive free molecules (called *free radicals*) capable of producing substances poisonous to the cell
> - Creation of new biologic molecules detrimental to the living cell
> - Injury to the cell that may manifest itself as abnormal function or loss of function
>
> *Each of these consequences is fully discussed in subsequent chapters.

- X-rays travel in straight lines and at the speed of light (300 million meters per second) until they interact with atoms.
- When passing through matter, x-rays will produce charged particles by interaction with atoms composing that matter, as well as cause an emission of light known as *fluorescence* in certain crystals.
- X-rays will darken photographic film, with the degree of darkening on portions of the film being associated with the intensity (amount or quantity) of the x-rays striking those portions.
- X-ray beams generally have within them a wide range of energies; that is, x-ray beams are normally heterogeneous instead of monoenergetic.

TEAM CONCEPT IN THE MEDICAL FIELD

In recent years, there has been an increasing awareness of the value of a "team approach" to patient care. In a team approach, various participants assume responsibility for their areas of expertise, and the importance of communication throughout the team is emphasized. The composition of the team will vary with the circumstances of the patient. It will include the physician of record, nursing and other medical assistants, and any specialty care physicians, including radiologists and their support group. This support group consists of radiologic technologists, radiologist assistants, and medical physicists. The team may also include physical therapists, respiratory therapists, dietary consultants, language interpreters, and a host of others. It is recognized that each member of the team brings his or her own unique contributions to a successful medical interaction with a patient and that teamwork reduces the rate of occurrence of medical errors. Such an organized collaborative approach can also have the benefit of increased radiation safety, both to patients and directly involved members of the imaging team. This model is becoming a standard part of the curriculum at all levels of training for medical schools, residencies, and medical professional training programs.[1-5] Organizations such as The American Registry of Radiologic Technologists, The American Society of Radiologic Technologists (ASRT), and The Joint Commission encourage health care providers to function as effective team members while establishing a culture of quality, patient safety, and high reliability.

CONTROL OF RADIANT ENERGY

By using the knowledge of radiation-induced hazards that has been gained over many years and by employing effective methods to limit or eliminate those hazards, humans can safely control the use of "radiant energy." An example of controllable radiant energy is the radiation produced from an x-ray tube (Fig. 1.1).

Radiologic technologists and radiologists:
- Are educated in the safe operation of x-ray–producing imaging equipment
- Use protective devices whenever possible
- Follow established procedures
- Select x-ray machine settings that significantly reduce radiation exposure to patients and to themselves

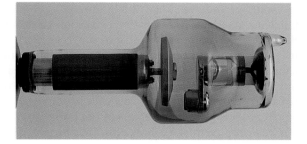

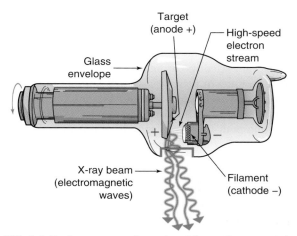

FIG 1.1 Radiant energy is emitted from the x-ray tube in the form of waves (or particles). This manmade energy can be controlled by the selection of equipment components and devices made for this purpose and by the selection of appropriate x-ray machine settings.

By adhering to these good practices, technologists and radiologists minimize the possibility of causing damage to healthy biologic tissue.

GOALS OF RADIATION PROTECTION

The goal of modern radiation protection programs is twofold: to protect persons from both short-term and long-term effects of radiation. Some of these effects occur in just specific organs and organ systems. Others, such as cancer and hereditary effects, affect the whole body and future generations.

CONCEPT OF RADIATION PROTECTION

Diagnostic imaging professionals have an ongoing responsibility to ensure radiation safety during all medical radiation procedures. They fulfill this obligation by following an established radiation protection program. **Radiation protection** may be defined simply as effective measures employed by radiation workers to safeguard patients, personnel, and the general public from *unnecessary* exposure to ionizing radiation. This refers to any radiation exposure that does not benefit a person in terms of diagnostic information obtained from images for the clinical management of medical needs. Effective protective measures take into consideration both human and environmental physical determinants, technical elements, and procedural factors. To comprehend that process more fully, this textbook has been designed to introduce its readers at appropriate times in the following chapters to the relevant scientific principles that underlie the tools and techniques of these measures. Scientific application of tools and techniques requires a common usage of quantities and units. Important examples of this are length and time with their corresponding units, meters, and seconds. Unfortunately, there is not just one unique set or system of these units for ionizing radiation. Rather, three such unit systems are currently in existence, and each one has a significant area of usage. Appendix A contains detailed lists of all the major units comprising each of the three systems and furthermore gives the numeric relationships among the corresponding units of each system.

Introduction to Radiation Quantities and Units of Measure

The science of radiation quantities and units is complex. An introduction is provided in this chapter to allow the reader to appreciate the relative magnitudes of sources of radiation exposure of humans to radiation. There are three main types of quantities to consider:
- Exposure
- Absorbed dose
- Effective dose

A brief explanation of these quantities and the units in which they are most commonly specified follows.

Exposure (coulomb per kilogram [C/kg] or milliroentgen [mR]).

The terms *exposure* and *exposed* are used in everyday speech to refer to any situation in which radiation is in contact with humans, as in "The patient was exposed to radiation to obtain a medical image." But there is a specific scientific meaning to the term *exposure*. **Exposure** is the amount of ionization produced in air when ionizing

radiation is present. The air at the surface of an x-ray room tabletop or the interior of a computed tomography (CT) scanner becomes ionized when the x-ray tube is energized. Devices called *ionization chambers* can measure this quantity directly and are used to determine the amount of radiation produced by x-ray equipment. Exposure is measured in **coulomb per kilogram (C/kg)** in the metric International System of Units (SI), or in **milliroentgens (mR)**, a subunit of the *roentgen*, a nonmetric unit likewise used for measuring the ionizing capability of radiation. A milliroentgen is equal to 1/1000 of a roentgen.

Absorbed Dose (milligray [mGy]).

The term *dose* is also employed in everyday speech, as in "We all receive a dose of radiation from sources in the environment." The exact meaning of **absorbed dose** is the amount of energy that is deposited in a material per unit mass of the material. More energy deposited is usually related to more disruption of biomolecules in living tissue. Less energy is related to less disruption. Absorbed dose is measured in **milligray (mGy)**, a subunit of the **gray (Gy)** in the SI. The milligray is equal to 1/1000 of a gray.

Effective Dose (millisievert [mSv]).

The term **effective dose** is an attempt to provide a quantity that is a measure of general harm in humans. It takes into account the amount of absorbed dose that is received by a human, the exact type of radiation (the effects of alpha, beta, protons, and neutrons are all somewhat different at the same absorbed dose levels), and the specific organs or organ systems irradiated. The effective dose is intended to be the best overall measure of the biologic effects of ionizing radiation. Effective dose is specified in **millisievert (mSv)**, a subunit of the **sievert (Sv)** in the SI. The millisievert is equal to 1/1000 of a sievert.

Need to Safeguard Against Adverse Biologic Effects of Ionizing Radiation

The need to safeguard against unnecessary radiation exposure is based on strong evidence that living tissue of animals and humans can be damaged by exposure to ionizing radiation. This type of damage is referred to as adverse **biologic effects**. In medicine, when radiation safety principles are correctly applied during imaging procedures, the energy deposited in living tissue by the radiation can be limited, thereby reducing the potential for adverse biologic effects. This book focuses on radiation protection for patients, diagnostic imaging personnel, and the general public.

JUSTIFICATION AND RESPONSIBILITY FOR IMAGING PROCEDURES

Benefit Versus Risk

Radiation exposure should *always* be kept at the lowest possible level for the general public. However, when illness or injury occurs or when a specific imaging procedure for health screening purposes is prudent, a patient may elect to assume a relatively small statistical risk to obtain essential diagnostic medical information. A prime example of such a voluntary assumption of risk occurs when women elect to undergo screening mammography to detect breast cancer in its early stages (Fig. 1.2). Because high-quality mammography continues to be the most effective tool for diagnosing breast cancer early, when the disease can best be treated,[6] its use contributes significantly to improving the life expectancy for women at risk. The realized benefits of this exposure to radiant energy far outweigh any slight chance of inducing a radiogenic malignancy or any genetic defects.

Diagnostic Efficacy

Diagnostic efficacy is the degree to which the diagnostic study accurately reveals the presence or absence of disease in the patient while adhering to radiation safety guidelines. It is maximized when essential images are produced with the least radiation exposure to the patient. Thus this concept of efficacy is a vital part of radiation protection in the healing arts. It provides the basis for determining whether an imaging procedure or practice is justified (Box 1.2). The referring physician carries the responsibility for determining this medical necessity for the patient.

BOX 1.2   Achievement of Diagnostic Efficacy

Imaging procedure or practice justified by referring physician → Minimal radiation exposure → Optimal image(s) produced

→ Presence or absence of disease revealed = Diagnostic efficacy

---

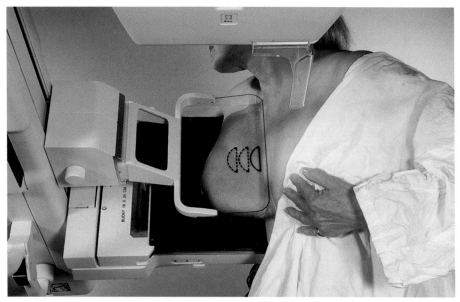

FIG 1.2 Mammography continues to be the most effective tool for diagnosing breast cancer. It can be used as a screening tool or a diagnostic procedure. In either instance, the realized benefits of exposure to radiant energy, in terms of medical information obtained, far outweigh any slight chance of possible biologic damage or genetic defects. (From Long BW, Rollins JH, Smith BJ: *Merrill's Atlas of Radiographic Positioning and Procedures*, ed 13, St. Louis, 2016, Elsevier.)

After ordering an x-ray examination or procedure, the referring physician must accept basic responsibility for protecting the patient from nonuseful radiation exposure. As health care professionals, radiographers accept a portion of the responsibility for the patient's welfare by being required to provide high-quality imaging services. The radiographer and radiologist together share in the responsibility of keeping the patient's medical radiation exposure at the lowest level possible. In this way imaging professionals help ensure that both occupational and nonoccupational doses remain well below maximum allowable levels. This can best be accomplished by producing optimal images with the *first* exposure. Repeated examinations made necessary by technical error or carelessness (Fig. 1.3) must be avoided because they increase radiation exposure to the patient and potentially to the radiation worker as well.

AS LOW AS REASONABLY ACHIEVABLE (ALARA) PRINCIPLE

ALARA is an acronym for "as low as reasonably achievable." This term is synonymous with the term optimization for radiation protection (ORP). The rationale for ALARA or ORP comes from evidence compiled by scientists over the past century.[7] At the time of this publication, radiation protection guidelines are rooted in the philosophy of ALARA. Therefore this dictum, *as low as reasonably achievable,* should be a main part of every health care facility's personnel radiation control program. In addition, because at this time no firm dose limits have been established for the amount of radiation that patients may receive for individual imaging procedures, the ALARA philosophy should be maintained and must show that all reasonable actions that will reduce doses to patients and personnel below required limits have been considered (Fig. 1.4). Radiation-induced cancer does not appear to have a fixed threshold, that is, a dose level below which individuals would have no chance of developing this disease, so the selection of exposure factors should always follow ALARA for all medical imaging procedures.

For many radiation regulatory agencies the ALARA principle provides a method for comparing the amount of radiation used in various health care facilities in a particular area for specific imaging procedures.

Cardinal Rules of Radiation Protection

The three cardinal (basic, central) principles of radiation protection are as follows:

- Time
- Distance
- Shielding

These principles can be applied to the patient and the radiographer. To reduce the exposure to the patient:

- Reduce the amount of the x-ray "beam-on" time.
- Use as much distance as warranted between the x-ray tube and the patient for the examination.
- Always shield the patient with appropriate gonadal and/or specific area shielding devices.

Occupational radiation exposures of imaging personnel can be minimized by the use of these cardinal principles:

- Shorten the length of time spent in a room where x-radiation is produced.
- Stand at the greatest distance possible from an energized x-ray beam.
- Interpose a radiation-absorbent shielding material between the radiographer and the source of radiation.

Responsibility for Maintaining ALARA in the Medical Industry

Both employers of radiation workers and the workers themselves have a responsibility for radiation safety in the medical industry. For the welfare of patients and workers, facilities providing imaging services must have an effective radiation safety program in place. This requires a firm commitment to radiation safety by all participants. It is the responsibility of the employer to provide the necessary resources and appropriate environment in which to execute an ALARA program. A written policy statement describing this program and identifying the commitment of management to keeping all radiation exposure ALARA must be available to all employees in the workplace. In a hospital setting, an individual called the *Radiation Safety Officer (RSO)* is expressly charged by the hospital administration with being directly responsible for the execution, enforcement, and maintenance of the ALARA program.

To determine how radiation exposure in the workplace may be lowered, management should perform periodic exposure audits.[8] Radiation workers with appropriate education and work experience must function with awareness of rules governing the work situation. They are required to perform their occupational practices in a manner consistent with the ALARA principle (Box 1.3). When radiation is safely and prudently used in the imaging of patients, the benefit of the exposure can be maximized while the potential risk of biologic damage is minimized.

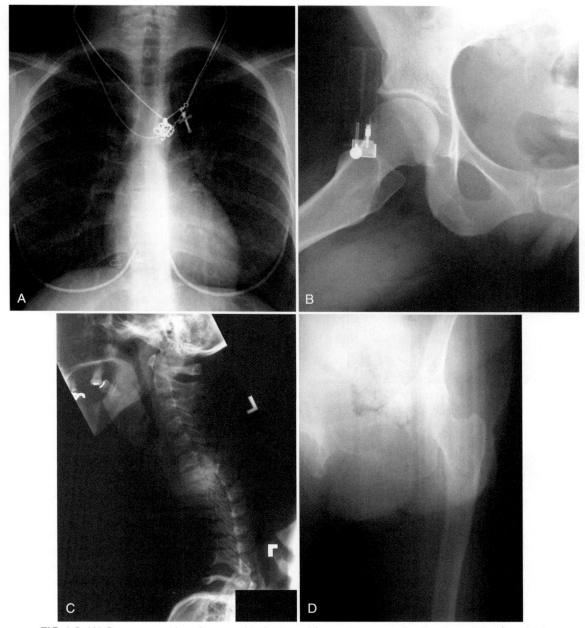

FIG 1.3 (A) Posteroanterior chest projection requiring repeat examination because of multiple external foreign bodies (several necklaces and an underwire bra) that should have been removed before the x-ray examination. (B) Anteroposterior projection of a right hip requiring a repeat examination because of poor collimation and the presence of an external foreign body (a cigarette lighter) overlying the anatomy of concern. The patient's slacks with the pocket containing the lighter should have been removed before the x-ray examination. (C) Double exposure (two lateral projections of the cervical spine) requiring a repeat examination. (D) A conventional radiograph of a left hip demonstrating an "off-level" grid error. This occurs when the patient's weight is not evenly distributed on the grid, thus causing the grid to tilt so that it is not properly aligned with the x-ray tube.

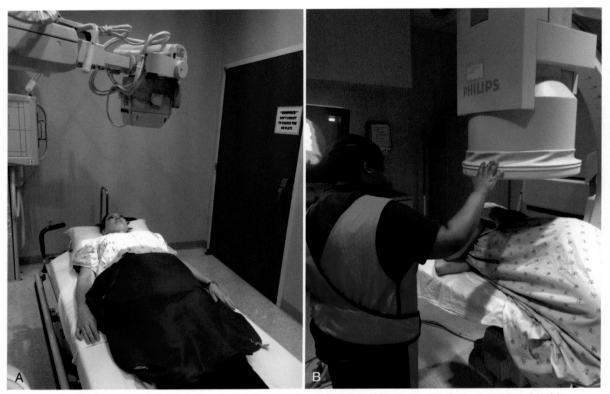

FIG 1.4 (A) Patient protection. (B) Radiographer protection. Medical radiation exposure should always be kept as low as reasonably achievable (ALARA) for the patient and for imaging personnel.

Employers' Responsibilities
- Implement and maintain an effective radiation safety program in which to execute ALARA* by providing the following:
  - Necessary resources
  - Appropriate environment for ALARA program
- Make a written policy statement describing the ALARA program and identifying the commitment of management to keep all radiation exposure ALARA available to all employees in the workplace.
- Perform periodic exposure audits to determine how to lower radiation exposure in the workplace.

Radiation Workers' Responsibilities
- Be aware of rules governing the workplace.
- Perform duties consistent with ALARA.

*ALARA, As low as reasonably achievable.

PATIENT PROTECTION AND PATIENT EDUCATION

Educating Patients About Imaging Procedures

Facilities that provide imaging services have a responsibility to ensure the highest quality of service. An important aspect is education of patients about imaging procedures. Patients not only should be made aware of what a specific procedure involves and what type of cooperation is required, but also they must be informed of what needs to be done, if anything, as a follow-up to their examination. Through appropriate and effective communication, patients can be made to feel that they are active participants in their own health care (Fig. 1.5).

Risk of Imaging Procedure Versus Potential Benefit

In general terms, risk can be defined as the probability of injury, ailment, or death resulting from an activity. In

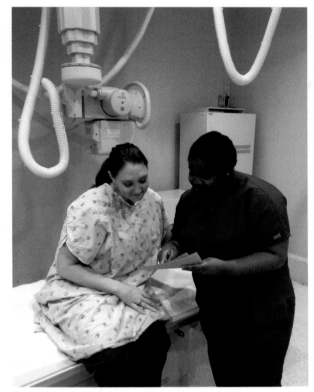

FIG 1.5 Effective communication is an important part of the patient–radiographer relationship. Patients need to be educated about imaging procedures so that they can understand what the procedure involves and what type of cooperation is required. The radiographer must answer patient questions about the potential risk of radiation exposure honestly. To create understanding and reduce fear and anxiety for the patient, the radiographer can provide an example that compares the amount of radiation received for a specific procedure with natural background radiation received over a given period.

the medical industry with reference to the radiation sciences, risk is the possibility of inducing adverse biologic effects such as injury to the skin or induction of cancer or a genetic defect after irradiation. Typically, people are more willing to accept a risk if they perceive that the potential benefit to be obtained is greater than the risk involved. Regarding exposure to ionizing radiation, patients who are educated to understand the medical benefit of an imaging procedure are more likely to suppress any radiation phobia and be willing to assume a small chance of possible biologic damage. A significant

understanding of biologic effects associated with diagnostic radiology was acquired throughout the twentieth century. The medical imaging industry currently continues to build on this knowledge. This information, coupled with improved designs of medical imaging equipment and more stringent radiation safety standards, has greatly reduced risk from imaging procedures for both patients and radiographers.

Background Equivalent Radiation Time

Besides a normal explanation of a medical imaging procedure, another way that radiographers can improve understanding and reduce fear and anxiety for the patient is to use the background equivalent radiation time (BERT) method. On occasion, a radiographer will receive the question "Are x-rays safe?" Radiologic technologists are responsible for giving an honest and understandable answer to the patient. An example of this is telling patients that for normal diagnostic examinations, such as the one they are about to undergo, there are no existing data of any unsafe effects from the x-rays used in the examination. A second potential question about the amount of radiation that the patient will receive from the procedure is difficult to answer in a way that an ordinary patient will understand because (1) the received dose is specified in a number of different units of measure and (2) the scientific units for radiation dose are normally not comprehensible by a patient. The intent of this dialog with the patient is not to provide high scientific accuracy but to relieve anxiety about radiation by giving an understandable and reasonably correct answer. The BERT method compares the amount of radiation received, for example, from a patient's chest x-ray examination or from radiography of any other part of the anatomy, with natural background radiation received over a specified period such as days, weeks, months, or years (Table 1.1). This method is also recommended by the US National Council on Radiation Protection and Measurements (NCRP).[9] As an example of its usage, consider a patient who is having a chest x-ray study and asks the radiographer, "How much radiation will I receive from this x-ray?" The radiographer can then respond by using an estimation based on the comparison of radiation received from the x-ray to natural background radiation received, for example, over a certain number of days. Thus the radiographer can say, "The radiation received from having a chest x-ray is equivalent to what would be received while spending approximately 10 days in your natural surroundings" (see Table 1.1).

TABLE 1.1 **Typical Adult Patient Effective Dose (EfD) and Background Equivalent Radiation Time (BERT) Values**

Radiologic Procedure	EfD (mSv)	BERT (AMOUNT OF TIME TO RECEIVE THE SAME EfD FROM NATURE)
Dental, intraoral	0.06	1 wk
Chest radiograph	0.08	10 days
Cervical spine	0.1	2 wk
Thoracic spine	1.5	6 mo
Lumbar spine	3.0	1 yr
Upper GI series	4.5	1.5 yr
Lower GI series	6.0	2 yr
Skull	0.07	11 day
Hip	0.3	7 wk
Pelvis	0.7	4 mo
Abdomen	0.7	4 mo
Limbs and joints (except hip)	<0.01	<1.5 days
CT brain	2.0	1 yr
CT chest	8.0	3.6 yr
CT abdomen/pelvis	10.0	4.5 yr

CT, Computed tomography; *GI*, gastrointestinal; *mSv*, millisievert.

Adapted from Wall BF: *Patient Dosimetry Techniques in Diagnostic Radiology*, York, 1988, Institute of Physics and Engineering in Medicine, pp 53, 117; Cameron JR: Are X-rays Safe?, *Med Phys World*, 15:20, 1999; Stabin MG: *Radiation Protection and Dosimetry: An Introduction to Health Physics*, New York, 2008, Springer.

BERT is based on an annual US population exposure of approximately 3 millisieverts per year.

Using the BERT method in this context has the following advantages:

- BERT does not imply radiation risk; it is simply a means for comparison.
- BERT emphasizes that radiation is an innate part of our environment.
- BERT provides an answer that is easy for the patient to comprehend.

Patients may mistakenly think that manmade radiation is more dangerous than an equal amount of natural radiation. Most patients are unaware that most of their background radiation comes from natural radioactivity in their own body. In summary, radiation phobia can be greatly reduced by explaining the diagnostic radiation dose to the patient by using the BERT method. BERT is not a radiation quantity. It is a method of explaining radiation to the public. Its name is never used in the explanation.[10]

Increased Radiation Sensitivity of Children

Although radiation dose is important for all patients, there are clear indications that children are significantly more radiation sensitive than are adults, and that exposure to radiation early in life, at levels found in computed tomography and even lower, leads to a measurable increase in cancer incidence as these individuals age into their 50s and 60s. A study from the Radiation Effects Research Foundation published in March 2008, in which a particular number of individuals were followed, showed that exposure in utero ($n = 2452$, where n is the number of individuals followed from childhood exposure from the atomic bombs of Hiroshima and Nagasaki) and as a child (≤ 6 years old, $n = 15,288$) was associated with a significantly increased risk of fatal cancer in adulthood.[11] Even older children were affected. A study of patients with scoliosis (in which the mean age at exposure was 10.6 years, the mean dose received was 0.11 Gy, and the number of persons exposed was 4822) who were followed up into adulthood found 70 cases among the exposed individuals when 35 cases were expected from comparison with a control group.[12] The National Academy of Science's most recent report on the biologic effects of ionizing radiation summarized the available data as follows[13]: The same radiation in the first year of life for boys produces three to four times the cancer risk as exposure between the ages of 20 and 50 years. For girls, the difference is six to eight times. For children in general, the risk is approximately three times greater than for adults.

Alliance for Radiation Safety in Pediatric Imaging

The Alliance for Radiation Safety in Pediatric Imaging was founded in 2007. It is a partnership of medical societies whose overall common purpose is to reduce the radiation dose for pediatric patients. Its first goal is to raise awareness among nonradiology users (e.g., emergency room physicians, referring physicians, orthopedists, neurosurgeons, etc.) of potentially high radiation exposure from computed tomography. If a child receives a dose of radiation in a CT scan where adult protocols are used, the child, because of being smaller in size, will receive a higher effective dose than would an adult, but the image produced will appear to be of acceptable quality—it will not appear overexposed, as would an image formed on a radiographic film. Radiologists have been aware of this for some time, and many practices have altered their protocols for pediatric patients. However, as of 2007, many referring physicians and nonradiology owners of CT scanners were not aware of the problem. Since 2007 the Alliance for Radiation Safety in Pediatric Imaging has continued in their pursuit to raise awareness of the need for dose reduction protocols by promoting pediatric-specific scan protocols to be used for both radiology and nonradiology users of CT. A study was performed to determine the general prevalence of the use of CT in the pediatric emergency department from 2003 to 2010. Although an increase in prevalence was demonstrated during that period, it was also demonstrated "in areas where alternative non-radiation-based modalities were options, there were decreased trends in CT use and increased use of alternative non-radiation-based modalities."[14]

Image Gently Campaign

On January 22, 2008, the alliance initiated the Image Gently Campaign. The campaign includes dissemination of information on pediatric CT dose reduction among the various medical specialties that refer patients for computed tomography examinations or even operate their own CT scanners. It also included the establishment of the Image Gently website. The website (www.imagegently.org) delivers the message that CT saves children's lives but that patient dose should be lowered by "child sizing" the kV and mA x-ray machine settings, by scanning only the indicated area (e.g., if ultrasound demonstrates a possible dermoid in the upper abdomen and a follow-up CT is ordered, there is rarely a need to scan the entire abdomen and pelvis) and by removing multiphase scans from the pediatric protocol (e.g., precontrast, postcontrast, and delayed CT scans rarely add more information in children yet can double or triple the dose). The website also contains a downloadable worksheet that allows a medical physicist to determine the technique factors that will ensure the pediatric dose on different manufacturers' scanners is no higher than the adult dose. Input for the worksheet is a series of measurements made on a CT scanner by a medical physicist. With the use of these techniques, the pediatric dose may be reduced by as much as 50% with no reduction in image quality. Even greater dose reductions are possible if the viewer is willing to tolerate an increase in noise, or grainy appearance, in the image. A high-contrast imaging situation (a more black-and-white image with fewer shades of gray) such as bone imaging or verification of tube placement may be successfully interpreted in the presence of increased noise.

Radiology departments or individual radiologic technologists can "pledge" to image gently. The pledge includes the following:

- Make the image gently message a priority in staff communications each year.
- Review the protocol recommendations, and, where necessary, implement adjustments to practice processes.
- Communicate openly with parents.

The Alliance for Radiation Safety in Pediatric Imaging consists of more than 24 medical societies, including the American Society of Radiologic Technologists and the American Association of Physicists in Medicine. Therefore it represents more than 600,000 physicians, medical physicists, and technologists. The alliance has held summit meetings with all the major vendors of CT equipment and has lobbied for features that encourage the use of dose reduction techniques, more training of the vendor's application specialists in dose reduction techniques, and display of patient dose for patients of all sizes.

Image Wisely Campaign

The American College of Radiology (ACR) and the Radiological Society of North America (RSNA) formed the Joint Task Force on Adult Radiation Protection to address concerns about the increase of public exposure to ionizing radiation from medical imaging. The Joint Task Force collaborated with the American Association of Physicists in Medicine (AAPM) and the American Society of Radiologic Technologists (ASRT) to create the Image Wisely Campaign with the objectives of lowering the amount of radiation used in medically necessary imaging studies and eliminating unnecessary procedures.

Image Wisely offers resources and information as guidance to radiologists, medical physicists, other imaging practitioners, and patients. The Image Wisely website (http://www.ImageWisely.org) serves as an excellent resource for this information.[15]

Monitoring and Reporting Radiation Dose

There is a trend toward more rigorous reporting of patient dose in radiology. In computed tomography and in interventional procedures, various added measures related to patient dose recording are becoming the norm. For example, many states now require that a log of maximum skin dose to each patient be kept as part of the patient record for each interventional procedure. Also, the US Food and Drug Administration mandates that measures of dose in CT be available as part of the record of each examination.

The Joint Commission is an independent, not-for-profit organization that accredits hospitals and free-standing imaging centers for reimbursement from Medicare and Medicaid. Most major private health care insurance companies also accept their guidelines for reimbursement. The Joint Commission endorses and certifies nearly 21,000 health care organizations and programs in the United States. Although at the present time it only requires monitoring of patient dose in CT and in interventional procedures, there are indications of it also moving toward requirements for all modalities in radiology. The Joint Commission specifies that all imaging equipment that uses ionizing radiation be regularly tested by qualified personnel and properly maintained. In particular, for CT The Joint Commission requires[16]:

- Annual education of staff in dose reduction techniques
- Minimum qualifications for medical physicists
- Documentation of CT radiation doses
- Management of CT protocols to minimize radiation dose

The NEXT Program and Reference Values

Various groups have compiled reference values for patient dose. These values are usually based upon large-scale surveys of actual measurements of x-ray machines in hospitals. The Nationwide Evaluation of X-ray Trends (NEXT) project[17] is conducted by the FDA and the Conference of Radiation Control Program Directors[18] and most state health departments to provide data on systems as they exist in the United States as of the date of the latest survey. Reference levels are set at some fraction, for example, 75% of the maximum of the distribution of dose values measured. These levels may then be used to allow individual institutions to determine where they stand with regard to standard practices at the majority of institutions. Because practice patterns such as age and health status of the patient population served vary widely from one institution to another, there are no prescribed values for patient exposures for different examinations and procedures.[19,20] But such data allow institutions to gauge the need and justification for their

exposure of patients to ionizing radiation. Another method for setting reference levels is used by the American College of Radiology to provide x-ray information based upon measurements made in plastic phantoms as part of their accreditation programs.[21,22]

Protocols for Dose Alerts

Facilities often have protocols for alert levels. When patient dose is predicted to or has actually substantially exceeded present dose levels, the staff radiologist is notified. In some cases a medical physicist may be called upon to estimate patient doses such as effective dose, peak skin dose, or fetal dose.

It is the technologist's responsibility to make sure that the radiologist and/or medical physicist has the information needed to carry out the dose estimate. The information needed might include patient size, pregnancy status, technical factors used for the examination, the anatomic regions imaged, and any dose measurements available through the electronic information system. If the examination involves prolonged fluoroscopy, information such as the amount of time that specific areas of the patient remained in view as opposed to having the field of view move through those regions is helpful in the assessment of radiation dose.

SUMMARY

- Radiation is the transfer of kinetic energy from one location to another.
- X-rays have several unique properties.
- X-rays are a form of ionizing radiation.
- Ionizing radiation has both a beneficial and a destructive potential.
- A team approach to patient care is an organized collaborative approach that can also have the benefit of increased radiation safety to patients and directly involved members of the imaging team.
- Radiant energy can be controlled by using the knowledge of radiation-induced hazards that has been gained over many years and by employing effective methods to limit or eliminate those hazards.
- Radiologic technologists and radiologists should adhere to good radiologic practices that minimize the possibility of causing damage to healthy biologic tissue.
- The goal of modern radiation protection programs is twofold: to protect persons from both short-term and long-term effects of radiation.

- To safeguard patients, personnel, and the general public from unnecessary exposure to ionizing radiation, effective radiation protection measures should always be employed when diagnostic imaging procedures are performed.
- Healthy normal living tissue of animals and humans can be damaged by exposure to ionizing radiation; therefore it is necessary to safeguard against unnecessary exposure to ionizing radiation.
- The realized benefits of exposing patients to ionizing radiation should far outweigh any slight chance of inducing radiogenic cancer or any genetic defects.
- Referring physicians should justify the need for every radiation procedure and accept basic responsibility for protecting the patient from nonuseful radiation exposure.
- Radiographers should select the smallest radiation exposure that produces the best radiographic results and should avoid errors that result in repeated radiographic exposures.
- Radiation exposure should always be kept ALARA to minimize the probability of any potential damage to people.
- The three basic principles of radiation protection are time, distance, and shielding.
- Imaging facilities must have an effective radiation safety program in place that provides patient protection and patient education.
- A significant understanding of biologic effects of ionizing radiation, improved designs of medical x-ray equipment, and more stringent radiation safety standards have greatly reduced the risk from imaging procedures for both patients and radiographers.
- BERT is a method used to compare the amount of radiation a patient receives from a radiologic procedure with natural background radiation received over a specific period.
- Children are significantly more radiation sensitive than are adults, and exposure to radiation early in life at levels found in CT and even lower leads to a measurable increase in cancer incidence as these individuals age into their 50s and 60s.
- The goal of the Alliance for Radiation Safety in Pediatric Imaging is to increase awareness of the need to reduce radiation dose for pediatric patients, especially in CT imaging.
- The Image Gently Campaign advocates lowering patient dose by "child sizing" the kV and mA x-ray machine

settings, scanning only the indicated areas, and removing multiphase scans from pediatric protocols.
- The objectives of the Image Wisely Campaign are lowering the amount of radiation used in medically necessary imaging studies and eliminating unnecessary procedures for adults.
- In CT and in interventional procedures various added measures related to patient dose recording are becoming the norm. The FDA mandates that measures of dose in CT be available as part of the record of each examination. The Joint Commission requires monitoring of patient dose in CT and in interventional procedures, and there are indications of it also moving toward requirements for all modalities in radiology.
- Reference values for patient dose are usually based upon large-scale surveys of actual measurement of x-ray machines in hospitals.
- Alert levels are sometimes used when patient dose is predicted to or has actually substantially exceeded preset dose levels.

REFERENCES

1. Leasure EL, et al: There is no "i" in teamwork in the patient-centered medical home: defining teamwork competencies for academic practice. *Acad Med* 88(5):585–592, 2013.
2. Interprofessional Education Collaborative Expert Panel: *Core competencies for interprofessional collaborative practice: report of an expert panel*, Washington, DC, 2011, Interprofessional Education Collaborative, IPEC sponsors:
American Association of Colleges of Nursing
American Association of Colleges of Osteopathic Medicine
American Association of Colleges of Pharmacy
American Dental Education Association
Association of American Medical Colleges
Association of Schools of Public Health, https://ipecollaborative.org/uploads/IPEC-2016-Updated-Core-Competencies-Report_final_release_.PDF
3. Sexton JB, Thomas EJ, Helmreich RL: Error, stress, and teamwork in medicine and aviation: cross sectional surveys. *Br Med J* 320:745, 2000. doi: http://dx.doi.org/10.1136/bmj.320.7237.745 (Published 18 March 2000).
4. Havyer RDA, et al: Teamwork assessment in internal medicine. *J Gen Intern Med* 29(6):894–910, 2014.
5. Kohn LT, Corigan JM, Donaldson MS, editors: *To err is human: building a safer health system*, Washington, DC, 1999, National Academies Press.

6. Mammogram Facts Sheet – National Cancer Institute. http://www.cancer.gov/types/breast/mammograms-fact-sheet#q1.
7. Health Risks from Exposure to Low Levels of Ionizing Radiation, BEIR VII PHASE 2, Committee to Assess Health Risks from Exposure to Low Levels of Ionizing Radiation, Board on Radiation Effects Research, Division on Earth and Life Studies, National Research Council of The National Academies, The National Academies Press, Washington, DC. www.nap.edu, ISBN: 978-0-309-09156-5, doi:10.17226/11340, 2006.
8. Gollnick DA: *Basic radiation protection technology*, ed 4, Altadena, Calif, 2000, Pacific Radiation Corporation.
9. National Council on Radiation Protection and Measurements (NCRP): *Research needs for radiation protection, Report No. 117*, Bethesda, MD, 1993, NCRP, p 51.
10. Ng K-H, Cameron JR: Using the BERT concept to promote understanding of radiation, international conference on the radiological protection of patients organized by the International Atomic Energy Agency, Malaga, Spain, 26-30 March 2011. C&S Paper Series 7/P, Austria, Vienna. 784-787.
11. Preston DL, et al: Solid cancer incidence in atomic bomb survivors exposed in utero or as young children. *J Natl Cancer Inst* 100:428, 2008.
12. Doody MM, et al: Breast cancer mortality after diagnostic radiography: findings from the U.S. Scoliosis Cohort Study. *Spine* 25:2052, 2000.
13. National Academy of Sciences Committee on Biological Effects of Ionizing Radiation: *Report VII: health risks from exposure to low levels of ionizing radiation*, Washington, DC, 2005, National Academy Press.
14. Menoch MJA, et al: Trends in computed tomography utilization in the pediatric emergency department. *Pediatrics* 129:e690, 2012. originally, published online February 13, 2012. doi:10.1542/peds.2011-2545. http://pediatrics.aappublications.org/content/129/3/e690.full.html.
15. Image Wisely. http://www.imagewisely.org/.
16. The Joint Commission: 601 13th Street, NW, Suite 560 South, Washington, DC 20005. http://www.jointcommission.org/diagnosticimaging standards/.
17. Nationwide Evaluation of X-Ray Trends (NEXT). http://www.fda.gov/radiation-emittingproducts/radiationsafety/nationwideevaluationofx-raytrendsnext/default.htm.
18. Conference of Radiation Control Program Directors (CRCPD), 1030 Burlington Lane, Suite 4B, Frankfort, KY 40601. http://crcpt.org/contact_information.aspx.
19. Hausleiter J, et al: Estimated radiation dose associated with cardiac CT angiography. *JAMA* 301(5):500–507, 2009.
20. Hricak H, et al: Managing radiation use in medical imaging: a multifaceted challenge. *Radiology* 258(3):889–905, 2011.
21. Image Wisely Website Guide to Diagnostic Reference Levels. http://www.imagewisely.oirg/~/media/ImageWisely%20Files/Medical%20Physicist%20Articles/IW%20McCullough%20Diagnostic%20Reference%20Levels.pdf.
22. American College of Radiology, 1891 Preston White Dr., Reston, VA 20191, 703-648-8900. http://www.ncradiation.net/xray/documents/acrreflevelsfluoro.pdf.

GENERAL DISCUSSION QUESTIONS

1. What are the consequences of ionization in the human cell?
2. When is medical radiation exposure considered unnecessary?
3. How can the background equivalent radiation time (BERT) method be used to eliminate a patient's fears about medical radiation exposure?
4. Describe how radiographers can use the ALARA concept in the performance of their daily responsibilities.
5. Why is a team approach of significant value in patient care?
6. How will a patient benefit from monitoring and reporting of radiation dose?
7. Why should the ALARA philosophy be maintained as a main part of every health care facility's radiation safety program?
8. When are patients more likely to suppress any radiation phobia and be willing to assume a small chance of possible biologic damage?
9. On what premise is BERT based?
10. In the medical industry with reference to the radiation sciences, how is risk defined?
11. What is the goal of the Alliance for Radiation Safety in Pediatric Imaging?
12. Describe the Image Wisely Campaign and Image Gently Campaign.

REVIEW QUESTIONS

1. A patient may elect to assume a relatively small statistical risk of exposure to ionizing radiation to obtain essential diagnostic medical information when:

1. Illness occurs
2. Injury occurs
3. A specific imaging procedure for health screening purposes is prudent

A. 1 and 2 only
B. 1 and 3 only
C. 2 and 3 only
D. 1, 2, and 3

2. Effective measures employed by radiation workers to safeguard patients, personnel, and the general public from unnecessary exposure to ionizing radiation defines:

A. Diagnostic efficacy
B. Optimization
C. Radiation protection
D. Reference values

3. Which of the following is a method that can be used to answer patients' questions about the amount of radiation received from a radiographic procedure?

A. ALARA concept
B. BERT
C. BRET
D. EPA

4. The term *optimization for radiation protection* (ORP) is synonymous with the term:

A. As low as reasonably achievable (ALARA)
B. Background equivalent radiation time (BERT)
C. Effective dose (EfD)
D. Diagnostic efficacy (DE)

5. Monitoring and reporting of patient dose for computed tomography and interventional procedures can lead to:

A. An invasion of patient privacy
B. An increase in patient radiation dose
C. A reduction in patient radiation dose
D. Elimination of the need for imaging equipment radiation safety features

6. The amount of ionization produced in the air when ionizing radiation is present is known as:

A. Absorbed dose
B. Effective dose
C. Efficacy
D. Exposure

7. The degree to which the diagnostic study accurately reveals the presence or absence of disease in the patient while adhering to radiation safety guidelines defines which of the following terms?

A. Radiation protection
B. Radiographic pathology
C. Effective diagnosis
D. Diagnostic efficacy

8. The millisievert (mSv) is equal to:

A. $\frac{1}{10}$ of a sievert
B. $\frac{1}{100}$ of a sievert
C. $\frac{1}{1000}$ of a sievert
D. $\frac{1}{10,000}$ of a sievert

9. An effective radiation safety program requires a firm commitment to radiation safety by:

1. Facilities providing imaging services
2. Radiation workers
3. Patients

A. 1 and 2 only
B. 1 and 3 only
C. 2 and 3 only
D. 1, 2, and 3

10. If a child receives a dose of radiation in a CT scan where adult protocols are used, the child, because of being smaller in size, will receive a:

A. Lethal dose of radiation
B. Higher effective dose than would an adult, but the image produced will be of acceptable quality
C. Lower effective dose than would an adult, and the image produced will be of acceptable quality
D. Severe radiation burns

2

Radiation: Types, Sources, and Doses Received

OBJECTIVES

After completing this chapter, the reader will be able to perform the following:

- Define all key terms.
- Give some examples of different types of radiation.
- Draw a diagram to illustrate the electromagnetic spectrum, and explain how the spectrum can be divided for the purpose of studying radiation protection.
- List the different forms of electromagnetic and particulate radiations, and identify those forms that are classified as ionizing radiation.
- Identify the unit of measure in which radiation absorbed dose is most commonly specified.
- Explain the concepts of equivalent dose and effective dose, and identify the unit of measure in which each of these radiation quantities is most commonly specified.
- Explain how ionizing radiation can cause biologic damage in body tissue.
- List and describe three sources of natural background ionizing radiation and seven sources of manmade, or artificial, ionizing radiation.
- Discuss the local and global consequences of radiation exposure resulting from accidents in nuclear power plants.
- Discuss the general responsibility for radiation safety and the need for radiation protection in medical imaging.
- Discuss the modalities used in medical imaging that have caused an increase in radiation dose for patients from 1980 until the present time.

CHAPTER OUTLINE

Radiation
    Types of Radiation
    The Electromagnetic Spectrum
    Ionizing and Nonionizing Radiation
    Particulate Radiation

An Introduction to the Concept of Radiation Dose
Biologic Damage Potential
Sources of Radiation
Summary

KEY TERMS

absorbed dose
biologic damage
cellular damage
effective dose (EfD)
electromagnetic radiation
electromagnetic spectrum
electromagnetic wave
equivalent dose (EqD)

ionization
isotopes
manmade, or artificial, radiation
milligray (mGy)
millisievert (mSv)
natural background radiation
organic damage
particulate radiation

radiation
radiation dose
radioactive decay
radioisotope
radionuclides
radon

Radiation has different types and sources. Some types of radiation produce damage in biologic tissue, whereas others do not. Some sources of radiation are considered *natural* because they are always present in the environment. However, other sources are created by humans for specific purposes and therefore are classified as *manmade*. This chapter presents an overview of the various types and sources of radiation, as well as the doses that are typically received from both natural and manmade sources.

RADIATION

Types of Radiation

In the simplest terms, energy is the ability to do work, that is, to move an object against resistance. Energy in motion is called *kinetic energy*. Radiation is kinetic energy and exists in many forms. For objects with mass, kinetic energy is written as $KE = \frac{1}{2}mv^2$. However, photons, which don't have mass, have energy related to their frequency. Higher frequency photons carry more energy. Some examples of different types of radiation are presented in Box 2.1.

The Electromagnetic Spectrum

The full range of frequencies and wavelengths of electromagnetic waves is known as the **electromagnetic spectrum**. Each grouping on this scale represents a type or category of radiation generated by varying electric and magnetic fields. Table 2.1 shows the electromagnetic spectrum in terms of *frequency* (given in units of hertz [Hz] i.e., cycles per second), *wavelength* (in meters), and *energy* (specified in electron volts [eV], a unit of energy equal to the quantity of kinetic energy an electron acquires as it moves through a potential difference of 1 volt). Each frequency within the spectrum has a characteristic wavelength and energy. Some of the practical uses of these different frequency ranges are listed. Note that higher frequencies are associated with shorter wavelengths and higher energies; therefore as the wavelength ranges from largest to smallest, frequencies and energy cover the corresponding smallest to largest ranges. Precise frequency intervals attributed to different parts of the electromagnetic spectrum may vary in different references, and there is substantial overlap of ranges (note that FM radio falls completely within the television range). Box 2.2 demonstrates the calculation of the wavelength and energy of electromagnetic radiation. All forms of electromagnetic

Example 1. Mechanical Vibrations of Materials
Such mechanical vibrations can travel through the air or other materials to interact with structures in the human ear and produce the sensation we call *sound*. *Ultrasound* is the mechanical vibration of a material in which the rate of vibration does not stimulate the human ear sensors and therefore is beyond the range of human hearing.

Example 2. the Electromagnetic Wave
Radio waves, *microwaves*, *visible light*, and *x-rays* are all representatives of the **electromagnetic wave**. In these waves, electric and magnetic fields fluctuate rapidly as they travel through space. A limited range of frequencies of this fluctuation is interpreted by its interaction with the human system as visible light. Within this range, small variations in frequency—the number of cycles or wavelengths of a simple harmonic motion per unit of time—are interpreted as different colors. However, frequencies both above and below the visible range exist and have many uses. Electromagnetic waves are also characterized by their wavelength, which is simply the physical distance between successive maximum values of oscillating wavelike electric and magnetic fields.

At the beginning of the 20th century, leading scientists first realized that electromagnetic radiation appears to have a dual nature, referred to as *wave–particle duality*. This means that this form of radiation travels or propagates through space in the form of a wave but can interact with matter as a particle of energy called a *photon*. For this reason, x-rays may be described as both waves and particles.

radiation have one common characteristic: their velocity. It is equal to the speed of light. The speed of light (or any type of electromagnetic radiation) is 3×10^8 meters per second in empty space (a vacuum) and is slightly less in transparent materials such as glass or plastic.

Ionizing and Nonionizing Radiation

For our purposes in the study of radiation protection, the electromagnetic spectrum (Fig. 2.1) can be divided into two parts:
1. Ionizing radiation
2. Nonionizing radiation

Of the entire span of types of radiation included in the electromagnetic spectrum, only the following radiations are classified as ionizing radiations[1]:

TABLE 2.1   The Electromagnetic Spectrum*

Use	Frequency	Wavelength	Energy
AM radio	0.54–1.6 MHz	0.6–0.2 km	2–7 neV
FM radio	88–108 MHz	3.4–3 m	370–440 neV
Television	54 MHz–0.8 GHz	5.6–0.4 m	220 neV–3.3 µeV
Microwaves	0.1–100 GHz	3 m–3 mm	0.4 eV–0.4 meV
Infrared	100 GHz–400 THz	3 mm–0.7 m	0.4 meV–1.6 eV
Visible	400–700 THz	0.7–0.4 m	1.6–2.8 eV
Ultraviolet	1–100 PHz	300–3 nm	4–400 eV
X-rays	100 PHz–100 EHz	3 nm–3 am	0.4–400 keV
Gamma rays	100 EHz–infinity	3–0 am	400 keV–infinity

*Frequency (in units of hertz [Hz] or cycles per second), wavelength (in meters), and energy (in electron volts [eV]). Each member of the spectrum has a characteristic wavelength and frequency. Some of the uses of different frequency ranges are listed. Note that higher frequencies are associated with shorter wavelengths and higher energies. The values shown here are typical representations. See Appendix B for an explanation of the abbreviations (M, G, T, P, µ, etc.).

BOX 2.2   Calculation of the Wavelength and Energy of Electromagnetic Radiation

The speed of light (c), wavelength (λ), and frequency (v) are related by the following equation:

$$c = \lambda v$$

where $c = 3 \times 10^8$ m/sec.

Therefore if the frequency of an electromagnetic wave is known, the wavelength may be calculated as follows:

$$\lambda = \frac{c}{v}$$

Example: Find the wavelength of a 0.5-MHz radio wave.

$$\lambda = \frac{3 \times 10^8 \text{ m/sec}}{0.5 \times 10^6 \text{ sec}^{-1}} = 6.0 \times 10^2 \text{ m} = 0.6 \times 10^3 \text{ m} = 0.6 \text{ km}$$

The energy (in electron volts, eV) of an electromagnetic wave may be calculated using the frequency (v) and Planck's constant (h) as follows:

$$E = hv$$

where $h = 4.14 \times 10^{-15}$ eV-sec.

Example: Find the energy of an x-ray having a wavelength of 1 picometer (1 pm = 10^{-12} m).

Solution: The energy is given by the following relation:

$$E = hv = hc/\text{wavelength}$$
$$= (4.14 \times 10^{-15} \text{ eV-sec})(3 \times 10^8 \text{ m/sec})/(1 \times 10^{-12} \text{ m})$$
$$= 12.42 \times 10^5 \text{ eV}$$
$$= 1.242 \times 10^6 \text{ eV}$$
$$= 1.24 \text{ MeV}$$

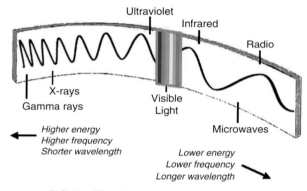

FIG 2.1 The electromagnetic spectrum.

- X-rays
- Gamma rays
- Ultraviolet radiation with energy greater than 10 eV

Because they do not have sufficient kinetic energy to eject electrons from the atom, the following radiations are considered nonionizing:

- Ultraviolet radiation with energy less than 10 eV
- Visible light
- Infrared rays
- Microwaves
- Radio waves

If **electromagnetic radiation** is of a high enough frequency, it can transfer sufficient energy to some orbital electrons to remove them from the atoms to which they were attached. As mentioned in Chapter 1, this process, called **ionization,** is the foundation of the interactions of x-rays with human tissue. It makes them valuable for creating images but has the undesirable result of potentially producing some damage in the biologic material.

Particulate Radiation

In addition to electromagnetic radiation, there is another category of ionizing radiation, called **particulate radiation.** This form of radiation includes the following:

- Alpha particles
- Beta particles
- Neutrons
- Protons

All these are subatomic particles that are ejected from the nucleus of atoms at very high speeds. They possess sufficient kinetic energy to be capable of causing ionization by direct atomic collision. However, no ionization occurs when the subatomic particles are at rest.

Alpha particles, also known as *alpha rays,* are emitted from nuclei of very heavy elements such as uranium and plutonium during the process of radioactive decay. **Radioactive decay** is a naturally occurring process in which unstable nuclei relieve that instability by various types of nuclear spontaneous emissions, one of which is the emission of charged particles. Alpha particles contain two protons and two neutrons. They are simply helium nuclei, or helium atoms minus their electrons. Alpha particles have a large mass that is approximately four times the mass of a hydrogen atom and a positive charge twice that of an electron. This permits them to have the potential of transferring very substantial amounts of kinetic energy to orbital electrons of other atoms.[2]

Particulate radiations vary in their ability to penetrate matter. Compared with beta particles, which are just fast electrons, alpha particles are much less penetrating. Because they lose energy quickly as they travel a short distance—for example, into the superficial layers of the skin—they are considered virtually harmless as an external source of radiation. Several pieces of ordinary paper can significantly attenuate them and therefore serve as a shield. However, as an internal source of radiation, the reverse is true. If emitted from a radioisotope that was deposited in the body—for example, in the lungs—alpha particles will be absorbed in the relatively radiosensitive epithelial tissue and be extremely damaging to that tissue. The process is in a way analogous to what a bowling ball does to a set of pins.

Beta particles, also known as *beta rays,* are identical to high-speed electrons except for their origin. Electrons originate in atomic shells outside of the nucleus, whereas beta particles, like alpha particles, are emitted from within the nuclei of radioactive atoms. This process of *beta decay* occurs when a nucleus relieves instability by a neutron transforming itself into a combination of a proton and an energetic electron (called a *beta particle*). There is also emission of another particle called a *neutrino,* which has negligible mass and no electric charge but carries away any excess energy. Beta particles are 8000 times lighter than alpha particles and have only one unit of electrical charge (−1) as compared with the alpha's two units of electrical charge (+2). These attributes mean that beta particles will not interact as strongly with their surroundings as alpha particles do. Therefore they are capable of penetrating biologic matter to a greater depth than alpha particles with far less ionization along their paths. Not all high-speed electrons, however, are beta radiation. Alternative sources of high-speed electrons are produced in a radiation oncology treatment machine called a *linear accelerator.* These electrons are most often used to treat superficial skin lesions in small areas or to deliver radiation boost treatments to breast tumors at tissue depths typically not exceeding 5 to 6 cm. Such very high-energy electrons require either millimeters of lead or multicentimeter-thick slabs of wood to absorb them. As previously stated, alpha rays can be absorbed by a few pieces of ordinary paper because they interact so readily with matter and consequently lose their kinetic energy quite rapidly. Beta rays, however, with a noticeably lesser probability of interaction with atoms of matter, will penetrate more deeply and therefore cannot be stopped by ordinary pieces of paper. For energies of less than 2 MeV, either a 1-cm-thick piece of wood or a 1-mm-thick lead shield would be sufficient for absorption.

Protons are positively charged components of an atom. An isolated proton, which is simply identical to an ionized hydrogen atom, has a relatively small mass that exceeds the mass of an electron by a factor of 1800. The number of protons in the nucleus of an atom constitutes its atomic number, or "Z" number. The atomic number identifies an element and determines its placement in the periodic table of elements (see Appendix C).

Neutrons are the electrically neutral components of an atom and have approximately the same mass as a proton. If two atoms have the same number of protons but a different number of neutrons in their nuclei, they are referred to as **isotopes.** If one of these combinations of Z protons and some number of neutrons leads to an unstable nucleus, then that combination is called a radioisotope.

An Introduction to the Concept of Radiation Dose

In the remainder of this chapter, radiation doses that humans can receive and have received are described. To appreciate the relative magnitude of these exposures, it is necessary to discuss the quantities and units that are used to specify radiation dose. The purpose of this section is to provide a very brief introduction to this topic.

The radiation quantity, absorbed dose (sometimes just shortened to "dose"), refers to the amount of kinetic energy per unit mass that has been absorbed in a material due to its interaction with ionizing radiation. It is usually measured in units of milligray (mGy).

The amount of energy absorbed by human tissue is an important determinant of the extent of biologic harm that may occur. However, other factors must be considered when attempting to predict how much actual biologic harm might be caused by radiation dose. The equivalent dose (EqD) takes into account the type of ionizing radiation that was absorbed. In diagnostic radiology, this absorption is caused by x-rays. But exposure to radioisotopes in the environment or to radioactive materials released from nuclear reactors involves other types of ionizing radiation, such as neutrons, protons, electrons, etc. The equivalent dose provides an overall dose value that includes the different degrees of tissue interaction that could be caused by the different types of radiation. The most common unit of measure of equivalent dose is the millisievert (mSv).

Another factor that plays a role in determining the degree of biologic damage that may be caused by ionizing radiation is the organ or organ systems irradiated. For example, irradiation of internal organs has very different, and generally much more severe, consequences than irradiation of extremities. Therefore the contribution of radiation absorbed dose that affects different organs and organ systems, as well as the type of ionizing radiation that caused the dose, is considered in deriving the effective dose (EfD). The effective dose is intended to be the best estimate of overall harm that might be produced by a given dose of radiation in human tissue. It takes into account both the type of radiation and the part of the body irradiated. The unit of effective dose is the same as the unit of equivalent dose, the millisievert (mSv). This implies that when a dose value is given in millisieverts, the radiation quantity that is being expressed needs to be identified.

Biologic Damage Potential

While penetrating body tissue ionizing radiation produces biologic damage primarily by ejecting electrons from the atoms comprising the tissues. Destructive radiation interaction at the atomic level results in molecular change, and this in turn can cause cellular damage, leading to abnormal cell function or even entire loss of cell function. If excessive cellular damage occurs, the living organism will have a significant possibility of exhibiting genetic or somatic changes such as the following:

- Mutations
- Cataracts
- Leukemia

Changes in blood count are classic examples of organic damage that results from nonnegligible exposure to ionizing radiation. An EqD of 250 mSv delivered to the *whole body* may cause a substantial decrease within a few days in the number of lymphocytes or white blood cells that are the body's primary defense against disease. Table 2.2 provides some basic information on the known

TABLE 2.2 Radiation Equivalent Dose and Subsequent Biologic Effects Resulting From Acute Whole-Body Exposures*

RADIATION EqD	
Sv	**Subsequent Biologic Effects**
0.25	Blood changes (e.g., measurable hematologic depression, substantial decreases within a few days in the number of lymphocytes or white blood cells that are the body's primary defense against disease)
1.5	Nausea, diarrhea
2.0	Erythema (diffuse redness over an area of skin after irradiation)
2.5	If dose is to gonads, temporary sterility
3.0	50% chance of death; lethal dose for 50% of population over 30 days (LD 50/30)
6.0	Death

*Radiation exposures are delivered to the entire body over a time period of less than a few hours.
Adapted from *Radiologic health*, unit 4, slide 17, Denver, Multi-Media Publishing (slide program).

biologic effects that result when radiation exposures of various EqDs are delivered to the whole body over a time period of less than a few hours (acute exposures). This emphasizes that the use of ionizing radiation should be limited whenever possible.

Sources of Radiation

Human beings are continuously exposed to sources of ionizing radiation. Sources of ionizing radiation may be one of the following:
- Natural
- Manmade (artificial)

Table 2.3 summarizes current estimates of the radiation received on average by individuals in the United States per year. Note that the dose from natural background and the dose from manmade sources are both roughly 3 mSv. The total dose per year is approximately 6 mSv. Fig. 2.2 shows a pie chart that gives the percentage contributions of the various sources of background radiation.

Natural Radiation. Natural sources of ionizing radiation have always been a part of the human environment. They are a consequence of our planet's geology and its location relative to the sun and our solar system's location in the galaxy. Ionizing radiation from planetary and extraplanetary sources is called natural background radiation and has the following three components:
- Terrestrial radiation from radioactive materials in the crust of the earth
- Cosmic radiation from the sun (solar) and beyond the solar system (galactic)
- Internal radiation from radioactive atoms, also known as radionuclides, which make up a small percentage of the body's tissue

If radiation from any of these natural sources grows larger because of accidental or deliberate human actions such as mining radioactive elements, the sources are termed *enhanced natural sources.*

Terrestrial radiation. Long-lived radioactive elements such as uranium-238, radium-226, and thorium-232 (all emitters of densely ionizing radiations) are present in variable quantities in the crust of the earth. These sources of ionizing radiation are classified as *terrestrial radiation.* The quantity of terrestrial radiation present in any area depends on the composition of the soil or rocks in that geographic region. The most recently available data show that 37% of natural background radiation exposure comes primarily from the gaseous radionuclide, radon, and to a much lesser degree from the radionuclide *thoron** (see Fig. 2.2). Both these gases emit alpha radiation. Radon initially does not cling to or interact with the atoms of other particles. Because of this property, it is sometimes referred to as a *noble gas.* It behaves as a free agent that floats around in the soil. As a consequence, the natural flow of air can draw radon gas into the lower levels of homes through cracks or holes in the foundation, and then the gas may permeate upward as it decays and becomes solid particles.[3,4]

Geologic formations or soils containing granite, shale, phosphate, and pitchblende produce higher concentrations of radon than other commonly encountered materials. Radon is by far the largest contributor to background radiation. The average US resident receives approximately

TABLE 2.3 Average Annual Radiation Equivalent Dose for Estimated Levels of Radiation Exposure for Humans

Category	Type of Radiation	DOSE mSv
Natural	Radon	2.0
	Cosmic	0.3
	Terrestrial and internally deposited radionuclides	0.7
	Total	3.0
Medical imaging	CT scanning	1.5
	Radiography	0.6
	Nuclear medicine	0.7
	Interventional procedures	0.4
	Total	3.2
Other manmade		0.1
	Total annual EqD from all sources	6.3

CT, Computed tomography; EqD, equivalent dose.
Adapted from Bushong SC: *Radiologic Science for Technologists: Physics, Biology, and Protection,* ed 10, St. Louis, 2013, Mosby.

---

*Thoron is a radioactive decay product of an isotope of radon, namely radon-220, with a half-life of 54.5 seconds as compared with the much longer 3.8 day half-life of radon. It is given the name thoron because radon-220 was itself derived from the radioactive decay of thorium-232, a naturally occurring material.

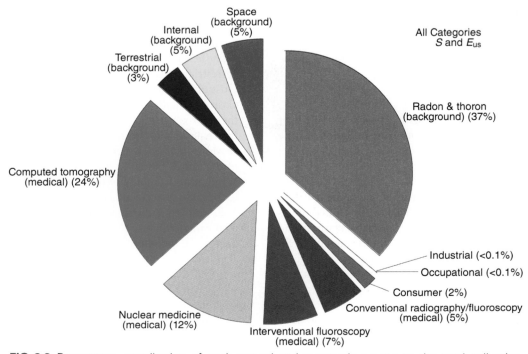

FIG 2.2 Percentage contribution of each natural and manmade source to the total collective effective dose for the population of the United States, 2006. (From National Council on Radiation Protection and Measurements [NCRP]: *Ionizing radiation exposure of the population of the United States, Report No. 160,* Bethesda, 2009, NCRP.)

2.0 mSv per year from indoor and outdoor levels of radon. Radon is the first decay product of radium, a metallic chemical element, and is produced as radium decays in soil. It is a colorless, odorless, invisible, heavy radioactive gas that, along with its own decay products, polonium-218 (^{218}Po) and ^{214}Po (solid form), is always present to some degree in the air. Radon has a half-life of 3.825 days.[4] To summarize, in homes, radon may gain access through the following areas (Fig. 2.3):

- Crawl spaces under the living areas
- Floor drains
- Sump pumps
- Porous cement block foundations

In many cases, a pressure gradient exists between a house and the soil on which it rests so that the house draws on the ground like a vacuum cleaner. Commonly used building materials such as bricks, concrete, and gypsum wallboard contain radon. These construction materials are classified as earth-based materials.[2]

Radon concentrations in a particular structure vary across days and seasons. In the cooler months, when homes and buildings are tightly closed, radon levels are usually higher. This is the best time to perform tests for radon.*

High indoor concentrations of radon and radon decay products, which are actually solid particles that have attached themselves to dust, have the potential to cause serious health hazards for humans.[3] After being inhaled, these airborne radioactive gases and decay products produce daughter radioactive isotopes that remain for lengthy periods in the epithelial tissue of the lungs. As these secondary isotopes decay, they give off alpha radiation that will injure lung tissues, thereby increasing the risk for lung cancer. The severity of this risk depends on

---

*Detection kits are relatively easy to use and may be purchased at retail stores or obtained at minimal cost from the National Safety Council in Washington, DC, by calling 1-800-SOS-RADON.

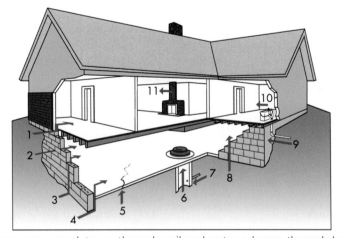

FIG 2.3 Radon gas can percolate up through soil and enter a home through holes or cracks in its framework, crawl spaces under the living areas, floor drains, sump pumps, and porous cement block foundations. *1*, Spaces behind brick veneer on top of block foundation; *2*, pores and cracks in concrete block foundation; *3*, open top of block foundation walls; *4*, floor to wall joints; *5*, cracks in concrete floor; *6*, exposed soil as in basement sump; *7*, weeping drain tile draining into open sump; *8*, mortar joints; *9*, loose-fitting pipe wall penetration; *10*, well water from some wells; *11*, building materials such as stone. (From US Environmental Protection Agency, Washington, DC.)

the concentration of the radon and the length of time to which the person is exposed to the gas and solid particles.[5] Smokers exposed to high radon levels face a higher risk of lung cancer than do nonsmokers. One reason for this may be that smokers have already been exposed to higher concentrations of radioactivity from the lead-210 (^{210}Pb) and polonium-210 (^{210}Po) isotopes contained in tobacco and tobacco smoke. The Environmental Protection Agency (EPA) considers radon to be the second leading cause of lung cancer in the United States. Radon is responsible for approximately 20,000 cancer deaths per year. The EPA recommends that action be taken to reduce elevated levels of radon to a concentration *less than* 4 picocuries* per liter (pCi/L) of air (the number of radioactive emissions per second that occur on average in 1 L of air). A radon air activity density of 4 pCi/L results in a yearly EqD to the lung of approximately 0.05 mSv.[6] A presence of radon below this level is considered statistically safe by the EPA. The EPA estimates that 1 in every 15 homes in the United States exceeds the recommended action limit of 4 pCi/L.[7] Hence,

accurate radon testing and appropriate structural repair, if required, are essential to reducing the risk of lung cancer from radon. In actuality, radiation exposure to radon cannot be entirely eliminated, but with suitable structural correction, it can be significantly reduced.

Cosmic radiation. Cosmic rays are of extraterrestrial origin and result from nuclear interactions that have taken place in the sun and other stars. The amount of cosmic rays varies with altitude relative to the earth's surface. The greatest intensity occurs at high altitudes where there is less attenuation due to the low atmospheric density, whereas the lowest intensity occurs at sea level. The great reduction at sea level happens because the cosmic rays that are not deflected by the earth's magnetic field must traverse the entire thickness and steadily increasing density of the earth's atmosphere before reaching the surface. The average US inhabitant received an EqD of approximately 0.3 mSv per year from extraterrestrial radiation (see Table 2.3). Cosmic radiations consist predominantly (about 90%[†]) of high-energy protons that have an estimated mean energy of 300 MeV. As a result of

---

*1 picocurie = 10^{-12} curie. 1 Ci = 3.7 $(10)^{10}$ nuclear disintegrations per second. So 1 pCi = .04 dps.

[†]The remaining 10% are composed mostly of alpha particles and heavier nuclei.

interactions with molecules in the earth's atmosphere, these protons may be accompanied by alpha particles, atomic nuclei, mesons*, gamma rays, and high-energy electrons as they approach the earth's surface. These other forms of radiation are collectively referred to as *secondary cosmic radiation.* The gamma rays among them can be energetic enough to penetrate several meters of lead.

Terrestrial and internal radiation. The tissues of the human body contain many naturally existing radionuclides that have been ingested in minute quantities from various foods or inhaled as particles in the air. The types of ionizing radiation released by these radionuclides may include the following:
- Alpha particles (helium nuclei)
- Beta particles (electrons)
- Gamma rays (similar to x-rays, but usually of higher energy, in the range of a million electron volts [MeV])
- Some types of radioactive decay also affect the distribution of electrons around the atom and result in the emission of x-rays.

Examples of radioactive nuclides that exist in small quantities in the human body are as follows:
- Potassium-40 (^{40}K)
- Carbon-14 (^{14}C)
- Hydrogen-3 (^{3}H; tritium)
- Strontium-90 (^{90}Sr)

Radionuclides in the soil and air also add to the human radiation dose burden. The average member of the general population received approximately 0.7 mSv per year from combined exposure to radiations from the earth's surface (terrestrial) and radiation within the human body. Radon (2.00 mSv), cosmic ray radiations (0.3 mSv), terrestrial, and internally deposited radionuclides (0.7 mSv) that comprise the natural background radiation in the United States result in an estimated average annual individual EqD of approximately 3.0 mSv (see Table 2.3).

Manmade (Artificial) Radiation. Ionizing radiation created by humans for various uses is classified as manmade, or artificial, radiation. Sources of artificial ionizing radiation include the following:

- Consumer products containing radioactive material
- Air travel
- Nuclear fuel for generation of power
- Atmospheric fallout from nuclear weapons testing
- Nuclear power plant accidents
- Nuclear power plant accidents as a consequence of natural disasters
- Medical radiation

Manmade radiation contributes about 3.3 mSv to the average annual radiation exposure of the US population. Of this EqD, 0.6 mSv resulted from medical radiographic procedures, 0.7 mSv resulted from nuclear medicine imaging, 1.5 mSv resulted from computed tomography (CT) scanning, 0.4 mSv resulted from interventional procedures, and 0.1 mSv resulted from other manmade radiation sources (see Table 2.3). These figures represent an "average share" of dose to members of the population that would be true if the total medical radiation dose were shared equally among all individuals in the population. A qualified medical physicist can calculate an individual's actual medical radiation exposure from x-ray examinations if he or she is provided with the essential technical details (e.g., x-ray tube voltage used, exposure time, tube current [mA], patient dimensions, etc.) pertaining to the studies.

Consumer products containing radioactive material. Consumer products containing radioactive material include the following:
- Airport surveillance systems
- Electron microscopes
- Ionization-type smoke detector alarms
- Industrial static eliminators

These products contribute a very small fraction of the total average EqD to each member of the general population. As a result of technologic advances since the 1970s and strict regulations imposed within the United States by the Food and Drug Administration regarding such devices, the radiation exposure of the general public from consumer products may now be considered negligible.

Air travel. Commercial airline flights bring many humans to higher elevations and therefore in closer contact with high-energy extraterrestrial radiation (e.g., cosmic radiation) and consequently increase their exposure. A flight on a typical commercial airliner results in an EqD rate of 0.005 to 0.01 mSv/hour.

Sunspots sometimes play a role in increasing radiation exposure during air travel. Sunspots are dark spots

---

*Mesons are short-lived (only a few hundredths of a microsecond) subatomic particles smaller in size than a proton and are generated as by-products from very high-energy collisions between protons and protons or between protons and neutrons. They can carry an electric charge of the same value as that of an electron or be neutral.

that every so often appear on the surface of the sun. They indicate regions of increased electromagnetic field activity and are occasionally responsible for ejecting particulate radiation into space. This radiation normally constitutes a small fraction of our dose from cosmic radiation here on Earth. However, the solar contribution to the cosmic ray background increases substantially during periods of high sunspot activity and will contribute nonnegligible added radiation dose to airplane passengers and crew. If a person spends 10 hours flying aboard a commercial aircraft during a period of normal sunspot activity, that individual will receive a radiation EqD that is about equal to the dose received from one chest x-ray examination. During a *solar flare*, "a tremendous explosion on the surface of the sun,"[8] however, this dose can be 10 to as much as 100 times higher. Awareness of these potentially large increases in radiation exposure at high altitudes is important information for pilots and airline crews and the general public. An increase in radiation exposure carries an immeasurably small health risk for those individuals who travel by air infrequently. However, for pilots, flight attendants, and the general public who are "frequent flyers," the possibility exists that they "may unknowingly be exposed to excessively large doses of radiation."[9] With adequate knowledge, a person choosing air travel during periods of high sunspot activity and solar flares can make an intelligent decision about whether the potential benefit of the air travel outweighs any increased health risk.

A commercial flight crew's (pilot, flight attendants, etc.) actual radiation exposure sometimes exceeds that of workers at nuclear power plants. The Federal Aviation Administration and other organizations maintain ongoing programs of monitoring and evaluation of radiation risks to maintain the safety of occupational exposed airline workers.[9]

Nuclear fuel for the generation of power. Nuclear power plants that produce nuclear fuel for the generation of power do not contribute significantly to the annual EqD of the US population during their normal operating cycles. The nuclear fuel cycle, along with other manmade radiations, contributes only a very small portion of 0.1 mSv to the total average annual EqD for persons living in the United States.

Atmospheric fallout from nuclear weapons testing. An accurate estimate of the total annual EqD from fallout cannot be made because actual radiation measurements do not exist. The *dose commitment*, a dose that may ultimately be delivered from a given intake of radionuclide,[10] may be estimated by using a series of approximations and simplistic models that are subject to considerable speculation. The actual radiation dose to the global population from atmospheric fallout from nuclear weapons testing is not received all at once. It is instead delivered over a period of years at changing dose rates. The changes in the dose rates depend on factors such as characteristics of the fallout field and the elapsed time since the test occurred. No atmospheric nuclear testing has occurred since 1980.

When spread over the inhabitants of the United States, fallout from nuclear weapons tests (Fig. 2.4) and other environmental sources along with other manmade radiation contributes only a small portion of 0.1 mSv to the EqD of each person. This annual EqD is still considered to have a negligible impact on the US population.

Nuclear power plant accidents. Although nuclear power benefits humans by creating a needed supply of electricity, unfortunate accidents involving nuclear reactors can occur. This can lead to substantial unplanned radiation exposure for humans and the environment. Examples of two nuclear power plant accidents are addressed in the discussions that follow.

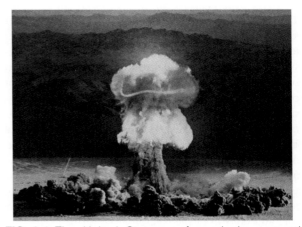

FIG 2.4 The United States performed aboveground nuclear weapons tests before 1963. During the Priscilla Test, this atomic cloud resulted when a 37-kiloton testing device exploded from a balloon at the Nevada test site on June 24, 1957. The atomic cloud top, which contained manmade ionizing radiation, ascended approximately 43,000 feet. (From US Department of Energy, Nevada Operations Office, Las Vegas, Nevada.)

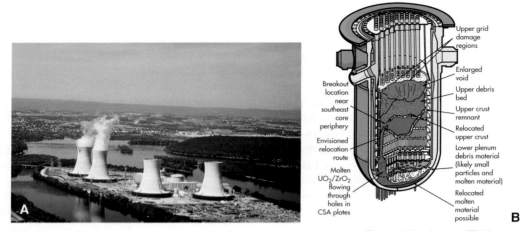

FIG 2.5 (A) Nuclear power stations, such as the one located on Three Mile Island (TMI) near Harrisburg, Pennsylvania, house nuclear reactors. The large round containment buildings holding the reactors retain radioactive liquids and gases even in a high-pressure environment. (B) TMI-2 end-state core conditions illustrating the damage to the radioactive nuclear reactor core after the loss of coolant accident on March 28, 1979. Some of the original core mass formed an upper layer of debris. A hard crust supports this material. Zones of previously molten material and standing fuel rod segments account for some of the core mass lying beneath the upper debris bed. The lower reactor vessel head contains some of the melted core material. Closed-circuit television, mechanical probing, and core-boring operations contributed to assessing the TMI-2 end-state core conditions. (A, From Pennsylvania State University Engineering Library. B, US Department of Energy, Nevada Operations Office, Las Vegas, Nevada.)

Three Mile Island Unit 2. On March 28, 1979, the Three Mile Island Unit 2 (TMI-2) pressurized water reactor, situated on an island in the Susquehanna River located about 15 miles southeast of Harrisburg, Pennsylvania (Fig. 2.5A), underwent a loss of coolant that resulted in severe overheating of the radioactive reactor core at a temperature greater than 5000°F Consequently, significant melting of the core occurred. The US Department of Energy estimated that about 40% of the material in the TMI-2 nuclear reactor core reached a molten state. Approximately 15% of the melted uranium dioxide fuel of the core actually flowed through the undamaged portions of the core and settled on the bottom of the reactor vessel. This melted material in the nuclear reactor core and bottom of the reactor vessel formed crusts on its outside surfaces and in time cooled to resolidified debris (Fig. 2.5B). Although significant melting of the core and flowing of the molten radioactive material into intact portions of the reactor vessel occurred, fortunately no "melt-through" of the reactor vessel resulted. The accident did, however, result in the destruction of the reactor.

Even though the potential existed for the release of significant amounts of radioactive material, according to the General Public Utilities Nuclear Corporation, the quantity of radiation that actually escaped during the accident, which was approximately 15 curies of iodine-131 [^{131}I]* was, as dispersed, not sufficient to cause health problems for persons occupationally exposed or for the 2 million people living within 50 miles of the plant. The average dose received by the exposed population living within a 50-mile radius of the TMI nuclear power station was determined to be 0.08 mSv, which is well below the average annual background radiation level.

According to conventional methods of risk assessment, if 0.08 mGy is used as an upper limit dose of ionizing radiation, it can be predicted that no more than one additional case of fatal cancer may occur in this population as a result of radiation exposure from this accident.[11]

---

*^{131}I is a radioactive isotope that emits both particles (fast electrons) and energetic gamma rays, with the most common beta emissions (89.3%) having 192 keV mean energy and the most common gamma emission (81.2%) having 365 keV energy.

Therefore detection of excess cancer deaths in this population as a consequence of the radiation dose it received is not expected.

Additional malignant deaths in the population exposed to radiation during the entire time of the TMI incident can be evaluated in another way. This is by applying the average dose received by the population as the "population dose" for persons living within a 100-mile radius of the nuclear power plant at the time of the accident. During this time, these residents received an average radiation exposure of 15 microgray.* If this dose is used as the population dose, then no more than two additional resulting cancer deaths can be predicted in the exposed inhabitants as a consequence of radiation exposure.[2]

Beginning at the time of the accident and continuing through 1992, the University of Pittsburgh followed more than 32,000 people who lived within 5 miles of TMI and were exposed to the low-level radioactivity released by the accident. Researchers found no link between radiation released (primarily xenon and iodine radioisotopes) during the TMI accident and cancer deaths among persons residing in the area. During the 13-year study of the people who lived within 5 miles of TMI at the time of the accident, only a single death occurred as a consequence of thyroid cancer, and this death was not attributed to radiation exposure.[11]

Because most radiation-induced cancers have a latent period of 15 years or more, continued monitoring of the health of the exposed residents is needed. Studies are expected to continue to obtain the necessary data to evaluate the mortality experience further.

Since the TMI-2 nuclear power plant accident, more than 35 years have passed. There has been no significant increase in cancer-related deaths reported among the population living near the TMI nuclear power station. Psychological stress at the time of the accident and shortly thereafter has been identified as the only detectable effect.[2,12] The Nuclear Regulatory Commission (NRC) reported that the TMI-2 pressurized water reactor is "permanently shut down and all of its fuel has been removed. The reactor coolant system is fully drained, the radioactive water decontaminated and evaporated. The accident's radioactive waste was shipped off-site to an appropriate disposal area, and the reactor fuel and core debris was shipped to the Department of Energy's Idaho Laboratory."[13] Long-term monitored storage of TMI-2 is expected to continue "until the operating license for the TMI-1 plant expires at which time both plants will be decommissioned."[13] "In 2009 the TMI-1 operating license was renewed, extending its life by 20 years to 2034."[14]

Chernobyl. On April 26, 1986, an explosion at a nuclear power plant in Chernobyl (Fig. 2.6), located near Kiev in the Ukraine in the former Soviet Union, resulted in the release of a number of radioactive nuclides, including 46 megacuries of ^{131}I, 136 megacuries of xenon radioisotopes, and 2.3 megacuries of cesium-137 (^{137}Cs)[†]. This is far more than 1 million times the amount of radioactive material released at TMI or "30 to 40 times as much radioactivity as the Hiroshima and Nagasaki atomic bombs combined in 1945."[15] More than 200 people working at the Chernobyl plant received a whole-body EqD exceeding 1 Sv. More than 2 dozen workers died as a result of explosion-related injuries and the effects of receiving doses greater than 4 Sv. The average EqD to the approximately quarter of a million individuals living within 200 miles of the reactor was 0.2 Sv. In some individuals, thyroid doses resulting from drinking milk contaminated with radioactive iodine actually exceeded several sieverts. Adverse health effects from radiation exposure are expected to occur for many years as a consequence of the total collective EqD received by the affected population, and "the number of people who could eventually die as a result of the Chernobyl accident is highly controversial."[16]

The ETHOS project. Beginning in 1996, a 3-year pilot research project called the ETHOS Project[16] was launched in the Republic of Belarus. This project was supported by the radiation project research program of the European Commission (DG XII). In the aftermath of the Chernobyl accident, the local citizens of the contaminated territories were empowered to make their own decisions to facilitate reconstruction of their overall quality of life. They were given the authority to manage their radiologic risk in the same way that the rural communities manage natural risk.[17,18]

---

*Gray (Gy) is the SI unit for measuring exposure. A milligray is a subunit of the Gy. It is equal to one thousandth of a Gy. The microgray is also a subunit of the Gy. It is equal to one millionth of a Gy.

[†]The half-life of cesium-137 is 30 years with a very energetic gamma ray emission of 662 KeV. When this radioisotope enters the bloodstream in the human body, it distributes itself rather uniformly throughout organs and muscle tissue and consequently causes radiation exposure to the whole body.

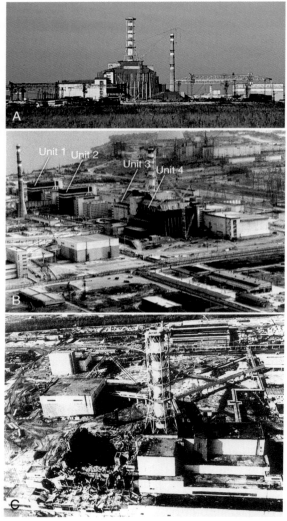

FIG 2.6 (A) Nuclear power plant in Chernobyl, former Soviet Union, site of the 1986 radiation accident. (B) Aerial view of the four identical units of the Chernobyl nuclear power plant before the accident. Graphics point out each of the reactors. (C) Chernobyl nuclear power plant after the explosion of unit 4 on April 26, 1986. (A, Ken Graham Photography. B and C, US Department of Energy, Nevada Operations Office, Las Vegas, Nevada.)

The aim of the ETHOS Project was to rebuild acceptable living conditions by actively involving the local population in the reconstruction process. This process encompassed dealing with the aspects of daily living that had been changed or threatened as a consequence of

radioactive contamination. One example was the establishment of guidelines for the amount of ash that is allowed to build up in wood stoves and fireplaces before cleaning is recommended. The ash is residue that remains after burning wood from trees that have taken up radioactive materials from the soil. The ash contains radioactive materials and is more compact than the piles of wood from which it came. The elimination of use of wood from the surrounding forests would have posed an unreasonable economic hardship on the population and was unnecessary as long as appropriate guidelines were set. Through this program, local citizens have been engaging in cooperative problem-solving as they reconstruct their environment.

Thyroid cancer, leukemia, and breast cancer as a result of the Chernobyl event. Thyroid cancer continues to be the main adverse health effect of the 1986 Chernobyl nuclear power accident. Children and adolescents living in the Ukraine region of Russia, where the dose was heaviest after the disaster, continue to be the focus of the disease. More than 1700 cases of thyroid cancer were diagnosed between 1990 and 1998.[19] Most of these cases are attributed to the radiation dose delivered when ^{131}I was taken up by the thyroid gland, although previous studies of atomic bomb survivors and Pacific Island inhabitants exposed to fallout predicted only 10 or so extra cases of thyroid cancer.[20] "The 2005 report prepared by the Chernobyl Forum, led by the International Atomic Energy Agency (IAEA) and the World Health Organization (WHO),* attributed 56 direct deaths (47 accident workers, and 9 children with thyroid cancer), and estimated that there may be 4000 extra deaths due to cancer among the approximately 600,000 most highly exposed and 5000 among the 6 million living nearby."[22,23]

Since the time of the Chernobyl accident, there has also been an increase in the incidence of breast cancer directly attributed to the radiation exposure.[24,25] The WHO Expert Group revealed that "reports indicate a

---

*The World Health Organization is the authority that directs and coordinates for health within the United Nations system. One of their greatest concerns is worldwide public health security. In situations such as a nuclear power plant accident, the mandate of the WHO is to determine and respond to public health risks. This organization also "conducts a program on radiation and health that aims to promote safe and appropriate use of radiation to protect patients, workers and the general public in planned, existing and emergency exposure situations."[21]

small increase in the incidence of pre-menopausal breast cancer in the most contaminated areas, which appear to be related to radiation dose."[26] However, follow-up epidemiologic studies are still necessary to confirm these findings. Some early research indicated no other increases in the effects that are generally associated with radiation exposure (leukemia, congenital abnormalities, or adverse pregnancy outcomes).[27] For example, the WHO found no increase in leukemia incidence by 1993 in the population hit hardest by fallout from Chernobyl.[28] Later studies began to show some of the expected effects. It was reported that there has been about a 50% increase in leukemia cases in children and adults in the Gomel region since the Chernobyl disaster.[29,30] Also reported in June 2001 at the Third International Conference on Health Effects of the Chernobyl accident held in Kiev, the Russian liquidators who worked during 1986 and 1987 at the Chernobyl power station complex had a statistically significant rise in the number of leukemia cases.[31,32] The WHO reported that "recent investigations suggest a doubling of the incidence of leukaemia* among the most highly exposed Chernobyl liquidators."[26] Furthermore, this organization also revealed that "no such increase has been clearly demonstrated among children or adults in any of the contaminated areas."[28] More time will be required before all the implications of these findings are clearly understood.

During the 6 months after the Chernobyl nuclear power plant disaster, a large concrete shelter known as the "sarcophagus" (Fig. 2.7) was constructed by the Soviets atop the remains of the reactor 4 building so that the other reactors could continue operating to provide nuclear power. Unfortunately, within 10 years after the shelter's construction the walls weakened, leaving the sarcophagus in danger of collapsing. Radiation leaks from the entombed reactor building also became apparent and caused great concern in the scientific community. During 1998 and 1999, some major repair work was carried out on the massive structure to strengthen the roof and structural pillars and stabilize the ventilation stack. In spite of the efforts made to enhance the strength and stability of the sarcophagus, the integrity of the structure remained questionable. Furthermore, lethal radiation levels inside

*"Leukaemia" is a variation of the spelling of "leukemia" that is used in some countries and by the WHO. This European spelling can differ from the US spelling, as in, for example, "aluminum" (US spelling) and "aluminium" (British spelling).

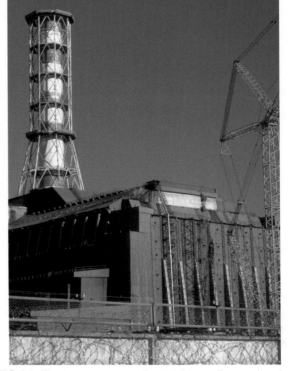

FIG 2.7 The large concrete "sarcophagus," encasing the remains of Chernobyl reactor unit 4. The structure is in danger of collapsing. (© Clive Shirley/Signum/Greenpeace.)

the shelter both complicated and limited opportunities for repair and maintenance.

Plans were made to cover the remains of Chernobyl reactor unit 4 and the concrete sarcophagus that entombs it with a weatherproof, massive steel vault (Fig. 2.8). Construction of this structure began in April 2012, with the now estimated completion date expected to be at the end of 2017.[33] The arch-shaped steel vault with a 100-year designed lifetime, referred to as the *New Safe Confinement structure*, is being built on site and, when completed, will be moved in place on rails and then slid over the collapsing sarcophagus. After this task has been accomplished, the concrete sarcophagus will be dismantled. The new shelter will provide protection so that highly radioactive fuel and damaged reactor remains can be better confined to protect the environment and the population more effectively.

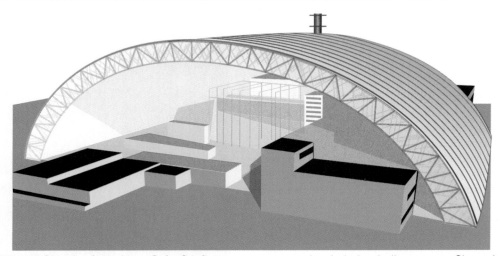

FIG 2.8 Sketch of the New Safe Confinement structure that is being built to cover Chernobyl reactor unit 4 and the concrete sarcophagus that entombs it.

Nuclear power plant accidents as a consequence of natural disasters. Accidents can occur in nuclear power plants as a consequence of natural disasters. This devastation can result in widespread environmental and health effects on the affected population of the surrounding area.

Fukushima Daiichi Nuclear Plant crisis. On March 11, 2011, a 9.0-magnitude earthquake that began approximately 96.6 kilometers (60 miles) off the northeast coast of Japan triggered a tsunami that slammed into the island's coast and bombarded it with 914-cm (30-foot)-high waves that actually traveled as far as 9.66 kilometers (6 miles) inland and devastated everything in their path within minutes.[34]

The Tokyo Electric Power Company's Fukushima Daiichi Nuclear Plant, housing six reactors, is located in the town of Naraha 93 miles southwest of the epicenter. As a consequence of the earthquake, the entire Japanese coastline dropped as much as 90 centimeters (3 feet). This left the shutdown nuclear power plant, in which the reactor cores had been automatically taken offline by sensors, much more vulnerable to the seismic waves of the tsunami that were racing toward it. Even though the plant had survived the earthquake, its 549-centimeter (18-foot) protection walls were not high enough to stop 914-centimeter (30-foot) waves from flooding the diesel generators cooling the nuclear reactor cores. Eventually even the backup batteries that kept the pumps going failed.

With the reactors in lockdown and no power being generated to operate the cooling pumps, a critical situation was created as temperatures continued to rise in the reactors. This led to a significant overheating of the fuel rods that resulted in the production of hydrogen gas, which eventually exploded. In desperation, an attempt was made to cool the reactors by dumping seawater on them. Unfortunately, this procedure did not work. Destruction of some reactors and severe damage to others occurred, leading to the release of a considerable amount of radiation (e.g., ^{137}Cs) in the atmosphere and surrounding area.[34] Because it is extremely difficult to measure the amounts of radiation people received, the long-term effects such as an increased incidence of cancer in the exposed population cannot be accurately determined.[35] However, since the time of the earthquake and following tsunami that resulted in the Fukushima nuclear plant disaster, the WHO has estimated that the lifetime risk for development of some cancers may be somewhat higher "above baseline rates in certain age and sex groups that were in areas with the highest estimated doses."[36] Increased health risks are not expected to be observed beyond the borders of Japan.[36] Areas of Fukushima Prefecture that were less affected by radiation exposure from the accident are also not expected to demonstrate an increase in cancer risk as a consequence of the combined accident.[36]

Sometime after the nuclear power plant accident, some hospitals in Japan noticed strange-looking "black

TABLE 2.4	**Medical Radiation Exposure: 2006**				
Modalities	Number of Procedures	Percentage (%)	Collective Dose (Person-Sv)	Percentage (%)	Per Capita (mSv)
Computed tomography	67 million	16	440,000	49	1.50
Nuclear medicine	18 million	4	231,000	26	0.80
Radiography and fluoroscopy	324 million	76	99,000	11	0.30
Interventional	17 million	4	129,000	14	0.40
Total	**~426 million**		**899,000**		**~3.0**

spots" on digital images. These spots were attributed to radioactive particulate fallout from the accident. However, the black spots on the digital images did not have any effect on the health of people but did possibly increase the fear of radiation exposure among the general population. In actuality, the spots proved to be somewhat of an annoyance during radiologic interpretation of digital images.[37]

Medical radiation. As mentioned earlier in this chapter, NCRP Report No. 160 was released on March 3, 2009. Data from this report are presented in Table 2.4. The previous report, NCRP Report No. 93 published in 1987, used data on medical usage from 1980 to 1982. The number of medical procedures involving the use of ionizing radiation had increased dramatically since the 1980s. Because of this trend, exposure of the US population from medical sources has also increased significantly.

Medical radiation exposure results from the use of diagnostic x-ray machines and radiopharmaceuticals in nuclear medicine. Diagnostic x-ray radiation (which includes CT scanning, interventional fluoroscopy, and conventional radiography or fluoroscopy) and nuclear medicine procedures are the two largest sources of artificial radiation, and they collectively accounted for 48% of the total collective EfD of the US population as of 2006 (see Fig. 2.2). The main reason for the increase is the enormously expanded use of CT. With the advent of multislice spiral (helical) computed tomography the use of this imaging modality in areas such as emergency medicine increased dramatically. In 1980 the CT usage resulted in a collective dose of 3700 person-sieverts. By 2006 that number had risen to 440,000 person-sieverts (see Table 2.4).[38]

Of course, modern CT offers tremendous medical benefit with regard to the diagnosis of disease and trauma, and the risk-to-benefit ratio is still very small when CT examinations are ordered for appropriate reasons.

Medical radiation accounts for approximately 3.2 mSv of the average annual individual EfD of ionizing radiation received (see Table 2.3). The total average annual EfD from manmade and natural radiation, including radon, is not associated with any measurable level of harm.[38]

Although the amount of natural background radiation remains fairly constant from year to year at 3.0 mSv, the frequency of exposure to manmade radiation in medical applications *continues to increase rapidly* among all age groups in the United States for a number of reasons. Among the main instigators of this are medicolegal considerations. Physicians, to protect themselves from often frivolous malpractice lawsuits, in general rely more and more on unneeded expensive sophisticated technology to assist them in making diagnoses for patient care rather than much less expensive and much lower radiation dose procedures such as basic x-ray projections that may well be just as informative. To reduce the possibility of genetic damage in future generations, this increase in frequency of radiation exposure in medicine must be counterbalanced by controlling the amount of patient exposure in individual imaging procedures. This can best be accomplished by limiting the widespread substitution of unnecessary CT scans and/or repetitive CT scans by many emergency departments for convenience in place of using alternative, less costly diagnostic procedures. In other areas such as interventional procedures, radiation doses to the public can be kept in check through efficient application of radiation protection measures (e.g., pulsed not continuous operation, lesser mA, last image hold and therefore less radiation beam on time) on the part of the radiographer, radiologist, and physicians using fluoroscopy. Because of the large variety of radiologic equipment and differences in imaging procedures and in individual radiologist and radiographer technical skills, the patient dose for each examination varies according to the facility providing imaging services. The amount of radiation actually received by a patient from a

TABLE 2.5   Representative Entrance Skin Exposures, Bone Marrow Dose, and Gonadal Dose From Various Diagnostic X-Ray Procedures

Examination	Exposure Factors (kVp/mAs)	Entrance Skin Dose (mGy$_t$)*	Bone Marrow Dose (mGy$_t$)	Gonad Dose (mGy$_t$)
Skull	76/50	2.0	0.10	<1
Chest	110/3	0.1	0.02	<1
Cervical spine	70/40	1.5	0.10	<1
Lumbar spine	72/60	3.0	0.60	2.25
Abdomen	74/60	4.0	0.30	1.25
Pelvis	70/50	1.5	0.20	1.50
Extremity	60/5	0.5	0.02	<1
CT (head)	125/300	40.0	0.20	0.50
CT (pelvis)	125/400	20.0	0.50	20

CT, Computed tomography.
*Milligray in tissue.
Adapted from Bushong SC: *Radiologic Science for Technologists: Physics, Biology, and Protection*, ed 10, St. Louis, 2013, Mosby.

diagnostic x-ray procedure may be indicated in terms such as the following:

1. Entrance skin exposure (ESE), which includes skin and glandular dose
2. Bone marrow dose
3. Gonadal dose

In pregnant women, fetal dose also may be estimated. Table 2.5 provides some examples of patient ESEs (skin and glandular), bone marrow, and gonadal doses, and Table 2.6 provides some representative fetal doses for several different radiologic examinations.

Because humans are unable to control natural background radiation, exposure from artificial sources that can be controlled must be limited to protect the general population from further biologic damage.

TABLE 2.6   Representative Fetal Doses for Radiographic Examinations

Examination	Fetal Dose (mGy)
Skull (lateral)	0
Cervical spine (AP)	0
Shoulder	0
Chest (PA)	0
Thoracic spine (AP)	0.1
Lumbosacral spine (AP)	0.8
Abdomen (AP)	0.7
Intravenous urogram (IVP)	0.6
Hip*	0.5
Extremity	0

AP, Anteroposterior projection; *IVP*, intravenous urogram; *PA*, posteroanterior projection.
*Gonadal shields should be used if possible.
Adapted from Bushong SC: *Radiologic Science for Technologists: Physics, Biology, and Protection*, 10 ed, St. Louis, 2013, Mosby.

■ SUMMARY

- Radiation is kinetic energy and exists in many forms.
- For radiation protection purposes, the electromagnetic spectrum can be divided into two categories: ionizing radiation and nonionizing radiation.
- X-rays, gamma rays, and ultraviolet radiation with energy greater than 10 eV are classified as ionizing radiations.
- Low-energy ultraviolet radiation, visible light, infrared rays, microwaves, and radio waves are classified as nonionizing radiations.
- X-rays are classified as electromagnetic radiation.

- The process of ionization is the foundation of the interaction of x-rays with human tissue. It makes the x-rays valuable for creating images but has the undesirable result of potentially producing some damage in biologic material.
- Alpha particles, beta particles, neutrons, and protons are particulate radiations. They vary in their ability to penetrate matter.
- Radiation absorbed dose is usually measured in units of milligray (mGy).

- Equivalent dose (EqD) takes into account the type of radiation that was absorbed. It provides an overall dose value that includes the different degrees of tissue interaction that could be caused by the different types of radiation. The millisievert (mSv) is the most common unit of measure of equivalent dose.
- Equivalent dose enables the calculation of the effective dose.
- The effective dose (EfD) is intended to be the best estimate of overall harm that might be produced by a given dose of radiation in human tissue. It takes into account both the type of radiation and the part of the body irradiated. The millisievert (mSv) is also the unit of measure for the effective dose.
- Ionizing radiation produces electrically charged particles that can cause biologic damage on molecular, cellular, and organic levels in humans.
- Sources of ionizing radiation may be natural or manmade.
- Natural sources include radioactive materials in the crust of the earth, cosmic rays from the sun and beyond the solar system, internal radiation from radionuclides deposited in humans through natural processes, and terrestrial radiation in the environment.
- Manmade sources include consumer products containing radioactive material, air travel, nuclear fuel, atmospheric fallout from nuclear weapons testing, nuclear power plant accidents whatever their origin, and medical radiation from diagnostic x-ray machines and radiopharmaceuticals in nuclear medicine procedures.
- Although there has not been much change in the amount of natural background radiation to the US population since 1987, there have been significant increases in the amount of radiation exposure resulting from medical imaging procedures such as CT scanning, cardiac nuclear medicine examinations, and interventional procedures.
- The most recently available data show that 37% of natural background radiation exposure comes primarily from the gaseous radionuclide, radon, and to a much lesser degree from the radionuclide thoron.
- The EPA considers radon to be the second leading cause of lung cancer in the United States.
- The recommended action limit for radon in homes is 4 pCi/L of air.
- Natural background radiation in the United States results in an estimated average annual individual EqD of 3.0 mSv.
- Manmade radiation exposure contributes about 3.3 mSv to the average annual radiation exposure on the US population.
- The total average annual EfD from natural background and manmade radiations combined is about 6.3 mSv.
- Thyroid cancer continues to be the main adverse health effect of the 1986 Chernobyl nuclear power plant accident.
- The amount of ionizing radiation actually received by a patient from a diagnostic x-ray procedure may be indicated in terms such as entrance skin exposure (ESE), bone marrow dose, and gonadal dose. In pregnant women, fetal dose also may be estimated.

REFERENCES

1. Environmental Protection Agency: Ionizing and non-ionizing radiation. Available at: http://www.epa.gov/radiation/understand/.
2. Bushong SC: *Radiologic science for technologists: physics, biology, and protection*, ed 10, St. Louis, 2013, Mosby.
3. Broadhead B: *The health effects of radon in layman's terms*, 2008, WPB Enterprises, Inc. Available at: www.wpb.radon.com.
4. Broadhead B: *Thoron measurements and health risk*, 2008, WPB Enterprises, Inc. Available at: http://wpb-radon.com/Thoron_measurement.html.
5. Read AB: Radon gas: the invisible threat. *RT Image* 5:12, 1992.
6. National Council on Radiation Protection and Measurements (NCRP): *Exposure of the population in the United States and Canada from natural background radiation, Report No. 94*, Washington, DC, 1987, NCRP.
7. News Release: Surgeon General Release National Health Advisory on Radon, Contact: HHS Press Office, (202) 690-6343. Available at: adph.org/radon/assets/surgeon.general.radon.pdf. (13 January 2005).
8. National Aeronautics and Space Administration (NASA): Solar flares. Available at: http://solarscience.msfc.nasa.gov/flares.shtml. (14 August 2012).
9. Pratt L, Strekel A: Prepare for take-off: the risk of cosmic radiation associated with air travel. *RT Image* 20:34, 2007.
10. National Council on Radiation Protection and Measurements (NCRP): *Ionizing radiation exposure of the population of the United States, Report No. 93*, Bethesda, Md, 1987, NCRP.
11. Talbott EO, et al: Mortality among the residents of the Three Mile Island accident area: 1979-1992, Research

Triangle Park, NC. *Environ Health Perspect* 108:545, 2000.

12. Three Mile Island: 1979, March 2001. Available at: www.world-nuclear.org/info/inf36.html.

13. United States Nuclear Regulatory Commission Fact Sheet, Background on the Three Mile Island Accident. Available at: www.nrc.gov/reading-rm/doc-collections/facts/3mile-isle.html. Last updated: 12 December 2014.

14. United States Nuclear Regulatory Commission, NRC News, NRC Renews Operating License for Three Mile Island Nuclear Power Plant for an Additional 20 Years, No. 09-176. Available at: http://pbadupws.nrc.gov/docs/ML0929/ML092950481.pdf. (22 October 2009).

15. Putting a lid on Chernobyl. Available at: http://www.washingtonpost.com/wp-dyn/article/A49461-2002Dec28.html.

16. The Chernobyl disaster, 2005. Available at: http://news.bbc.co.uk/2/shared/spl/hi/guides/456900/456957/html/nn3page1.stm. Publication date is 2005 June 20.

17. Dubreuil GH, et al: Chernobyl post-accident management: the ETHOS project. *Health Phys* 77:361, 1999.

18. Ollagnon H: *Approche patrimoniale de gestion du risque naturel*, Paris, 1992, Etude de CEMAGREFF.

19. United Nations Scientific Committee on the Effects of Atomic Radiation (UNSCEAR): *2000 report to the General Assembly, with Scientific Annexes, UNSCEAR 2000: sources and effects of ionizing radiation*, New York, 2000, United Nations.

20. Lazole E: Thoughts and lessons from the Chernobyl accident. *Health Phys Soc Newsl* 28:10, 2000.

21. World Health Organization: Health risk assessment from the nuclear accident after the 2011 Great East Japan Earthquake and Tsunami based on a preliminary dose estimation, Preface p 10, ISBN: 978 92 4 15013 0 (NLM classification: WN 665) World Health Organization Press, World Health Organization, 20 Avenue Appia, 1211 Geneva 27, Switzerland, 2013.

22. Chernobyl: the true scale of the accident. 2005. Available at: http://www.who.int/mediacentre/news/releases/2005/pr38/en/.

23. International Atomic Energy Agency (IAEA): Revisiting Chernobyl: 20 years later. Available at: www.iaea.org/NewsCenter/Focus/Chernobyl/. Last access date was March 4, 2017.

24. Fifteen years after the Chernobyl accident: lessons learned, Executive Summary, Kiev, April 2001.

25. Swiss Agency for Development and Cooperation: Chernobyl.info. Available at: www.chernobyl.info/.

26. World Health Organization: Health effects of the Chernobyl accident: an overview. Fact Sheet No. 303, April 2006. Available at: http://www.who.int/ionizing_radiation/chernobyl/backgrounder/en/index.html.

27. Stone R: Living in the shadow of Chernobyl. *Science* 292:420, 2001.

28. Walker SJ: *Permissible dose: a history of radiation protection in the twentieth century*, Berkeley, 2000, University of California Press.

29. Otto Hug Strahleninstit: Information, Ausgabe 9/2001 K, 2001.

30. Chernobyl Children's Project International. Available at: http://www.chernobyl-international.org/documents/chernobylfacts2.pdf.

31. Conclusions of 3rd international conference, health effects of the Chernobyl accident. *Int J Radiation Med* 3:3–4, 2001.

32. Romanenko A, Bebeshko V, et al: The Ukrainian-American study of leukemia and related disorders among Chornobyl cleanup workers from Ukraine: I. Study methods. *Radiat Res* 170(6):691–697, 2008. doi:10.1667/RR1402.1.

33. World Nuclear News: Chernobyl confinement reaches final stage, but funds need boost. March 17, 2015. Available at: http://www.world-nuclear-news.org/WR-Chernobyl-Confinment-reaches-final-stage-but-funds-need-boost-17031502.html.

34. Nova: Japan's killer quake, An eyewitness account and investigation of the epic earthquake, tsunami, and nuclear crisis. Aired on February 29, 2012, on PBS, originally aired March 30, 2011. Available at: http://www.pbs.org/wgbh/nova/earth/japan-killer-quake.html.

35. Ritter M: Japan nuclear disaster released higher radiation levels than previously reported, study finds. Huff Post World, October 28, 2011. Available at: http://www.huffingtonpost.com/2011/10/27/japan-nuclear-disaster-fukushima-tsunami-earthquake-chernobyl_n_1062605.html.

36. Ionizing radiation, Frequently asked questions on health risk assessment. 2013, Available at: www.who.int/ionizing_radiation/pub_meet/faqs_fukushima_risk_assessment/en/.

37. Kashimura Y, Chida K: Clinical perspective: nuclear reactor accident fallout artifacts: unusual black spots on digital radiographs. *Am J Roentgenol* 205:1240–1243, 2015. doi:10.2214/AJR.15.14557.

38. National Council on Radiation Protection and Measurements (NCRP): *Ionizing radiation exposure of the population of the United States, Report No. 160*, Bethesda, Md, 2009, NCRP.

GENERAL DISCUSSION QUESTIONS

1. What form of energy is radiation?
2. How do electromagnetic and particulate radiations differ?
3. When inhaled into the lungs of a human, why is radon more dangerous than thoron?
4. What is a solar flare?
5. Explain the use of the radiation quantity "equivalent dose" (EqD).
6. What are enhanced natural sources of radiation?
7. How does radon affect the epithelial tissue of the lungs in humans?
8. How can a flight on a typical commercial airliner result in radiation exposure for a passenger?
9. What consumer products contain radioactive materials?
10. Give four examples of radioactive nuclides that exist in small quantities in the human body.
11. Following the Fukushima Daiichi nuclear plant disaster, what were the black spots in digital images seen in some hospitals attributed to?
12. Since the time of the earthquake and tsunami that resulted in the Fukushima nuclear plant disaster in 2011, what has the World Health Organization estimated the lifetime risk for development of some cancers to be in the areas where the most exposure occurred?

REVIEW QUESTIONS

1. The amount of radiation actually received by a patient from a diagnostic x-ray procedure may be indicated in terms such as:
   1. Entrance skin exposure (ESE)
   2. Bone marrow dose
   3. Gonadal dose
   A. 1 and 2 only
   B. 1 and 3 only
   C. 2 and 3 only
   D. 1, 2, and 3
2. Which of the following processes is the foundation of the interaction of x-rays with human tissue?
   A. Ionization
   B. Linear acceleration
   C. Particle emission
   D. Radioactive decay

3. Why are the long-term effects, such as an increased incidence of cancer in the exposed population living near Japan's Fukushima Daiichi Nuclear Plant, unable to be accurately determined?
   A. After the tsunami, winds carried all the radiation back out to sea.
   B. It was extremely difficult to measure the amounts of radiation people received.
   C. Radiation from the crippled reactors was negligible.
   D. Radiation levels exceeded the reading scales on the instruments used to measure population exposure.
4. According to the most recent available data, what percentage of natural background radiation exposure comes from radon and thoron?
   A. 10
   B. 29
   C. 37
   D. 48
5. Which of the following are natural sources of ionizing radiation?
   A. Medical x-radiation and cosmic radiation
   B. Radioactive elements in the crust of the earth and in the human body
   C. Radioactive elements in the human body and a diagnostic x-ray machine
   D. Radioactive fallout and environs of atomic energy plants
6. An equivalent dose as low as 250 mSv delivered to the whole body may cause which of the following within a few days?
   A. An increase in the number of lymphocytes in the circulating blood
   B. A substantial decrease within a few days in the number of lymphocytes or white blood cells that are the body's primary defense against disease
   C. A drop immediately to zero in the lymphocyte count
   D. A large increase in the number of platelets
7. How is actual radiation dose to the global population from atmospheric fallout from nuclear weapons testing received?
   A. It is received all at once within a short period of time after such a test.
   B. It is received in large quantities within a period of 2 years after such a test.

C. It is not received all at once but instead is delivered over a period of years at changing dose rates.

D. No fallout from such testing is ever received.

8. Which of the following is the total average annual radiation equivalent dose from manmade and natural radiation?

A. 1.8 mSv per year

B. 3.0 mSv per year

C. 3.2 mSv per year

D. 6.3 mSv per year

9. The Russian liquidators who worked during 1986 and 1987 at the Chernobyl power complex demonstrated a statistically significant rise in the number of:

1. Breast cancer cases
2. Leukemia cases
3. Prostate cancer cases

A. 1 only

B. 2 only

C. 3 only

D. 1, 2, and 3

10. Which of the following is recognized as the main adverse health effect from the 1986 Chernobyl nuclear power accident?

A. Increase in the incidence of leukemia in adults

B. Increase in the incidence of leukemia in children

C. Increase in the incidence of thyroid cancer in adults

D. Increase in the incidence of thyroid cancer in children and adolescents

3

Interaction of X-Radiation With Matter

OBJECTIVES

After completing this chapter, the reader will be able to perform the following:

- Define all key terms.
- Explain the meaning and significance of peak kilovoltage (kVp) and milliampere-seconds (mAs) as technical exposure factors.
- Describe the process of absorption, and explain why absorbed dose in atoms of biologic matter should be kept as small as possible.
- Differentiate among the following: primary radiation; exit, or image-formation, radiation; and scattered radiation.
- List two types of x-ray photon transmission, and explain the difference between them.
- Discuss the way x-rays are produced, and detail the range of energies present in the x-ray beam.

- Catalog the events that occur when x-radiation passes through matter.
- Explain what determines the probability of photon interaction with matter.
- Describe and illustrate by diagram the x-ray photon interactions with matter that are important in diagnostic radiology.
- List the x-ray photon interactions with matter that occur above the energy range used in diagnostic radiology.
- Explain how the introduction of positive contrast media affects the appearance and the absorbed dose of body structures that contain it.
- Describe the effect of kVp on radiographic image quality and patient absorbed dose.

CHAPTER OUTLINE

Significance of X-Ray Absorption in Biologic Tissue
X-Ray Beam Production and Energy
    Production of Primary Radiation
    Energy of Photons in a Diagnostic X-Ray Beam
Attenuation
    Direct and Indirect Transmission X-Ray Photons
    Primary, Exit, and Attenuated Photons
Probability of Photon Interaction With Matter

Processes of Interaction
    Coherent Scattering
    Photoelectric Absorption
    Compton Scattering
    Pair Production
    Photodisintegration
Summary

KEY TERMS

absorbed dose (D)
absorption
attenuation
Auger effect
characteristic photon

characteristic x-ray
coherent scattering
Compton scattered electron, or
    secondary, or recoil, electron
Compton scattering

contrast media
effective atomic number (Zeff)
exit, or image-formation, photons
fluorescent radiation
fluorescent yield

mass density	photodisintegration	radiographic contrast
milliampere-seconds (mAs)	photoelectric absorption	radiographic fog
pair production	photoelectron	radiographic image receptor
peak kilovoltage (kVp)	primary radiation	small-angle scatter

In this chapter, fundamental physics concepts that relate to radiation absorption and scatter are reviewed. The processes of interaction between radiation and matter are emphasized because a basic understanding of the subject is necessary for radiographers to optimally select the following technical exposure factors:

- peak kilovoltage (kVp), the highest energy level of photons in the x-ray beam, equal to the highest voltage established across the x-ray tube
- milliampere-seconds (mAs), the product of electron tube current and the amount of time in seconds that the x-ray tube is activated

Peak kilovoltage controls the quality, or penetrating power, of the photons in the x-ray beam and to some degree also affects the quantity, or number of photons, in the beam. The product of milliamperes (mA), which is the x-ray tube current, and time (seconds [s] during which the x-ray tube is activated) is the main determinant of how much radiation is directed toward a patient during a selected x-ray exposure. Because the level of energy (beam quality) and the number of x-ray photons are controlled by technique factors selected by the radiographer, the radiographer is responsible for the radiation dose the patient receives during an imaging procedure. With a suitable understanding of these factors, radiographers will be able to select appropriate techniques that can minimize that dose to the patient while producing optimal-quality images.

SIGNIFICANCE OF X-RAY ABSORPTION IN BIOLOGIC TISSUE

X-rays are carriers of manmade electromagnetic energy. If x-rays enter a material such as human tissue, they may:

1. Interact with the atoms of the biologic material in the patient and be absorbed
2. Interact with the atoms in the biologic material and be scattered, causing some indirect transmission
3. Pass through without interaction

If an interaction occurs, electromagnetic energy is transferred from the x-rays to the atoms of the patient's biologic material. This process is called absorption (Fig. 3.1), and the amount of energy absorbed per unit mass is referred to as the absorbed dose (D). The more electromagnetic energy that is received by the atoms of the patient's body, the greater is the possibility of biologic damage in the patient. Therefore the amount of electromagnetic energy transferred should be kept as small as possible. However, without absorption and the differences in the absorption properties of various body structures, it would not be possible to produce diagnostically useful images, that is, images in which different anatomic structures could be perceived and distinguished. So some small amount of radiation dose is necessary. The radiographer also benefits when the patient's dose is minimal because less radiation is scattered from the patient.

X-RAY BEAM PRODUCTION AND ENERGY
Production of Primary Radiation

A diagnostic x-ray beam is produced when a stream of very energetic electrons bombards a positively charged target in a highly evacuated glass tube. In general radiography, this target, also known as the *anode,* is usually made of tungsten or an alloy of tungsten and rhenium. These materials have:

- High melting points
- High atomic numbers (tungsten [74] and rhenium [75])

As the electrons interact with the atoms of the tube target, x-ray photons are produced. Photons are particles associated with electromagnetic radiation that have neither mass nor electric charge and travel at the speed of light. X-ray photons exit from the tube target with a broad range, or spectrum, of energies and leave the x-ray tube through a glass window. The glass window permits passage of all but the lowest-energy components of the x-ray spectrum. It therefore acts as a filter by removing diagnostically useless, very-low-energy x-rays. In addition

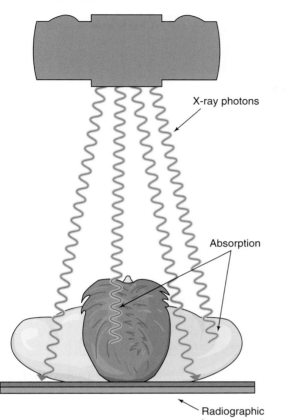

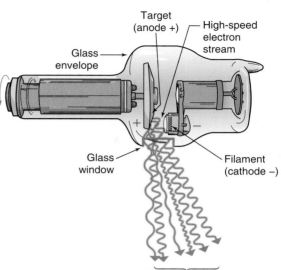

FIG 3.2 Primary radiation emerges from the x-ray tube target and consists of x-ray photons of various energies. It is produced when the positively charged target is bombarded with a stream of high-speed electrons and these electrons interact with the atoms of the target.

FIG 3.1 X-ray photons can interact with atoms of the patient's body and transfer energy to the tissue. This transference of electromagnetic energy to the atoms of the material is called *absorption*.

to this, a certain thickness of added aluminum is placed within the collimator assembly to intercept the emerging x-rays before they reach the patient. This aluminum "hardens" the x-ray beam (i.e., raises its effective energy) by removing low-energy components that would serve only to increase patient dose. The combination of the x-ray tube glass wall and the added aluminum placed within the collimator may be called the *permanent inherent filtration* of the x-ray unit. This filtered x-ray photon beam is collectively referred to as **primary radiation** (Fig. 3.2).

Energy of Photons in a Diagnostic X-Ray Beam

Although all photons in a diagnostic x-ray beam do not have the same energy, the most energetic photons in the beam can have no more energy than the electrons that bombard the target. The energy of the electrons inside the x-ray tube is generally specified in terms of the electrical voltage applied across the tube. In diagnostic radiology, this voltage is expressed in thousands of volts, or kilovolts (kV). Because the voltage across the tube fluctuates, it is usually characterized by the kilovolt peak value (kVp).

If an electron is drawn across an electrical potential difference of 1 volt, we say that it has acquired energy of 1 electron volt (eV). Therefore a technique factor of 100 kVp means that the electrons bombarding the target have a maximum energy of 100,000 eV, or 100 keV. X-rays of various energies are produced, but the most energetic x-ray photon can have no more energy than 100 keV. For a typical diagnostic x-ray unit, the mean photon energy in the x-ray beam is about one-third the energy of the most energetic photon. Therefore a 100-kVp beam contains photons having energies of 100 keV or less, with an average or effective energy of approximately 33 keV. In summary, the units kVp or kV refer to the voltage on the x-ray tube, and keV refers to the energy of specific x-rays.

ATTENUATION

Direct and Indirect Transmission X-Ray Photons

When an x-ray beam passes through a patient, it goes through a process called **attenuation**. Attenuation is simply the reduction in the number of primary photons in the x-ray beam through absorption (a total loss of radiation energy) and scatter (a change in the direction of travel that may also involve a partial loss of radiation energy) as the beam passes through the patient in its path. Some primary x-ray photons also traverse the patient without interacting. This outcome is called *direct transmission*. These non-interacting x-ray photons reach the **radiographic image receptor** (IR), which may be one of the following:

• Phosphor plate
• Digital radiography receptor
• Radiographic film

Other primary photons can undergo what are called *Compton* and/or *coherent interactions* (these processes are discussed later in this chapter) and as a result may be scattered or deflected with a potential loss of energy. Such photons may still traverse the patient and strike the IR. This process is termed *indirect transmission*. The optimal x-ray image is formed when only direct transmission x-ray photons reach the IR. In clinical situations, however, with either conventional or digital radiography, because the image receptor covers a broad area, scattered photons do reach the IR and as a result degrade or lessen the contrast of the recorded image. Several methods have been devised to limit the presence of indirectly transmitted x-ray photons.

Primary, Exit, and Attenuated Photons

Fig. 3.3 illustrates the passage of four x-ray photons through a patient. Before the four photons produced by the x-ray source enter human tissue, they are referred to as *primary photons*. Only two photons emerge from the tissue and strike the x-ray detector below it. They are referred to as **exit, or image-formation, photons**. The two that miss the detector are classified as attenuated. The term *attenuation* is rather broad. With respect to x-rays, attenuation may be used to refer to any process decreasing the intensity of the primary photon beam (i.e., the number of photons crossing unit area per second) directed toward a particular destination. In Fig. 3.3 that end point is the image receptor. Therefore photon 3,

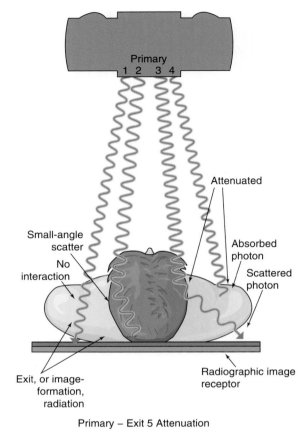

FIG 3.3 Primary, exit, and attenuated photons. Primary photons (photons 1, 2, 3, and 4) are photons that emerge from the x-ray source. Exit, or image-formation, photons (photons 1 and 2) are photons that pass through the patient being radiographed and reach the radiographic image receptor. Attenuated photons (photons 3 and 4) are photons that have interacted with atoms of the patient's biologic tissue and been scattered or absorbed such that they do not reach the radiographic image receptor.

which has deviated from its path (i.e., it has been "scattered") to the extent that it will not strike the detector is said to have been attenuated. Photon 4 seems to disappear. It has transferred all its kinetic energy to the atoms of the patient and has therefore been eliminated. This occurs because a photon has no mass, only kinetic energy, which implies that it ceases to exist when it gives up its kinetic energy. *Attenuation,* then, refers to both absorption and scatter processes that prevent photons from reaching a predefined location. Fig. 3.3 shows that the path of photon 2 was bent, but not so much that the photon missed its target. Because photon 2 reaches the IR, it is part of the exit, or image-formation, radiation, but the bending of its path represents what is called small-angle scatter. Scattered photons in this category have essentially the same energy as the incoming, or "incident," photons. As was mentioned previously, small-angle scatter degrades the appearance of a completed radiographic image by blurring the sharp outlines of dense structures. Because many billions of such scatter events happen, a greater overall exposure of the IR occurs than is needed. This additional, undesirable exposure is called radiographic fog. It interferes with the radiologist's ability to distinguish different structures in the image. Reducing the amount of tissue irradiated decreases the amount of fog produced and is therefore another method of limiting the number of indirectly transmitted photons. The radiographer can achieve this by confining, or collimating, the x-ray beam as much as possible to include only the region of interest (Fig. 3.4).

PROBABILITY OF PHOTON INTERACTION WITH MATTER

Because the interaction of photons with biologic matter is random, it is impossible to predict with certainty what will happen to a single photon when it enters human tissue. When dealing with a large number of photons, however, it is possible to predict what will happen on the average, and this is more than adequate to determine the characteristics of the image that results from these numerous interactions (Table 3.1). An example is provided in Box 3.1.

Table 3.2 shows the factors that influence the probability of interactions in matter. In the remainder of this chapter, the different interactions of photons with individual atoms and the effect of a particular type of interaction on the radiographic image are examined.

PROCESSES OF INTERACTION

Five types of interactions between x-radiation and matter are possible:
1. Coherent scattering
2. Photoelectric absorption
3. Compton scattering
4. Pair production
5. Photodisintegration

BOX 3.1 Probability of Photon Interaction With Matter

In an ordinary beam of x-ray photons (which consists of a vast number of such particles) a 50-keV photon, on average, has a 66% probability of interaction when it travels through 5 cm of soft tissue (see Appendix D); 34% of the time such photons will be likely to just pass through the tissue. As an illustration of this process, consider that in a randomly chosen group of 1000 50-keV photons traveling through 5 cm of soft tissue, 666 interactions may be expected to occur. Of the 666 interactions, 11% (73 of the 666 interactions) should be of a type called *photoelectric*. In the photoelectric interaction, a photon is completely absorbed by the atoms of the tissue (i.e., removed from the beam). If this were the only interaction possible, irradiating 5 cm of soft tissue with 50-keV photons would create a lighter area on a radiographic image, which would be the result of fewer photons reaching that portion of the image receptor. In reality, the process is much more complicated because several additional effects occur, and a typical x-ray beam is composed of photons with a continuous range of energies rather than a single energy.

BOX 3.2 Importance of Various Interactions of X-Radiation With Matter

Interaction	Where Important
Coherent scattering	Not important in any energy range
Photoelectric absorption	Diagnostic radiology
Compton scattering	Diagnostic radiology and therapeutic radiology
Pair production	Therapeutic radiology
Photodisintegration	Therapeutic radiology

Of these, only two are important in diagnostic radiology:
1. Compton scattering
2. Photoelectric absorption

Box 3.2 presents an overview of the various interactions between x-radiation with matter and where they are important.

Coherent Scattering

Coherent scattering is sometimes also called by the following names:

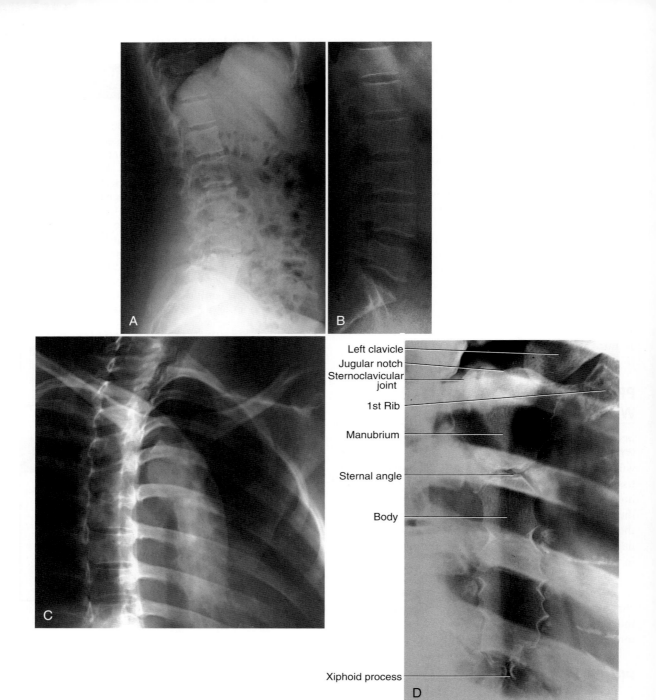

FIG 3.4 (A) Lateral image of the lumbar vertebrae showing improper collimation, which results in the production of radiographic fog and a consequent lack of radiographic clarity. (B) Lateral image of the lumbar vertebrae showing adequate collimation, which eliminates radiographic fog and consequently increases radiographic clarity. (C) Posterolateral (PA) oblique projection (right anterior oblique [RAO] position) of the sternum, demonstrating poor collimation. (D) PA oblique projection (RAO position) of the sternum, demonstrating good collimation. (D, From Long BW, Rollins JH, Smith BS: *Merrill's Atlas of Radiographic Positioning & Procedures,* ed 13, St. Louis, 2016, Elsevier.)

TABLE 3.1 Interaction of X-Radiation With Soft Tissue: Overview

X-Ray Photon Energy Range	Site of Interaction	X-Ray Photon	Typical Interaction	By-Products of Interaction
1–50 kVp	An atom	Energy: unchanged; direction after interaction: slight change (<20 degrees)	Coherent scattering*	None
1–50 kVp	Inner-shell electron (usually K or L shell)	Energy: absorbed; direction after interaction: not applicable	Photoelectric absorption[†]	Photoelectron (characteristic photon)
60–90 kVp	Outer-shell electron	Energy: reduced; direction after interaction: changed (x-ray photon energy partially absorbed)	Compton scattering[‡] Photoelectric absorption[†]	Compton scattered electron Compton scattered photon
90–120 kVp	Outer-shell electron	Energy: reduced after interaction: changed (x-ray photon energy partially absorbed)	Compton[‡] scattering Photoelectric absorption[†]	Compton scattered electron Compton scattered photon
200 kVp–2 MeV	Outer-shell electron	Energy: reduced; direction after interaction: changed	Compton scattering[§‖]	Compton scattered electron Compton scattered photon
Begins at about 1.022 MeV; becomes important at 10 MeV; becomes predominant at 50 MeV and greater	Nucleus of atom	Energy: disappears after interaction with nucleus; transformed into two new particles that annihilate each other; after interaction: energy reappears in the form of two 0.511-MeV photons moving in opposite directions	Pair production	Positive electron (positron); ordinary electron (negatron); two 0.511-MeV photons
Greater than 10 MeV	Nucleus of atom	Energy: absorbed by nucleus after collision with high-energy photon; excess energy in nucleus creates instability that is usually alleviated by emission of a neutron; other emissions possible	Photodisintegration	Neutron; other types of emissions possible if sufficient energy is absorbed by the nucleus: proton or proton–neutron combination (deuteron) or even an alpha particle

*This scattering occurs mostly in this energy range, but it is still much less probable than photoelectric absorption.
[†]The interaction most responsible for radiation dose in this energy range.
[‡]Both Compton and photoelectric interactions occur in this energy range.
[§]Compton interaction is predominantly responsible for radiation dose in this energy range.
[‖]In this energy range, the scattered particles go on to produce many more Compton and photoelectric interactions on their own.

TABLE 3.2 Factors That Influence the Probability of Interaction of Photons With Energy E in Materials With Density ρ

Interaction	Photon Energy	Atomic Number	Electron Density ρ_e (e/g)	Physical Density ρ (g/cm³)
Photoelectric	$1/E^3$	Z^3	Independent	ρ
Compton	$1/E$	Independent	ρ_e	ρ
Pair production	E	Z	Independent	ρ

- Classical scattering
- Elastic scattering
- Unmodified scattering

It is a simple process that results in no loss of energy as x-rays scatter.

Process of Coherent Scattering. When a low-energy (typically less than 10 keV) photon interacts with an atom, it may transfer its energy by causing some or all of the electrons of the atom to momentarily vibrate. This is analogous to the behavior of electrons in the antenna of a receiver intercepting a radio signal. Because they are charged particles, each of the atom's vibrating electrons radiates energy in the form of electromagnetic waves. These waves combine with one another to form a scattered wave, or photon. Because the wavelengths of both incident and scattered waves are the same, no net energy has been absorbed by the atom (see Appendix E). However, a small change in the direction of the emitted photon is very likely. In general, this change in direction is less than 20 degrees with respect to the initial direction of the original photon. This is the net effect of coherent, or unmodified, scattering. Although coherent scattering is most likely to occur at less than 10 keV (energies that will be eliminated by the inherent filtration), some of this unmodified scattering occurs throughout the diagnostic energy range and may result in small amounts of radiographic fog (Fig. 3.5). This source of fog, however, is not significant in general diagnostic imaging. In mammography, which of necessity involves many low-energy photons, coherent scattering also does not contribute noticeably to radiographic fog because during this imaging procedure, breast tissue is gently but firmly compressed. As a result of this compression, the breast becomes relatively thin. This eliminates the production of a large amount of scatter radiation.

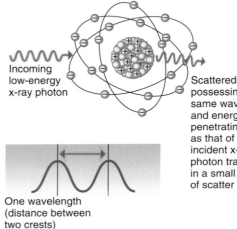

FIG 3.5 Coherent Scattering. The incoming low-energy x-ray photon interacts with an atom and transfers its energy by causing some or all of the electrons of the atom to momentarily vibrate. The electrons then radiate energy in the form of electromagnetic waves. These waves nondestructively combine with one another to form a scattered wave, which represents the scattered photon. Its wavelength and energy, or penetrating power, are the same as those of the incident photon. Generally, the emitted photon may change in direction less than 20 degrees with respect to the direction of the original photon. (Wavelength is the distance from one crest to the next.)

Small angle coherent scattering does not have much of an effect on radiographic imaging, but it does have a noticeable effect on visible light. This is why the sky is blue and sunsets are red.[1] Much longer wavelengths than those of x-rays, especially "visible" wavelengths such as those belonging to blue light, are far more likely to be scattered and to scatter over a greater angle. Therefore

BOX 3.3   Summary of the Process of
Coherent Scattering

The process of coherent scattering is of no importance
in any energy range. When the low-energy x-ray photon
interacts with an atom of human tissue, it does not lose
kinetic energy. The emitted photon merely changes
direction by 20 degrees or less. No ionization of the
biologic atom occurs.

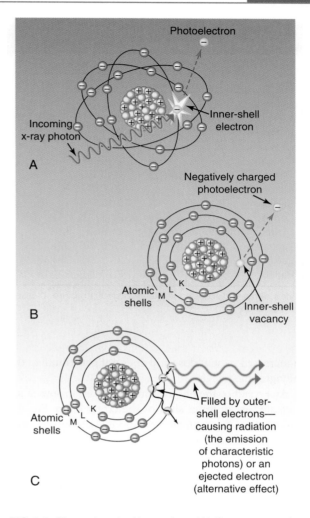

when you look up in the sky in any direction, you tend
to see the blue light scattered toward you. At sunset,
looking toward the sun, the blue light is mainly scattered
away from you, so the sun appears to consist of mostly
longer wavelength visible light, that is, mostly red.

A summary of facts about the process of coherent
scattering is presented in Box 3.3 for quick reference.

Photoelectric Absorption

Within the energy range of diagnostic radiology (23 to
150 kVp), which also includes mammography, photoelectric absorption is the most important mode of
interaction between x-ray photons and the atoms of the
patient's body for producing useful images.

Process of Photoelectric Absorption. Photoelectric
absorption is an interaction between an x-ray photon and
an inner-shell electron (usually in the K or L shells [Fig.
3.6, Table 3.3; for a detailed explanation see Appendix F]).
To dislodge an inner-shell electron from its atomic orbit,
the incoming x-ray photon must be able to transfer a
quantity of energy as large as or larger than the amount of
energy that holds the electron in its orbit. On interacting
with an inner-shell electron, the x-ray photon surrenders
all its energy to the orbital electron and ceases to exist.
The electron escapes from its inner shell, thus creating
a vacancy. The now unbound orbital electron, called
a **photoelectron,** possesses kinetic energy equal to the
energy of the incident photon minus the binding energy
of the electron shell. This photoelectron may interact with
other atoms in the vicinity, thereby causing excitation
(promotion of electrons from lower energy shells to higher
energy shells) or ionization (complete ejection of the
electron from an atom), until all of its kinetic energy
has been spent. The photoelectron is usually absorbed
within a few micrometers of the medium through which
it travels. In the human body, this energy transfer results

FIG 3.6 Photoelectric Absorption. (A) On encountering
an inner-shell electron, usually in the K or L shell, the
incoming x-ray photon surrenders all its energy to the
electron, and the photon ceases to exist. (B) The atom
responds by ejecting the electron, called a *photoelectron,*
from its inner shell, thus creating a vacancy in that shell.
(C) To fill the opening, an electron from an outer shell
drops down to the vacated inner shell by releasing energy
in the form of a characteristic photon. Then, to fill the
new vacancy in the outer shell, another electron from
the shell next farthest out drops down and another
characteristic photon is emitted and so on until the atom
regains electrical equilibrium. There is also some probability that instead of a characteristic photon, an Auger
electron will be ejected.

TABLE 3.3   Electron Shell Occupancies for Some Common Atoms*

Atom	Symbol	Atomic Number	K	L	M	N	O	P
Hydrogen	H	1	1					
Helium	He	2	2					
Lithium	Li	3	2	1				
Carbon	C	6	2	4				
Oxygen	O	8	2	6				
Sodium	Na	11	2	8	1			
Aluminum	Al	13	2	8	3			
Calcium	Ca	20	2	8	8	2		
Copper	Cu	29	2	8	18	1		
Molybdenum	Mo	42	2	8	18	13	1	
Tungsten	W	74	2	8	18	32	12	2
Lead	Pb	82	2	8	18	32	18	4
Radon	Rn	86	2	8	18	32	18	8

*For a detailed discussion of electron shell structure, please see Appendix F.

in increased patient dose and does not contribute to the radiographic image.

As a result of the photoelectric interaction, a vacancy is created in an inner shell of the target atom. For the ionized atom, this represents an unstable energy situation. The instability is alleviated by filling the vacancy in the inner shell with an electron from an outer shell, which spontaneously "falls down" into this opening. To do this, the descending electron must lose energy, that is, must pass from a less tightly bound atomic state (farther from the nucleus) to a more tightly held status (closer to the nucleus). The amount of energy loss involved is simply equal to the difference in the binding, or "holding," energies associated with each electron shell. For a large atom such as an atom of the element lead, this energy can be in the kiloelectron volt range, whereas for the small or low atomic number atoms that make up most of the human body, the energy is on the order of 10 eV. The "released" energy is carried off in the form of a photon that is called a **characteristic photon,** or **characteristic x-ray,** because its energy is directly related to the shell structure of the atom from which it was emitted. Those photons generated from photoelectric interactions within human tissue are low enough in energy that they are predominantly absorbed within the body. In general, ensuing vacancies in other electron

shells are successively filled, and associated characteristic photons are emitted until the atom achieves an electronic equilibrium.

One additional process can occur as a result of photoelectric interactions. It is called the **Auger effect** (pronounced "awzhay"), named after the French scientist, Pierre Victor Auger, who discovered it in 1925. When an inner electron is removed from an atom in a photoelectric interaction, thus causing an inner-shell vacancy, the energy liberated when this vacancy is filled can be transferred to another electron of the atom, thereby ejecting that electron, instead of emerging from the atom as characteristic radiation. Such an emitted electron is called an *Auger electron.* Its energy is equal to the difference between that released by an outer electron in filling the initial created vacancy and the binding energy of the emitted or Auger electron. Because this process does not include any x-ray emission, it is called a *radiationless effect.* It reduces the total amount of characteristic radiation produced by photoelectric interactions. The term **fluorescent yield** refers to the number of x-rays emitted per inner-shell vacancy. Because the Auger effect is more prevalent in materials with higher atomic number atoms, the fluorescent yield per photoelectron is generally lower in such materials than for substances with low atomic numbers (see Fig. 3.6C).

In summary, the by-products of photoelectric absorption include the following:
1. Photoelectrons (those induced by interaction with external radiation and the internally generated Auger electrons)
2. Characteristic x-ray photons (**fluorescent radiation**)

When the energy of these by-products is locally absorbed in human tissue, both the dose to the patient and the potential for biologic damage increase.

A summary of facts about the process of photoelectric absorption is presented in Box 3.4 for quick reference.

Probability of Occurrence of Photoelectric Absorption. The probability of occurrence of photoelectric absorption per atom within a particular material depends on the energy (E) of the incident x-ray photons and the atomic number (Z) of the atoms comprising the irradiated object; it increases markedly as the energy of the incident photon decreases and the atomic number of the irradiated atoms increases. Experimentally, the probability is observed to vary approximately as Z^3/E^3. Thus in the radiographic kilovoltage range, compact bone with an effective atomic

BOX 3.4 Summary of the Process of Photoelectric Absorption

Photoelectric absorption is the most important mode of interaction between x-radiation and the atoms of the patient's body in the energy range used in diagnostic radiology because this interaction is responsible for both the patient's dose and contrast in the image. During the process of photoelectric absorption, the total energy of the incident photon is completely absorbed as it interacts with and ejects an inner-shell electron of biologic tissue from its orbit. The newly ejected photoelectron possesses kinetic energy and can ionize other atoms it encounters until its energy is spent. After losing an electron, the original ionized atom is unstable and attempts to resta-bilize. This occurs as an electron from a higher shell drops down and fills the vacancy in the inner shell by releasing energy as a characteristic photon. This cascading effect of electrons dropping down to fill existing shell vacancies continues until the original atom regains its stability.

number* of 13.8 undergoes much more photoelectric absorption than an equal mass of soft tissue (Z_{eff} approximately = 7.4) and air (Z_{eff} = 7.6). Consequently, because of the greater "x-ray shadow" that it casts, bone can be exceptionally well delineated from soft tissue and air in diagnostic imaging.

Because air has only a slightly higher effective atomic number than soft tissue, the photoelectric interaction occurrence probability for either substance is virtually identical. Thus this interaction alone will not yield an imaging difference between the two media.

Mass Density and Effective Atomic Number of Different Body Structures. Since the density of air is approximately 1000 times smaller than that of soft tissue, a given volume of air will interact with far fewer x-ray photons than adjacent regions of soft tissue, thereby permitting more radiation to reach the image receptor. This results in a greater exposure to the phosphor plate or the digital radiography receptor or to radiographic film than from the denser expanses of tissue. The outcome is more

---

*Effective atomic number [Z_{eff}] is a composite Z value by weight for a material that is composed of multiple chemical elements.

adequate image contrast. As discussed with "air," dissimilar densities (**mass density** measured in grams per cubic centimeter) of different body structures influence attenuation. A density increase leads to a corresponding increase in the number of atoms in a given volume with which x-ray photons can interact and therefore to an increased probability of photon absorption. Therefore in any given sample of biologic material, both density and atomic number are important in determining attenuation and ultimately imaging contrast. As an example, if radiography is performed on an equal thickness of bone and soft tissue, the bone, which is approximately twice as dense as soft tissue, would absorb twice as much radiation just due to the density difference alone. Furthermore, bone would absorb 6.5 times as much radiation because of the difference in effective atomic numbers since $(13.8)^3 / (7.4)^3 = 6.5$. So, for equal thicknesses of bone and soft tissue, bone will absorb 13 times as many x-ray photons as soft tissue in the diagnostic energy range (Fig. 3.7A).

Body Part Thickness and Density Differences. Thickness of body parts also plays a role in absorption. The thickness factor is approximately linear. If two structures have the same density and atomic number but one is twice as thick as the other, the thicker structure will absorb twice as many photons. Consider now the situation where you have different thickness and density values for adjacent structures: if a 2-cm-thick bone sample is radiographed next to a 4-cm-thick tissue sample, because the bone is half as thick in this example but is approximately twice as dense, the density and thickness factors will cancel each other out (Fig. 3.7B). The effective atomic number difference remains, however, so that there will be 6.5 times as many x-ray photons absorbed in the bone, and it will still cast a noticeable "shadow."

Effects of Attenuation on Radiographic Images. The less a given structure attenuates radiation, the darker (i.e., more radiographically dense) its radiographic image will be and vice versa. A radiograph must have a sufficient amount of variation in densities to clearly visualize anatomic structures of interest. These principles are illustrated in Fig. 3.8.

In Fig. 3.9, two posteroanterior (PA) hand projections illustrate age-related changes in bone density resulting from changes in calcium content.
1. Image A exhibits substantial quantities of calcium in the bones of a young person.

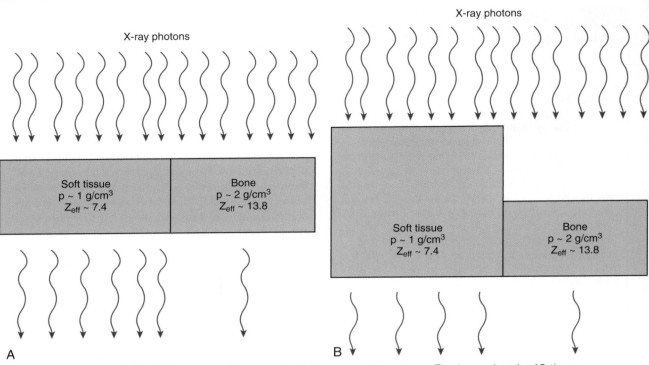

FIG 3.7 (A) Equal thickness of bone and soft tissue are shown here. The bone absorbs 13 times as many photons as the soft tissue. A factor of 2 is the result of bone's being approximately twice as dense as soft tissue. A factor of 6.5 is the result of the higher atomic number of bone compared with that of soft tissue. Both factors together result in 2 × 6.5 = 13 times more absorption in this sample of bone. (B) In the example shown here, the soft tissue is twice as thick as the bone. This thickness difference approximately cancels out the density difference between the bone and soft tissue. However, because the difference in atomic number still exists, in this example the bone would absorb 6.5 times as many photons as the soft tissue.

2. Image B exhibits the demineralized bones of an elderly person. The lack of x-ray absorption results from the decrease in bone calcium. Hence the elderly person's bones are almost transparent in radiographic appearance. Pathologic conditions such as degenerative arthritis also contribute to differences in absorption. Technical radiographic exposure factors must be adjusted to compensate for such changes.

Impact of Photoelectric Absorption on Radiographic Contrast. Within the energy range of diagnostic radiology, the greater the difference there is in the amount of photoelectric absorption, the greater the contrast in the radiographic image will be between adjacent structures of differing atomic numbers. However, as absorption by

structures increases, so does the potential for biologic damage. To ensure both radiographic image quality and patient safety, the radiographer should choose the technical factors that permit adequate radiographic contrast while delivering the smallest dose to the patient. Usually, the selection of technique factors is predetermined by the equipment manufacturer. However, the manufacturer's technical factors are only a guide for the radiographer. Ultimately, the radiographer must make the decision as to what technical factors to use for a particular patient based on patient conditions such as existing disease processes. Often, with the aid of an experienced radiographer and a medical physicist, the manufacturer's protocols can be modified at the time of commissioning of a new x-ray unit. Even with this, there will be some

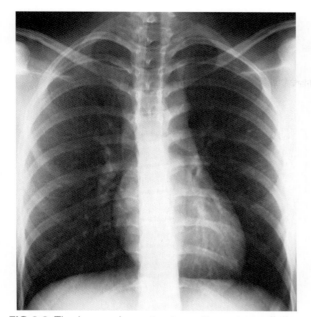

FIG 3.8 The less a given structure attenuates radiation, the darker its radiographic image will be and vice versa. Thus compact bone, with a higher effective atomic number and greater mass density than either soft tissue or air cavities, absorbs more radiation and appears light on a radiographic image, whereas soft tissue presents a gray image, and air-containing structures such as the lungs appear black.

occasions when the radiographer may be called upon to manually adjust techniques. One of the simplest and best ways of reducing patient dose through technique adjustment is to raise the kVp (never the opposite, which would substantially increase patient dose). The higher energy x-ray beam will be more penetrating, thereby permitting a lower mAs setting. This higher energy will, however, lead to a slight but workable lessening of image contrast because of a decrease in the amount of photoelectric interactions at the higher beam energy.

Use of Contrast Media to Ensure Visualization of Anatomic Structures. If tissues or structures that are similar in atomic number and mass density must be distinguished, the photoelectric interaction by itself will not be sufficient to produce the imaging differences needed in those tissues or structures to visually

differentiate them in the radiographic image. To resolve the problem, the use of contrast media has been adopted. Very simply, positive contrast media consist of solutions (e.g., barium or iodine based) containing elements having a higher atomic number than surrounding soft tissue. These solutions are either swallowed or injected into the tissues or structures to be visually enhanced. The high atomic number of the contrast media (barium, Z = 56; iodine, Z = 53) significantly increases the occurrence of photoelectric interaction relative to adjacent similar structures that do not have the contrast media. In addition, the inner-shell electrons of iodine and barium have a binding energy that is in the energy range of the x-ray photons that are most commonly used in general-purpose radiography (30 to 40 keV). This means that photoelectric absorption of the photons in the x-ray beam is further increased. In the radiographic image, positive contrast–enhanced structures therefore appear lighter than adjacent structures that did not receive the contrast. Fig. 3.10A presents an anteroposterior (AP) projection of the abdomen without the aid of a positive contrast medium to visualize the urinary system, whereas Fig. 3.10B presents an AP projection of the abdomen with a positive contrast medium that shows each contrast-filled structure in the urinary system to be distinguished.

Caution must be exercised in the use of contrast media because some patients may not be able to tolerate its presence. The use of a positive contrast medium also leads to an increase in absorbed dose in the body structures that contain it. A negative contrast medium such as air or gas can be used for some radiologic examinations. These negative agents, which are far easier to penetrate, result in areas of increased brightness on the radiographic image.

Compton Scattering

Compton scattering is also known by the following terms:
- Incoherent scattering
- Inelastic scattering
- Modified scattering

It is responsible for most of the scattered radiation produced during radiologic procedures (Fig. 3.11). This scatter may be directed forward as small-angle scatter, to the rear as backscatter, and laterally as side scatter. The intensity of radiation scatter in various directions is a major factor in planning protection for medical imaging personnel during a radiologic examination (Fig. 3.12).

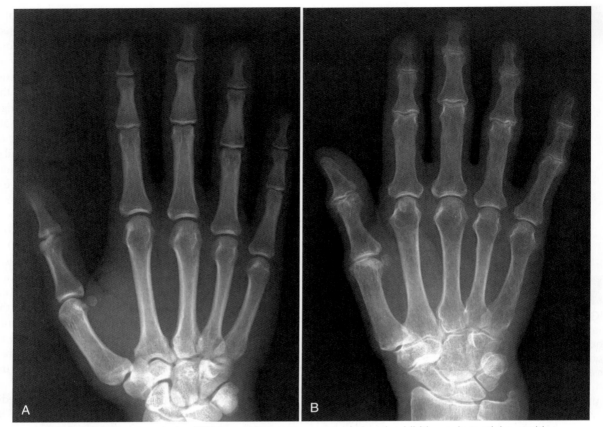

FIG 3.9 (A) Posteroanterior (PA) image of a young person's hand exhibiting substantial quantities of calcium in the bones. (B) PA image of an elderly person's hand exhibiting demineralized bone as a consequence of a decrease in bone calcium. This and other degenerative changes account for the almost transparent appearance of the bones.

Process of Compton Scattering in a Patient. In a Compton interaction event within a patient, an incoming x-ray photon interacts with a loosely bound outer electron of an atom (Fig. 3.13). On encountering the electron, the incoming x-ray photon surrenders a portion of its kinetic energy in dislodging the electron from its outer-shell orbit, thereby ionizing the biologic atom (see Appendix G for an extended discussion of this type of interaction). The freed electron, called a **Compton scattered electron, or secondary, or recoil, electron,** possesses excess kinetic energy and thus is potentially capable of ionizing other biologic atoms. In general it loses its kinetic energy by a series of collisions with nearby atoms and finally recombines with an atom that needs another electron.

This usually occurs within a few micrometers of the site of the original Compton interaction.

The incident x-ray photon that surrendered some of its kinetic energy (see Appendix G) to free the loosely bound outer-shell electron from its orbit continues on its way, but in a new direction, and is now called a *Compton scattered photon.* It has the potential to interact with other atoms either by the process of photoelectric absorption or by subsequent Compton scattering. The photons can also emerge from the patient, possibly contributing to degradation of the radiographic image by adding to it an additional multidirectional off-focus exposure (radiographic fog). In fluoroscopy, these deflected exit photons expose personnel who are present

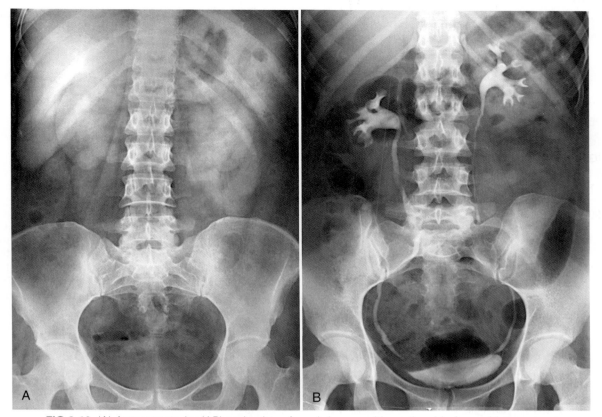

FIG 3.10 (A) Anteroposterior (AP) projection of an abdomen without the aid of a positive contrast medium. Parts of the urinary system other than the kidneys, which have their own unique density, are not radiographically demonstrated. (B) AP projection of an abdomen, following intravenous injection of an appropriate positive contrast medium that permits visualization of the entire urinary system, thereby allowing each contrast-filled structure to be distinguished. (A, From Ballinger PW, Frank ED: *Merrill's Atlas of Radiographic Positions & Radiologic Procedures*, ed 10, St. Louis, 2003, Mosby. B, Frank ED, Long BW, Smith BS: *Merrill's Atlas of Radiographic Positioning & Procedures*, ed 12, St. Louis, 2012, Mosby.)

in the room to scattered radiation. This scattering mandates that such personnel wear protective lead shielding. The Compton interaction's probability of occurrence has no explicit dependence on atomic number. Instead, it shows something of an energy and density dependence. Density dependence just means that the more atoms or targets per unit volume, the greater the likelihood of an interaction occurring in that volume. With increasing x-ray photon energy, the chance for a billiard ball–like interaction between the photon and an outer atomic electron decreases. What must be emphasized, however, is that the Compton interaction's lack of Z dependence

implies that it does not differentiate between *equal amounts* of bone and soft tissue and thus does not serve as a useful contrast mechanism for radiographic imaging. Fortunately, as long as the radiographer selects appropriate kVp technical factors, the photoelectric interaction will provide that mechanism.

In diagnostic radiology, the probability of occurrence of Compton scattering relative to that of the photoelectric interaction increases as the energy of the x-ray photon increases. Compton scattering and photoelectric absorption in tissue are equally probable at approximately 35 keV. Therefore in a 100-kVp x-ray beam, when the photons

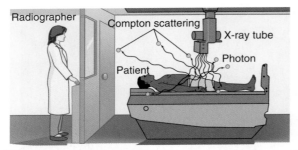

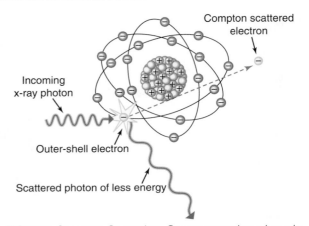

FIG 3.11 Compton interactions are responsible for most of the scattered radiation produced during a radiologic procedure. (From *Radiobiology and Radiation Protection: Mosby's Radiographic Instructional Series,* St. Louis, 1999, Mosby.)

FIG 3.13 Compton Scattering. On encountering a loosely bound outer-shell electron, the incoming x-ray photon surrenders a portion of its kinetic energy to dislodge the electron from its orbit. The energy-degraded x-ray photon then continues on its way, but in a new direction. The high-speed electron ejected from its orbit is called a *Compton scattered electron, or secondary, or "recoil" electron.*

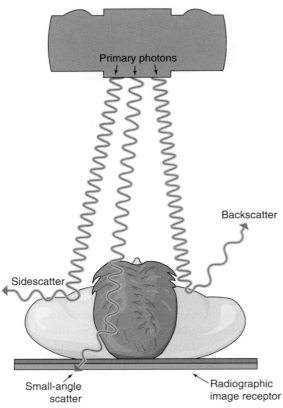

FIG 3.12 Compton scattering results in all-directional scatter. This scatter may be directed forward as small-angle scatter, to the rear as backscatter, and laterally as side scatter. The intensity of radiation scatter in various directions is a major factor in planning the protection for medical imaging personnel during a radiologic examination.

have an average energy in the range of 30 to 40 keV, significant numbers of Compton events occur.

A summary of facts about the process of Compton scattering is presented in Box 3.5 for quick reference.

Pair Production

Pair production is a process that does not occur unless the energy of the incident x-ray photon is at least 1.022 million electron volts (MeV). Although this energy range is far higher than that used in diagnostic radiology, a brief description of the pair production interaction is included in this chapter to provide the reader with a broad-scale understanding of the possible interactions of x-radiation with matter.

Process of Pair Production. In pair production, the incoming x-ray photon strongly interacts with the electric field surrounding the nucleus of an atom of the irradiated biologic tissue and disappears (Fig. 3.14). In the process, the energy of the photon is absorbed and transformed into matter composed of two particles: a negatron (an ordinary electron) and a positron (a positively charged electron). The negatron and the positron have the same mass and magnitude of charge; the only difference is in the "sign" of their electrical charges. The incoming

BOX 3.5   Summary of the Process of Compton Scattering

Compton scattering is important in the energy range used in diagnostic radiology. Because the scattered x-ray photon produced from the interaction of the incoming photon with an outer-shell electron of an atom of human tissue results only in a partial transfer of kinetic energy to that biologic atom, the scattered photon now traveling in a different direction can become a potential health hazard for imaging personnel by increasing their occupational radiation exposure. In the event that Compton scattered photons reach the image receptor, they can decrease contrast of the image by adding an undesirable additional exposure called *radiographic fog*. Because its energy dependence decreases much more slowly with increasing energy than does the photoelectric interaction, Compton scattering is very important even at therapeutic energies.

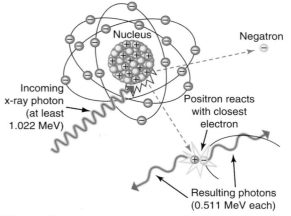

FIG 3.14 Pair Production. Pair production occurs when incoming x-ray photons with energy of at least 1.022 MeV interact with the nucleus of an atom. The end result of this interaction is the annihilation of a positron and an electron with their rest masses converted into energy, which appears in the form of two 0.511-MeV photons, each moving in the opposite direction.

photon must have enough energy to supply the combined rest mass* of these two particles. The minimum energy required to produce an electron–positron pair is 1.022 MeV (see Box 3.6). For this reason pair production does not occur at lower energies. The electron of the pair loses kinetic energy by exciting and ionizing atoms in its path. It eventually loses enough energy that it may be captured by an atom in need of another electron. Regarding the generated positron, as far as is known, no large quantities of positrons freely exist in the universe. A positron is classified as a form of *antimatter* because it

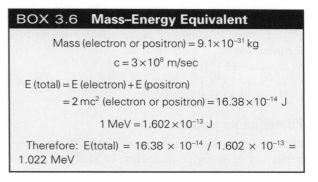

BOX 3.6   Mass–Energy Equivalent

$$\text{Mass (electron or positron)} = 9.1 \times 10^{-31} \text{ kg}$$

$$c = 3 \times 10^8 \text{ m/sec}$$

$$\text{E (total)} = \text{E (electron)} + \text{E (positron)}$$

$$= 2\,mc^2 \text{ (electron or positron)} = 16.38 \times 10^{-14} \text{ J}$$

$$1 \text{ MeV} = 1.602 \times 10^{-13} \text{ J}$$

$$\text{Therefore: E(total)} = 16.38 \times 10^{-14} / 1.602 \times 10^{-13} = 1.022 \text{ MeV}$$

*Rest mass is a term associated with the mass a particle possesses or would be measured to have when it is at rest relative to a frame of reference. According to the theory of special relativity, the mass of an object is not a fixed value but rather is dependent on the magnitude of its velocity "v" according to the relation:

$$m = m_0 / (1 - v^2/c^2)$$

where m_0 is the rest mass value of the particle and c is the speed of light in a vacuum. As can be seen from this expression, if the speed of the object is zero, then its mass is equal to m_0, but if the speed is not zero, then the mass of the particle will be increasing as its speed approaches the speed of light. The expression also shows that a particle with a nonzero rest mass can never be brought to the speed of light, for then its mass would be infinite, and the amount of energy required to do this would also be infinite.

is seen to interact destructively with any nearby ordinary matter that it may be attracted to, such as an atomic electron. During this interaction, the positron and the electron will annihilate each other, in the process converting matter into energy. This is the reverse of a pair production event in which energy is converted to matter. Both types of processes happen in accordance with Albert Einstein's famous concept of mass–energy equivalence, mathematically expressed as $E = mc^2$ (c is the speed of light in a vacuum). The energy that appears from the annihilation of the electron and positron does not disappear but rather is carried off by two 0.511-MeV photons moving in opposite directions. Although pair production does not occur unless the energy of the incoming photon is at least 1.022 MeV, its probability of occurrence starts to become significant (i.e., noticeably greater than zero) at 10-MeV x-ray energies and higher.

Use of Annihilation Radiation in Positron Emission Tomography. Annihilation radiation is used in an imaging modality employed in nuclear medicine called *positron emission tomography (PET)*. Briefly, in the PET scanning of patients, the source of the positrons are injected radionuclides, whose atomic nuclei are unstable because they contain too many protons relative to their number of neutrons. To relieve this instability, a surplus proton is converted in the nucleus into a neutron, and a positron and another particle called a *neutrino* are ejected from the nucleus. Within a very short distance (several micrometers or less), the emitted positron interacts with a local electron, and the two mutually annihilate, yielding a pair of photons emerging in opposite directions from the electron–positron interaction site. These *annihilation photons* are intercepted by a ring of detectors surrounding the patient. The positional information from these detectors is then used to build a cross-sectional image of the radioactivity within the patient. Some examples of radionuclides used in PET scanning are:

- Fluorine-18 (^{18}F)
- Carbon-11 (^{11}C)
- Nitrogen-13 (^{13}N)

Photodisintegration

Photodisintegration is another interaction that becomes important at energies exceeding 10 MeV during the operation of high-energy radiation therapy treatment machines. Because this energy range is also far higher than useful diagnostic energies, only a brief account of this interaction process of radiation with matter is included. With this discussion and those directly preceding it, the reader will have been introduced to all of the important types of radiation and matter encounters.

Process of Photodisintegration. In photodisintegration, a high-energy photon collides with the nucleus of an atom, which directly absorbs all the photon's energy. This energy excess in the nucleus creates an instability that in most cases is alleviated by the emission of a neutron by the nucleus. Other types of emissions—a proton or proton–neutron combination (deuteron) or

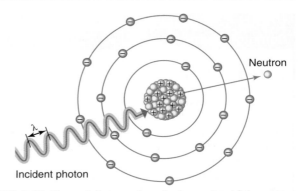

FIG 3.15 Photodisintegration. An incoming high-energy photon collides with the nucleus of an atom and absorbs all the photon's energy. This energy excess in the nucleus creates an instability that is usually alleviated by the emission of a neutron. In addition, if sufficient energy is absorbed by the nucleus, other types of emissions will be possible, such as a proton or proton–neutron combination (deuteron), or even an alpha particle.

even an alpha particle—are possible if sufficient energy is absorbed by the nucleus. Because emission of charged and/or uncharged particles has occurred from a previously inactive nucleus, we can say that the photodisintegration interaction has made a nucleus radioactive (Fig. 3.15).

▌ SUMMARY

- Peak kilovoltage (kVp) controls the quality, or penetrating power, of the photons in the x-ray beam and to some degree also affects the quantity, or number of photons, in the beam.
- Because radiographers select the technical exposure factors, they are responsible for the radiation dose the patient receives during an imaging procedure.
- The amount of energy absorbed by the patient per unit mass is called the *absorbed dose*.
- Biologic damage in the patient may result from the absorption of x-ray energy. However, some small amount of radiation dose is necessary to produce a diagnostic image.
- Variations in x-ray absorption properties of various body structures make radiographic imaging of human anatomy possible.
- Radiographers receive less radiation exposure when the patient's dose is minimal because less radiation

is scattered from the patient during an imaging procedure.

- The anode of an x-ray tube is usually made of tungsten or an alloy of tungsten and rhenium.
- The units kVp and kV refer to the voltage on the x-ray tube, and keV refers to the energy of specific x-rays.
- Attenuation results when, through the processes of absorption and scatter, the intensity of the primary photons in an x-ray beam decreases as it passes through matter.
- Scattered radiation can result in diminished contrast of the image by adding additional undesirable exposure to the IR (radiographic fog). In fluoroscopy, Compton scattered photons may expose personnel who are present in the room to scattered radiation.
- Two interactions of x-radiation are central in diagnostic radiology: photoelectric absorption and Compton scattering. The photoelectric absorption is the basis of useful radiographic imaging, whereas Compton scattering is its bane.
- For each radiographic procedure, an optimal peak kilovoltage (kVp) and milliampere-seconds (mAs) combination exists that minimizes the dose to the patient and produces an acceptable image.
- Within the energy range of diagnostic radiology (23 to 150 kVp), which also includes mammography, when kVp is decreased, the number of photoelectric interactions increases and the number of Compton interactions decreases; however, the patient absorbs more energy, and therefore the dose to the patient increases.
- When kVp is increased, the patient receives a lower dose, but image quality may be compromised.
- kVp selection is usually based on type of procedure and body part imaged.
- Radiographers must balance other variables such as the type of image receptor used, patient thickness, and degree of muscle tissue to arrive at technical exposure factors that will provide an acceptable image yet stay within the standards of radiation protection.
- Coherent scattering is most likely to occur at less than 10 keV; pair production and photodisintegration occur far above the range of diagnostic radiology.

REFERENCE

1. Hendee WR, Ritenour ER: *Medical imaging physics*, ed 4, Chicago, 2002, John Wiley & Sons.

GENERAL DISCUSSION QUESTIONS

1. Why is it necessary for radiographers to have a basic understanding of the processes of interaction between radiation and matter?
2. How is an x-ray beam produced?
3. Why is tungsten or tungsten and rhenium used in the target of the x-ray tube?
4. Explain the function of permanent inherent filtration in a diagnostic x-ray tube.
5. What is attenuation?
6. Why do human bones appear lighter in a completed diagnostic image?
7. Describe the interactions between x-radiation and matter that occur within the diagnostic radiology range.
8. In the mathematical expression $E = mc^2$, what does c represent?
9. What type of radiation is used in positron emission tomography?
10. When a high-energy photon collides with the nucleus of an atom during the process of photodisintegration, how much of the photon's energy is directly absorbed by the nucleus?
11. Define the term *effective atomic number* (Z_{eff}).
12. What is small-angle scatter?

REVIEW QUESTIONS

1. Exit, or image-formation, radiation is composed of which of the following?
   A. Primary photons and wide-angle Compton scattered photons
   B. Non-interacting and small-angle scattered photons
   C. Very low energy photons
   D. Auger electrons
2. Which of the following contributes *significantly* to the exposure of the radiographer?
   A. Positrons
   B. Electrons
   C. Compton scattered photons
   D. Compton scattered electrons
3. Which of the following defines attenuation?
   A. Absorption and scatter
   B. Absorption only
   C. Scatter only
   D. Weakened only

4. In the radiographic kilovoltage range, which of the following structures undergoes the *most* photoelectric absorption?
   A. Air cavities
   B. Compact bone
   C. Fat
   D. Soft tissue
5. In which of the following x-ray interactions with matter is the energy of the incident photon *partially* absorbed?
   A. Compton
   B. Photoelectric
   C. Coherent
   D. Pair production
6. When a high atomic number solution is either swallowed or injected into human tissue or a structure to visualize it during an imaging procedure, which of the following occurs?
   A. Photoelectric interaction becomes greatly decreased, resulting in an increase in the absorbed dose in the body tissues or structures that contain the contrast medium.
   B. Photoelectric interaction becomes significantly enhanced, leading to an increase in the absorbed dose in the body tissues or structures that contain the contrast medium.
   C. Photoelectric interaction becomes greatly decreased, resulting in a decrease in the absorbed dose in the body tissues or structures that contain the contrast medium.
   D. Photoelectric interaction becomes significantly enhanced, leading to a decrease in the absorbed dose in the body tissues or structures that contain the contrast medium.

7. Which of the following characteristics primarily differentiates the probability of occurrence of the various interactions of x-radiation with human tissue?
   A. Energy of the incoming photon
   B. Direction of the incident photon
   C. X-ray beam intensity
   D. Exposure time
8. Which of the following influences attenuation?
   1. Effective atomic number of the absorber
   2. Mass density
   3. Thickness of the absorber
   A. 1 and 2 only
   B. 1 and 3 only
   C. 2 and 3 only
   D. 1, 2, and 3
9. A decrease in contrast of the image by adding an unwanted additional exposure (radiographic fog) results from which of the following interactions between x-radiation and matter?
   1. Compton scattering
   2. Pair production
   3. Photoelectric absorption
   A. 1 only
   B. 2 only
   C. 3 only
   D. 1, 2, and 3
10. The interactions of x-ray photons with any atoms of biologic matter are:
   A. Able to be preplanned to selective atoms to limit radiation exposure to those atoms
   B. Important only in therapeutic radiology
   C. Random, so the effects of such interactions cannot be predicted with certainty
   D. Unimportant in diagnostic radiology, thus making radiation protection unnecessary

4

Radiation Quantities and Units

OBJECTIVES

After completing this chapter, the reader will be able to perform the following:

- Define all key terms.
- Explain how x-rays were discovered.
- Describe some of the early acute biologic damage to humans that resulted from exposure to x-rays.
- Explain the concepts of skin erythema dose, tolerance dose, and threshold dose.
- Differentiate between somatic and genetic (hereditary) effects.
- List five examples of radiation responses recognized in modern times as early tissue reactions, three examples of late tissue reactions, and two examples of stochastic effects.
- Differentiate among the following radiation quantities: exposure, air kerma, absorbed dose, equivalent dose, and effective dose, and identify the appropriate symbol for each quantity.
- List and explain the International System (SI) units for radiation exposure, air kerma, absorbed dose, equivalent dose, and effective dose.
- Define the term *dose area product (DAP)*.

- State the formula for determining the equivalent dose.
- Determine the equivalent dose in terms of SI units when given the radiation weighting factor and the absorbed dose for different ionizing radiations.
- Describe the function of a tissue weighting factor.
- State the formula for determining the effective dose.
- Given the absorbed dose of radiation to an organ, the radiation weighting factor for the energy and type of radiation in question, and the tissue weighting factor, determine the effective dose to that organ.
- Explain the concept of effective dose when used for radiation protection purposes.
- State the purpose of the radiation quantity, collective effective dose, and list its SI unit.
- Explain the importance of linear energy transfer as it applies to biologic damage resulting from irradiation of human tissue.
- State the whole-body total effective dose equivalent (TEDE) for occupationally exposed personnel and for the general public.

CHAPTER OUTLINE

Absorbed Dose
Equivalence of Radiation-Produced Damage From
   Different Sources of Ionizing Radiation
Equivalent Dose

Effective Dose
Collective Effective Dose
Total Effective Dose Equivalent
Summary

KEY TERMS

absorbed dose (D)
air kerma
collective effective dose (ColEfD)
committed effective dose
   equivalent (CEDE)
coulomb (C)
coulombs per kilogram (C/kg)
dose area product (DAP)
early tissue reactions

effective dose (EfD)
equivalent dose (EqD)
exposure (X)
genetic, or heritable, effects
gray (Gy)
International System of Units (SI)
late tissue reactions
linear energy transfer (LET)
occupational exposure

radiation weighting factor (W_R)
sievert (Sv)
somatic damage
stochastic effects
tissue weighting factor (W_T)
total effective dose equivalent
   (TEDE)

As the potentially harmful effects of ionizing radiation became known, the medical community sought to reduce these effects throughout the world by developing standards for measuring and limiting radiation exposure. To be able to control patient and personnel exposure in a consistent and uniform manner, diagnostic imaging personnel must become familiar with the radiation quantities and units discussed in this chapter.

HISTORICAL EVOLUTION OF RADIATION QUANTITIES AND UNITS

Discovery of X-Rays

On November 8, 1895, as he was working in a modest laboratory at the University of Wurzburg in Bavaria, German physics professor Wilhelm Conrad Roentgen (Fig. 4.1) discovered a mysterious ray. During an experiment investigating the nature of cathode rays and fluorescent materials, Roentgen passed electricity through a partially evacuated pear-shaped glass tube known as a *Crookes tube* that he had covered with a shield made of black cardboard (Fig. 4.2). As he passed a charge through it, he observed light emanating (a fluorescence effect) from a piece of paper coated with a material compound of barium, platinum, and cyanide that was lying on a bench several feet away. Roentgen hypothesized that some type of radiant energy, or "rays," had been emitted from the Crookes tube that caused the barium platinocyanide to glow. To determine whether any object had the ability to obstruct the mysterious rays, he held various items

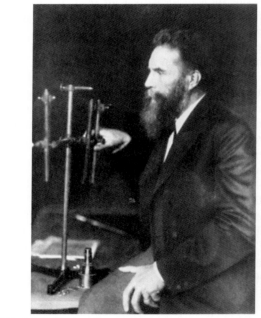

FIG 4.1 Wilhelm Conrad Roentgen, the discoverer of x-rays. (US National Library of Medicine.)

between the Crookes tube and the fluorescent-coated paper. He found that most materials would allow some degree of transmission. Roentgen called his momentous discovery *x-rays*. Very soon thereafter Roentgen produced an x-ray image on a glass plate "coated with a light-sensitive

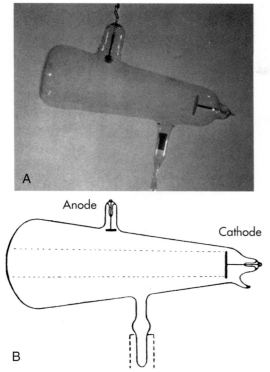

A

Anode

Cathode

B

FIG 4.2 Photograph (A) and diagram (B) of the original type of x-ray tube. The cathode stream produced x-rays by impinging on the large area of the glass wall of the tube. (Courtesy Carestream Health, Inc.)

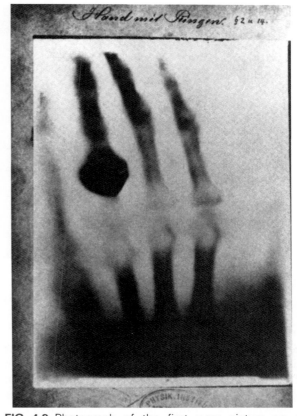

FIG 4.3 Photograph of the first x-ray picture on a glass plate: Mrs. Roentgen's hand. (From Glasser O: *William Conrad Roentgen and the Early History of the Roentgen Rays,* London, 1933, John Bale, Sons and Danielsson, Ltd.)

emulsion of silver salts. The emulsion consisted of silver halide crystals dispersed in gelatin."* Glass plates used to produce x-ray images only had emulsion on one side to avoid blurring of the image. The first x-ray image Roentgen produced was an image of his wife's hand that clearly showed her bones (Fig. 4.3). In December 1895 he announced his scientific findings in an abbreviated manuscript titled "On a New Kind of Ray, a Preliminary Communication," which was presented to the Physical Medical Society of Würzburg.

First Reports of Injury

In the months that followed the announcement of Roentgen's findings, unguarded experimentation with the new "wonder rays" unfortunately resulted in acute

---

*Personal communication, Dr. Uwe Busch, Director, Deutsches Roentgen Museum, Schwelmer Str. 41, Remscheid D - 42897, Germany, 03/16/2017 and 03/17/2017.

biologic damage to some investigators and their human subjects. Cases of somatic damage (from the Greek term *soma,* meaning "of the body") were reported in Europe as early as 1896. In the United States, Clarence Madison Dally (Fig. 4.4A), glass blower, tube maker, assistant, and long-time friend of fluoroscope inventor, Thomas A. Edison (Fig. 4.4B), became the first American radiation fatality. Dally died of radiation-induced cancer in October 1904 at the age of 39 years. Because of Clarence Dally's severe injuries and death, Thomas Edison discontinued his x-ray research.

Among physicians, cancer deaths attributed to x-ray exposure were reported as early as 1910. As a result of occupational exposure, that is, radiation exposure received in the course of exercising their professional

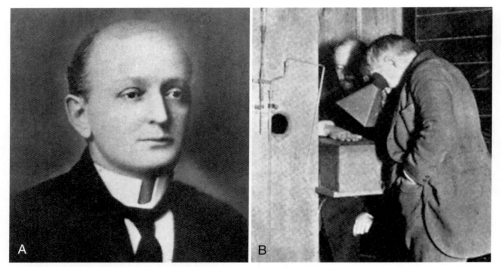

FIG 4.4 (A) Clarence Madison Dally (1865–1904), the first American radiation fatality. (B) Dally, assistant to Thomas A. Edison, is seen holding his hand over a box containing an x-ray tube while Edison examines the hand through a fluoroscope that he invented. (A, From Brown P: *American Martyrs to Science Through the Roentgen Rays,* Springfield, IL, 1936, Charles C Thomas. B, From Eisenberg RL: *Radiology: An illustrated history,* St. Louis, 1995, Mosby-Year Book.)

responsibilities, many radiologists and dentists using the new penetrating rays developed a reddening of the skin called *radiodermatitis.* A substantial number of these skin lesions on the hands and fingers of these radiation workers eventually became cancerous as a consequence of continued exposure to what was soon found to be ionizing radiation (Fig. 4.5). Blood disorders such as aplastic anemia, which results from bone marrow failure, and leukemia, an abnormal overproduction of white blood cells, were also seen to be much more common among early radiologists than among nonradiologists.

Investigation of Methods for Reducing Radiation Exposure

Alarmed by the increasing number of radiation injuries reported, the medical community decided to investigate methods for reducing radiation exposure from all sources of radiation. In 1921 the British X-Ray and Radium Protection Committee was created to perform this task. The committee planned to formulate guidelines for the manufacture and use of radium and x-ray equipment and devices to reduce the chance of occupational injury. Even though the committee members recognized the danger of excessive radiation exposure, they were handicapped because they did not have accurate measurement techniques or adequate background knowledge of

radiobiology. Ultimately, because they could not agree on a workable unit of radiation exposure, the members of the committee were unable to fulfill their responsibility.

Skin Erythema Dose

From 1900 to 1930, the unit in use for measuring radiation exposure was called the *skin erythema dose,* defined as the received quantity of radiation that causes diffuse redness over an area of skin after irradiation. This amount of absorbed radiation corresponds roughly to a skin dose that would be specified as several gray today. The radiation unit, gray (Gy), is discussed later in this chapter. Because the amount of radiation required to produce an erythema reaction varied from one person to another, the skin erythema dose was often a crude and inaccurate way to quantify radiation exposure. Scientists felt compelled to continue searching for a more reliable unit. The new unit selected was to be based on some exactly assessable effect produced by radiation, such as ionization of atoms or energy absorbed in the irradiated object.

Early Definition of Quantities and Units

The First International Congress of Radiology was held in London, England, in 1925. This meeting allowed radiologists from all over the world to collaborate.

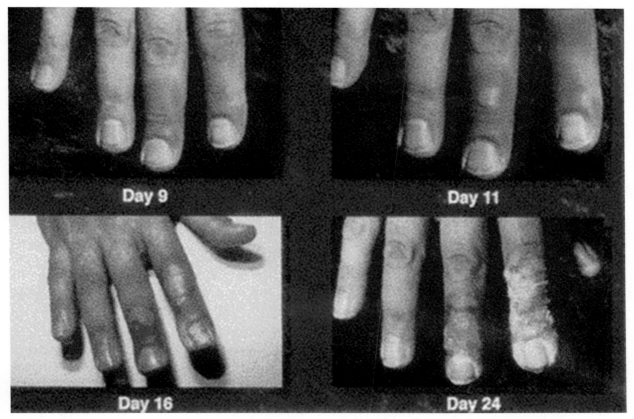

FIG 4.5 Lesions of the fingers induced by ionizing radiation. (From Gusev IA, Guskova AK, Mettler FA, Jr., editors. *Medical Management of Radiation Accidents*, 2nd ed, New York, 2001, CRC Press, Inc.)

Unfortunately, no definite decisions for quantifying the effects of ionizing radiation were made based on the recommendations presented. The International Commission on Radiation Units and Measurements (ICRU) was also formed in 1925. In 1928 a Second International Congress of Radiology was held in Stockholm, Sweden. Although at this time the "roentgen" was in place as a unit associated with a certain degree of exposure, it was not as yet by any means scientifically well defined. The 1928 congress charged the ICRU with precisely defining this unit of exposure. The congress also established the International X-Ray and Radium Protection Commission, predecessor of the International Commission on Radiological Protection (ICRP).

Since the early days of radiology, biologic effects in humans caused by exposure to ionizing radiation were only too apparent. These early tissue reactions (Box 4.1), which appeared within minutes, hours, days, or weeks of the time of radiation exposure, were believed to be preventable if doses to radiation workers were limited.

A *tolerance dose* is a radiation dose to which occupationally exposed persons could be continuously subjected without any apparent harmful acute effects, such as erythema of the skin. The general belief was that no adverse effects from radiation exposure would be demonstrated at doses lower than this level. Alternatively, this tolerance exposure level could be regarded as a *threshold dose,* that is, a dose of radiation lower than which an individual has a negligible chance of sustaining specific biologic damage. At the time of the 1928 International Congress, the tolerance dose was specified in *roentgen* units, which were then an imprecise measure of the quantity called *exposure.* Even with this uncertainty,

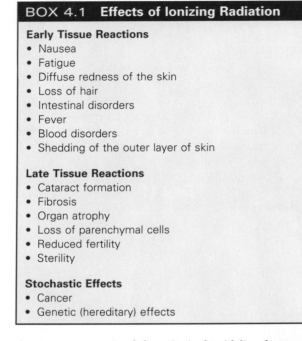

BOX 4.1   **Effects of Ionizing Radiation**

Early Tissue Reactions
- Nausea
- Fatigue
- Diffuse redness of the skin
- Loss of hair
- Intestinal disorders
- Fever
- Blood disorders
- Shedding of the outer layer of skin

Late Tissue Reactions
- Cataract formation
- Fibrosis
- Organ atrophy
- Loss of parenchymal cells
- Reduced fertility
- Sterility

Stochastic Effects
- Cancer
- Genetic (hereditary) effects

nuclei of radioactive substances). In 1962 the roentgen was conceptually revisited and more rigorously defined in scientific terms.

In 1946 the US Advisory Committee on X-Ray and Radium Protection became known as the National Committee on Radiation Protection. The name of this radiation standards organization underwent another change in 1956 and again in 1964, when it became the National Council on Radiation Protection and Measurements (NCRP).

The General Conference of Weights and Measures, which was responsible for the development and international unification of the metric system, assigned its International Committee for Weights and Measures the responsibility of developing guidelines for the units of measurement in 1948. To fulfill this responsibility, the committee developed the **International System of Units (SI)**, from the French "Système International d'Unités." This system makes possible the interchange of units among all branches of science throughout the world.

The Modern Era of Radiation Protection

By the early 1950s, maximum permissible dose (MPD) replaced the tolerance dose for radiation protection purposes. MPD essentially indicated the largest dose of ionizing radiation that an occupationally exposed person was allowed within a certain period that was not anticipated to result in major adverse biologic effects according to the best available data. However, the concept of an MPD did not mean that some small risk of damage would not exist with radiation doses at the MPD level. MPD was initially expressed in a unit called *rem*[†] (an acronym for *radiation equivalent man,* also historically known as *Roentgen equivalent man*), the traditional British unit used for radiation protection purposes at that time. The rem has since been replaced by the SI unit sievert. Please refer to Appendix A for all relationships between original, or traditional, units and the current standard SI units.

Removing the notion of "tolerance dose" and adopting the statistical MPD concept in its place ultimately meant that *no amount* of radiation was considered *completely*

the roentgen remained the principal guideline for occupational radiation exposure tolerance levels during the 1930s. Neither tolerance dose nor threshold dose is presently used for the purposes of radiation safety.

In 1934 the International X-Ray and Radium Protection Commission recommended a tolerance dose daily limit of 0.2 roentgen. In the United States, the Advisory Committee on X-Ray and Radium Protection, which was formed in 1931 to formulate recommendations for radiation control, also recommended a tolerance dose equal to 0.2 roentgen per day.

In 1936 the committee reduced this dose to 0.1 roentgen per day. As scientists began to recognize the late tissue reactions and stochastic effects of ionizing radiation that appeared months or years after exposure and the possibility of genetic, or heritable, effects, they began to focus on finding ways to minimize the risk of sustaining such damage (see Box 4.1). The search was on for a more reliable unit to replace the tolerance dose.

In 1937 the ICRU finished its assignment from the Second International Congress of Radiology, and, although still not accurately defined but now much better quantified, the roentgen became internationally adopted as the unit of measurement for exposure to x-radiation and gamma radiation (short-wavelength, higher-energy electromagnetic waves emitted by the

---

[†]One rem is defined as the dose that is equivalent to any type of ionizing radiation that produces the same biologic effect as 1 rad (radiation absorbed dose) of x-radiation. One rad corresponds to an energy transfer of 100 ergs per gram to an irradiated object. The rad is identical to the subunit centigray or cGY.

safe. The probability of long-term harm, such as the development of cancer, was expected to decrease as the dose decreased, but *it was not expected to become zero at any dose level!* This raised a dilemma: If no amount of radiation exposure was safe, and if it was impossible to design a work environment where the dose was zero (and still be able to perform procedures that unavoidably included some degree of exposure), then *what would determine the maximum allowed occupational exposure?* The solution was to compare rates of death and accident among various occupations. Insurance companies had been using this actuarial method of comparison for many years to determine insurance rates. Some occupations are very hazardous. Examples of such occupations are:

- Deep sea diving
- Professional mountaineering
  Some nonhazardous occupations are:
- Trade
- Government desk work

However, even in nonhazardous occupations, there is still a small risk of fatality or serious injury (approximately 1 chance in 10,000 each year[1]). With this in mind, the decision was made to base recommendations for dose limits on the concept that the probability of harm associated with typical dosimeter readings should be no more than the amount of harm in industries that are generally considered reasonably safe.

By the 1970s dosimetry and risk analysis had become quite sophisticated. Radiation units were developed that contained factors that accounted for the varied bioeffects of different types of radiation, namely:

- Alpha
- Beta
- Gamma
- X-radiation
- Neutrons

There was also growing recognition that the consequences from radiation exposure to the health of a human as a whole depended on which organs and organ systems had been irradiated. For example, irradiation of the bone marrow was found to be much more significant to the whole-body health of an individual than irradiation of the skin. Equal doses of radiation to bone marrow and to skin had very different penalties! In the late 1970s, using these concepts of different organ radiosensitivities expressed numerically in terms of tissue-specific weighting factors, dose limits were calculated and established to ensure that the overall risk from radiation exposure acquired on the

job did not exceed risks encountered in "safe" occupations, such as clerical work, in which the risk is approximately 10^{-4} (one chance in 10,000) per year.[1]

In 1991 the ICRP revised the values of the tissue radiosensitivity weighting factors. The revision was based on data from more recent epidemiologic studies of the atomic bomb survivors. The ICRP also adopted the term **effective dose (EfD)**. Based on the energy deposited in biologic tissue by ionizing radiation, it takes into account both of the following:

1. The type of radiation (e.g., x-radiation, gamma, neutron)
2. The variable sensitivity of the tissues exposed to the radiation

This quantity, EfD, is therefore actually a measure of the overall risk arising from the simultaneous irradiation of various biologic tissues and organs within an individual. EfD is expressed in the SI unit, **sievert (Sv)**, or in subunits of the sievert. The sievert is discussed further in the next section.

Quantities and Units in Use Today

In 1980 the ICRU adopted SI units, a unified system of metric units, for use with ionizing radiation and urged full implementation of the units as soon as possible. Many developed countries, particularly in Europe, have already made a complete transition to SI units. In the United States, SI units, such as the gray (Gy) and the centigray (cGy), are now used routinely in therapeutic radiology to specify absorbed dose. Even though the NCRP adopted the internationally accepted SI units for use in 1985, traditional units, older special units associated with radiation protection and dosimetry, such as the roentgen (R)* and its subunit the milliroentgen (mR), are being broadly utilized. In addition, the rem, the traditional unit for the radiation quantity equivalent dose currently remains a much used quantity. This is especially so in radiation dosimetry reports for occupationally exposed personnel. In the SI system of units, the sievert (Sv) has replaced the rem for radiation protection purposes. Like the rem, it provides a common scale whereby varying degrees of biologic damage caused by equal absorbed doses of different types of ionizing radiation can be

---

*One roentgen is the photon exposure that under standard conditions of pressure and temperature produces a total positive or negative ion charge of 2.58×10^{-4} coulombs per kilogram of dry air.

compared with the degree of biologic damage caused by the same amount of x-radiation or gamma radiation. One sievert is the same as 100 rem.

Fluoroscopic patient entrance radiation levels are now specified in milligray per minute (mGy_{-a}/min), but in many facilities they are still measured as exposure rates in roentgens per minute (R/min), and essentially all radiation survey instruments, even the newer SI-oriented devices, continue to also provide readings in traditional units. Furthermore, many regulatory criteria are given in terms of traditional units. In this text, in an effort to advance the full conversion to SI units, we shall present all dosimetry information as much as possible in terms of SI units. Appendix A contains a complete discussion of both SI and traditional units and the relationship between them. Examples of conversion between various units are also included.

Box 4.2 presents an overview of the important dates in the historical evolution of radiation quantities and units and an overview of terminology used in a given time period to describe radiation dose limitation.

The SI unit of absorbed dose, the **gray (Gy)**, was named after the English radiobiologist Louis Harold Gray (1901–1965), who was instrumental in developing what is arguably the most important theory in all of radiation dosimetry. The Bragg–Gray theory (1936) relates the ionization produced in a small cavity within an irradiated medium or object to the energy absorbed in that medium as a result of its radiation exposure. With the use of appropriate correction factors, the theory essentially links the determination of the absorbed radiation dose in a medium to a relatively simple measurement of ionization charge.

RADIATION QUANTITIES AND THEIR SI UNITS OF MEASURE

Diagnostic imaging professionals must have a clear understanding of the following basic radiation quantities:
- Exposure (X)
- Air kerma
- Absorbed dose (D)
- Equivalent dose (EqD)
- Effective dose (EfD)

Introduction

In everyday usage, we say that "exposure" has occurred when ionizing radiation strikes an object such as a human body. However, the quantity, "exposure," has a rigorous scientific meaning related to ionization produced in air. Absorbed dose is the deposition of energy per unit mass in any material from exposure to ionizing radiation. Equivalent dose (EqD) is a quantity that builds upon absorbed dose but then takes into account the type of radiation striking an object. Different types of radiation affect molecules and cells of the body in different ways. Effective dose (EfD) builds upon equivalent dose by adding an attempt to take into account the different harmful degrees of radiation effects on the parts of the body that are being irradiated to arrive at an index of overall harm to a human (Box 4.3). Each radiation quantity has its own special unit of measure. These quantities and units are discussed in detail in the following sections.

Exposure

When a volume of air is irradiated with x-rays or with gamma rays, the interaction that occurs between the radiation and neutral atoms in the air causes some electrons to be liberated from those air atoms as they are ionized. Consequently, the ionized air can function as a conductor and carry electricity because of the negatively charged free electrons and positively charged ions that have been created. As the intensity of x-ray exposure of the air volume increases, the number of electron–ion pairs produced also increases. Thus the amount of radiation responsible for the ionization of a well-defined volume of air may be determined by measuring the number of electron–ion pairs, or charged particles of either sign, in that volume of air. This radiation ionization in air is termed *exposure*.

Exposure (X) is defined as the total electrical charge of one sign, either all plus or all minus, per unit mass that x-ray and gamma ray photons with energies up to 3 million electron volts (MeV) generate in dry (i.e., nonhumid) air at standard temperature and pressure (760 mm Hg or 1 atmosphere at sea level and 22°C). It is a radiation quantity "that expresses the intensity of radiation delivered to a specific area, such as the surface of the human body."[2]

As it is defined, the exposure quantity, X, is based on a response produced when radiation interacts with air. For a precise measurement of X, the total amount of ionization (charge) an x-ray beam produces in a known mass of air must be obtained. This type of *direct* measurement is normally accomplished in an accredited dosimetry calibration laboratory (ADCL) by using a

BOX 4.2	**Historical Evolution of Radiation Quantities and Units**

Year	Event
1895	X-rays are discovered, and the discovery is announced.
1896	Initial cases of somatic damage caused by exposure to ionizing radiation are reported in Europe.
1900	Skin erythema dose becomes the unit for measuring radiation exposure.
1904	Clarence Madison Dally becomes the first American radiation fatality.
1910	First cancer deaths among physicians that are attributed to x-ray exposure are reported.
1921	The British X-Ray and Radium Protection Committee is formed to investigate methods for reducing radiation exposure.
1925	The First International Congress of Radiology is held in London, England; radiologists from all over the world collaborate, but no definite system for measuring ionizing radiation exposure is identified. The International Commission on Radiation Units and Measurements (ICRU) is formed.
1928	The ICRU is charged by the Second International Congress of Radiology (Stockholm, Sweden) with defining a unit of exposure. The International X-Ray and Radium Protection Commission (predecessor of the ICRP) is established by the Second International Congress of Radiology.
1930s	Tolerance dose is used for radiation protection purposes.
1931	The US Advisory Committee on X-Ray and Radium Protection is formed to formulate recommendations for radiation control.
1934	A tolerance dose of 0.2 R per day is recommended.
1936	The tolerance dose is reduced to 0.1 R per day.
	The Bragg–Gray theory is introduced.
1937	The roentgen (R) becomes internationally accepted as the unit of measurement for exposure to x-radiation and gamma radiation.
1946	The US Advisory Committee on X-Ray and Radium Protection becomes known as the National Committee on Radiation Protection and Measurements (NCRP).
1948	The International System of Units (SI) is developed.
Early 1950s	Maximum permissible dose (MPD) replaces the tolerance dose for radiation protection purposes.
1962	The roentgen (R) is redefined to increase accuracy and acceptability.
1963	The National Committee on Radiation Protection and Measurements becomes the National Council on Radiation Protection (NCRP).
1977	The International Commission on Radiological Protection (ICRP) recommends that the dose equivalent limit or effective dose equivalent replace the MPD.
1980	The ICRU adopts SI units for use with ionizing radiation.
1985	The National Council on Radiation Protection (NCRP) adopts SI units for use.
1991	The ICRP replaces effective equivalent dose with the term *effective dose (EfD)*.

History of Terminology Used to Determine Radiation Dose Limitation

1900–1930	Skin erythema dose (SED)
1930–1950	Tolerance dose (TD)
1950–1977	Maximum permissible dose (MPD)
1977–1991	Effective dose equivalent
1991–present	Effective dose (EfD)

standard, or free-air, ionization chamber (Fig. 4.6). The chamber contains a known quantity of air with precisely measured temperature, pressure, and low humidity. If in that specified volume of dry air the total charge of all the ions of one sign (either all plus or all minus) produced is collected and measured, the total amount of radiation exposure may be accurately determined. Lastly, the free-air chamber response is modified to correspond to standard temperature and pressure of dry air in accordance with the definition of exposure.

BOX 4.3 **Difference Between Equivalent Dose and Effective Dose**

The quantity *equivalent dose* uses radiation weighting factors (W_R) to adjust the value of the *absorbed dose* to reflect the different capacity for producing biologic harm by various types and energies of ionizing radiation.

The quantity *effective dose* uses tissue weighting factors (W_T) to adjust the quantity *equivalent dose* to reflect the difference in harm to the person as a whole depending on the tissues and organs that have been irradiated. Therefore effective dose takes into account both the type of radiation and the part of the body irradiated.

Such an instrument, however, is not a practical device at locations other than a standardization laboratory. As a result, much smaller and less complicated instruments have been developed for use away from the laboratory. Although very convenient, these instruments must be periodically recalibrated in an ADCL against a free-air chamber.

The coulomb (C) is the basic unit of electrical charge. It is equal to the "amount" of electrical charge moving past a point in a conductor in 1 second when an electrical current amounting to 1 ampere is used. The *ampere*** is the SI unit of electrical current. Current consists of moving electrical charges, the most common of which is the electron (the charge carried by an electron is equal to -1.6×10^{-19} C). Essentially, the ampere quantifies the flow rate of electric charge.

In the International System, the exposure unit is coulombs per kilogram (C/kg). No special name for this SI quantity has been assigned. This exposure unit is simply equal to an electrical charge of 1 C produced in a kilogram of dry air by ionizing radiation. Appendix A provides examples of numeric conversions between coulomb per kilogram and the roentgen traditional unit. Both of these

---

**The ampere is precisely defined as follows: Between two very long and very thin parallel wires carrying moving electric charges (i.e., a current), there is observed to be either a force of attraction or repulsion depending on the relative directions of motion of the charges in the wires. One ampere is defined to be that amount of constant wire current that leads to a force of 2×10^{-7} newtons per meter of wire length when the wires are situated in a vacuum and separated by 1 meter.

---

remain very useful for x-ray equipment calibration because x-ray output intensity is measured directly with an ionization chamber.

Air Kerma

Air kerma is another SI quantity that is used to express how energy is transferred from a beam of radiation to a material such as the patient's skin. It is in the process of replacing the traditional quantity exposure. Because of this, "x-ray tube output and inputs to image receptors are sometimes given in air kerma."[3] A standard, or free-air, ionization chamber is the instrument that can be calibrated to read air kerma.[2] "A conversion factor can also be used to change between air kerma and exposure values."[2]

"Kinetic energy released in air," "kinetic energy released in material," and "kinetic energy released per unit mass" all use the word *kerma* as an acronym. In simple terms, *air kerma* is the total kinetic energy released in a unit mass (kilogram) of air and is expressed in metric units of joule per kilogram (J/kg).[2] In a similar way one can define *tissue kerma* as the total kinetic energy released in a unit mass of tissue. Tissue kerma is also given in units of joules per kilogram. This unit for kerma is in fact the same radiation unit, the gray (Gy), which was previously defined as the SI unit for the radiation quantity, absorbed dose. With respect to radiographic and fluoroscopic units, however, "air" kerma, not "tissue" kerma, is the primary concept because in these situations we are concerned with exposure and the patient's resulting entrance dose.

Modern radiographic and fluoroscopic units have incorporated an ability to determine the entire amount of energy delivered to the patient by the x-ray beam. This quantity is often referred to as the dose area product (DAP). It is essentially the sum total of air kerma over the exposed area of the patient's surface or, in other words, a measure of the amount of radiant energy that has been thrust into a portion of the patient's body surface. DAP is usually specified in units of mGy-cm². As an illustration of this concept, consider a patient whose irradiated surface receives an air kerma dose of 20 mGy. If the area of the irradiated surface is 100 cm², then the DAP will be 20 mGy $\times$ 100 cm² = 2000 mGy-cm².

Absorbed Dose

As ionizing radiation passes through an object such as a human body, some of the energy of that radiation is

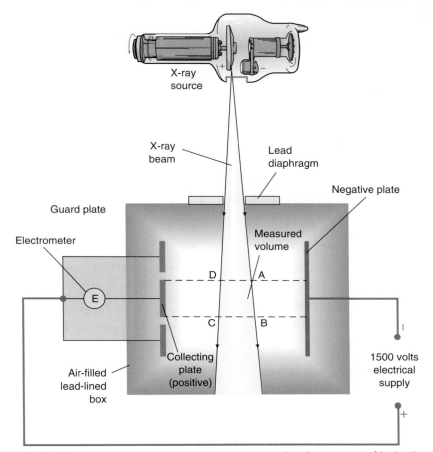

FIG 4.6 This device determines radiation exposure by measuring the amount of ionization (charge) an x-ray beam produces within its air collection volume. The instrument consists of a box containing a known quantity of air, two oppositely charged metal plates, and an electrometer, an instrument that measures the total amount of charge collected on the positively charged metal plate. The chamber measures the total amount of electrical charge of all the electrons produced during the ionization of a specific volume of air at standard atmospheric pressure and temperature. The electrical charge is measured in units called *coulombs (C)* (charge of an electron = -1.6×10^{-19} C). A collected electrical charge of 2.58×10^{-4} C/kg of irradiated air constitutes an exposure of 1 roentgen (R).

absorbed by the body and stays within it. The quantity **absorbed dose (D)** is defined as the amount of energy per unit mass absorbed by an irradiated object. Therefore absorbed dose indicates the energy that the patient actually receives from an exposure to ionizing radiation. This absorbed energy is what may cause damage in biologic tissues of the patient.

Because many x-ray examinations require relatively small radiation doses, smaller units, which are only a fraction of a specific unit, may frequently be used to indicate absorbed dose values. Examples of some of these subunits are provided in Box 4.4. Box 4.5 demonstrates conversion between decimal values of gray and the numerically smaller units: centigray (cGy) and milligray (mGy). It is also easy to convert milligray or centigray to gray. This is done just by dividing the number of milligray by 1000 or the number of centigray by 100. SI subunits can also facilitate conversion from traditional units of absorbed dose to SI units of absorbed dose, especially in therapeutic radiology (see Appendix A for an example).

BOX 4.4   Subunits of the Gray

Smaller fractions of measured quantities such as the gray (Gy) will have a prefix. Examples follow.

Prefix	Subunit	Symbol	Fraction	Factor
centi-	centigray (cGy)	c	$\frac{1}{100}$	10^{-2}
milli-	milligray (mGy)	m	$\frac{1}{1000}$	10^{-3}
micro-	microgray (μGy)	μ	$\frac{1}{1,000,000}$	10^{-6}

BOX 4.5   How to Convert Gray to Milligray and to Centigray

Rule: Number of gray × 1000 = Number of milligray
Example: 0.010 Gy × 1000 = 10 mGy
Rule: Number of gray × 100 = Number of centigray
Example: 0.100 Gy × 100 = 10 cGy

TABLE 4.1   Quality Factors for Different Types of Ionizing Radiation

Type of Ionizing Radiation	Quality Factor
X-ray photons	1
Beta particles	1
Gamma photons	1
Thermal neutrons	5
Fast neutrons	20
High-energy external protons	1
Low-energy internal protons*	20
Alpha particles	20
Multiple charged particles of unknown energy	20

*Protons produced as a result of neutrons interacting with the nuclei of tissue molecules.
Data from National Council on Radiation Protection and Measurements (NCRP): *Limitation of exposure to ionizing radiation, Report No. 116*, Bethesda, MD, 1993, NCRP.

Equivalence of Radiation-Produced Damage From Different Sources of Ionizing Radiation

Equal absorbed doses of different types of radiation produce different amounts of biologic damage in body tissue. For example, in laboratory experiments it has been shown that a 1-Gy absorbed dose of fast neutrons causes much more biologic damage than a 1-Gy absorbed dose of x-rays. A 1-Gy dose of neutrons would kill a laboratory rat, but a 1-Gy dose of x-rays would not. The concept of dose equivalence takes this varied biologic impact into consideration by using a specific modifying factor termed a *quality factor* to adjust the absorbed dose value. Quality factor (Q) is an adjustment multiplier that is employed in the calculation of dose equivalence to detail the ability of a dose of any kind of ionizing radiation to cause biologic damage.

X-rays, beta particles (high-speed electrons), and gamma rays produce virtually the same biologic effect in body tissue for equal absorbed doses. In terms of quality factor, these radiations have been given a numeric adjustment value of 1 (i.e., Q = 1) and are the basis, or standard, against which to compare the effectiveness of other types of ionizing radiation in producing biologic damage. The quality factors of different kinds of ionizing radiations are listed in Table 4.1. The concept of linear energy transfer (LET) helps explain the need for a quality, or modifying, factor. LET is the amount of energy transferred on average by incident radiation to an object per unit length of track, or passage, through the object and is expressed in units of kiloelectron volts per micrometer (keV/μm) (see Appendix B). Radiation with a high LET transfers a large amount of energy into a small area and can therefore do more biologic damage than radiation with a low LET. As a result, a high-LET radiation has a quality factor that is greater than the quality factor for a low-LET radiation.

Equivalent Dose

Equivalent dose (EqD) is the product of the average absorbed dose in a tissue or organ in the human body and its associated radiation weighting factor (W_R) chosen for the type and energy of the radiation in question. X-radiation and gamma radiation have a W_R of 1, whereby 1 Gy equals 1 Sv. Other types of radiation have different radiation weighting factors.

The radiation weighting factor (W_R) takes into consideration the fact that some types of radiation are more efficient at causing biologic damage than other types of radiation for a given dose. Values for the radiation weighting factors are selected by national and international scientific advisory bodies (NCRP, ICRP) and are based on quality factors and LET. The NCRP, in Report No. 116, described the radiation weighting factor as "a dimensionless factor" (a multiplier) that was chosen for radiation protection purposes to account for differences in biologic impact among various types of ionizing radiations.[1] This factor places risks associated with biologic effects on a common scale. Each type and energy of

TABLE 4.2   **Radiation Weighting Factors for Different Types and Energies of Ionizing Radiation**

Radiation Type and Energy Range	Radiation Weighting Factor (W_R)
X-ray and gamma ray photons and electrons (every energy)	1
Neutrons, energy <10 keV	5
10 keV–100 keV	10
>100 keV–2 MeV	20
>2 MeV–20 MeV	10
>20 MeV	5
Protons	2
Alpha particles	20

Data adapted from International Commission on Radiological Protection (ICRP): *Recommendations*, ICRP Publication No. 60, New York, 1991, Pergamon Press.

BOX 4.6   **Subunits of the Sievert**

Smaller fractions of measured quantities such as the sievert (Sv) will have a prefix. Examples follow.

Prefix	Subunit	Symbol	Fraction	Factor
centi-	centisievert (cSv)	c	$\frac{1}{100}$	10^{-2}
milli-	millisievert (mSv)	m	$\frac{1}{1000}$	10^{-3}
micro-	microsievert (µSv)	µ	$\frac{1}{1,000,000}$	10^{-6}

radiation has a specific radiation weighting factor, the numeric value of which may be found in Table 4.2. The radiation weighting factor actually has the same numeric value as the quality factor that was previously used for determining dose equivalence.

EqD is used for radiation protection purposes when a person receives exposure from various types of ionizing radiation. EqD is expressed in sieverts or in a subunit of the sievert (Box 4.6). Equivalent dose is obtained by multiplying the absorbed dose (D) by the radiation weighting factor (W_R) as follows:

$$EqD = D \times W_R$$

which in terms of units corresponds to:

$$Sv = Gy \times W_R$$

An example of determining and expressing equivalent dose using gray and sievert is provided in Box 4.7. Because

BOX 4.7   **Determining and Expressing Equivalent Dose Using Gray and Sievert**

Example: An individual received the following absorbed doses: 0.1 Gy_t of x-radiation, 0.05 Gy_t of fast neutrons, and 0.2 Gy_t of alpha particles. What is the total equivalent dose (EqD)?

$$EqD = (D \times W_R)_1 + (D \times W_R)_2 + (D \times W_R)_3$$

(The radiation weighting factor for each radiation in question may be obtained from Table 4.2.)
  Answer:

Radiation Type	D	×	W_R	=	EqD
X-radiation	0.1 Gy_t	×	1	=	0.1 Sv
Fast neutrons	0.05 Gy_t	×	20	=	1.0 Sv
Alpha particles	0.2 Gy_t	×	20	=	4.0 Sv
	Total EqD			=	5.1 Sv

radiation doses for radiation workers employed in diagnostic radiology are normally relatively small, they may be specified in terms of millisievert. To change sievert to millisievert, multiply the number of sievert by 1000, whereas millisievert can be converted to sievert by dividing the number of millisievert by 1000.

Effective Dose

EfD provides a measure of the overall risk of exposure to humans from ionizing radiation. The NCRP, in Report No. 116, defines it as "the sum of the weighted equivalent doses for all irradiated tissues or organs."[1] EfD incorporates both the effect of the type of radiation used (e.g., x-radiation, gamma, neutron, alpha) and the variability in radiosensitivity of the specific organ or body part irradiated through the use of appropriate weighting factors. These factors quantify the overall potential harm to those biologic components and the risk of developing a radiation-induced cancer or, for the reproductive organs, the risk of genetic damage. The term that specifically takes into account the relative detriment to each specific particular organ and tissue is called the **tissue weighting factor** (W_T). More precisely, each W_T value (Table 4.3) denotes the percentage ratio of the summed stochastic (cancer plus genetic) risk stemming from irradiation of a specific tissue or organ to the all-inclusive risk when the entire body is irradiated in a uniform fashion. As a result, EfD accounts for the risk to the entire organism brought on by all types of irradiation of individual tissues and organs. The ICRP originally introduced the tissue

TABLE 4.3 Organ or Tissue Weighting Factors

Organ or Tissue	Weighting Factor (W$_T$)
Gonads	0.20
Red bone marrow	0.12
Colon	0.12
Lung	0.12
Stomach	0.12
Bladder	0.05
Breast	0.05
Liver	0.05
Esophagus	0.05
Thyroid	0.05
Skin	0.01
Bone surface	0.01
Remainder*†	0.05

*The remainder takes into account the following additional tissues and organs: adrenals, brain, small intestine, large intestine, kidney, muscle, pancreas, spleen, thymus, and uterus.

†In extraordinary circumstances in which one of the remainder tissues or organs receives an equivalent dose in excess of the highest dose in any of the 12 organs for which a weighting factor (W$_T$) is specified, a W$_T$ of 0.025 should be applied to that tissue or organ and a W$_T$ of 0.025 to the average dose in the other remainder tissues or organs.
Data from National Council on Radiation Protection and Measurements (NCRP): *Limitation of exposure to ionizing radiation, Report No. 116,* Bethesda, Md, 1993, NCRP. Reprinted with permission of the National Council on Radiation Protection and Measurements, http://NCRPonline.org.

BOX 4.8 Determining and Expressing Effective Dose in Sievert

Example: The W$_R$ for alpha particles is 20 (see Table 4.2), and the W$_T$ for the lung is 0.12 (see Table 4.3). If the lungs receive an absorbed dose (D) of 0.5 Gy$_t$ from exposure to alpha radiation, what is the effective dose (EfD) in Sv?

Answer:

$$EfD = D \times W_R \times W_T$$
$$= 0.5 \times 20 \times 0.12$$
$$= 1.2\, Sv$$

TABLE 4.4 Typical Values for Radiation Doses Associated With an Anteroposterior Lumbar Spine Examination

Absorbed dose to skin at entrance surface	6.4 mGy
Absorbed dose to bone marrow	0.6 mGy
Absorbed dose to a fetus	3.5 mGy
Equivalent dose to a fetus	3.5 mSv
Effective dose to a fetus	3.3 mSv

weighting factor concept because uniform, whole-body irradiation seldom occurs, causing different organs and body tissues to vary considerably in the amount of absorbed dose received and, consequently, the intensity of their response.

To determine EfD, an absorbed dose (D) is multiplied by a radiation weighting factor (W$_R$) to obtain EqD and that product is multiplied by a tissue weighting factor (W$_T$) to give:

$$EfD = D \times W_R \times W_T$$

EfD is expressed in sievert or millisievert. An example of determining and expressing EfD in sievert is provided in Box 4.8.

EfD can be used to compare the average effective amount of radiation received by the entire body from a specific radiologic examination with that from natural background radiation (see Table 1.1). By using the background equivalent radiation time (BERT) method as discussed in Chapter 1, it is possible to describe the examination's significant radiation dose in terms of the length of time it would take to acquire a comparable amount from environmental sources.

Table 4.4 gives some typical values for radiation doses that are associated with a radiographic examination of the lumbar spine, and it illustrates some of the principles of the different ways to specify radiation dose. The dose to the patient is highest at the "entrance skin surface," the surface of the patient that is toward the x-ray tube. This surface will be exposed to the unattenuated primary beam of x-rays. Absorbed doses to various organs may be calculated from standard tables. Two organ absorbed doses are given in Table 4.4, namely, bone marrow and fetus. The EqD to the fetus is also given and is the same as the absorbed dose to the fetus because the radiation weighting factor is 1. Finally, the EfD to the fetus is given. It was calculated from the various tissue weighting factors and organ absorbed doses for organs in the field of view of this examination.

TABLE 4.5 SI Unit Equivalents

1 SI exposure unit equals	$\dfrac{1}{(2.58\times10^{-4})}$R
1 coulomb equals	1 ampere-second
1 coulomb per kilogram of air equals	1 SI unit of exposure $C/kg = \dfrac{1}{(2.58\times10^{-4})}$R
1 gray equals	1 J/kg
	100 cGy
	1000 mGy
	1 J/kg (for x-radiation, Q = 1)
1 sievert equals	100 centisievert (cSv)
	1000 mSv
	10^{-7} J
	10^{7} erg
1 erg equals	1 newton-meter
1 joule equals	6.24×10^{18} eV

Collective Effective Dose

In addition to EqD and EfD, another dosimetric quantity has been derived and implemented for use in radiation protection. It takes into account both internal and external dose measurements. **Collective Effective Dose (ColEfD)** represents an attempt to describe the radiation exposure of a population or group from low doses of different sources of ionizing radiation. It is determined as the product of the average EfD for an individual belonging to the exposed population or group and the number of persons exposed. The radiation unit for this quantity is *person-sievert*. An example using this unit is provided in Box 4.9. With respect to the validity of this concept, the ICRP states: "Collective effective dose is an instrument for optimization, for comparing radiological technologies and protection procedures. Collective effective dose is not intended as a tool for epidemiological studies, and it is inappropriate to use it in risk projections. This is because the assumptions implicit in the calculation of collective effective dose (e.g., when applying the LNT[‡] model) conceal large biological and statistical uncertainties. Specifically, the computation of cancer deaths based on collective effective doses involving trivial exposures to large populations is not reasonable and should be avoided."[4]

Total Effective Dose Equivalent

Total Effective Dose Equivalent (TEDE) is a radiation dosimetry quantity that was defined by the Nuclear Regulatory Commission (NRC) to monitor and control human exposure to ionizing radiation. Essentially, as described by NRC regulations, it is the sum of effective dose equivalent from external radiation exposures and a quantity called **Committed Effective Dose Equivalent**

(CEDE)[¶] from internal radiation exposures. Thus TEDE is designed to take into account all possible sources of radiation exposure. It is a particularly useful dose monitor for occupationally exposed personnel such as nuclear medicine technologists and interventional radiologists, who are likely to receive possibly significant radiation exposure during the course of a year. Traditionally, the whole-body TEDE regulatory limit is 0.05 Sv for occupationally exposed personnel and 0.001 Sv for the general public. Radiation monitoring services such as Landauer, Inc., and Global Dosimetry Solutions can provide annual TEDE values for individuals.

Tables 4.5 and 4.6 summarize radiation quantities, units, and equivalents. An additional table emphasizing relationship between traditional units and SI units is also found in Appendix A.

[‡]LNT, which stands for linear nonthreshold, is a dose model that implies there is no dose value below which there is no risk of biologic damage and that the degree of risk is directly proportional to the dose at any level.

[¶]The "committed dose" in radiation protection is a measure of the probabilistic health effect on an individual as a result of an intake of radioactive material into the body. A "committed dose" from an internal source is intended to carry the same effective risk as the same amount of equivalent dose applied uniformly to the whole body from an external source of radiation. This is the origin of the name "committed effective dose equivalent." For nuclear medicine technologists who, through certain procedures (e.g., thyroid ablations, using iodine-131), have a possibility of radioisotope absorption and consequent internal exposure, committed dose is certainly an appropriate measure.

TABLE 4.6 Summary of Radiation Quantities and Units

Type of Radiation	Quantity	SI Unit	Measuring Medium	Radiation Effect Measured
X-radiation or gamma radiation	Exposure (X)	Coulombs per kilogram (C/kg)	Air	Ionization of air
	Air kerma	Gray (Gy_a)		
All ionizing radiations	Absorbed dose (D)	Gray (Gy_t)	Any object	Amount of energy per unit mass absorbed by object
	Air kerma	Gray (Gy_t)		
All ionizing radiations	Equivalent dose (EqD)	Sievert (Sv)	Body tissue	Biologic effects
All ionizing radiations	Effective dose (EfD)	Sievert (Sv)	Body tissue	Biologic effects

SUMMARY

- German physics professor Wilhelm Conrad Roentgen discovered "x-rays" on November 8, 1895, during an experiment investigating the nature of cathode rays and fluorescent materials.
- Many individuals who were exposed to substantial doses of x-rays in the early years after their discovery developed somatic damage from the exposure.
- Skin erythema dose was used from 1900 to 1930 as the unit for measuring radiation exposure. Eventually a tolerance dose was established for occupationally exposed individuals that could be regarded as a threshold dose. MPD replaced the tolerance dose in the early 1950s. In 1977 dose equivalent or effective dose equivalent replaced the MPD. In 1991 the ICRP replaced effective dose equivalent with the term *effective dose,* which is still currently in use today.
- Effective dose is based on the energy deposited in biologic tissue by ionizing radiation. It takes into account both the type of radiation and the variable sensitivity of the tissues exposed to the radiation. EfD is expressed in the SI unit sievert (Sv) or in subunits of the sievert.
- In 1980 the ICRU adopted SI units for use with ionizing radiation. Many developed countries, particularly in Europe, have already made a complete transition to SI units. In the United States, this transition is not as yet fully complete and some conventional units are still in use.
- SI radiation units are preferred for specifying radiation quantities because the traditional system of units does not fit into the metric system that provides "one unified system of units for all physical quantities."[2]
- Coulomb per kilogram (C/kg) is used for specifying x-ray or gamma ray exposure in air only. This exposure unit is equal to an electrical charge of 1 coulomb produced in a kilogram of dry air by ionizing radiation.
- Air kerma is an SI quantity that is used to express radiation concentration transferred to a point, which may be at the surface of a patient's or radiographer's body.
- DAP is essentially the sum total of air kerma over the exposed area of the patient's surface.
- Absorbed dose (D) is the amount of energy per unit mass absorbed by an irradiated object.
- The gray (Gy) is used for measuring absorbed dose in air (Gy_a) or for measuring absorbed dose in tissue (Gy_t).
- The number of gray times 1000 equals the number of milligray. The number of gray times 100 equals the number of centigray.
- LET is the amount of energy transferred on average by incident radiation to an object per unit length of track, or passage, through the object and is expressed in units of kiloelectron volts per micrometer (keV/μm).
- Equivalent dose (EqD) and effective dose (EfD) are the quantities of choice for measuring biologic effects when all types of radiation must be considered.
- EqD specifies how the potential for biologic damage from different types and doses of radiation will be equivalent if correct weighting factors are included. To calculate equivalent dose: $EqD = D \times W_R$.
- EfD describes the total biologic damage to a human that is caused by equivalent doses received by specific organs. To calculate effective dose: $EfD = D \times W_R \times W_T$.
- In the SI system, sievert (Sv) or the subunits millisievert and microsievert are used to specify EqD and EfD. These units are used for occupational radiation exposure.
- ColEfD represents an attempt to describe the radiation exposure of a population or group from low doses of

different sources of ionizing radiation. Person-sievert is the radiation unit used to calculate this quantity. According to the ICRP it is not a valid method for computing the potential number of deaths from cancer.

- The radiation dosimetry quantity, TEDE, is designed to take into account all possible sources of radiation exposure and is used for dose monitoring for occupationally exposed personnel (e.g., nuclear medicine technologists and interventional radiologists) who are likely to receive possibly significant radiation exposure during the course of a year. The whole-body TEDE regulatory limit for exposed personnel is 0.05 sievert and 0.001 sievert for the general public.
- The CEDE in radiation protection is a measure of the probabilistic health effect on an individual resulting from an intake of radioactive material into the body.

REFERENCES

1. National Council on Radiation Protection and Measurements (NCRP): *Limitation of exposure to ionizing radiation, Report No. 116*, Bethesda, MD, 1993, NCRP.
2. Sprawls P: Radiation quantities and units, sprawls educational foundation. The physical principles of medical imaging online. Available at: http://www.sprawls .org/ppmi2/RADQU/.
3. Carlton RR, Adler AM: *Principles of radiographic imaging: an art and a science*, ed 5, New York, 2013, Delmar, Cengage Learning.
4. The 2007 Recommendations of the International Commission on Radiological Protection, ICRP publication 103 Ann. Elsevier Publishing, www.elsevier.com, ICRP 37 (2-4), 2007.

GENERAL DISCUSSION QUESTIONS

1. Why should diagnostic imaging personnel be familiar with standardized radiation quantities and units?
2. When, where, and how did Wilhelm Conrad Roentgen discover x-rays?
3. What types of medical problems did early radiation workers develop as a consequence of their occupational exposure?
4. What is the benefit of using the International System of Units of measurement for ionizing radiation?
5. What is a threshold dose?
6. In 1991 the International Commission on Radiological Protection (ICRP) revised tissue weighting factors. On what data was this revision based?

7. What radiation quantities are currently in use, and what SI units are used to relate these quantities?
8. What instrument can be calibrated to read air kerma?
9. What factors determine the amount of x-ray energy absorbed by a human anatomic structure?
10. When a person receives exposure from various types of ionizing radiation, what radiation quantity and what SI unit should be used to specify this exposure?
11. How is centigray converted to gray?
12. How were radiation dose limits calculated and established?

REVIEW QUESTIONS

1. Which of the following was used as the *first* measure of exposure for ionizing radiation?
   A. Air kerma
   B. Skin erythema
   C. Sievert
   D. Roentgen
2. A radiation weighting factor (W_R) has been established for each of the following ionizing radiations: x-rays ($W_R = 1$), fast neutrons ($W_R = 20$), and alpha particles ($W_R = 20$). What is the *total* equivalent dose (EqD) in sieverts for a person who has received the following exposures: 0.2 Gy_t of x-rays, 0.07 Gy_t of fast neutrons, and 0.3 Gy_t of alpha particles?
   A. 9.4 Sv
   B. 7.6 Sv
   C. 4.3 Sv
   D. 1.9 Sv
3. Which of the following is the unit of collective effective dose (ColEfD)?
   A. Coulombs per kilogram-sievert
   B. Gray-sievert
   C. Person-sievert
   D. Rad-sievert
4. The concept of tissue weighting factor (W_T) is used to do which of the following?
   A. Account for the risk to the entire organism brought on by irradiation of individual tissues and organs
   B. Eliminate the need for determining effective dose
   C. Measure absorbed dose from all different types of ionizing radiations
   D. Modify the radiation weighting factor for different types of ionizing radiation

5. To convert the number of gray into milligray, the number of gray must be:
   A. Divided by 100
   B. Divided by 1000
   C. Multiplied by 100
   D. Multiplied by 1000
6. What is the SI radiation unit coulomb per kilogram used to specify?
   A. Equivalent dose
   B. Absorbed dose in biologic tissue
   C. Radiation exposure in air only
   D. Speed at which x-ray photons travel
7. Which of the following radiation quantities accounts for some biologic tissues being *more* sensitive to radiation damage than other tissues?
   A. Absorbed dose
   B. Exposure
   C. Equivalent dose
   D. Effective dose

8. The radiation weighting factor for alpha particles is 20, and the tissue weighting factor for the lungs is 0.12. If the lungs receive an absorbed dose of 0.2 Gy_t from exposure to alpha particles, what is the effective dose in sievert?
   A. 0.48 Sv
   B. 4.8 Sv
   C. 48.0 Sv
   D. 480.0 Sv
9. If 100 people received an average effective dose of 0.35 Sv, what is the collective effective dose?
   A. 17.5 person-sieverts
   B. 35 person-sieverts
   C. 70 person-sieverts
   D. 285 person-sieverts
10. How is the SI unit for dose area product (DAP) usually specified?
    A. Coulomb
    B. Erg-sec
    C. $mGy-cm^2$
    D. Sievert

5

Radiation Monitoring

OBJECTIVES

After completing this chapter, the reader will be able to perform the following:

- Define all key terms.
- State the reason why a radiation worker should wear a personnel dosimeter, and explain the function and characteristics of such devices.
- Identify the appropriate location on the body where the personnel dosimeter(s) should be worn during the following procedures or conditions: (1) routine radiographic procedures, (2) fluoroscopic procedures, (3) special radiographic procedures, and (4) pregnancy.
- Describe the various components of the optically stimulated luminescence (OSL) dosimeter, thermoluminescent dosimeter (TLD), pocket

ionization chamber, and the personnel digital ionization dosimeter, and explain the use of each of these devices as personnel monitors.

- Explain the function of radiation survey instruments.
- List three gas-filled radiation survey instruments.
- Explain the requirements for radiation survey instruments.
- Give the useful operating regions of the following instruments: (1) ionization chamber–type survey meter (cutie pie), (2) proportional counter, and (3) Geiger–Müller (GM) survey meter.
- Identify the radiation survey instrument that can be used to calibrate radiographic and fluoroscopic x-ray equipment.

CHAPTER OUTLINE

Personnel Monitoring
  Requirement for Personnel Monitoring
  Purpose of Personnel Dosimeters
  Placement of Personnel Dosimeters
  Extremity Dosimeter
  Record of Radiation Exposure
Personnel Dosimeters
  Characteristics
  Types

Radiation Survey Instruments for Area Monitoring
  Radiation Detection and Measurement
  Types of Instruments
  Requirements
  Gas-Filled Radiation Survey Instruments
Instruments Used to Measure X-Ray Exposure in Radiology
Summary

KEY TERMS

control monitor
extremity dosimeter
Geiger–Müller (GM) survey meter
glow curve

ionization chamber–type survey meter (cutie pie)
optically stimulated luminescence (OSL) dosimeter

personnel digital ionization dosimeter
personnel dosimeter
personnel dosimetry

To ensure that occupational radiation exposure levels are kept well below the annual effective dose (EfD) limit, some means of monitoring personnel exposure must be employed. The radiographer and other occupationally exposed persons should be aware of the various radiation exposure monitoring devices and their functions. This chapter provides an overview of both personnel and area monitoring. In addition, because radiation dosimetry reports still report radiation exposure for workers in traditional units and subunits, traditional units' numerical values are identified in parentheses after SI units' numerical values.

PERSONNEL MONITORING

Requirement for Personnel Monitoring

Personnel dosimetry refers to the monitoring of equivalent dose to any person occupationally exposed on a regular basis to ionizing radiation, which is recommended. It is *required*, however, whenever radiation workers are likely to risk receiving 10% or more of the annual occupational EfD limit of 50 mSv (5 rem) in any single year as a consequence of their work-related activities. In keeping with the as low as reasonably achievable (ALARA) concept, most health care facilities issue dosimetry devices when personnel could receive approximately 1% of the annual occupational EfD limit (50 mSv [5000 mrem]) in any month, or approximately 0.5 mSv (50 mrem). Radiation exposure monitoring is accomplished by wearing personnel dosimeters.

Purpose of Personnel Dosimeters

The personnel dosimeter:
- Provides an indication of the working habits and working conditions of diagnostic imaging personnel
- Determines occupational exposure by detecting and measuring the quantity of ionizing radiation to which the dosimeter has been exposed over a period of time

- Does not protect the wearer from exposure because the instrument is only capable of detecting and measuring the amount of ionizing radiation to which it has been exposed

Placement of Personnel Dosimeters

During Routine Radiographic Procedures. A personnel monitoring device records only the exposure received in the area where the device is worn. During routine radiographic procedures, when a protective apron is not being used, the primary personnel dosimeter should be attached to the clothing on the front of the body at collar level to approximate the location of maximal radiation dose to the following (Fig. 5.1):
- Thyroid
- Head
- Neck

Consistency of location in wearing the dosimeter is necessary and is the responsibility of the individual wearing the device. A list of the types of personnel monitors available to diagnostic imaging personnel is found in Box 5.1. Discussion of each of the personnel monitoring devices follows.

When a Protective Apron Is Worn. Fluoroscopy, surgery, and special radiographic procedures produce the highest occupational radiation exposure for diagnostic imaging personnel. When a protective lead apron is used during such procedures, the dosimeter should be worn outside the apron at collar level on the anterior surface of the body because the unprotected head, neck, and lenses of the eye receive 10 to 20 times more exposure than the protected body trunk. When the dosimeter is located at collar level, it also provides a reading of the approximate equivalent dose to the thyroid gland and eyes of the occupationally exposed person. If the lead apron's shielding integrity is not compromised, a dosimeter reading that is within acceptable limits outside of the apron ensures a minimal reading under the apron.

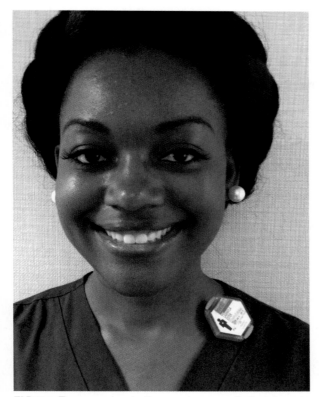

FIG 5.1 To approximate the maximum radiation dose to the thyroid and the head and neck during routine radiographic procedures, the primary personnel monitor should be attached to the clothing on the front of the body at collar level.

BOX 5.1   Personnel Monitoring Devices Currently Available

1. Optically stimulated luminescence (OSL) dosimeter
2. Extremity dosimeter (thermoluminescent dosimeter [TLD] ring)
3. Thermoluminescent dosimeter (TLD)
4. Pocket ionization chamber (pocket dosimeter)
5. Personnel digital ionization dosimeter

As a Second Monitor When a Protective Apron Is Worn. During lengthy interventional fluoroscopy procedures (e.g., cardiac catheterization), some health care facilities may prefer to have diagnostic imaging personnel wear two separate monitoring devices. As mentioned previously, the first, or primary, dosimeter is to be worn outside the protective apparel at collar level, whereas the second dosimeter should be placed beneath a wraparound-style lead apron at waist level to monitor the approximate equivalent dose to the lower body trunk. Commercially available lead aprons typically have either 0.5-mm or 0.25-mm lead equivalent shielding. Another version is also available with 0.35-mm lead equivalent in the front and 0.25-mm shielding in the back. For those occupationally exposed personnel who use two radiation dosimeters as described earlier, it is useful to have some knowledge of what the difference in equivalent dose readings between those dosimeters could be. For a primary beam at 100 kVp and 250 mAs incident at a distance of 100 cm (40 in.) on a 0.5-mm lead apron, the transmission through the apron has been measured as approximately 3.2%, corresponding to a disparity between the outer and inner dosimeter readings of a factor of 30. For a similar situation with the lighter apron in the front, the transmission was approximately 8.5% (factor of 12) and in the rear approximately 10.5% (a factor of 9.5).

As a Monitor for the Embryo-Fetus. In addition to a primary dosimeter worn at collar level, pregnant diagnostic imaging personnel may be issued a second monitoring device to record the radiation dose to the abdomen during gestation. This monitor, therefore, can provide an estimate of the equivalent dose to the embryo-fetus. Many facilities do provide pregnant radiographers with a second dosimeter for this purpose.

Extremity Dosimeter

An **extremity dosimeter**, which is commonly a **thermoluminescent dosimeter (TLD)** ring (Fig. 5.2), may be used by an imaging professional as a second monitor when performing fluoroscopic procedures that require the hands to be near the primary x-ray beam. Even though ring badges are worn under gloves to avoid contamination, such extremity monitors have a laser-etched cover to ensure the retention of permanent identification. The reusable TLD element of the dosimeter is encapsulated within its engraved cover.

Record of Radiation Exposure

A record of radiation exposure should be part of the employment record of all radiation workers. Table 5.1 gives occupational exposures (gathered from personnel dosimeter readings) for a typical year. The listed values

TABLE 5.1	Occupational Exposure Values for a Typical Year				
	NUMBER OF WORKERS (THOUSANDS)		AVERAGE ANNUAL EFFECTIVE DOSE (mSv)		Collective Effective
Category	All	Exposed	All	Exposed	Dose (Person-Sv)*
Medicine	584	277	0.7	1.5	416
Industry	350	156	1.2	2.4	380
Nuclear power	151	91	3.6	5.6	550
Flight crews, flight attendants	97	97	1.7	1.7	165
Other[†]					789
				Total	2300

*See NCRP Report No. 101, p 60.
[†]Includes workers in the US government (Department of Energy, US Public Health Service), uranium mining, well logging, miscellaneous workers, visitors to facilities, and so forth.
Data from National Council on Radiation Protection and Measurements (NCRP): *Exposure of the U.S. population from occupational radiation, Report No. 101,* Bethesda, MD, 1989, NCRP, pp 65–70.

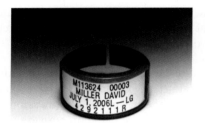

FIG 5.2 An extremity dosimeter (thermoluminescent dosimeter [TLD] ring badge) can be used to monitor the equivalent dose to the hands. (From Landauer, Inc., Glenwood, IL.)

represent the corresponding average annual EfD to the whole body and the related collective effective dose.

PERSONNEL DOSIMETERS

Characteristics

A personnel dosimeter should be lightweight and easy to carry and be made of materials durable enough to tolerate normal daily use. The dosimeter must be able to detect and record both small and large exposures in a consistent and reliable manner. Outside influences such as very warm weather, humidity, and ordinary mechanical shock should not affect the performance of the instrument. Because many employees in a health care facility may be assigned to wear radiation monitors, the monitors

are required to be reasonably inexpensive to purchase and maintain. This permits health care facilities to use large numbers of monitors in a cost-effective manner.

Types

Four types of personnel dosimeters are currently widely used to measure individual exposure of the body to ionizing radiation:

- Optically stimulated luminescence (OSL) dosimeters
- Thermoluminescent dosimeters (TLDs)
- Pocket ionization chambers
- Personnel digital ionization dosimeters

TLD ring badges, previously discussed, are extremity dosimeters that are used for monitoring of the hands only.

Optically Stimulated Luminescence Dosimeter. The optically stimulated luminescence (OSL) dosimeter for personnel monitoring provides the best features of TLDs (discussed later in this chapter) and the discontinued traditional film badges while eliminating some of their disadvantages (Fig. 5.3). This radiation monitor is the most common type of device used for monitoring of occupational exposure in diagnostic imaging. It has replaced its predecessor, the film badge, for personnel monitoring in essentially all health care facilities.

The OSL dosimeter shown in Fig. 5.3 contains an aluminum oxide (Al_2O_3) detector (thin layer). The dosimeter is "read out" by using laser light at selected frequencies. When such laser light is incident on the

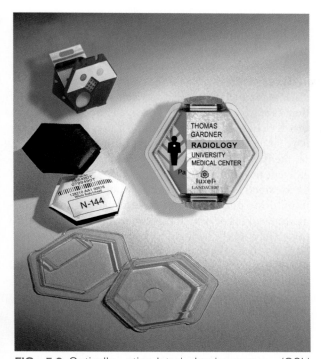

FIG 5.3 Optically stimulated luminescence (OSL) dosimeter. Disassembled OSL dosimeter demonstrating components of the monitor: sensing material holder, preloaded packet incorporating an Al_2O_3 strip sandwiched within a three-element filter pack that is heat sealed within a light-tight black paper wrapper that has been laminated to the white paper label. The front of the white paper packet may also be color-coded to facilitate correct usage and placement of the dosimeter on the body of occupationally exposed personnel. (All components are sealed inside a tamperproof plastic blister pack.) (From Landauer, Inc., Glenwood, IL.)

sensing material, it becomes luminescent in proportion to the amount of radiation exposure received.

Although the OSL dosimeter can be worn for up to 1 year, it is common practice to wear it for a period of 1 to 3 months. Like traditional film badge monitors, OSL dosimeters are usually shipped to the monitoring company for reading and dose determination, a task that requires some time for the result of a reading to be communicated. A company such as Landauer, Inc. (Glenwood, IL) manufactures and sells an in-house reader called *microStar* that may be purchased. In this way, occupational exposure doses can be determined on the day of occurrence.

Energy discrimination. As can be seen in Fig. 5.3, three different filters are incorporated into the detector packet of the OSL dosimeter. The filters are, respectively, made of:
- Aluminum (Al)
- Tin (Sn)
- Copper (Cu)

Each filter blocks a portion of the radiation-sensitive aluminum oxide and causes a different degree of attenuation for any radiation striking the dosimeter, depending on its energy. The aluminum filter offers the least absorption, whereas the copper filter attenuates the most. When the exposed aluminum oxide layer is read out by a laser, the degree of luminescence detected in the areas from beneath the filters is a measure of radiation dose occurring within different energy ranges. Thus a situation in which high-energy radiation strikes the dosimeter would show a similar reading through all the filters. Conversely, if the dosimeter had been subjected to only very low-energy radiation, then the laser readout would be much more pronounced in the region covered by the aluminum filter than in the other filter-blocked portions. Somewhat more energetic radiation would also enhance the intensity of the region beneath the tin filter. This is the way that radiation energy discrimination is achieved by the OSL dosimeters. The different energy ranges are typically classified as "deep," "eye," and "shallow" and physically correlate with different penetration depths and therefore different effective radiation energies, with "deep" being the most penetrating at a cm or more, "eye" at 0.3 cm, and "shallow" at the surface, or below 0.01 cm.

In the latest type of OSL dosimeter from one manufacturer[1] a "bare" or unfiltered portion of the aluminum oxide is used to detect dynamic exposures, that is, those received during rapid motion between the source of radiation and the dosimeter. Examination of the glow curves from this bare region demonstrates a shift or spread in their light frequency that can be correlated with motion (technically classifiable as a Doppler shift*).

Doppler shift refers to the apparent change in frequency of a light wave as observer and light source move toward or away from each other. This is similar to the increase in pitch of a train whistle experienced by a pedestrian as the locomotive moves toward him or her and its decrease in pitch noted by the pedestrian as the train moves away from him or her.

Optically stimulated luminescence dosimeter sensitivity. The OSL dosimeter provides an accurate reading as low as 10 µSv (1 mrem) for x-ray and gamma ray photons with energies ranging from 5 keV to greater than 40 MeV. Because of this, the OSL dosimeter is actually more sensitive than a TLD dosimeter, discussed later in this chapter. However, when compared with the pocket ionization chamber that is only used in selective personnel monitoring situations (also discussed later in this chapter), the OSL is actually the second most sensitive of the four personnel monitoring devices. The OSL's maximum equivalent dose measurement for x-ray and gamma ray photons is 10 Sv (1000 rem). For beta particles with energies from 150 keV to in excess of 10 MeV, dose measurement ranges from 100 µSv to 10 Sv (10 mrem to 1000 rem). For neutron radiation with energies of 40 keV to greater than 35 MeV, the OSL has a dose measurement range from 200 microsieverts to 250 microsieverts (20 mrem to 25 mrem).

Control monitor. The monitoring company that supplies a health care facility with OSLs provides a control monitor with each batch of dosimeters. This control serves as a basis for comparison with the remaining OSL badges after they have been returned to the company for processing. The control monitor is supposed to be kept in a radiation-free area within an imaging facility so that its response should be zero. After processing, if a control monitor reading greater than zero is obtained, then the associated batch of OSLs may have been exposed to radiation while in transit. To ensure that false readings are not recorded, the control monitor reading is reported to the health care facility. This reading, if different from zero, must be subtracted from each of the remaining OSLs in the batch to ensure accuracy in exposure reporting.

Advantages of the OSL dosimeter. The OSL is lightweight, durable, and easy to carry. It contains an integrated, self-contained, preloaded packet. Color-coding, graphic formats, and body location icons provide easy identification. Unlike its film badge predecessor, the OSL's tamperproof blister packet is not affected by heat, moisture, and pressure. This device offers complete reanalysis in the event a health care facility believes that an error in reading the dosimeter has occurred. Because of the OSL dosimeter's sensitivity down to as low as 10 µSv (1 mrem) for x-ray and gamma ray photons in the energy range 5 keV to 40 MeV, it is an excellent and practical monitoring device for employees working in low-radiation environments and for pregnant workers. In addition,

when compared with the discontinued film badge and the thermoluminescent dosimeter described later, the OSL can be worn for longer periods of time (up to 1 year) to record occupational exposure.

Disadvantages of the OSL dosimeter. As is true with other personnel monitoring devices, occupational radiation exposure is recorded only in the body area where the device is worn. In addition, if the facility does not have an in-house reader, exposure cannot be determined on the day of occurrence. The OSL dosimeter is not an efficient monitoring device if it is not worn.

Personnel monitoring report. Results from personnel monitoring programs must be recorded accurately and maintained for review to meet state and federal regulations. To comply with such requirements, health care facilities use established dosimetry services. These monitoring services process various types of personnel dosimeters, such as the OSL dosimeter and the TLD and then supply written **personnel monitoring reports** to the health care facility (Fig. 5.4A). These statements, typically one for each hospital department that is being monitored, list the deep, eye, and shallow occupational exposure of each covered person on a monthly, quarterly, year to date, and lifetime equivalent basis. In addition, if requested, the total effective dose equivalent for persons of interest can be supplied at year's end. Information on the report is arranged in a series of columns. These columns include the items listed in Box 5.2.

The cumulative columns shown in Fig. 5.4A provide a continuous audit of actual absorbed radiation equivalent dose. These totals can be compared with allowable values established by regulatory agencies. Whenever the letter *M* appears under the current monitoring period or in the cumulative columns, it signifies that an equivalent dose below the minimum measurable radiation quantity was recorded during that time. The minimal reporting levels vary according to the dosimeter type and radiation quality as follows:

X-ray, gamma	10 µSv (1 mrem)
Beta	100 µSv (10 mrem)
Neutron	200 µSv (20 mrem) *fast*, 100 µSv (10 mrem) *thermal*
Fetal	10 µSv (1 mrem)
Rings	300 µSv (30 mrem)

Change in employment by radiation worker. When changing employment, the radiation worker must convey the data pertinent to accumulated permanent equivalent

SAMPLE ORGANIZATION
RADIATION SAFETY OFFICER
1000 HIGH TECH AVENUE
GLENWOOD, IL 60425

LANDAUER®

Landauer, Inc. 2 Science Road Glenwood, Illinois 60425-1586
Telephone: (708) 755-7000 Facsimile: (708) 755-7016
www.landauerinc.com

luxel®

RADIATION DOSIMETRY REPORT

ACCOUNT NO.	SERIES CODE	ANALYTICAL WORK ORDER	REPORT DATE	DOSIMETER RECEIVED	REPORT TIME IN WORK DAYS	PAGE NO.
103702	RAD	9920800151	06/11/04	06/07/04	4	1

PARTICIPANT NUMBER	NAME: ID NUMBER	BIRTH DATE	SEX	DOSIMETER	USE	RADIATION QUALITY	DOSE EQUIVALENT (MREM) FOR PERIODS SHOWN BELOW			QUARTERLY ACCUMULATED DOSE EQUIVALENT (MREM)			YEAR TO DATE DOSE EQUIVALENT (MREM)			LIFETIME DOSE EQUIVALENT (MREM)			RECORDS FOR YEAR	INCEPTION DATE (MM/YY)
							DEEP DDE	EYE LDE	SHALLOW SDE	DEEP DDE	EYE LDE	SHALLOW SDE	DEEP DDE	EYE LDE	SHALLOW SDE	DEEP DDE	EYE LDE	SHALLOW SDE		
FOR MONITORING PERIOD:							05/01/04 - 05/31/04			QTR 2			2004							
0000H	CONTROL CONTROL CONTROL			Ja Pa U	CNTRL CNTRL CNTRL		M M	M M	M M M										5	07/97 07/97 07/97
00191	ADDISON, JOHN		M	Ja	WHBODY	PN P NF	90 60 30	90 60 30	90 60 30	90 60 30	90 60 30	90 60 30	100 70 30	100 70 30	100 70 30	200 170 30	200 170 30	200 170 30	5	07/97
00192	JORGENSON, MIKE		M	Pa U	WHBODY RFINGR		M	M	M M	M	M	M M	M	M	M 70	M	M	M 100	5	07/97 07/97
00193	THOMAS, LEE		M	Pa U	WHBODY RFINGR		ABSENT ABSENT			M	M	M M	M	M	M M	M	M	M M	5	07/97 07/97
00196	WALKER, JANE		F	Pa	WHBODY		3	3	3	12	11	11	12	11	11	22	21	21	5	11/97
00197	EDWARD, CHRIS		M	Pa	WHBODY		M	M	M	M	M	M	M	M	M	M	M	M	5	01/98
00198	ZERR, ROBERT		M	Pa	WHBODY NOTE		40 CALCULATED	40	40	160	160	160	200	200	200	240	240	240	5	07/98
00199	ADAMS, JANE		F	Pa	WHBODY		M	M	M	M	M	M	9	10	12	9	10	12	5	07/98
00200	MEYER, STEVE		M	Pa Pa U	COLLAR WAIST ASSIGN NOTE RFINGR	PL	105 M 4 ASSIGNED DOSE BASED ON EDE 1 CALCULATION	105 M 105	105 M 105 140	6	162	165 400	11	327	334 690	51	1247	1284 2180	5	08/98 08/98 08/98
00202	HARRIS, KATHY		F	Pa U	WHBODY RFINGR		M	M	M M	M	M	M M	M	M	M 30	M	M	M 30	4	02/99 02/99

QUALITY CONTROL RELEASE: VS   20 - PR 6774 - RPT130 - N1   - 02013

M: MINIMAL REPORTING SERVICE OF 1 MREM
ELECTRONIC MEDIA TO FOLLOW THIS REPORT

NVLAP®
NVLAP LAB CODE 100518-0**

A

FIG 5.4 (A) The personnel monitoring report must include the items of information shown here. *Continued*

B - FORM 5 A NI L 1 17 M INCEPTION DATE: 01/01/87

FIG 5.4, cont'd (B) Modified report showing a summary of occupational exposure. (From Landauer, Inc., Glenwood, IL.)

BOX 5.2 Information Found on a Personnel Monitoring Report

1. Personal data: participant's identification number, name, (and may also include) birth date, and sex.
2. Type of dosimeter: *P* represents Luxel optically stimulated luminescence (OSL) dosimeter* for x-ray, beta, and gamma radiation; *J* represents Luxel OSL dosimeter for x-ray, beta, gamma, and fast neutron radiation; *U* represents a finger badge used to monitor x-radiation and gamma and beta radiation.
3. Radiation quality (e.g., x-rays, beta particles, neutrons, combined radiation exposure).
4. Equivalent dose data, including current deep, eye, and shallow recorded dose equivalents (millirem) for the time indicated on the report (e.g., from the first day of a given month to the last day of that month).
5. Cumulative equivalent doses for deep, eye, and shallow radiation exposures for specific time period, the year to date, and lifetime radiation.
6. Inception date (month and year) that the monitoring company began keeping dosimeter records for a given dosimeter for an individual listed on the account who is wearing a monitoring device.

*Luxel OSL dosimeter is manufactured by Landauer, Inc., Glenwood, IL.

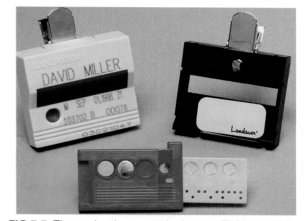

FIG 5.5 Thermoluminescent dosimeter (TLD) containing the sensing material lithium fluoride (LiF).

dose to the new employer so that this information can be placed on file. Fig. 5.4B is an example of an appropriate summary of an occupational exposure report. A copy of such a report should be given to the radiation worker on termination of employment.

In health care facilities that have a well-structured radiation safety program, personnel monitoring reports are received and reviewed by the radiation safety officer (RSO). Such a process should be an integral component of the facility's radiation safety program. This practice is compatible with the ALARA policy.

Thermoluminescent Dosimeter (TLD). The exterior of this type of dosimeter may resemble that of a traditional film badge (Fig. 5.5). However, its interior differs completely. This light-free device usually contains a crystalline form (powder or, more frequently, small chips) of lithium fluoride (LiF), which functions as the sensing material of the TLD.

Ionizing radiation causes the LiF crystals in the TLD to undergo changes in some of their physical properties. When irradiated, some of the electrons in the crystalline

lattice structure* of the LiF molecule absorb energy and are "excited" to higher energy levels or bands. The presence of impurities in the crystal causes electrons to become trapped within these bands. When the LiF crystals are passed through a special heating process, however, these trapped electrons receive enough energy to rise above their present locations into a region called the *conduction band*. From there, the electrons can return to their original or normal state with the emission of energy in the form of visible light. The energy emitted is equal to the difference between the electron-binding energies of the two orbital levels. The intensity of the light is proportional to the amount of radiation that interacted with the crystals.

A device called a **TLD analyzer** measures the amount of ionizing radiation to which a TLD badge has been exposed by first heating the crystals to free the trapped, highly energized electrons and then recording the amount of light emitted by the crystals (which is proportional to the badge exposure) (Fig. 5.6). A graphical plot is constructed that demonstrates the relationship of light output, or emitted thermoluminesence intensity, to temperature variation. The plot known as a **glow curve** represents a unique signature of the exposure received by the TLD dosimeter.

Advantages of the thermoluminescent dosimeter over the traditional film badge. The TLD has several advantages over the film badge. The LiF crystals interact with

---

*A geometric arrangement of the points in space at which the atoms, molecules, or ions of a crystal occur. Also called *space lattice*.

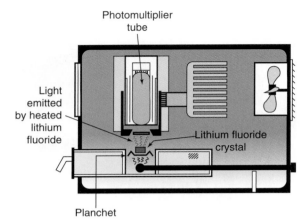

Photomultiplier tube

Light emitted by heated lithium fluoride

Lithium fluoride crystal

Planchet

FIG 5.6 Diagram of a typical analyzer. The analyzer measures the amount of ionizing radiation to which a badge has been exposed by heating the irradiated lithium fluoride (LiF) crystals of the exposed badge with linearly rising temperatures produced by hot gas. This represents a departure from the previously used heating method, which relied on physical contact between the crystals and a heated plate. The newer method is a technical improvement because it eliminates any need for contact readjustments.

ionizing radiation as human tissue does*; hence this monitor determines dose more accurately. Exposures as low as 1.3×10^{-6} C/kg (5 mR)[†] can be measured precisely. Humidity, pressure, and normal temperature changes do not affect the TLD. Unlike the film in a monthly film badge, which could possibly fog if the badge were to be worn for more than 1 month, the TLD badge may be used for up to 3 months. After a reading has been obtained, the crystals can be reused. This makes the device somewhat more cost effective, even though the initial cost is high.

Disadvantages of the thermoluminescent dosimeter. TLDs have some disadvantages in addition to their high cost. They can be read only once. The readout process destroys the stored information; TLDs may be reused, but once the crystal is heated, the record of any previous exposure is gone. The necessity of using calibrated dosimeters with TLDs is also a disadvantage because the calibrated dosimeters must be prepared and read with each group, or batch, of TLDs when they are processed.

---

*The effective atomic number of LiF is equal to 8.2, which is similar to that of soft tissue (Z = 7.4).
[†]1 R = $2.58 \times (10)^{-4}$ C/kg by definition.

Pocket Ionization Chamber. The pocket ionization chamber (pocket dosimeter) is the most sensitive type of personnel dosimeter (Fig. 5.7). However, the use of these monitors in diagnostic imaging is uncommon. Externally, the pocket dosimeter resembles an ordinary fountain pen, but it contains a slender cylindrical (thimble) ionization chamber that measures radiation exposure. A clip on the eyepiece end allows the dosimeter to be attached to an individual's apparel (e.g., a pen in a laboratory coat pocket).

Types. Two types of pocket ionization chambers exist: the self-reading type, which contains a built-in electrometer (a device that measures electrical charge), and the non–self-reading type, which requires a special accessory electrometer to read the device. The self-reading pocket dosimeter has largely replaced the non–self-reading type for most operations. The operating principle of both types is similar to that of the gold leaf electroscope, which detects the presence and sign of an electric charge.

Components. The pocket ionization chamber contains two electrodes: one positively charged (the central electrode) and one negatively charged (the outer electrode). A quartz fiber may form part of the positive electrode and also function as the indicator on a transparent reading scale. In such a system, the quartz fiber casts a shadow onto a lit scale so that the exiting quantity of charge on the positively charged electrode determines the position of the shadow along the scale. At full charge, the dosimeter's scale readout is set up so that the quartz fiber shadow is aligned with the zero scale marking. When the device is exposed to gamma or x-radiation, the air surrounding the precharged central electrode (+) becomes ionized. The negative ions in the air are attracted to the positively charged central electrode, neutralizing some of the charge there. This has the effect of discharging the mechanism in direct proportion to the amount of radiation to which it has been exposed. Visually, this is demonstrated by a linear displacement of the fiber shadow along the scale. The scale is usually labeled in milliroentgens so that the new location of the fiber represents the net exposure reading in milliroentgens.

Special charging unit. A special charging unit is required for pocket ionization chambers. Each dosimeter must be charged to a predetermined voltage before use so that the quartz fiber indicator shows a zero reading. Pocket chambers generally used in medical imaging are sensitive to exposures ranging from 0 to 5.2×10^{-5} C/kg (0 to 200 mR).

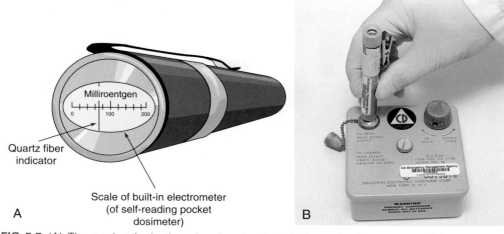

FIG 5.7 (A) The pocket ionization chamber (pocket dosimeter), the most sensitive personnel dosimeter, looks like a fountain pen on the outside but contains an ionization chamber that measures radiation exposure. Viewed through an eyepiece, the quartz fiber indicator of the built-in electrometer of the self-reading pocket dosimeter generally used in radiology indicates exposures over the range of 0 to 5.2×10^{-5} C/kg (0 to 200 mR). Before being used, each pocket dosimeter should be charged to a predetermined voltage by a special charging unit (B) so that the charges of the positive and negative electrodes are balanced and the quartz fiber indicator reads zero.

Advantages. Historically, the pocket ionization chamber was used to provide immediate exposure readouts for radiation workers who worked in high-exposure areas (e.g., a cardiac catheterization laboratory). Such individuals could read the dosimeter on site to determine the dose received at the completion of a given assignment and, if necessary, alter their working habits. Furthermore, pocket ionization chambers were compact, easy to carry, and convenient to use. Reasonably accurate and sensitive, they were useful monitoring devices for procedures of relatively short duration. Currently, however, in many institutions a device such as the Landauer-manufactured microStar system (a portable reader of the OSL dosimeter) has been substituted.

Disadvantages. Pocket ionization chambers are fairly expensive, costing $150 or more per unit. If not read each day, the dosimeter may give an inaccurate reading because the electric charge tends to escape (i.e., the fiber indicator drifts with time; thus a false high reading may be obtained from a dosimeter read too late). Pocket ionization chambers can also discharge if they are subjected to mechanical shock, which again would result in a false high reading. Because these devices provide no permanent legal record of exposure, health care facilities that use this method to record personnel exposure must delegate someone to keep such a record. This task is generally

the responsibility of the radiation safety officer (RSO), an individual such as a medical physicist or radiologist, qualified through training and experience and approved by the Nuclear Regulatory Commission and the state to ensure that internationally accepted guidelines for radiation protection are followed in the facility.

Digital Ionization Dosimeter. The personnel digital ionization dosimeter is a fairly new device that provides radiation workers with an immediate measurement of radiation exposure while including features such as long-term exposure tracking. It is small in size and is similar in appearance to a flash drive (Fig. 5.8). The device contains a small ionization chamber that responds to radiation exposure by producing a small collection of electrical charge. The charge is delivered to a semiconductor component that can store small amounts of electrical charge.[2] When connected to a computer, a small voltage delivered to a transistor "gate" provides a digital signal "readout" that reflects the radiation exposure of the dosimeter. Built-in memory chips may be used to store data on the user and the facility. The dosimeter provides an instant readout of dose information when connected to a computer via a connector such as a universal serial bus (USB). When a user wishes to obtain a reading, he

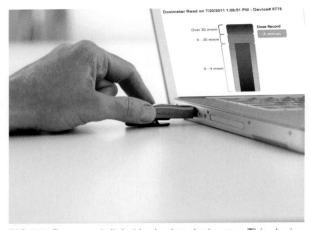

FIG 5.8 Personnel digital ionization dosimeter. This device is relatively small and resembles a flash drive in appearance. It provides an instant readout of dose information when connected to a computer via a connector such as a USB. (Photo courtesy of Mirion Technologies, Inc.)

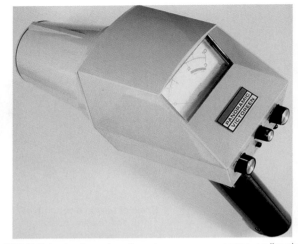

FIG 5.9 Ionization chamber–type survey meter, or "cutie pie." (From Victoreen, Inc., Cleveland, OH.)

or she simply logs in to his or her account, plugs in the dosimeter, and activates the dosimetry vendor's software. Once complete, a graphical representation of the current dose will load on the screen.

A variety of reports may then be generated, including:
• Radiation Exposure Summary Report
• History Detail Report
• Who Has Not Read Their Device

Global positioning system (GPS) or microchip-containing devices may be able to add data concerning the location of exposure events. Advantages of the personnel digital ionization dosimeter include instant access to reports and no wait time for mailing dosimeters. It is also lightweight and durable and can be dropped or scratched with little chance of harm to the device.

Summary of Advantages and Disadvantages of Personnel Monitoring Devices. Table 5.2 provides a summary of the advantages and disadvantages of the personnel monitoring devices discussed in this chapter.

RADIATION SURVEY INSTRUMENTS FOR AREA MONITORING

Radiation Detection and Measurement

Radiation survey instruments fall into several categories. The most common of these have as their detector a Geiger–Müller (GM) tube, the operation of which is

described later in this chapter. Such instruments can be used in multiple ways, depending on their level of calibration ("the adjustment of an instrument to accurately read the radiation level from a reference source"[3]) and associated components. The simplest version, lacking any readout scale but possibly having adjustable sensitivity levels, is only a "detector" used to just indicate the presence of any radiation above background. It can do this by emitting a repetitive sound whose loudness or repetitive frequency is directly associated with the intensity of radiation. Other versions, more fully equipped, have calibrated readout scales as well as audible indicators and are typically used either as area or room monitors or as portable survey instruments for measuring exposure rates at any location or object of interest. These instruments, however, do not directly supply a cumulative radiation exposure reading. Finally, there are ionization chamber–based instruments, which are described in more detail later in this chapter. The most common type of survey meter that incorporates an ionization chamber as its radiation detector is called the *cutie pie* (Fig. 5.9). It acquired this nickname sometime during 1943 or 1944 "due to its diminutive size."[4] This instrument, when properly calibrated, is capable not only of measuring radiation exposure rates over a very wide range but also of determining cumulative radiation exposure for whatever period of time the instrument is irradiated. In this regard, it can be considered a dosimeter, as are all properly calibrated ionization chamber–based devices.

TABLE 5.2   Advantages and Disadvantages of Personnel Dosimeters

Monitoring Device	Advantages	Disadvantages
Optically stimulated luminescence dosimeter (OSL)	Lightweight, durable, easy to carry Contains an integrated, self-contained, preloaded packet Color-coding, graphic formats, and body location icons provide easy identification Heat, moisture, and pressure will not affect the tamperproof blister packet Has extended wear frequencies Offers complete reanalysis Has increased sensitivity Gives accurate readings as low as 10 µSv (1 mrem) for x-ray and gamma ray photons with energies from 5 keV to 40 MeV Can be used for up to 1 year Excellent monitoring device for employees working in low-radiation environments and for pregnant workers Reasonably inexpensive to purchase and maintain Control monitor indicates whether group dosimeters were exposed in transit	Records occupational exposure only in the body area where the device is worn If the facility does not have an "in-house reader," exposure is not determinable on day of occurrence Not effective as a monitoring device if not worn
Thermoluminescent dosimeter (TLD)	Not affected by humidity, pressure, or normal temperature changes Can be worn up to 3 months After a reading has been obtained, TLD crystals can be reused, making the device somewhat cost effective	Readings may be lost if not carefully recorded Readout process destroys information stored in TLD, thus preventing the "read" TLD from serving as a permanent legal record of exposure Calibrated dosimeters must be prepared and read with each group of TLDs as they are processed Not effective as a monitoring device if not worn
Pocket ionization chamber	Small, compact, easy to carry and use Reasonably accurate and sensitive Can be used for procedures that last a short time Immediate exposure readout	Not cost effective for large numbers of personnel Readings may be lost if not carefully recorded Dosimeter must be calibrated to zero, or its initial reading must be noted each day it is used Mechanical shock can cause false high readings No permanent, legal record of exposure Records only exposure received in body area where worn Initial cost is greater than other personnel monitoring devices Not effective as a monitoring device if not worn
Personnel digital ionization dosimeter	Is lightweight and durable Provides instant access to reports Has no waiting time for mailing dosimeters Can be dropped or scratched with little chance of harm to the device	Not effective as a monitoring device if not worn

Types of Instruments

When in contact with ionizing radiation, survey instruments respond because of the charged particles that are produced by the radiation interacting with and subsequently ionizing the gas (usually air) in the detector. These instruments measure either the total quantity of electrical charge resulting from the ionization of the gas or the rate at which the electrical charge is produced.

Three different gas-filled radiation detectors serve as field instruments:

- Ionization chamber–type survey meter ("cutie pie")
- Proportional counter
- GM survey meter

All three detect the presence of radiation and, when properly calibrated, give a reasonably accurate measurement. The first two measure both exposure and exposure rate, whereas the GM meter typically gives only exposure rate. Each of these instruments has its own special use, and they are not all equally sensitive in the detection of ionizing radiation.

Requirements

Radiation survey instruments for area monitoring should meet the following requirements:

1. They must be portable so that one person can carry and operate the device in an efficient manner for a period of time.
2. They must be durable enough to withstand normal use, including routine handling that occurs during standard operating procedures.
3. They must be reliable; only in such a case can radiation exposure or exposure rate in a given area be accurately assessed.
4. They should interact with ionizing radiation similarly to the way human tissue reacts. This permits dose to be determined more accurately.
5. They should be able to detect all common types of ionizing radiation. Such a capability increases their usefulness.
6. The energy of the radiation should not significantly affect the response of the detector, and the direction of the incident radiation should not affect the performance of the unit. Such characteristics ensure consistency in unit operation among individual users.
7. They should be cost effective. The initial cost and subsequent maintenance charges should be as low as possible.
8. They should be calibrated annually to ensure accurate operation.

Gas-Filled Radiation Survey Instruments

As mentioned earlier, three types of gas-filled radiation survey instruments exist: the ionization chamber–type survey meter (cutie pie), the proportional counter, and the GM detector.

Ionization Chamber–Type Survey Meter (Cutie Pie).

The ionization chamber–type survey meter (cutie pie) is both a rate meter device (for exposure rate) used for area surveys and an accurate integrating or cumulative exposure instrument (see Fig. 5.9). It measures x-radiation and gamma radiation, and, if equipped with a suitable window, it can also record beta radiation.

Sensitivity ranges and uses. In the rate mode, the cutie pie can measure radiation intensities ranging from 10 to several thousand microgray per hour (1 mR/hr to several thousand milliroentgens per hour); in the integrate mode, it can sum exposures from as little as 10 μGy_{-a} to several Gy_{-a} (1 mR to several R). This device is useful for monitoring radiographic x-ray installations when exposure times of a second or more are chosen and for measuring fluoroscopic and computed tomography scatter radiation exposure rates at a second or more. It is usually the instrument of choice when determining exposure rates from patients containing therapeutic doses of radioactive materials and when assessing the exposure rates in radioisotope storage facilities. Finally, it is especially valuable when quantifying the cumulative exposures received outside of protective barriers associated with radiation oncology treatment rooms.

Advantages and disadvantages. Among the advantages of the cutie pie is its ability to measure a wide range of radiation exposures within a few seconds over a broad expanse of radiation energies, exhibiting essentially the same response or sensitivity. The delicate detector of the unit, however, may be considered a disadvantage. Another caveat is that without adequate warm-up time, its meter will drift on its most sensitive scales and thereby potentially produce an inaccurate reading. This device cannot be used to accurately measure exposures or exposure rates produced by typical diagnostic procedures because the exposure times are too short to permit the meter to respond appropriately.

Counter.

The proportional counter serves no useful purpose in diagnostic imaging. It is generally used in a laboratory setting to detect alpha and beta radiation and small amounts of other types of low-level radioactive contamination. The proportional counter can discriminate between alpha and beta particles. Because alpha radiation travels only a short distance in air, the operator of the proportional counter must hold the unit's probe close to the surface of the object being surveyed to obtain an accurate reading of the alpha radiation emitted by the object.

Geiger–Müller Survey Meter

Sensitivity and use. The Geiger–Müller (GM) survey meter serves as the primary portable radiation survey instrument for area monitoring in nuclear medicine facilities (Fig. 5.10). With the exception of alpha particle emission, the unit is sensitive enough to detect individual particles (e.g., electrons emitted from certain radioactive nuclei) or photons. Hence it can easily detect any area contaminated by radioactive material. Because the GM survey meter allows rapid monitoring, it can be used to locate a lost radioactive source or low-level radioactive contamination. By using its audio mode, the GM survey meter may also be employed to scan radiation barriers for any shielding defects.

Components. The GM survey meter has an audible sound system (an audio amplifier and speaker) that alerts the operator to the presence of ionizing radiation. Metal encloses the counter's gas-filled tube or probe, which is the unit's sensitive ionization chamber. When the shield covering the probe's sensitive chamber is open, very low-energy x-radiation and beta and gamma radiation can be detected. Meter readings are usually obtained in milliroentgens per hour. Because GM tubes tend to lose their calibration over time, the instrument generally has a "check source" of a weak, long-lived radioisotope located on one side of its external surface to verify its constancy daily.

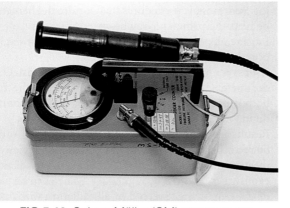

FIG 5.10 Geiger–Müller (GM) survey meter.

Disadvantages. The scale reading of a GM survey meter is not independent of the energy of the incident photons. This means that photons of widely different energies cause the instrument to respond quite differently. The cutie pie (ionization chamber–type survey meter), as mentioned previously, exhibits a much flatter, or more constant, response, with varying photon energies. In addition, the GM survey meter is likely to saturate or jam when it is placed in a pulsed (i.e., noncontinuous) high-intensity radiation area (e.g., that associated with a linear accelerator used in radiation therapy), thereby giving a false reading.

INSTRUMENTS USED TO MEASURE X-RAY EXPOSURE IN RADIOLOGY

Ionization chambers can be used to measure the radiation output from both radiographic and fluoroscopic x-ray equipment. As described previously, a cutie pie ionization chamber may also be used for radiation protection surveys. If a cutie pie ionization chamber operating in "rate" mode were to be placed in the beam emanating from an x-ray tube during a radiographic exposure, the electrical signal produced during the very brief (usually a fraction of a second) exposure duration would be too small to be recorded and measured reliably. An ionization chamber device specifically designed for such measurement conditions consists of an ion chamber connected to an electrometer, a very fast-responding electrical instrument that can measure tiny electrical currents with high precision and accuracy. Such a combination is shown in Fig. 5.11. Both the ionization chamber and the electrometer system must be calibrated periodically to meet state and federal requirements. Several regional calibration laboratories offer this service. A current listing of calibration laboratories is available from the American Association of Physicists in Medicine.*

Medical physicists use ionization chambers connected to electrometers to perform the annual standard measurements required by state, federal, and health care accreditation organizations for radiographic and fluoroscopic devices. These annual measurements (sometimes referred to as physics survey) include x-ray output in Gy or mGy, fluoroscopic radiation entrance rates in mSv/min or R/min, kVp setting accuracy, exposure timer exactness, and half-value layers or beam quality. From these measurements important x-ray machine performance values such

*1631 Prince Street, Alexandria, VA 22314 or www.aapm.org.

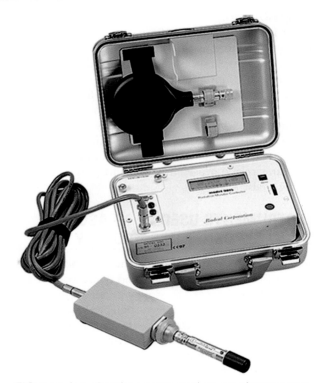

FIG 5.11 Ion chamber connected to an electrometer. Ionization chamber (probe with black sensitive element containing electrodes at its end) and electrometer (in carrying case) that may be used for measurement of x-ray machine output. Also shown (stored in the lid of the carrying case) is a larger, more sensitive disk-shaped ionization chamber that may be used for measurement of scattered radiation. (Photo from RadCal Corp.)

as µSv/mAs or mR/mAs as a function of selected kVp and linearity of machine radiation output are obtained. Data that can be utilized for determining radiation dose to patients are another by-product of this survey. It is to be noted that such a measurement device as described earlier but equipped with a specially calibrated parallel plate chamber may be used for similar measurements for mammography x-ray units.

■ SUMMARY

- Personnel monitoring ensures that occupational radiation exposure levels are kept well below the annual effective dose (EfD) limit.

- Personnel monitoring is required whenever radiation workers are likely to risk receiving 10% or more of the annual occupational EfD limit of 50 mSv (5 rem) in any 1 year as a consequence of their work-related activities.
- To keep radiation exposure ALARA, most health care facilities issue dosimeter devices when personnel could receive approximately 1% of the annual occupational EfD limit in any month, or approximately 0.5 mSv (50 mrem).
- The working habits and conditions of diagnostic imaging personnel can be assessed over a designated period through the use of the personnel dosimeter.
- Even when a protective apron is not normally required, a radiation worker should still wear a personnel monitoring device attached to the clothing on the front of the body at collar level during routine radiographic procedures to detect any potential radiation dose to the thyroid and the head and neck.
- During high-level radiation procedures, imaging professionals are required to wear both a thyroid shield and a protective lead apron, with the dosimeter worn outside the front of the garment at collar level, so as to provide a reading of the approximate equivalent dose to the thyroid gland and eyes.
- Commercially available lead aprons typically have either 0.5-mm or 0.25-mm lead equivalent shielding.
- Pregnant radiation workers may wear a second dosimeter beneath a lead apron to monitor the abdomen during gestation to provide an estimate of the equivalent dose to the embryo-fetus. Many facilities provide pregnant radiographers with a second dosimeter for this purpose.
- An extremity dosimeter, which is commonly a TLD ring, may be used as a second monitor when performing fluoroscopic procedures that require the hands to be near the primary x-ray beam.
- In general, personnel dosimeters must be lightweight, portable, durable, and cost efficient.
- Four types of personnel monitoring devices exist: OSL dosimeters, TLDs (both extremity and for the full body), pocket ionization chambers, and personnel digital ionization dosimeters.
- Results from personnel monitoring programs must be recorded accurately and maintained for review to meet state and federal regulations. A record of radiation exposure is required by regulatory agencies to be part of the employment record of all radiation workers.

- Personnel monitoring reports list the deep, eye, and shallow occupational exposure of each covered person on a monthly, quarterly, year-to-date, and lifetime equivalent basis.
- Whenever the letter *M* appears under the current monitoring period or in the cumulative columns on a radiation monitoring report, it signifies that an equivalent dose below the minimum measurable radiation quantity was recorded during that time.
- In health care facilities that have a well-structured radiation safety program, personnel monitoring reports are received and reviewed by the RSO.
- Area monitoring can be accomplished through the use of radiation survey instruments that fall into several categories.
- When in contact with ionizing radiation, survey instruments respond because of the charged particles that are produced by the radiation interacting with and subsequently ionizing the gas (usually air) in the detector. These instruments measure either the total quantity of electrical charge resulting from the ionization of the gas or the rate at which the electrical charge is produced.
- Three different types of gas-filled radiation detectors serve as field instruments. They include the ionization chamber–type survey meter ("cutie pie"), the proportional counter, and the GM survey meter.
- Radiation survey instruments for area monitoring must be durable and easy to carry, be able to detect all common types of ionizing radiation, and not be substantially affected by the energy of the radiation or the direction of the incident radiation.
- Ionization chambers can be used to measure the radiation output from both radiographic and fluoroscopic x-ray equipment.
- Medical physicists use ionization chambers connected to electrometers to perform the annual standard measurements required by state, federal, and health care accreditation organizations for radiographic and fluoroscopic devices.

REFERENCES

1. Landauer, Inc., 2 Science Road, Glenwood, Ill. Available at: www.landauer.com.
2. Wernli C, Kahilainen J: *Direct ion storage dosimetry systems* (vol 96) nos. 1-3. 2001, Nuclear Technology Publishing, pp 255–259.
3. Gollnick DA: *Basic Radiation Protection Technology*, ed 4, Altadena, CA, 2000, Pacific Radiation Corporation.
4. Frame P: The nicknames of early survey meters, Oak Ridge, TN, 1999, Oak Ridge Associated Universities. Available at: http://www.orau.org/ptp/collection/surveymeters/nicknamessurveymeters.htm.

GENERAL DISCUSSION QUESTIONS

1. How is personnel exposure monitoring accomplished?
2. Why should a personnel dosimeter be worn outside a protective apron at collar level on the anterior surface of the body during a fluoroscopic procedure?
3. What should a personnel dosimeter provide an indication of?
4. Why does a monitoring company supply a control monitor with every new batch of dosimeters?
5. What information is included in personnel monitoring programs to meet state and federal regulations?
6. When changing employment, what responsibility does a radiation worker have for his or her personal data that is pertinent to his or her accumulated permanent equivalent dose?
7. How sensitive to x-radiation and gamma radiation is an OSL dosimeter?
8. What are some of the requirements that radiation survey instruments must meet if they are to be used for area monitoring?
9. How does a GM survey meter alert the operator to the presence of ionizing radiation?
10. What type of diagnostic x-ray equipment would ionization chambers be used to calibrate?
11. How does a user of a personnel digital ionization dosimeter obtain a readout from the device?
12. How many electrodes does a pocket ionization chamber contain?

REVIEW QUESTIONS

1. When laser light is incident on the sensing material in an OSL dosimeter, the material:
   A. Becomes luminescent in proportion to the amount of radiation exposure received
   B. Fluoresces in proportion to the amount of radiation exposure received and then emits beta particles

C. Phosphoresces in proportion to the amount of radiation exposure received and then darkens

D. Turns ice blue in color and fluoresces in proportion to the amount of radiation exposure received

2. Which of the following chemical compounds functions as the sensing material in a thermoluminescent dosimeter?
   A. Barium sulfate
   B. Calcium tungstate
   C. Lithium fluoride
   D. Sodium iodide

3. During routine radiographic procedures, when a protective apron is *not* being worn, the primary personnel dosimeter should be attached to the clothing on the front of the body at:
   A. Collar level to approximate the location of maximal radiation dose to the thyroid and the head and neck
   B. Chest level to approximate the location of maximal radiation dose to the heart and lungs
   C. Hip level to approximate the location of maximal radiation dose to the reproductive organs
   D. Waist level to approximate the location of maximal radiation dose to the small intestine

4. Which of the following requirements should radiation survey instruments fulfill?
   1. Instruments must be reliable so that radiation exposure or exposure rate in a given area can be accurately assessed.
   2. Instruments must be durable enough to withstand normal use.
   3. Instruments should interact with ionizing radiation similar to the way in which human tissue reacts.
   A. 1 only
   B. 2 only
   C. 3 only
   D. 1, 2, and 3

5. During diagnostic imaging procedures, how may the radiation dose to the abdomen of a pregnant radiographer be monitored during gestation?
   A. It may be estimated from the radiation dose recorded by the primary monitor worn at collar level.
   B. It may be obtained from the primary radiation monitor worn at the abdominal level.

C. It may be obtained from a second radiation monitor worn at the abdominal level.

D. It is not necessary to monitor the radiation dose to the embryo-fetus that results from occupational exposure of a pregnant radiographer during gestation.

6. When a radiologic procedure requires the hands of a radiation worker to be near the primary beam, the equivalent dose to the hands of that individual may be determined through the use of:
   A. The primary personnel monitor worn at collar level
   B. A pocket ionization chamber attached to the wristwatch of the radiation worker
   C. A TLD ring worn on the hand of the radiation worker
   D. A cutie pie

7. Which of the following instruments is used to calibrate radiographic and fluoroscopic x-ray equipment?
   A. Proportional counter
   B. GM survey meter
   C. Ionization chamber with electrometer
   D. Pocket ionization chamber

8. For x-ray and gamma ray photons with energies from 5 keV to greater than 40 MeV, the _____ gives an accurate reading as low as 10 μSv (1 mrem).
   A. Personnel digital ionization dosimeter
   B. OSL dosimeter
   C. Pocket ionization chamber
   D. TLD

9. Which of the following instruments should be used to locate a lost radioactive source or detect low-level radioactive contamination?
   A. GM survey meter
   B. Proportional counter
   C. Ionization chamber–type survey meter (cutie pie)
   D. TLD analyzer

10. Which of the following instruments should be used in an x-ray installation to measure the fluoroscopic scatter radiation exposure rate?
    A. Geiger detector
    B. Cutie pie
    C. Proportional counter
    D. TLD

6

Overview of Cell Biology

OBJECTIVES

After completing this chapter, the reader will be able to perform the following:
- Define all key terms.
- State the purpose for acquiring a basic knowledge of cell structure, composition, and cell function as a foundation for understanding the effects of radiation in biology.
- Identify and describe some important roles of the major classes of organic and inorganic compounds that exist in the cell.
- List the essential tasks of water in the human body.
- Name and describe a landmark event pertaining to the human genome that occurred in 2001, and explain the progress that has been made since then as a result of this project.
- Describe the molecular structure of deoxyribonucleic acid, and explain the way it operates in the cell.
- Describe the structural differences between DNA and RNA.
- List the various cellular components, and identify their physical characteristics and functions.
- Distinguish between the two types of cell divisions, mitosis and meiosis, and describe each process.

CHAPTER OUTLINE

The Cell
Cell Chemical Composition
  Protoplasm
  Organic Compounds
  Inorganic Compounds

Cell Structure
  Cell Membrane
  Cytoplasm
  Cytoplasmic Organelles
  Nucleus

Cell Division
  Mitosis
  Meiosis
  Summary

KEY TERMS

amino acids
anaphase
carbohydrates
cell division
cell membrane
centrosome
chromosomes
cytoplasm
cytoplasmic organelles
deoxyribonucleic acid (DNA)
endoplasmic reticulum (ER)
genes

human genome
inorganic compounds
interphase
lipids
meiosis
messenger RNA (mRNA)
metaphase
mitochondria
mitosis (M)
nucleic acids
nucleus
organic compounds

osmosis
oxidation
prophase
proteins
protein synthesis
protoplasm
ribonucleic acid (RNA)
ribosomal RNA (rRNA)
ribosomes
saccharides
telophase
transfer RNA (tRNA)

93

Biology is a science that explores living things and life processes. Cells are the basic units of all living matter and are essential for life. The cell is the fundamental component of structure, development, growth, and life processes in the human body. Before imaging professionals can comprehend the effects of ionizing radiation on the human body, they must acquire a basic knowledge of how cells are put together, what they are made of, and how they operate. This chapter is designed to provide an understanding of cellular biology, which ultimately will help the learner in appreciating the effects of radiation in the body.

THE CELL

The human body is composed of trillions of cells. These cells exist in a multitude of different forms and perform many diverse functions for the body such as the following:

- Conduction of nerve impulses
- Contraction of muscles
- Support of various organs
- Transportation of body fluids such as blood

Some cells are freely moving, independent units (e.g., leukocytes), whereas others remain in one position as part of the tissues of larger organisms throughout their lifetimes (e.g., bone marrow cells). Every mature human cell is highly specialized and has predetermined tasks to perform in support of the body.

Cells:

- Move
- Grow
- React
- Protect themselves
- Repair damage
- Regulate life processes
- Reproduce

To ensure efficient cell operation, the body must provide food as a source of raw material for the release of energy, supply oxygen to help break down the food, and have enough water to transport inorganic substances such as calcium and sodium into and out of the cell. In turn, proper cell function enables the body to maintain homeostasis or equilibrium, which is the ability to operate in a normal manner despite any changes the body may undergo because of outside influences such as stress, exercise, injury, or disease.

In summary, cells are engaged in an ongoing process of obtaining energy and converting it to support their vital functions. They absorb molecular nutrients through the cell membrane and use these nutrients to produce energy and synthesize molecules. If exposure to outside influences such as ionizing radiation damages the components involved in molecular synthesis beyond repair, then cells either behave abnormally or die.

CELL CHEMICAL COMPOSITION

Protoplasm

Cells are made of **protoplasm**, the chemical building material for all living things. This substance carries on the:

- Complex process of metabolism
- Reception and processing of food and oxygen
- Elimination of waste products

Metabolism enables the cell to synthesize proteins and produce energy.

Protoplasm consists of:

- Organic compounds (those compounds that contain carbon, hydrogen, and oxygen)
- Inorganic materials (compounds that do not contain carbon)

These are either dissolved or suspended in water.

The biomolecules that constitute protoplasm are formed from many elements, among which there are four primary elements:

- Carbon
- Hydrogen
- Oxygen
- Nitrogen

When combined with phosphorus and sulfur, they comprise the essential major *organic* compounds:

- Proteins
- Carbohydrates
- Lipids
- Nucleic acids

These compounds are discussed later in this chapter. The most important *inorganic* substances are:

- Water
- Mineral salts (electrolytes)

Water plays a fundamental role in sustaining life and is the most abundant inorganic compound in the body. The essential functions of water are listed in Box 6.1 and are also discussed later in this chapter. Depending on cell type, water normally accounts for 80% to 85% of protoplasm (Fig. 6.1). Mineral salts exist in smaller quantities but are of vital importance in sustaining cell

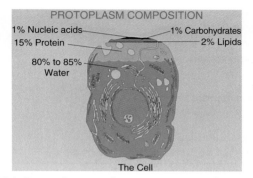

PROTOPLASM COMPOSITION

1% Nucleic acids — 1% Carbohydrates
15% Protein — 2% Lipids
80% to 85% Water

The Cell

FIG 6.1 Depending on cell type, water normally accounts for 80% to 85% of protoplasm. (From *Radiobiology and Radiation Protection: Mosby's Radiographic Instructional Series*, St. Louis, 1999, Elsevier.)

BOX 6.1   Life-Sustaining Role of Water in the Human Body

- Acts as the medium in which acids, bases, and salts are dissolved
- Functions as a solvent by dissolving chemical substances in the cell
- Functions as a transport vehicle for material the cell uses or eliminates
- Maintains a constant body core temperature of 98.6°F (37°C)
- Provides a cushion for vital organs such as the brain and lungs
- Regulates concentration of dissolved substances
- Lubricates the digestive system
- Lubricates skeletal articulations (joints)

BOX 6.2   Major Classes of Organic Compounds That Compose the Cell

Proteins	Lipids (fats)
Carbohydrates	Nucleic acid

---

life. They help produce energy and aid in the conduction of nerve impulses. Mineral salts are also responsible for the prevention of muscle cramping.

Organic Compounds

The four major classes of **organic compounds** (proteins, carbohydrates, lipids [fats], and nucleic acids) all contain carbon (Box 6.2). Carbon is the basic constituent of all organic matter. By combining with:

- Hydrogen
- Nitrogen
- Oxygen

carbon makes life possible. Of the four classes of organic compounds, proteins contain the most carbon.

Proteins. Proteins are the most elementary building blocks of cells, and they constitute approximately 15% of cell content (see Fig. 6.1). They are essential for growth, the construction of new body tissue (including acellular tissue such as hair and nails), and the repair of injured or debilitated tissue. Proteins are formed when organic compounds called **amino acids** combine into long, chainlike molecular complexes. Amino acids are essentially made up of combinations of NH_2 (called *amine*) and COOH (carboxylic acid) molecules. Thus nitrogen, hydrogen, carbon, and oxygen are the key constituents of amino acids, of which approximately 500 different types are currently known, although humans require only 22 specific amino acids. To summarize, proteins are macromolecules (very large molecules) made up of strings of amino acids. When proteins are produced within a cell, a process known as **protein synthesis,** the order of arrangement of amino acids, determines the precise function of each protein molecule, and the types of proteins that any given cell contains determine the characteristics, or genetics, of that cell. Key components of genetic material, called *chromosomes* and *genes,* which organize the amino acids into different orderings to make different types of proteins, are discussed later in this chapter (Fig. 6.2).

Structural and enzymatic proteins. Structural proteins such as those found in muscle provide the body with its shape and form and are a source of heat and energy. Enzymatic proteins function as organic catalysts, that is, agents that affect the rate or speed of chemical reactions without being altered themselves. As a result of this, enzymatic proteins (sometimes just called *enzymes*) moderate or control the cell's various physiologic activities. They can cause an increase in cellular activity that in turn causes biochemical reactions to occur more rapidly to meet the needs of the cell in stressful situations. Hence proper cell functioning depends on enzymes.

Repair enzymes. Many of the proteins produced in the cell are enzymes, initiating vital chemical reactions within the cell at the appropriate time. Some of the enzymes produced, called *repair enzymes,* can also mend damaged molecules and are therefore capable of helping

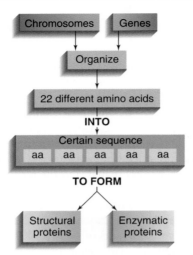

FIG 6.2 Chromosomes and genes organize the 22 different amino acids into certain sequences to form the different structural and enzymatic proteins.

the cell recover from a small amount of radiation-induced damage. Both the catalytic and repair capabilities of enzymes are of vital importance to the survival of the cell.

Repair enzymes work effectively in both diagnostic and therapeutic radiation energy ranges. However, if the radiation damage is excessive because of a large delivered equivalent dose, the damage will be too severe for repair enzymes to have enough positive effect. Thus when ionizing radiation is used for therapeutic purposes to destroy malignant cells, a very significant effort using the latest advances in imaging and computer treatment planning algorithms is also made to spare healthy surrounding tissue. In radiation therapy, this concept is referred to as a *therapeutic ratio,* wherein the intent is to deliver enough radiation to kill cancerous cells in a tumor (i.e., damage them sufficiently so that they are irreparable) while delivering a less-than-cell-killing equivalent dose to any surrounding noncancerous tissue structure. This stratagem is the foundation on which successful radiation therapy rests.

Hormones and antibodies. In addition to providing structure and support for the body, proteins may function as hormones and antibodies. Hormones are chemical secretions manufactured by various endocrine glands and carried by the bloodstream to influence the activities of other parts of the body. For example, hormones produced by the thyroid gland located in the neck control metabolism throughout the body. Hormones also regulate body functions such as growth and development.

BOX 6.3   Simple to Complex Carbohydrates

Monosaccharides
$C_6H_{12}O_6$

Disaccharides
$C_6H_{12}O_6 + C_6H_{12}O_6$

Polysaccharides
$C_6H_{12}O_6 + C_6H_{12}O_6 + C_6H_{12}O_6 + C_6H_{12}O_6 + \ldots\ldots$

Antibodies are protein molecules produced by specialized cells in the bone marrow called *B lymphocytes.* Lymphocytes are white blood cells involved in the body's immune reactions. Antibodies are produced when other lymphocytes in the body, known as *T lymphocytes,* detect the presence of molecules that do not belong to the body. These foreign objects (e.g., bacteria, flu viruses) are called *antigens.* Although the skin of the body is the initial barrier to any outside invasion by pathogens or the like, once it has been penetrated, the body's primary defense mechanism against infection and disease are the antibodies that chemically attack any foreign invaders.

Carbohydrates. Carbohydrates, also referred to as saccharides, make up approximately 1% of cell content (see Fig. 6.1). They include starches and various sugars. Carbohydrates range from simple to complex compounds (Box 6.3), even though they are composed of only carbon, hydrogen, and oxygen. Simple sugars such as glucose, fructose, and galactose have six carbon atoms and six molecules of water (e.g., glucose has the chemical formula $C_6H_{12}O_6$). Glucose is the primary energy source for the cell. Because it is a simple sugar, it is called a *monosaccharide.* Other sugars that have two units of a simple sugar linked together are called *disaccharides.* Sucrose (cane sugar) and lactose are examples of disaccharides. Both monosaccharides and disaccharides are relatively small molecules. *Polysaccharides* contain several or many molecules of simple sugar. Plant starches and animal glycogen* are the two most important polysaccharides.

*Glycogen, also known as animal glycogen, is a polysaccharide that is the main storage form for glucose in both animals and humans. In humans, it is mainly concentrated in the liver, comprising about 10% of the liver mass.

BOX 6.4 **Lipid Formation**

Fats or lipids

↑

1 molecule of glycerin + 3 molecules of fatty acid

↑

Carbon, oxygen, hydrogen

BOX 6.5 **Functions That Lipids Perform for the Body**

1. Act as reservoirs for the long-term storage of energy
2. Insulate and guard the body against the environment
3. Support and protect organs such as the eyes and kidneys
4. Provide essential substances necessary for growth and development
5. Lubricate the joints
6. Assist in the digestive process

Through the process of metabolism, the body breaks these down into simpler sugars for energy.

Carbohydrates, simply described as chains of sugar molecules, function as short-term energy warehouses for the body. Their primary purpose is to provide fuel for cell metabolism. Although carbohydrates are found throughout the human body, they are most abundant in the liver and in muscle tissue. They also are important structural parts of intercellular materials.

Lipids. Lipids can simply be defined as substances such as fats and fatty acids, oil, or wax that dissolve in alcohol but not in water. Lipids are organic macromolecules, in general containing carbon, hydrogen, and oxygen. In their simplest form, they are made up of a molecule of glycerin* and three molecules of fatty acid** (Box 6.4). Lipids are the structural parts of cell membranes constituting approximately 2% of cell content (see Fig. 6.1). Therefore lipids are present in all body tissue. The functions they perform for the body are listed in Box 6.5.

Nucleic Acids. Nucleic acids comprise approximately 1% of the cell (see Fig. 6.1). They are very large, complex macromolecules whose primary components are shown in Fig. 6.3. The much smaller structures that make up nucleic acids are called *nucleotides*. Each nucleotide is a unit formed from a nitrogen-containing *organic base*,* a five-carbon sugar molecule (deoxyribose), and a *phosphate molecule*.**

Deoxyribonucleic and ribonucleic acids. Cells contain two types of nucleic acids that are important to human metabolism:

- Deoxyribonucleic acid (DNA)
- Ribonucleic acid (RNA)

The DNA macromolecule is composed of two long sugar–phosphate chains, which twist around each other in a double-helix configuration and are linked by pairs of *nitrogenous organic bases*** at the sugar molecules of the chain to form a tightly coiled structure resembling a twisted ladder or spiral staircase. The sugar–phosphate compounds are the rails, and the pairs of nitrogenous bases, which consist of complementary chemicals, are the steps, or rungs, of the DNA ladder-like structure (Fig. 6.4). Hydrogen bonds attach the bases to each other and join the two side rails of the DNA ladder.

Nitrogenous organic bases in DNA. The four nitrogenous organic bases (see Fig. 6.3) in DNA macromolecules are as follows:

---

*Glycerin is a clear, odorless, syrupy liquid that is a simple sugar and alcohol compound. It has the chemical formula $C_3H_8O_3$.

**When glucose is broken down in the body during respiration, fats are among the generated intermediate products. When some of these fats combine with an acidic group of atoms (e.g., the carboxyl group, COOH), a fatty acid is formed. An example of a fatty acid is CH_3COOH, which is commonly known as *acetic acid*. Fatty acids are constituents of amino acids from which proteins are built.

*In general, a base is a substance that, among other characteristics, is slippery to the touch in aqueous solutions, tends to accept protons (i.e., ionized hydrogen atoms) from any proton donor, and reacts with acids to neutralize them, forming salts in the process. If the base contains one or more carbon and hydrogen bonded components, it may be classified as an organic base.

**A phosphate molecule has the chemical description PO_4 and therefore consists of one phosphorus atom bonded to four oxygen atoms. It is a negative ion carrying a charge of −3 produced by the dissolution of phosphoric acid H_3PO_4.

***If an organic base is covalently bonded to one or more nitrogen atoms, this chemical combination is called a *nitrogenous base*. A nitrogenous base may also contain oxygen atoms that form bonds with carbon.

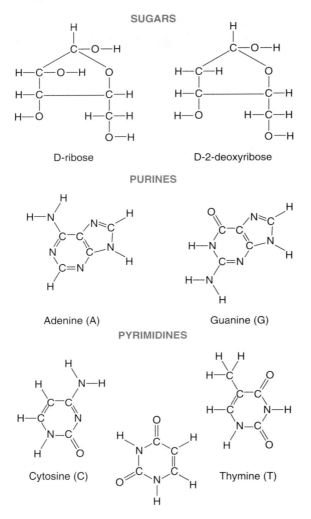

FIG 6.3 The components of nucleic acid (H, hydrogen; C, carbon; N, nitrogen; O, oxygen). Sugars are strung together with phosphate groups, and a base is attached to each sugar. DNA uses d-2-deoxyribose sugar, and RNA uses d-ribose. Both nucleic acids use the same two purines, but thymine (T) in DNA is replaced by uracil (U) in RNA.

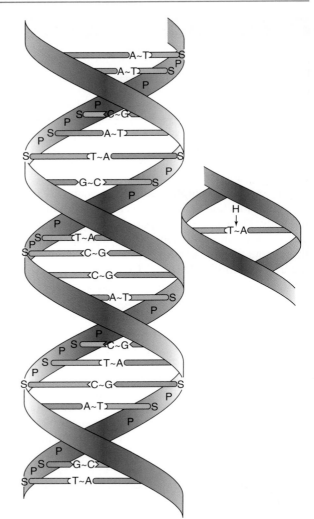

FIG 6.4 Diagram of a DNA macromolecule that illustrates its twisted ladder-like or spiral staircase–like configuration. Alternating sugar and phosphate molecules form the side rails of the ladder, and the nitrogenous organic bases, which consist of the complementary chemicals adenine (A), thymine (T), guanine (G), and cytosine (C), form the rungs, or steps. A hydrogen bond joins the bases together.

- Adenine (A)
- Cytosine (C)
- Guanine (G)
- Thymine (T)

Adenine and guanine are compounds called *purines*, and the compounds cytosine and thymine are classified as *pyrimidines*. As can be seen in the figure, a primary difference between the two classes of compounds is the number of carbon–hydrogen rings, with purines always having two rings and pyrimidines only one. A unique characteristic of these organic bases in DNA is that purines link with pyrimidines only in certain specific combinations; more precisely, adenine always bonds only with thymine, and cytosine bonds only with guanine. This property is the reason the two strands of DNA are described as complementary.

DNA: the master chemical substance. DNA may be regarded as the master chemical substance because it is a very large conglomeration of complex molecules that contain all of the information a cell needs to function.* It carries the genetic information necessary for cell replication and regulates all cellular activity needed to direct protein synthesis. DNA determines a person's characteristics by regulating the ordering of amino acids in the person's constituent proteins during the synthesis of these proteins. These arrangements of amino acids are determined by the succession of adenine–thymine and cytosine–guanine base pairs in the DNA macromolecules. Therefore the sequence of nitrogenous base pairs in the DNA molecule constitutes a genetic code. Different sequences of amino acids produce proteins with different functions. Protein characteristics determine cell characteristics, and cell characteristics ultimately determine the characteristics of the entire individual. All of the information necessary to construct and maintain a living organism is written in the "genetic code book" of DNA—the letters, words, and sentences are the arrangements and groupings of the nitrogenous organic bases. What makes one person's DNA different from another's? Small differences in base pair layouts are responsible for variations in human beings because such slightly altered base pair configurations lead to changes in the proteins produced, how much are produced, and when they are produced.

Structural differences between DNA and RNA. The nucleic acid polymer RNA plays an essential part in the translation of genetic information from DNA into protein products. RNA functions as a messenger between DNA and the ribosomes, or "protein factories," where synthesis occurs. RNA differs structurally from DNA in several ways, some of which are as follows:

- RNA is a single-strand macromolecular structure, whereas DNA is a double-strand macromolecular structure. Both have spiral ladder-like arrangements of their bases.
- RNA contains ribose,** whereas DNA contains deoxyribose.**

- RNA has the nitrogenous base uracil (see Fig. 6.3) as a component of its ladder steps, whereas DNA has thymine instead in its ladder steps. Both also contain the bases adenine, guanine, and cytosine as elements of their spiral structure. Unlike with DNA where thymine forms a bond with adenine, for RNA it will be uracil that links with an adenine base.
- RNA performs many different biologic functions (e.g., acts as an enzyme), but DNA carries the genetic information.
- RNA has a much shorter chain of nucleotides than DNA.

Messenger RNA. Because DNA is found mostly in the cell nucleus, it cannot directly influence cellular activity such as growth and differentiation, which occur in the cytoplasm (the part of the cell that lies outside the nucleus). Instead, DNA regulates cellular activity indirectly, transmitting its genetic information outside the cell nucleus by reproducing itself in the form of messenger RNA (mRNA), which is able to leave the cell nucleus. Once in the cytoplasm, mRNA directs the process of making proteins out of amino acids.

DNA serves as a prototype for mRNA, but mRNA differs from DNA in two important ways:

1. mRNA contains in its backbone the sugar molecule, ribose, which differs only in the presence of an extra O–H bond from the sugar molecule, deoxyribose, found in the backbone of DNA (Fig. 6.4).
2. In mRNA, the pyrimidine base *uracil* (U) replaces the thymine that is found in DNA (Fig. 6.5).

An mRNA macromolecule, as does any type of RNA, resembles one half of a DNA macromolecule. It appears as a single strand of the DNA ladder-like configuration, with the ladder being severed in half lengthwise (see Fig. 6.5).

Transfer RNA. Macromolecules of mRNA carry their genetic codes in their sequences of nitrogenous organic bases (e.g., U, U, C, C, A, U, G, etc.) from the cell nucleus to the *ribosomes.**

Proteins are manufactured in the ribosomes. Within the ribosome, both mRNA and transfer RNA (tRNA) macromolecules are present. The mRNA delivers its genetic code to tRNA. This encoded tRNA combines with

---

*By definition a chemical substance may be considered to be a chemical element or a combination of elements arranged in molecular combinations that maintains constant chemical composition and characteristic properties. DNA does this.

**Ribose is an organic compound classified as a simple sugar. Chemically, ribose is made up of a bonded pentagon-shaped arrangement of 5 carbon atoms, 10 hydrogen atoms, and 5 oxygen atoms. If a ribose molecule should lose one of its oxygen atoms, it is called *deoxyribose*.

---

*Ribosomes: small, spherical organelles (subunits of a cell that perform a specific function) that are the assembly sites (similar to an auto assembly line) where mRNA and tRNA combine amino acids into proteins. A further discussion of ribosomes is provided later in this chapter.

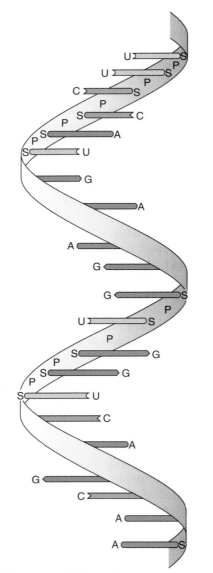

FIG 6.5 Messenger RNA (mRNA) resembles one half of a DNA macromolecule. It appears as a single strand (one side rail) of the DNA ladder-like configuration, with the ladder being severed in half lengthwise. Uracil (U) replaces thymine (T) as one of the nitrogenous organic bases in the mRNA molecule.

individual amino acids from different areas of the cell and attaches them to the ribosomes, where the amino acids are subsequently arranged in specific orders to form chainlike protein molecules. Each tRNA molecule is specifically coded for a particular amino acid. Because

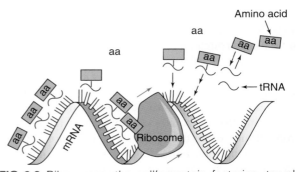

FIG 6.6 Ribosomes, the cell's protein factories, travel along the messenger RNA (mRNA) rails, linking transfer RNA (tRNA) and its corresponding amino acids in the proper sequences to produce the proteins appropriate for the needs of the cell.

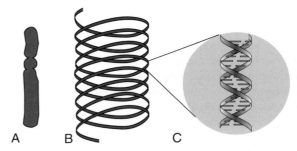

FIG 6.7 A chromosome viewed under a microscope appears rod shaped (A); when further magnified, a chromosome appears as a tightly wound spiral structure (B) composed of hundreds of genes—a segment of the DNA macromolecule (C).

each of the 22 different amino acids has an associated tRNA, at least 22 different types of tRNAs exist. The ribosomes travel along the mRNA and link tRNA and its corresponding amino acids in the correct order so that the proteins necessary to provide for the needs of the cell are produced (Fig. 6.6).

Ribosomal RNA. Ribosomal RNA (rRNA) is yet another type of RNA. Its function is to assist in the linking of mRNA to the ribosome to facilitate protein synthesis.

Chromosomes and genes. Chromosomes are tiny, rod-shaped bodies that under a microscope appear to be long, threadlike structures that become visible only in dividing cells (Fig. 6.7). Chromosomes are composed of:
• Protein
• The genetic material DNA

A normal human being has 46 different chromosomes composed of 23 pairs in each somatic (non-reproductive) cell. Individual male and female reproductive cells, also known as *germ cells,* do not have this pairing. Instead, each of these germ cells has only 23 chromosomes, which pair up to form a full set of 46 chromosomes when a sperm fertilizes an egg cell. The DNA that makes up every chromosome is divided into many hundreds of segments or subunits called **genes.** Each gene, because of the ordering of its nitrogenous base pairs, contains information responsible for or related to one or more of the following:

- Directing cytoplasmic activities
- Controlling growth and development of the cell
- Transmitting various aspects of hereditary information (e.g., hair color, blood type, general body characteristics, etc.)

Thus genes are the *basic units of heredity.* Taken as a whole, they control the formation of proteins in every cell through the intricate process of parentally shared genetic coding.

The human genome. The total amount of genetic material (DNA) contained within the chromosomes of a human being is called the **human genome.** The process of locating and identifying the genes in the genome is called *mapping.* A landmark event occurred in 2001, when after years of intense effort two rival groups succeeded in deciphering the human genome. Essentially they uncovered the entire sequence of DNA base pairs (i.e., all of the "rungs" of the DNA ladder structure) on all 46 chromosomes. This major milestone in biology and medicine was accomplished by Celera Genomics, a private company in Rockville, Maryland, and the International Human Genome Sequencing Consortium, a group of academic centers funded mostly by the National Institutes of Health and the Wellcome Trust of London.[1]

The groups found that there are 2.9 billion base pairs in the human genome and that these base pairs are arranged into approximately 30,000 genes. It is estimated that these genes are capable of producing at least 90,000 different proteins.

According to the National Institutes of Health (2010), the Human Genome Project has already led to the discovery of more than 1800 disease genes. In addition, with the knowledge gained from the project, today's researchers can find a gene suspected of causing an inherited disease in a matter of days, rather than the years it took before the genome sequence was in hand.

There are now more than 2000 genetic tests for human conditions. These tests enable patients to learn their genetic risks for disease and help health care professionals diagnose disease. In 2010 at least 350 biotechnology-based products resulting from the Human Genome Project are currently in clinical trials. Having the complete sequence of the human genome is similar to having all the pages of a manual needed to make the human body. The challenge now is to determine how to read the contents of these pages and understand how all of these many complex parts work together in human health and disease.[2]

Interpreting the map of the human genome is similar to that of a building contractor finding a list of all the things that are needed to build a house but not having a blueprint that shows how often or in what order to do things. Over the next few decades, the great tasks will be to answer questions such as the following:

1. What determines when genes will produce proteins and when genes will not?
2. In what order are various proteins produced during development and throughout life?
3. What genes cause some individuals to be susceptible to a certain disease?
4. Is it possible to learn how to deactivate those genes and turn on other genes that provide resistance?
5. Are there genes that make some people more or less sensitive to the effects of ionizing radiation?
6. Can we use our new insight into the human genome to both detect and properly correct the defective genes that are the root of genetically transmitted disease?

The Human Genome Project has provided data that allow work on problems in molecular biology such as those listed here. It is surprising, then, to realize that the primary stimulus for initiating the project[3] can be traced to an urgency to attack radiobiologic questions that were raised during a scientific conference held in March 1984 at Hiroshima, Japan. At this conference, participants repeatedly stressed the need to use molecular DNA tools to enable direct detection of radiation exposure–induced mutations that could be inherited from the survivors of the atomic bomb blasts. Another conference was held some 9 months later in Alta, Utah. At this meeting, it was concluded that available knowledge was still insufficient to detect such mutations, which could be as few as 30 per individual genome per generation, and that only a massive effort, designed to improve the technology by orders of magnitude, would suffice for unraveling the human genome to the required degree. The intense

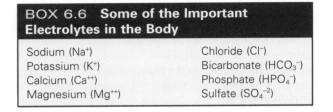

Sodium (Na$^+$)	Chloride (Cl$^-$)
Potassium (K$^+$)	Bicarbonate (HCO$_3^-$)
Calcium (Ca^{++})	Phosphate (HPO$_4^-$)
Magnesium (Mg^{++})	Sulfate (SO$_4^{-2}$)

discussions and ideas put forth at this meeting by the attendees were what ultimately led to the establishment of the Human Genome Project.

Inorganic Compounds

Inorganic compounds are compounds that do not contain carbon. The inorganic compounds found in the body occur in nature independent of living things and are made up of three categories:

- Inorganic acids
- Inorganic bases
- Salts (electrolytes)

Inorganic acids are hydrogen-containing compounds such as HNO$_3$ (nitric acid) that can attack and dissolve metal. *Inorganic bases* are alkali or alkaline-earth (see Appendix C, first 2 columns) OH compounds such as Mg(OH)$_2$ (otherwise known as *milk of magnesia*) that can neutralize acids. *Salts* are chemical compounds resulting from the action of an acid and a base on each other. Salts are sometimes referred to as *electrolytes.* Chemically, they "are substances that become ions in solution and acquire the capacity to conduct electricity. Electrolytes are present in the human body, and the balance of the electrolytes in our bodies is essential for normal function of our cells and our organs."[4] A list of some of the important electrolytes in the body may be found in Box 6.6.

Water is the primary inorganic substance contained in the human body; it comprises approximately 80% to 85% of the body's weight (Fig. 6.8). The quantity of water present in a cell is very important. If water content is insufficient, the cell will collapse, resulting in a lack of ability to continue normal biologic function. Conversely, if water content is excessive, the cell most likely will rupture. Therefore it is imperative that the correct amount of water in a cell be maintained.[5]

Function of Water Within and Outside of the Cell.

Within the cell, water is indispensable for metabolic activities because it is the medium in which the chemical

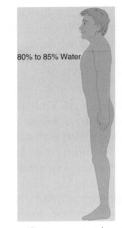

FIG 6.8 Water constitutes approximately 80% to 85% of the body's weight. (From *Radiobiology and Radiation Protection: Mosby's Radiographic Instructional Series,* St. Louis, 1999, Elsevier.)

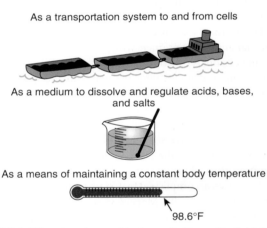

As a transportation system to and from cells

As a medium to dissolve and regulate acids, bases, and salts

As a means of maintaining a constant body temperature
98.6°F

FIG 6.9 Water's role outside the cell. (From *Radiobiology and Radiation Protection: Mosby's Radiographic Instructional Series,* St. Louis, 1999, Elsevier.)

reactions that are the basis of these activities occur. It also acts as a solvent, keeping compounds dissolved so that they can more easily interact and their concentration may be regulated. Outside the cell, water functions as a transport vehicle for materials the cell uses or eliminates. In addition, water is responsible for maintaining a constant body core temperature of 98.6°F (37°C) (Fig. 6.9) while at the same time serving to lubricate both the digestive system and skeletal articulations (joints). Organs such as the brain and lungs are also protected by a cushion of compounds composed primarily of water.

Function of Mineral Salts Within the Cell. Salts resulting from acid/base reactions, predominantly involving sodium (Na) and/or potassium (K) bases, keep the correct proportion of water in the cell. Because they are inorganic (i.e., no carbon is present) and have a crystalline atomic structure, these salts are classified as *mineral salts*. Their presence is vital for:
- Proper cell performance
- Creation of energy
- Conduction of impulses along nerves

Within an aqueous solution, these salts can be broken down, with their constituents existing as ions (particles carrying either a positive or negative electric charge) in the cell. The resulting medium is called a *solute*. The ions within the solute, via chemical reactions, cause materials to be altered, fragmented, and recombined to form new substances. Potassium (K) contributes most of the positive ions (also known as *cations*) present in cells, whereas phosphorus (P) contributes the majority of negative ions (*anions*). Potassium is of primary importance in maintaining adequate amounts of intracellular fluid. This is so because water, a solvent, will preferentially move across cell surfaces or membranes into areas with a high concentration of ions, also known as *high solute regions*. This motion is referred to as osmosis. Thus by controlling its concentration of potassium ions (as well as the ever-present sodium [Na] and chloride [Cl] ions resulting from the intake of table salt), the cell regulates the amount of water passing through its membrane and consequently the amount of fluid it contains. Osmotic pressure is the external pressure required to be applied so that there is no net movement of solvent, typically water, across the cell membrane. Retaining the correct proportion of water in the cell causes osmotic pressure to be maintained. Potassium also aids in maintaining acid–base balance, a state of equilibrium, or stability, between acids and bases.

CELL STRUCTURE

The normal cell has the following components (Fig. 6.10):
1. Cell membrane
2. Cytoplasm
3. Cytoplasmic organelles (organelles are subcellular structures)

   a. Endoplasmic reticulum
   b. Golgi apparatus or complex
   c. Mitochondria
   d. Lysosomes
   e. Ribosomes
   f. Centrosomes
4. Nucleus

Cell Membrane—A "Plastic Storage Bag" to Contain the Cell

The cell membrane is a frail, semipermeable, flexible structure encasing and surrounding the human cell.
- It is made up of lipids and proteins.
- It functions as a barricade to protect cellular contents from the outside environment.
- It controls the passage of water and other materials into and out of the cell.

Because the cell membrane allows penetration only by certain types of substances and regulates the speed at which these substances travel within the cell, it plays a primary role in the cell's transport system. When a substance moves through the cell membrane by osmosis, the transport system is classified as passive because the cell uses no energy to maintain the concentration. When the movement of a substance across a cell membrane is controlled more by the properties and powers of the cell membrane than it is by the relative concentrations of particles in fluid, the transport system is classified as active. In *active transport*, the cell must expend energy to pump substances into and out of it.

Cytoplasm

Cytoplasm is the protoplasm that exists outside the cell's nucleus. It is primarily composed of water, but also contains:
- Proteins
- Carbohydrates
- Lipids
- Salts
- Minerals

The cytoplasm makes up the majority of the cell and contains large amounts of all the cell's molecular components with the exception of DNA. All cellular metabolic functions occur in the cytoplasm. The major functions of the cytoplasm are listed in Box 6.7.

Cytoplasmic Organelles

The cytoplasm contains all the miniature cellular components that enable the cell to function in a highly

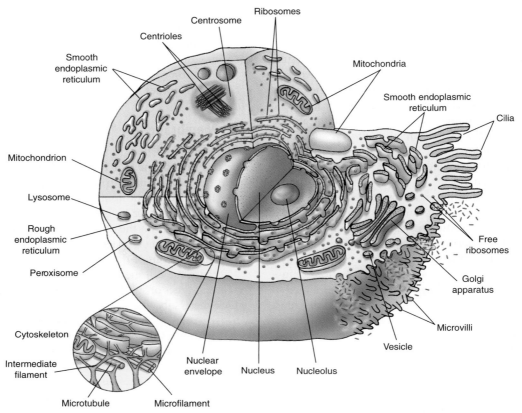

FIG 6.10 Diagram of a typical cell, demonstrating its basic components. (From Thibodeau A: *Anatomy and Physiology,* ed 9, St. Louis, 2016, Mosby.)

BOX 6.7   Major Tasks of the Cytoplasm

Behaving like a factory, the cytoplasm performs the following major tasks:

1. Accepts and builds up unrefined materials and assembles from these materials new substances such as carbohydrates, lipids, and proteins; the assembly of larger molecules from smaller ones is known as *anabolism*
2. Breaks down organic materials to produce energy (catabolism)
3. Packages substances for distribution to other areas of the cell or to various sites in the body through the circulation
4. Eliminates waste products

---

organized manner. These little organs of the cell are collectively referred to as **cytoplasmic organelles.** They consist of the following:

- Tubules (small tubes)
- Vesicles (small cavities or sacs containing liquid)
- Granules (small insoluble, nonmembranous particles found in cytoplasm)
- Fibrils (minute fibers or strands that are frequently part of a compound fiber)

Together these structures perform the major functions of the cell in a systematized way. DNA, which is located in the cell nucleus separated from the cytoplasm, determines the function of each cytoplasmic organelle; mRNA carries the DNA code from the nucleus into the cytoplasm.

Endoplasmic Reticulum—The "Highway" of the Cell. The **endoplasmic reticulum (ER)** is a vast, irregular network of tubules and vesicles spreading and interconnecting in all directions throughout the cytoplasm. It enables the cell to communicate with the extracellular environment and transfer food and molecules from one part of the cell to another. Thus the ER functions as the highway system of the cell. For example, mRNA travels from the nucleus to different locations in the cytoplasm through the ER, and lipids and proteins are also routed into and out of the nucleus through the ER tubular network.

Cells have two types of endoplasmic reticulum:
- Rough surfaced (granular)
- Smooth (agranular)

If numerous ribosomes (the small, spherical organelles that are the sites where mRNA and tRNA assemble amino acids into proteins) are present on the surface of the ER, the surface is rough or granular. If they are not present, the surface is smooth or agranular. The "smooth" or "rough" distinction refers to the ER's appearance when viewed with an electron microscope. The cell type determines the type of ER. For example, cells that actively manufacture proteins for export, such as the pancreatic cells, which produce insulin, need more ribosomes and therefore have an extensive rough or granular endoplasmic reticulum. A lesser amount of rough or granular ER is found in cells that synthesize proteins mainly for their own use.

Golgi Apparatus or Complex—Hauls "Freight" Within and Out of the Cell. The Golgi apparatus, bodies, or complex contains minute vesicles that extend from the nucleus to the cell membrane. The vesicles consist of tubes and a tiny sac located near the nucleus. This structure unites large carbohydrate molecules (i.e., various types of sugars) and then combines them with proteins, which are usually found floating in or around the membrane of cells, to form *glycoproteins*. Glycoproteins are involved in nearly every process in cells. They have diverse functions throughout the body such as within the immune system, in communication between cells, and in the reproductive systems. In addition, when the cell manufactures glycoproteins that function as enzymes and hormones, the Golgi apparatus concentrates, packages, and transports them through the cell membrane so that they can exit the cell, enter the bloodstream, and be carried to the areas of the body where they are required.

Mitochondria—The "Power-Generating Station" of the Cell. The large, double-membranous, oval or bean-shaped structures called mitochondria function as the "powerhouses" of the cell because they supply the energy for cells. They contain highly organized enzymes in their inner membranes that produce this energy for cellular activity by breaking down nutrients such as:
- Carbohydrates
- Fats
- Proteins

This breakdown of nutrients occurs through the process of oxidative metabolism. Oxidation is any chemical reaction in which atoms lose electrons. The substance that loses electrons is said to have been oxidized, and chemical energy is released in the process. The oxidation of iron, for example, which occurs in a moist environment in the presence of oxygen, produces iron oxide (Fe_2O_3) commonly known as *rust*. In the case of rust, the iron atoms give up electrons to oxygen atoms, creating a bond between iron and oxygen.

Destructive metabolism (also known as *catabolism*) is the breaking down of large molecules (e.g., polysaccharides, lipids, proteins) into smaller ones. Oxidative metabolism is the oxidation of these smaller molecules to release energy. Some of this energy is lost as heat, and the rest is primarily used with the assistance of the enzymes contained within the mitochondria to produce the compound *adenosine triphosphate (ATP)*.* ATP is the prime energy-containing molecule in the cell. It is essential for sustaining life and plays a major role in active transport within the cell. As mentioned previously, in active transport molecules are moved or pumped through cell membranes. This happens regardless of the relative concentrations of particles on either side of the membrane. This process will therefore often require energy. The needed energy is supplied by ATP. ATP works by losing its endmost phosphate group (Fig. 6.11) when instructed to do so by enzymes. This reaction releases a lot of energy, which the organism can then also use to build proteins, contract muscles, etc. When the organism is resting and energy is not

*The ATP molecule is composed of three molecular subgroups. At the center is a sugar molecule, ribose (the same sugar that forms the basis of RNA). Attached to one side of this is a *base* (a group consisting of linked rings of carbon and nitrogen atoms); in this case the base is adenine. The other side of the sugar is attached to a string or chain of phosphate groups. These phosphates are the key to the energy activity of ATP (see Fig. 6.11).

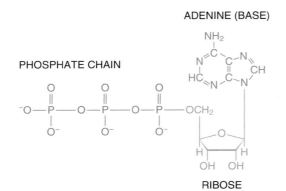

FIG 6.11 Molecular structure of adenosine triphosphate (ATP).

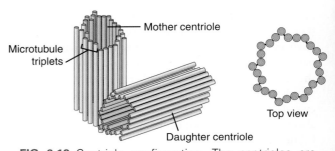

FIG 6.12 Centriole configuration. The centrioles are cylindrical-shaped cellular organelles that occur in pairs. Each centriole is made up of groups of microtubules that are arranged in a pattern, forming a ring of nine trio microtubules known as *triplets*. As shown, the centrioles are arranged at right angles to one another. In human cells, the centrioles facilitate the organizing and assembly of microtubules during the process of cell division.

immediately needed, the reverse reaction takes place and the phosphate group is reattached to the molecule using energy obtained from food or sunlight. Thus the ATP molecule acts as a chemical "battery," storing energy when it is not needed, but able to release it instantly when the organism requires it. The number of mitochondria in cells varies from a few hundred to several thousand. The greatest number is found in cells exhibiting the greatest activity.

Lysosomes—"Garbage Bags" With "Poison Pills."

Lysosomes are small, pealike sacs or single-membrane spherical bodies that are of great importance for digestion within the cytoplasm. They contain a group of different digestive enzymes that target proteins, and their primary function appears to be the breaking down of unwanted large molecules that either penetrate into the cell through microscopic channels or are drawn in by the cell membrane itself. If lysosomes fail in their cellular "garbage disposal" tasks, the resulting accumulation of large molecules may ultimately obstruct normal functions in organs. Lysosomes are sometimes referred to as *suicide bags*, because the enzymes they contain can break down and digest not only proteins and certain carbohydrates, but also the cell itself should the lysosome's surrounding membrane break. Exposure to radiation may induce such a rupture. When this occurs, the cell is likely to die.

Ribosomes—"Manufacturing Facilities" of the Cell.

Ribosomes are very small, spherical organelles that attach to the endoplasmic reticulum. They consist of:

- Two-thirds RNA
- One-third protein

Ribosomes are commonly referred to as the cell's *protein factories* because their job is to manufacture (synthesize) the various proteins that cells require by using the blueprints provided by mRNA. Their role in the assembly of amino acids into proteins is described earlier in this chapter.

Centrosomes—"Weavers of the Spindle."

Centrosomes are located in the center of the cell near the nucleus. They contain the *centrioles*, which in each centrosome are a pair of small, hollow, cylindrical structures (Fig. 6.12) oriented at right angles to each other and embedded in a material mass of more than 100 proteins.

Mitosis is a process where cells divide and make two new identical cells. Before mitosis can start, the cells need to make two copies of their DNA. Each one will go to a new cell so that the new cells have the exact, correct amount of DNA.

The centrosome and centrioles are crucial for this process. During cell division, two centrioles come together with some other special proteins and form the centrosome. Fig. 6.13 is an image of a centrosome, made of two centrioles and microtubules. The centrosome is an organelle that serves as the main microtubule-organizing center of the cell, as well as a regulator of cell-cycle progression.

The centrioles' pair duplicates within a cell, and the resultant two pairs migrate to the opposite ends of the

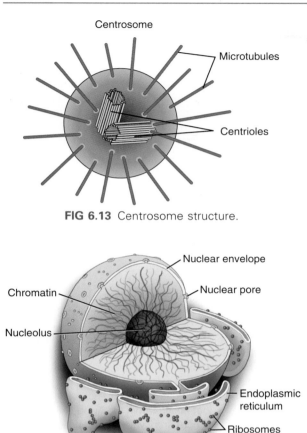

FIG 6.13 Centrosome structure.

FIG 6.14 Anatomy of the cell nucleus.

blueprints, or instructions, for building proteins in the cell), and proteins. These pores in the nuclear envelope allow molecules of specific types and sizes to pass back and forth between the nucleus and the cytoplasm.

The proteins and DNA within the nucleoplasm are arranged in long threads called *chromatin*. Chromatin is essentially a less condensed or less tightly packed form of the cell's DNA that, together with various proteins, during the division of a cell contracts into the tiny rod-shaped bodies that are called *chromosomes*. Within these chromosomes will be carried the genetic history of the cell in the segments of DNA called *genes*.

The nucleus also contains at least one very small, rounded body called the *nucleolus*. The nucleolus is the RNA copy center. This nuclear organelle manufactures and holds a large amount of RNA and protein. The nucleolus synthesizes ribosomes, which we have learned previously are protein-producing machines.

In summary, the nucleus controls cell division and multiplication and the biochemical reactions that occur within the cell. By directing protein synthesis, the nucleus plays an essential role in the following:

- Active transport
- Metabolism
- Growth
- Heredity

A summary of cell components is presented in Table 6.1.

CELL DIVISION

Cell division is the multiplication process whereby one cell divides to form two or more cells (Fig. 6.15). The two types of cell divisions that occur in the body are:

- Mitosis
- Meiosis

When somatic cells (all cells in the human body except the germ cells) divide, they undergo mitosis, a process in which the nucleus first divides, followed by the division of the cytoplasm. Genetic cells (the oogonium, or female germ cell, and the spermatogonium, or male germ cell) undergo meiosis, a process of reduction division.

Mitosis

Through the process of **mitosis (M)** (Fig. 6.16), a parent cell divides to form two daughter cells identical to the parent cell. This process results in an approximately equal distribution of all cellular material between the two

cell to form and organize the mitotic spindle.* The stages of cell division are discussed in detail later in this chapter.

Nucleus—Information-Processing and Administrative Center

Separated from the other parts of the cell by a double-walled membrane with pores, called the *nuclear envelope*, the **nucleus** is a highly specialized organelle that is the information-processing and administrative center of the living cell (Fig. 6.14). It consists of a spherical mass of semifluid protoplasm, known as *nucleoplasm*, which contains the genetic or hereditary material, DNA (the

---

*The mitotic spindle is essentially a protein machine that segregates chromosomes into two daughter cells during the cell division process.

TABLE 6.1 **Summary of Cell Components**

Component	Site	Activity
Cell membrane	Cytoplasm	*Plastic storage bag* – Functions as a barricade to protect cellular contents from their environment and controls the passage of water and other materials into and out of the cell; performs many additional functions such as elimination of wastes and refining of material for energy through breakdown of the materials.
Endoplasmic reticulum	Cytoplasm	*The highway* – Enables the cell to communicate with the extracellular environment and transfers food from one part of the cell to another.
Golgi apparatus	Cytoplasm	*Freight hauling* – Unites large carbohydrate molecules and combines them with proteins to form glycoproteins; transports enzymes and hormones through the cell membrane so that they can exit the cell, enter the bloodstream, and be carried to areas of the body in which they are required.
Mitochondria	Cytoplasm	*Power-generating stations* – Produce energy for cellular activity by breaking down nutrients through a process of oxidation.
Lysosomes	Cytoplasm	*Garbage bags with poison pills* – Dispose of large particles such as bacteria and food, as well as smaller particles; also contain hydrolytic enzymes that can break down and digest proteins, certain carbohydrates, and the cell itself if the lysosome's surrounding membrane breaks.
Ribosomes	Cytoplasm	*Manufacturing facilities* – Manufacture the various proteins that cells require.
Centrosomes	Cytoplasm	*Spindle weaver* – Plays an important role in organizing the formation of the mitotic spindle during cell division.
Nucleus	Nucleus	*Information-processing and administrative center of the cell* – Contains the genetic or hereditary material, DNA, and proteins. Also contains the nucleolus. The nucleus controls cell division and multiplication and the biochemical reactions that occur within the cell. Also directs protein synthesis.
DNA	Nucleus	*The blueprints* – Contains the genetic material; controls cell division and multiplication and biochemical reactions that occur within the living cell.
Nucleolus	Nucleus	*RNA copy center* – Holds a large amount of RNA and synthesizes ribosomes.

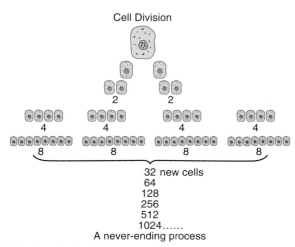

Cell Division

2 2
4 4 4 4
8 8 8 8

32 new cells
64
128
256
512
1024......
A never-ending process

FIG 6.15 Cell division is the multiplication process whereby one cell divides to form two or more cells. (From *Radiobiology and Radiation Protection: Mosby's Radiographic Instructional Series,* St. Louis, 1999, Elsevier.)

daughter cells. The entire cellular life cycle may be depicted as shown in Fig. 6.17. Different degrees of cell growth, maturation, and division occur in each phase. Four distinct chapters of the cellular life cycle are identifiable:

- G_1 (pre-DNA synthesis phase)
- S (synthesis phase)
- G_2 (post-DNA synthesis phase)
- M (mitosis phase)

In addition, the M phase can be divided into four subphases:

- Prophase
- Metaphase
- Anaphase
- Telophase

Mitosis is the division phase of the cellular life cycle. It is actually the last phase of the cycle. After it has commenced, it takes only about 1 hour to complete in all cells. Interphase, the period of cell growth that occurs before actual mitosis, consists of three intervals:

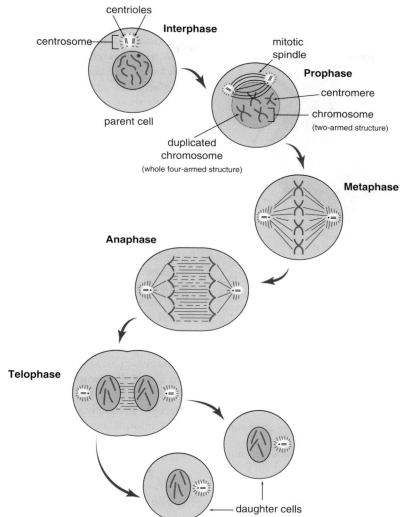

FIG 6.16 Diagram of mitosis. An animal cell with four chromosomes first multiplies (duplicates its DNA) and then divides, forming two new daughter cells, each of which contains exactly the same genetic material as the parent cell.

1. G_1
2. S
3. G_2

G_1 is the earliest phase among reproductive events. It is the gap in the growth of the cell that occurs between mitosis and DNA synthesis. Depending on the types of cells involved, this interval may take just a few minutes, or it may take several hours. G_1 is designated as the pre-DNA synthesis phase. During G_1, a form of RNA is synthesized in the cells that are to reproduce. This RNA

is needed before actual DNA synthesis can efficiently begin. S is the actual DNA synthesis period. While in S phase, each DNA molecule contained within the chromosome (Fig. 6.18A) is first copied (replicated) and then is divided into two individual sister components called *chromatids,** each containing DNA molecules. By the end

---

*A chromatid is a highly coiled strand; one of the two duplicated portions of DNA in a replicated chromosome that appear during cell division.

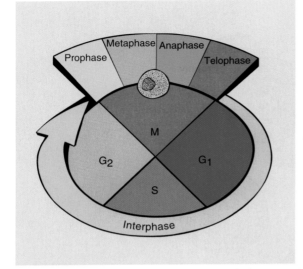

FIG 6.17 The entire cellular life cycle may be depicted as four distinct, identifiable phases: G_1, S, G_2, and M. M may be divided into four subphases: prophase, metaphase, anaphase, and telophase. (From Bushong SC: *Radiologic Science for Technologists: Physics, Biology and Protection*, ed 10, St. Louis, 2013, Elsevier.)

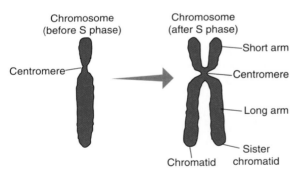

FIG 6.18 A single-strand chromosome gets duplicated during S phase, and the duplicates are joined together in an X-shape configuration to form a new chromosome. Each crossed arm of this new chromosome is called a *sister chromatid*.

of the S phase these chromatids will join together to form a new chromosome that has an X-shaped structure (see Fig. 6.18B). Thus each of the identical genetic pieces has now become one half of a new chromosome. The region of this chromosome where the two chromatids join together is called the *centromere* (see Fig. 6.18B).

During the anaphase of mitosis (described later), the paired sister chromatids separate from one another to form individual daughter chromosomes.

When compared with G_1 and G_2, the S phase is relatively long. It can take up to 15 hours. G_2 is the post-DNA manufacturing interval in the cellular life cycle. It is a relatively short period, occupying approximately 1 to 5 hours of the whole cycle. During this phase, cells manufacture certain proteins and RNA molecules needed to enter and complete subsequent mitosis. When G_2 has ended, cells enter the first phase of mitosis, the prophase, and the process of division commences.

Interphase. Interphase is the period of cell growth that occurs before actual mitosis. As previously stated, G_1, S, and G_2 are the phases of the cell cycle that comprise interphase. Cells are not yet undergoing division during this phase. If during interphase, a cell is viewed through a microscope with a DNA-specific stain applied, the nucleus looks somewhat odd. It appears as clumps of material shaped in different patterns. These patterns are seen throughout the nucleus, but individual chromosomes, however, are not visualized. During the synthesis portion of interphase (S), as we have seen, two sister chromatids form a new chromosome by attaching to each other at the centromere (see Fig. 6.18B). Hence, the cell's DNA molecules have duplicated in preparation for cell division. Genetic information also is transcribed into different kinds of RNA molecules such as mRNA and tRNA, which, after passing into the cytoplasm, translate the genetic information by promoting the synthesis of specific proteins.

The Four Phases of Mitosis. In the discussion which follows, it will be helpful to the reader to refer to Fig. 6.16, the figure entitled as "Diagram of Mitosis."

Prophase. During prophase, the first phase of cell division, the nucleus enlarges, the DNA complex (the chromatid network of threads) coils up more tightly, and the chromatids become more visible on stained microscopic slides. Chromosomes enlarge, and the DNA begins to take structural form. The nuclear membrane disappears, and the centrioles (small hollow, cylindrical structures) migrate to opposite sides of the cell and begin to regulate the formation of the *mitotic spindle*, the delicate fibers that are attached to the centrioles and extend from one side of the cell to the other across the equator of the cell.

Metaphase. As metaphase begins, the fibers collectively referred to as the *mitotic spindle* form between the centrioles. Each chromosome, which now consists of two chromatids, lines up in the center, or equator, of the cell attached by its centromere to the mitotic spindle. This configuration forms the equatorial plate (see Fig. 6.16). During metaphase, cell division can be stopped, and visible chromosomes can be examined under a microscope. Chromosome damage caused by radiation can then be evaluated.

Anaphase. Anaphase begins with the breakdown of a protein called *securin* that inhibits the action of a protein called *separase* whose function is to break down the protein *cohesin*. The latter is ultimately responsible for maintaining the integrity of the centromeres attached to the microtubules making up the mitotic spindle. With the breakdown of cohesin, the centromeres are severed and the sister chromatids move apart and are subsequently pulled toward opposite poles of the spindle. Along the way they take on a shape that is similar to a V placed on its side (see Fig. 6.16). This process causes the cell to stretch or elongate into an oval shape. The cell is now ready to begin the last phase of division.

Telophase. During telophase, the chromatids undergo changes in appearance by uncoiling and becoming long, loosely spiraled threads. Simultaneously, the nuclear membrane forms anew, and two nuclei (one for each new daughter cell) appear. The cytoplasm also divides (cytokinesis) near the equator of the cell to surround each new nucleus. After this cell division completes, each daughter cell has a complete cell membrane and contains exactly the same amount of genetic material (46 chromosomes) as the parent cell.

Meiosis

Meiosis is a special type of cell division that reduces the number of chromosomes in each daughter cell to half the number of chromosomes in the parent cell (Fig. 6.19). Box 6.8 provides terms associated with the female reproductive cell. Male and female germ cells, or sperm and ova, of sexually mature individuals each begin meiosis with 46 chromosomes. However, before the male and female germ cells unite to produce a new organism, the number of chromosomes in each must be reduced by one half to ensure that the daughter cells (called *zygotes*) formed when they unite will contain only the normal number of 46 chromosomes. Hence meiosis is really a process of reduction division (Fig. 6.20).

Meiosis begins with a doubling of the amount of genetic material. This doubling of the amount of DNA

BOX 6.8 Female Reproductive Cell Terms

Oogonium: One of the undifferentiated germ cells that can give rise to oocytes

Ovum: A female reproductive cell (i.e., egg cell) ultimately capable of developing into an individual after fertilization

Oocytes: An immature egg cell that matures during the menstrual cycle

Ootid: An egg cell that results from the second mitotic division of an oocyte

---

is called *replication* and occurs during interphase. As a result of DNA replication, each one-chromatid chromosome duplicates, thus forming a two-chromatid chromosome. This means that sperm and egg cells begin meiosis with twice the amount of genetic material as the original parent cell. Thus at the beginning of meiosis, the number of chromosomes increases from $2n$ to $4n$ ($n = 23$).

The various phases of meiosis are similar to those of mitosis. The major difference between the two types of cell division begins at the end of telophase. In meiosis, after the parent germ cell has formed two daughter cells, each of which (in human beings) contains 46 chromosomes, the daughter cells divide without DNA replication. Chromosome duplication does not occur at this phase of division. These two successive divisions result in the formation of four granddaughter cells, each of which contains only 23 chromosomes. This means that the proper number of 46 chromosomes will be produced when a female ovum containing 23 chromosomes is fertilized by a male sperm containing 23 chromosomes.

During meiosis, the sister chromatids exchange some chromosomal material (genes). This process, called *crossover,* results in changes in genetic composition and traits that can be passed on to future generations.

Multiple Births. Multiple births can occur during a pregnancy in one of two ways. The first way is if a fertilized ovum (zygote) splits after fertilization and two separate offspring develop. The two offspring would be referred to as *monozygotic* (coming from one zygote) *twins.* Monozygotic twins are also known as *identical twins* because they contain exact replicas of genetic material. Another way to achieve a multiple birth is if more than one ootid is available for fertilization and the separate ootids are fertilized by separate spermatozoa. In this case

MEIOSIS

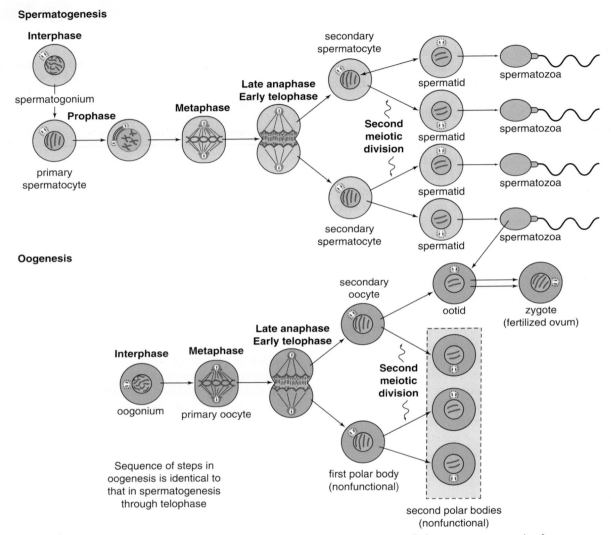

FIG 6.19 Diagram of meiosis. Four cells result from one germ cell. In spermatogenesis, four spermatids become mature spermatozoa. In oogenesis, one ootid may be fertilized, and three second polar bodies remain nonfunctional.

the children would have no more resemblance to each other than would other children born at different times from the same parents. Such dizygotic twins are also known as *fraternal twins*. More than two such twins would be known as *polyzygotic siblings*. Fraternal twins or multiple siblings, as with siblings born in different pregnancies, sometimes bear a striking resemblance to one another. However, unless they were monozygotic, they are not identical twins and do not have exact copies of all their chromosomes.

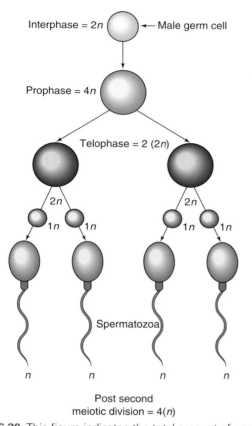

Interphase = 2n ○ ◄— Male germ cell

Prophase = 4n

Telophase = 2 (2n)

2n   2n

1n 1n   1n 1n

Spermatozoa

n   n   n   n

Post second
meiotic division = 4(n)

FIG 6.20 This figure indicates the total amount of genetic material at different stages of meiosis of a male germ cell. Twenty-three chromosomes, half the amount needed to produce a new human organism, are needed in the spermatozoa. If we refer to 23 chromosomes as an amount of genetic material n, then before meiosis (during interphase) the germ cell has 2n. During prophase, this number doubles to 4n. There then follows two reduction divisions to form the final 1n (23 chromosomes) in the spermatozoa. An egg cell, or ovum, undergoes a similar process, but only one of the four resulting germ cells at the end of the process is functional.

▌ SUMMARY

- The cell is the fundamental component of structure, development, growth, and life processes in the human body.
- Cells are made of protoplasm, which consists of proteins, carbohydrates, lipids, nucleic acids, water, and mineral salts (electrolytes).

- Proteins are essential for growth, the construction of new body tissue, and repair of injured or debilitated tissue; they may function as hormones and antibodies.
- The primary purpose of carbohydrates is to provide fuel for cell metabolism.
- Lipids act as a reservoir for long-term storage of energy, insulate and guard the body against the environment, and protect organs.
- Nucleic acids (DNA, RNA) carry genetic information necessary for cell replication.
- RNA has the nitrogenous base uracil as a component of its ladder steps, whereas DNA has thymine instead in its ladder steps.
- Genes are the basic units of heredity.
- The Human Genome Project has mapped the entire sequence of DNA base pairs on all 46 chromosomes. This project has led to the discovery of more than 1800 disease genes.
- There are 2.9 billion base pairs arranged into approximately 30,000 genes.
- Water, the primary inorganic substance contained in the human body, comprises approximately 80% to 85% of the body's weight, is essential to sustaining life, and serves as the transport vehicle for materials the cell uses or eliminates.
- Mineral salts keep the correct proportion of water in the cell, support proper cell function, assist in the creation of energy, aid in the conduction of impulses along nerves, and prevent muscle cramping.
- Cells have multiple components or subunits called *organelles.*
- The cell membrane surrounds the human cell, functions as a barricade, and controls passage of water and other materials into and out of the cell.
- Cytoplasm is the portion of a cell outside the nucleus in which all metabolic activity occurs.
- The endoplasmic reticulum transports food and molecules from one part of the cell to another. It functions as the highway system of the cell.
- The Golgi apparatus unites large carbohydrate molecules with proteins to form glycoproteins.
- Mitochondria, the powerhouses of the cell, contain enzymes that produce energy for cellular activity.
- Lysosomes break down unwanted large molecules; they may rupture when they are exposed to radiation, with resulting cell death.

- Ribosomes synthesize the various proteins that cells require.
- Centrosomes contain the centrioles.
- The nucleus controls cell division, multiplication, and biochemical reactions.
- Somatic cells divide through the process of mitosis.
- The cellular life cycle has four distinct phases: pre-DNA synthesis, actual DNA synthesis, post-DNA manufacturing, and division (mitosis).
- Mitosis has four subphases: prophase, metaphase, anaphase, and telophase.
- Genetic cells divide through meiosis.
- Meiosis is similar to mitosis, except no DNA replication occurs in telophase; the number of chromosomes in the daughter cell is reduced to half the number of chromosomes in the parent cell.

REFERENCES

1. Ventner JC: The sequence of the human genome. *Science* 291:1304–1351, 2001.
2. NIH Fact Sheet. http://report.nih.gov/NIHfactsheets/ViewFactSheet.aspx?csid=45&key=H#H.
3. Lee TF: *The Human Genome Project: Cracking the Genetic Code of Life*, New York, 1991, Plenum Press.
4. Stöppler MC: Electrolytes. Available at: www.medicinenet.com/electrolytes/article.htm.
5. Dowd SB, Tilson ER: *Practical Radiation Protection and Applied Radiobiology*, ed 2, Philadelphia, 1999, Saunders.

GENERAL DISCUSSION QUESTIONS

1. What are the essential functions of water in the human body?
2. What role do antibodies fulfill for the human body?
3. Describe the structure of a DNA (deoxyribonucleic) macromolecule.
4. Name the four nitrogenous base pairs in a DNA macromolecule.
5. How do genes control the formation of proteins in every cell?
6. Describe the Human Genome Project, and explain the progress that has been made as a result of it.
7. Why is potassium of primary importance to the human body?
8. List the components of the normal cell, and explain their function.
9. Describe the processes of mitosis and meiosis.
10. How can multiple births occur from one pregnancy?
11. What is the period of cell growth that occurs before actual mitosis called?
12. What are centrioles, and what is their function in the human cell?

REVIEW QUESTIONS

1. In a DNA macromolecule, the sequence of _____ determines the characteristics of every living thing.
   A. Sugars
   B. Phosphates
   C. Nitrogenous organic bases
   D. Hydrogen bonds
2. How many base pairs are there in the human genome?
   A. 2.58×10^4
   B. 2.58×10^{-4}
   C. 2.9×10^9
   D. 2.9×10^{-9}
3. Radiation-induced chromosome damage may be evaluated during which of the following processes?
   A. Prophase
   B. Metaphase
   C. Anaphase
   D. Telophase
4. If exposure to ionizing radiation damages the components involved in molecular synthesis beyond repair, cells do which of the following?
   A. Continue to function normally
   B. Function abnormally or die
   C. Repair themselves immediately because of the enzymatic proteins they contain
   D. Reproduce themselves in pairs
5. Which of the following produces antibodies?
   A. Erythrocytes
   B. Lymphocytes
   C. Thrombocytes
   D. Platelets
6. Water comprises approximately _____ of the weight of the human body.
   A. 50% to 55%
   B. 60% to 70%
   C. 80% to 85%
   D. 90% to 95%
7. Which of the following must the human body provide to ensure efficient cell operation?
   1. Food as a source of raw material for the release of energy

   2. Oxygen to help break down food
   3. Water to transport inorganic substances into and out of the cell
   A. 1 and 2 only
   B. 1 and 3 only
   C. 2 and 3 only
   D. 1, 2, and 3

8. Which human cell component controls cell division and multiplication as well as biochemical reactions that occur within the cell?
   A. Endoplasmic reticulum
   B. Mitochondria
   C. Lysosomes
   D. Nucleus

9. What term is used to describe chemical secretions that are manufactured by various endocrine glands and carried by the bloodstream to influence the activities of other parts of the body?
   A. Amino acids
   B. Antibodies
   C. Hormones
   D. Disaccharides

10. Somatic cells divide through the process of:
   A. Meiosis
   B. Mitosis
   C. Mapping
   D. Metabolism

7

Molecular and Cellular Radiation Biology

OBJECTIVES

After completing this chapter, the reader will be able to perform the following:
- Define all key terms.
- Explain how ionizing radiation damages living systems.
- List three characteristics of ionizing radiation that determine the extent to which different radiation modalities transfer energy into biologic tissue.
- List the three radiation energy transfer determinants, and explain their individual concepts.
- Explain why x-rays and gamma rays can also be referred to as a stream of particles called photons.
- Differentiate among the three levels of biologic damage that may occur in living systems as a result of exposure to ionizing radiation, and describe how the process of direct and indirect action of ionizing radiation on the molecular structure of living systems occurs.
- Draw a diagram to illustrate the various effects of ionizing radiation on a DNA macromolecule, and describe the effects of ionizing radiation on chromosomes, various types of cells, and ultimately the entire human body.
- Explain the target theory.
- List and explain six effects of irradiation on the entire cell that can result from damage to the cell's nucleus.
- Explain the purpose and function of survival curves for mammalian cells.
- List the factors that affect cell radiosensitivity.
- State and describe the law of Bergonié and Tribondeau.
- Describe effects of ionizing radiation on human blood cells, epithelial tissue, muscle tissue, nervous tissue, and male and female reproductive cells.

CHAPTER OUTLINE

KEY TERMS

apoptosis
cell survival curve
chromosome breakage
direct action
free radicals
indirect action

law of Bergonié and Tribondeau
linear energy transfer (LET)
mutation
oxygen enhancement ratio (OER)
point lesion
radiation weighting factor (W_R)

relative biologic effectiveness
  (RBE)
target theory
wave-particle duality

Radiation biology is the branch of biology concerned with the effects of ionizing radiation on living systems. Areas of study included in this science are the:
- Sequence of events occurring after the absorption of energy from ionizing radiation
- Action of the living system to make up for the consequences of this energy assimilation
- Injury to the living system that may be produced

The human body is a complex interconnected living system composed of very large numbers of various types of cells, most of which may be damaged by radiation. Because the potentially harmful effects of ionizing radiation on living systems occur primarily at the cellular level, the preceding chapter placed a strong emphasis on the basics of cell structure, composition, and function. This chapter provides the reader with an introduction to those aspects of molecular and cellular radiation biology that are relevant to the subject of radiation protection.

IONIZING RADIATION

Ionizing radiation damages living systems by ionizing (removing electrons from) the atoms comprising the molecular structures of these systems. X-ray and gamma-ray photons can impart energy to orbital electrons in atoms if the photons happen to pass near the electrons. High-energy charged particles such as alpha and beta particles and protons also may ionize atoms by interacting electromagnetically with orbital electrons. The alpha particle, which is composed of two protons and two neutrons and therefore carries an electric charge of +2, strongly attracts the negatively charged electrons as it passes by.

Biologic damage, then, begins with the ionization produced by various types of radiation. An ionized atom does not bond properly in molecules. If the molecule in question is necessary for the normal functioning of an

organism, then the entire organism may be adversely affected.

RADIATION ENERGY TRANSFER DETERMINANTS

Characteristics of ionizing radiation vary among different types of radiation. Characteristics include:
- Charge
- Mass
- Energy

These attributes determine the extent to which different radiation modalities transfer energy into biologic tissue. To understand the way ionizing radiation causes injury and how the effects can vary in biologic tissue, three important concepts must be studied:
1. Linear energy transfer
2. Relative biologic effectiveness
3. Oxygen enhancement ratio

Linear Energy Transfer

When passing through a medium, ionizing radiation may interact with it during its passage and as a result lose energy along its path (called a *track*). The average energy deposited per unit length of track is called **linear energy transfer (LET)** (Fig. 7.1). The energy average is calculated by dividing the total energy deposited in the medium by the total length of the track. LET is generally described in units of kiloelectron volts (keV) per micron (1 micron [μm] = 10^{-6} m). The rate of transfer of energy from ionizing radiation used for diagnostic purposes (x-rays) to soft biologic tissue is estimated to be 3 keV/μm. This is considered to be relatively low-LET radiation compared with other types of radiation, which can have much higher keV/μm values. Because the amount of ionization produced in an irradiated object is related to the amount of energy it absorbs, and because both chemical and

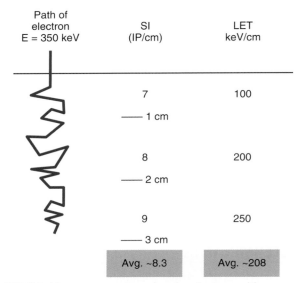

Path of electron E = 350 keV	SI (IP/cm)	LET keV/cm
	7	100
— 1 cm		
	8	200
— 2 cm		
	9	250
— 3 cm		
Avg. ~8.3		Avg. ~208

FIG 7.1 Linear energy transfer. An electron with energy (E) of 350 keV interacts in a tissue-like material. Its actual path is tortuous, changing direction a number of times, as the electron interacts with atoms of the material via excitations and ionizations. As interactions reduce the energy of the electron through excitation and ionization, the electron's energy is transferred to the material. The interactions that take place along the path of the particle may be summarized as specific ionization (SI; ion pairs/cm) or as linear energy transfer (LET; keV/cm) along the straight-line continuation of the particle's trajectory beyond its point of entry. (From Hendee WR, Ritenour ER: *Medical Imaging Physics*, ed 4, Chicago, 2002, John Wiley & Sons.)

biologic effects in tissue coincide with the degree of ionization experienced by the tissue, the LET value of the radiation involved is a very important factor in assessing potential tissue and organ damage from exposure to that type of ionizing radiation. When LET increases, the chance of producing a significant biologic response in the radiosensitive DNA macromolecule grows.

Radiation Categories According to Linear Energy Transfer. Radiation may be divided into two general categories according to its LET (Box 7.1):
• Low
• High
   Low–linear energy transfer radiation. Low-LET radiation is electromagnetic radiation, such as:

• X-rays
• Gamma rays (short-wavelength, high-energy waves emitted by the nuclei of radioactive substances)
and also charged particles with very low mass, such as:
• Electrons
   Due to a property known as **wave-particle duality**, x-rays and gamma rays, as we have seen in Chapter 3 and as discussed in Appendix E, can also be referred to as streams of particles called *photons*, each of which has no mass and no charge.
   Although this electromagnetic radiation can be quite penetrating, it is sparsely ionizing and interacts randomly along the length of its track. Consequently, it does not relinquish all its energy quickly. Thus when low-LET radiation interacts with biologic tissue, it causes damage to a cell primarily through an *indirect* action that involves the production of molecules called **free radicals.** These are solitary atoms, for example, a lone hydrogen atom [H], or most often a combination of atoms such as [OH] that behave as single entities and are very chemically reactive as a result of the presence of unpaired valence (outermost) electrons. In addition, but much less likely, the low-LET radiation may *directly* induce single-strand breaks in the ladder-like DNA structure. Because low-LET radiation generally causes sublethal damage to DNA, repair enzymes can usually reverse the cellular damage.
   High–linear energy transfer radiation. High-LET radiation includes particles that possess substantial:
• Mass
• Charge
   This type of radiation, unlike low-LET radiation, can produce dense ionization along its path and therefore is much more likely to interact significantly with biologic tissue. Some typical examples of high-LET radiation are:
• Alpha particles
• Ions of heavy nuclei

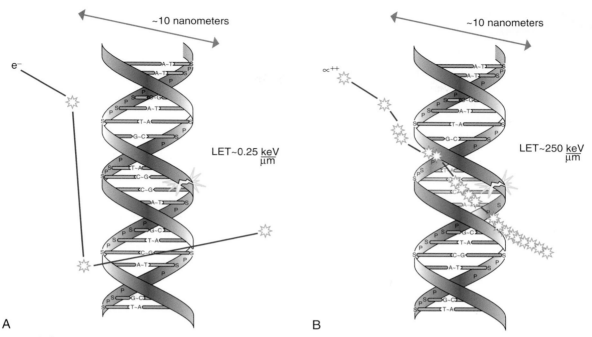

FIG 7.2 An electron and an alpha particle passing through the nucleus of a cell near a strand of DNA. (A) For an electron, several interactions may occur in the vicinity of a DNA strand and create a risk of damage to the DNA. (B) Because many interactions may occur in the vicinity of a DNA strand, some damage is likely.

- Charged particles released from interactions between neutrons and atoms

Low-energy neutrons, which carry no electrical charge, also are a form of high-LET radiation. Compared with low-LET radiation, all these types of high-LET radiation lose or deposit energy more rapidly because significantly more ionization per unit of distance traveled is produced. As a result, they exhaust their energy in a shorter length of track and unless they are of extremely high energies, cannot travel or penetrate as far as x-ray and gamma ray photons. Even so, it is clear that high-LET radiation can be very destructive to biologic matter.

Risk of damage to DNA. Fig. 7.2 shows an electron and an alpha particle passing through the nucleus of a cell in the vicinity of a strand of DNA. The size of the entire area is only approximately 10 nanometers (10 billionths of a meter). The electron is either a Compton scattered electron or a photoelectron generated by the interaction of a photon from a diagnostic x-ray beam. The alpha particle represents one of the particles ejected from the nucleus of an atom after radioactive decay of an element such as radon.

Probability of interaction with DNA. The presence of many more alpha particle interactions in the small region displayed is reflected in the finding that the LET for the alpha particle shown in Fig. 7.2 is 1000 times the LET of the electron. Each time the particle interacts, it loses some energy and slows down in the cell. When enough interactions have occurred, the particle will essentially be at rest, and interactions beyond this path penetration are unlikely. Because it does not interact as often, the electron, however, can travel significantly farther than the alpha particle. A Compton scattered electron or photoelectron set in motion in a patient exposed to diagnostic x-rays may travel through thousands of cells, having interactions in only some of them and with a low probability that any of these will occur in the DNA. Conversely, an alpha particle, such as the one shown, may travel through only a few cells, but will have a high probability of interacting with the DNA of a cell it encounters.

High–linear energy transfer radiation and internal contamination. For radiation protection, high-LET radiation is of greatest concern when internal contamination is possible, that is, when a radionuclide has been:

BOX 7.2 Mathematical Expression of Relative Biologic Effectiveness

$$RBE = \frac{\text{Dose in } Gy_t \text{ from 250-kVp x-rays (reference radiation)}}{\text{Dose in } Gy_t \text{ of test radiation}}$$

Example: A biologic reaction is produced by 2 Gy_t of a test radiation. It takes 10 Gy_t of 250-kVp x-rays to produce the same biologic reaction. What is the RBE of the test radiation?

$$\frac{10}{2} = 5$$

The RBE is 5, which means that the test radiation is five times as effective in producing this biologic reaction as are 250-kVp x-rays.

RBE, Relative biologic effectiveness.

BOX 7.3 Oxygen Enhancement Ratio

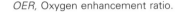

$$OER = \frac{\text{Radiation dose required to cause biologic response without } O_2}{\text{Radiation dose required to cause biologic response with } O_2}$$

OER, Oxygen enhancement ratio.

- Implanted
- Ingested
- Injected
- Inhaled

Then, the potential exists for irreparable damage because, with high-LET radiation, multiple-strand breaks in DNA are possible. For example, with a double-strand break in the same rung of the DNA ladder-like structure, complete **chromosome breakage** occurs (see Fig. 7.8A later in this chapter). Repair enzymes are not effective at undoing this damage, and hence cell death will most likely follow.

Relative Biologic Effectiveness

Biologic damage produced by radiation escalates as the LET of radiation increases. Identical doses of radiation of different LETs do not render identical biologic effects. The **relative biologic effectiveness (RBE)** describes the relative capabilities of radiation with differing LETs to produce a particular biologic reaction. RBE of the type of radiation being used is the ratio of the dose of a reference radiation (conventionally 250-kVp x-rays) to the dose of radiation of the type in question that is necessary to produce the same biologic reaction in a given experiment. The reaction is what is produced by a dose of the test radiation delivered under the same conditions. Box 7.2 demonstrates how RBE can be expressed mathematically.

Use of the Relative Biologic Effectiveness Concept for Specific Experiments.
The concept of RBE is used to refer to specific experiments with specific cells or animal

tissues (e.g., tumor cells in a Petri dish, skin of the left hind flank of a certain strain of laboratory rat). Because the various types of cells or tissues differ in their biologic response per unit quantity of absorbed dose, the concept of RBE is not practical for specifying radiation protection dose levels in humans. To overcome this limitation, a **radiation weighting factor** (W_R) is used to calculate the equivalent dose (EqD) to determine the ability of a dose of any kind of ionizing radiation to cause biologic damage. The W_R values are similar to the values of RBE for any particular type of radiation. For example, the W_R for x-radiation is 1, and the RBE for diagnostic x-rays is also 1. The W_R values for different types of ionizing radiation are listed in Table 4.2 in Chapter 4.

Oxygen Enhancement Ratio

When irradiated in an oxygenated, or aerobic, state, biologic tissue is more sensitive to radiation than when it is exposed to radiation under anoxic (without oxygen) or hypoxic (low-oxygen) conditions. This is known as the *oxygen effect*. The **oxygen enhancement ratio (OER)** describes this effect numerically.[1,2]

The OER is the ratio of the radiation dose required to cause a particular biologic response of cells or organisms in an oxygen-deprived environment to the radiation dose required to cause an identical response under normal oxygenated conditions. The OER formula is given in Box 7.3.

In general, x-rays and gamma rays, which are low-LET types of radiation, have an OER of approximately 3.0 when the radiation dose is high. The OER may be less (approximately 2.0) when radiation doses are lower than 2 Gy_t. This surprising result exists because a 2 Gy_t dose is associated with the linear (i.e., straight-line) portion of the linear-quadratic dose–response relationship for cell killing (see Fig. 9.3), whereas higher doses can fall on the curved (i.e., quadratic) portion of the dose–response curve.[3] The term *linear-quadratic* means that the equation that best fits the data has terms that depend on dose (linear dependency) and dose squared (quadratic dependency). Because high-LET radiation such as alpha particles produces its biologic effects from direct action—namely, direct ionization and disruption of biomolecules—the presence or absence of oxygen is of little or no consequence. Therefore the OER of high-LET radiation is approximately equal to 1. For low-LET radiation, a significant fraction of bioeffects is caused by indirect actions in which a *free radical* is formed. Because of their high reactivity, free radicals can dramatically increase the amount of biologic damage. Oxygen, if present in biologic tissues, will react with these chemical entities to produce organic peroxide compounds*. The latter represent nonrestorable changes in the chemical composition of the target material. Without oxygen, damage produced by the indirect action of radiation on a biologic molecule may be repaired, but when damage occurs through an oxygen-mediated process, the end result is lasting or fixed. This phenomenon has been called *the oxygen fixation hypothesis.*

MOLECULAR EFFECTS OF IRRADIATION

In living systems, biologic damage stemming from exposure to ionizing radiation is observed on three levels:
- Molecular
- Cellular
- Organic systems

Any visible radiation-induced injuries of living systems at the cellular or organic level always begin with damage at the molecular level. Molecular damage results in the formation of structurally changed molecules that may impair cellular functioning.

Effects of Irradiation on Somatic and Genetic Cells

Cells of the human body are highly specialized. Each cell has a predetermined task to perform, and each cell's function is governed and defined by the structures of its constituent molecules. Because energy from ionizing radiation can alter these structures, such exposure may disturb the cell's chemical balance and ultimately the way it operates. When this occurs, the cell no longer performs its normal tasks. If sufficient quantities of somatic cells (i.e., all cells in the body other than female

---

*An organic peroxide is any organic (carbon-containing) compound with two oxygen atoms joined together (-O-O-).

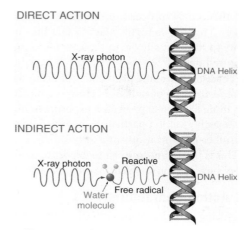

FIG 7.3 The action of radiation on the cell can be direct or indirect. It is direct when ionizing particles interact with a vital biologic macromolecule such as DNA. The action is indirect when ionizing particles interact with a water molecule, thus resulting in the creation of ions and reactive free radicals that eventually produce toxic substances that can create biologic damage. (From *Radiobiology and Radiation Protection: Mosby's Radiographic Instructional Series*, St. Louis, 1999, Mosby.)

and male germ cells) are affected, entire body processes can be disrupted. Conversely, if radiation damages the germ (reproductive) cells, the damage may be passed on to future generations in the form of genetic mutations.

Classification of Ionizing Radiation Interaction

When ionizing radiation interacts with a cell, ionizations and excitations (the addition of energy to a molecular system that raises it from a ground state to a higher-energy, or excited, state) are produced either in vital biologic macromolecules or in water (H_2O), the medium in which the cellular organelles are suspended. Based on the site of the interaction, the effect of radiation on the cell is classified as either (Fig. 7.3):
- Direct
- Indirect

As mentioned previously, in **direct action,** biologic damage occurs as a result of ionization of atoms on essential molecules produced by straight interaction with the incident radiation. **Indirect action,** instead, is always a multistage process that first involves the production of free radicals that are created by the interaction of the radiation with water (H_2O) molecules. These unstable agents, then, may proceed to interact with cellular molecules. They are so highly reactive that they have the capability to substantially disrupt master molecules, with resulting cell death.

Direct action has some probability of occurring after exposure to any type of radiation. However, direct action is much more likely to happen after exposure to high-LET radiation such as alpha particles, which produce a very large number of ionizations in a very short distance of travel. This is in glaring contrast to exposure to low-LET radiation, such as x-rays, which are only sparsely ionizing.

Direct Action Characteristics

When ionizing particles interact directly with vital biologic macromolecules such as:

- DNA
- Ribonucleic acid (RNA)
- Proteins
- Enzymes

damage to these molecules occurs from the absorption of energy through photoelectric and Compton interactions. The ionization or even the excitation of the atoms of the biologic macromolecules can often result in breakage of the macromolecules' intricate chemical bonds causing them to become abnormal structures. This change could in turn lead to inappropriate cellular chemical reactions. As an example, when enzyme molecules are damaged by interaction with ionizing particles, essential biochemical processes that depend on the facilitating action of the enzymes may not occur in the cell when needed. Should this happen during the process associated with the synthesis of a particular protein, the protein will not be manufactured, and if this protein was intended to perform a specific function, its failure to exist will hinder or prevent that function. In the event that other cell operations depend on the suppressed function, these operations will be compromised as well, and so a negative biologic sequence essentially occurs.

Radiolysis of Water

Ionization of Water Molecules. When x-ray photons interact with and ionize water molecules contained within the human body, this can result in their separation into other molecular components. For example, one type of interaction could create an ion pair consisting of a water molecule with a positive charge (HOH^+) and a solitary electron (e^-). After the original ionization of the water molecule, several other successive reactions are possible.

One such outcome is that the positively charged water molecule (HOH^+) may recombine with the electron (e^-) to reform a stable water molecule ($HOH^+ + e^- = H_2O$). If this happens, no damage will occur. Alternatively, the electron (the negative ion) may join with another water molecule to produce a negative water ion ($H_2O + e^- = HOH^-$). This result may have unfavorable consequences.

Production of Free Radicals. The positive water molecule (HOH^+) and the negative water molecule (HOH^-) are basically unstable. Hence they will soon break apart into smaller molecules. HOH^+ decomposes into a hydrogen ion (H^+) and the neutral oxygen–hydrogen combination called the *hydroxyl radical* (OH^*), whereas HOH^- becomes a hydroxyl ion (OH^-) and a hydrogen radical (H^*). The asterisk symbolizes a free radical. A free radical has no net electrical charge but because of having an unpaired valence electron, this entity typically exists as such for approximately 1 millisecond before pairing up with another electron, even if it has to break a chemical bond to do this. Hence the interaction of radiation with water ultimately results in the formation of an ion pair, H^+ and OH^- (hydrogen ion and hydroxyl ion), and two free radicals, H^* and OH^* (a hydrogen radical and a hydroxyl radical) (Fig. 7.4).

Production of Undesirable Chemical Reactions and Biologic Damage. Because the hydrogen and hydroxyl *ions* usually recombine to form a normal water molecule, the presence of these ions as free agents within the human body is insignificant in terms of biologic damage. The presence of hydrogen and hydroxyl *free radicals,* however, is not insignificant. They can produce undesirable chemical reactions, in the process transferring their excess energy to biologic molecules, thereby either breaking these molecules' chemical bonds or at the very least causing point lesions (i.e., altered areas caused by the breaking of a single chemical bond) in the molecule. Approximately two-thirds of all radiation-induced damage is believed to be ultimately caused by the hydroxyl free radical (OH^*). In addition, because the free radicals have this excess energy and can travel through the cell, they are capable of destructively interacting with other molecules located at some distance from the radicals' place of origin.

Production of Cell-Damaging Substances. Hydrogen and hydroxyl radicals are not the only destructive substances produced during the radiolysis of water. A hydroxyl

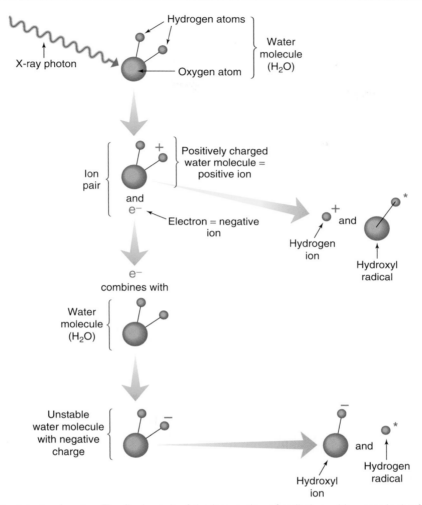

FIG 7.4 Radiolysis of water. The final result of the interaction of radiation with water is the formation of an ion pair (H+ and OH–) and two free radicals (H* and OH*).

radical (OH*) can bond with another hydroxyl radical (OH*) and form hydrogen peroxide (OH* + OH* = H$_2$O$_2$), a substance that is very poisonous to the cell. In addition, a hydroperoxyl radical (HO$_2$*) is formed when a hydrogen free radical (H*) combines with molecular oxygen (O$_2$). The hydroperoxyl radical and hydrogen peroxide are believed to be among the primary substances that produce biologic damage directly after the interaction of radiation with water.

Organic Free Radical Formation. Absorption of radiation can cause a normal organic molecule (for simplicity, let us call it *RH,* in which *H* stands for hydrogen and *R*

can be any organic molecule) to form the free radicals R* (an organic-neutral free radical) and H*. Without oxygen or a force to attract an electron, these radicals usually react with each other to reform the original organic molecule (RH). When oxygen is present, however, R* and H* may react with oxygen molecules (O$_2$) to form the radicals RO$_2$* and HO$_2$*. Hence the original organic molecule (RH) is destroyed and replaced by the radicals RO$_2$* and HO$_2$*. These radicals can react with other organic molecules to cause biologic damage. Thus a small-scale chain reaction of destructive events results when radiation deposits energy within tissue in the presence of oxygen.

Indirect Action Characteristics

To summarize, when free radicals previously produced by the interaction of radiation with water molecules act on a molecule such as DNA, the damaging action of ionizing radiation is indirect in the sense that the radiation is not the immediate cause of injury to the macromolecule. The by-products of the radiation, the free radicals, are the immediate cause of this damage. Because the human body is 80% water and less than 1% DNA, essentially all effects of low-LET irradiation in living cells result from indirect action.[1] Fig. 7.5 depicts a useful flow chart of the radiobiologic process of indirect action.

Effects of Ionizing Radiation on DNA

Single-Strand Break. If ionizing radiation interacts with a DNA macromolecule, the energy transferred could rupture one of its chemical bonds and possibly sever one of the sugar–phosphate chain side rails, or strands, of the ladder-like molecular structure (single-strand break) (Fig. 7.6). This type of injury to DNA is called a **point lesion.** Such a single alteration along the sequence of nitrogenous bases can result in a gene abnormality. Point lesions commonly occur with low-LET radiation. Repair enzymes, however, are often capable of reversing this damage.

Double-Strand Break. Further exposure of the affected DNA macromolecule to ionizing radiation will likely lead to additional breaks in the sugar–phosphate molecular chain(s). These breaks may also be repaired, but double-strand breaks (one or more breaks in each of the two sugar–phosphate chains) (Fig. 7.7) are not fixed as easily as single-strand breaks. If repair does not take place, further separation can occur in the DNA chains, threatening the life of the cell. Double-strand breaks happen more commonly with densely ionizing (high-LET) radiation and often are associated with the loss of one or more nitrogenous bases. Thus when high-LET radiation interacts with DNA molecules, the ionization interactions may be so closely spaced that, by chance, both strands of a DNA chain are broken. Should both strands be broken at the same nitrogenous base "rung" (Fig. 7.8A), the result will be the same as if both side rails of the ladder were cut at the same step, namely the DNA ladder would be chopped into two pieces. This situation will result in the associated chromosome to be broken itself. Thus some types of chromosomal damage that are specifically caused

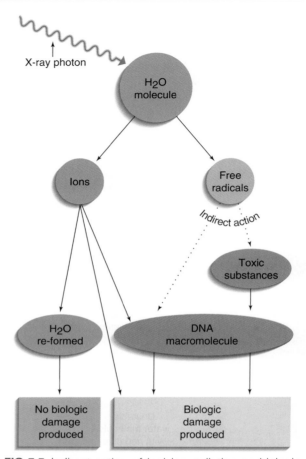

FIG 7.5 Indirect action of ionizing radiation on biologic molecules. X-ray photons interact directly with a water (H_2O) molecule. The H_2O molecule breaks down into ions and free radicals. The ions can recombine to form a water molecule, thereby creating no biologic damage. The free radicals can migrate to another molecule, such as a DNA molecule located at some distance from the site of the initial ionization, and destructively interact with it by ionizing it or rupturing some chemical bonds. This creates molecular or point lesions in the DNA macromolecule. Alternatively, free radicals can spread biologic damage by combining with other molecules to form toxic substances that also can migrate to distant DNA molecules and destructively interact.

by high-LET radiation are related to double-strand breaks of DNA. Because the chance of reversing this type of damage is very low, the possibility of a lethal alteration of nitrogenous bases within the genetic sequence is far greater.

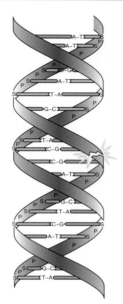

FIG 7.6 A single-strand break in the ladder-like DNA molecular structure.

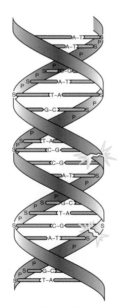

FIG 7.7 A widely spaced double-strand break in the DNA molecular structure.

Chromosome Effect After a Double-Strand Break in the Same Rung of DNA.

As mentioned earlier, when two interactions (hits), one on each of the two sugar–phosphate chains, occur within the same rung of the

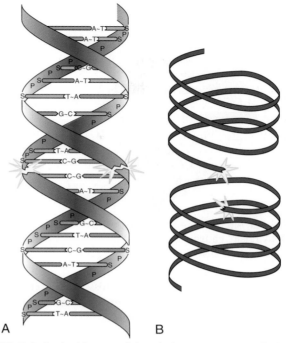

A   B

FIG 7.8 A double-strand break in same rung of the DNA molecular structure (A) causes complete chromosome breakage, resulting in a cleaved or broken chromosome (B).

DNA ladder-like configuration (see Fig. 7.8A), the result is a cleaved or broken chromosome (see Fig. 7.8B), with each new portion containing an unequal amount of genetic material. If this damaged chromosome divides, each new daughter cell will receive an incorrect amount of genetic material. This will culminate in either death or impaired functioning of the new daughter cell.

Mutation. Interactions of ionizing radiation with DNA molecules may cause the loss of or change in a nitrogenous base on the DNA chain. The direct consequence of this damage is an alteration of the base sequence (Fig. 7.9) within the DNA molecule. Because the genetic information to be passed on to future generations is contained in the strict sequence of these bases, the loss or change of a base in the DNA chain represents a mutation. It may not be reversible and may generate acute consequences for the cell, but, more important, if the cell remains viable, incorrect genetic information will be transferred to one of the two daughter cells when the cell divides.

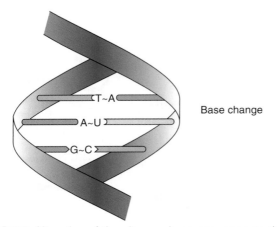

FIG 7.9 Alteration of the nitrogen base sequence on the DNA chain caused by the action of ionizing radiation directly on a DNA molecule.

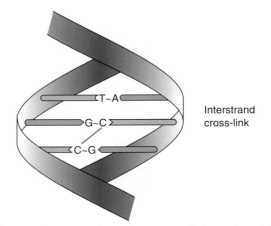

FIG 7.10 Interstrand covalent cross-link produced by high-LET radiation acting directly on a DNA molecule.

Covalent Cross-Links. Covalent cross-links are chemical unions created between atoms by the single sharing of one or more pairs of electrons. Covalent cross-links involving DNA comprise another effect directly initiated by high-LET radiation. With low-LET interactions, however, covalent cross-links are most likely caused by the process of indirect action. After irradiation, some molecules can fragment or change into small, spurlike molecules that become very interactive ("sticky") when they themselves are exposed to radiation. Such sticky molecules can facilitate cross-linking by attaching or connecting to other macromolecules or to other segments of the same macromolecule chain. Cross-linking can occur in many different patterns. For example, it can form between two places on the same DNA strand. This joining is termed an *intrastrand cross-link.* Cross-linking may also happen between complementary DNA strands (Fig. 7.10) or between entirely different DNA molecules. These joinings are termed *interstrand cross-links.* Finally, DNA molecules also may become covalently linked to a protein molecule.[4] All these linkages are potentially fatal to the cell if they are not properly repaired.

Effects of Ionizing Radiation on Chromosomes

Large-scale structural changes in a chromosome produced by ionizing radiation may be as grave for the cell as are radiation-induced changes in DNA. When changes occur in the DNA molecule, the chromosome exhibits the variation. Because DNA modifications are discrete, they do not inevitably result in observable structural chromosome revisions. However, if these discrete effects are numerous enough, such as may be brought about by exposure to very high-LET radiation, then an observable structural chromosome alteration is possible.

Radiation-Induced Chromosome Breaks. After irradiation and during cell division, some radiation-induced chromosome breaks may be viewed microscopically. These changes are manifested during the metaphase and anaphase of the cell division cycle, when the length of the chromosomes is visible. Because the events that precede these phases of cell division are not visible, they can only be assumed to have occurred. What can be seen, however, is the effect of these events—the gross or visible differences in the structure of the chromosome. Both somatic cells and reproductive cells are subject to chromosome breaks induced by radiation.

Chromosomal Fragments. After chromosome breakage, two or more chromosomal splinters are produced. Each of these has a fractured extremity. These broken ends are chemically very active and therefore have a strong tendency to adhere to another similar sticky end. The broken fragments can:
- Rejoin in their original configuration
- Fail to rejoin and create an aberration (lesion or anomaly)
- Join to other broken ends and thereby create new chromosomes that may not look structurally altered compared with the chromosome before irradiation

Chromosome Anomalies. Two types of chromosome anomalies have been observed at metaphase. They are called:

- Chromosome aberrations
- Chromatid aberrations

Chromosome aberrations result when irradiation occurs early in interphase, before DNA synthesis takes place. In this situation, the break caused by ionizing radiation is in a single strand of chromatin, which is the original chromosome. During the DNA synthesis that follows, the resultant break is replicated when this strand of chromatin lays down an identical strand adjacent to itself (called the *sister chromatid*) if repair is not complete before the start of DNA synthesis. This situation leads to a chromosome aberration in which both chromatids (the arms of the new chromosome) exhibit the break. The break is visible at the next mitosis. Each daughter cell generated will have inherited a damaged chromatid as a consequence of a failure in the repair mechanism. Solitary chromatid aberrations, conversely, result when irradiation of individual chromatids occurs later in interphase, after DNA synthesis has taken place. Then only one chromatid of the X-shaped pair may undergo a radiation-induced break. Therefore only one daughter cell is affected.

Summary of Structural Changes Caused by Ionizing Radiation. Ionizing radiation interacts randomly with matter, giving up energy in the process. Because of this energy transfer, exposure to radiation can lead to the occurrence of a variety of deleterious effects in biologic tissue, including the following in cell nuclei:

- A single-strand break in one chromosome
- A single-strand break in one chromatid
- A single-strand break in separate chromosomes
- A strand break in separate chromatids
- More than one break in the same chromosome
- More than one break in the same chromatid
- Chromosome stickiness, or clumping together

Consequences to the Cell From Structural Changes Within the Nucleus

1. *Restitution,* whereby the breaks rejoin in their original configuration with no visible damage (Fig. 7.11). In this case, no injury to the cell occurs because the chromatid has been restored to the condition it was in before irradiation. The process of healing by restitution is believed to be the way in which 95% of single-chromosome breaks mend.[4]
2. *Deletion,* whereby a part of the chromosome or chromatid is lost at the next cell division, thus creating

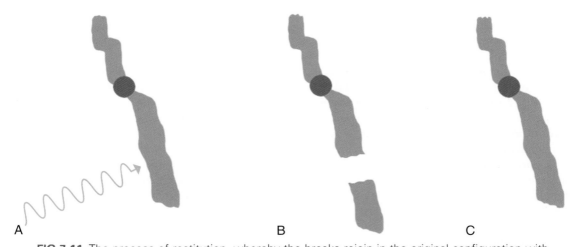

A   B   C

FIG 7.11 The process of restitution, whereby the breaks rejoin in the original configuration with no visible damage. (A) The chromatid (single-strand chromosome) break occurs because of a photon interaction. (B) The fragment is fully separated from the rest of the chromatid. This same type of damage could occur to a metaphase or X-shaped chromosome if S phase had already occurred. (C) The broken fragment has reattached in its original location through the action of repair enzymes.

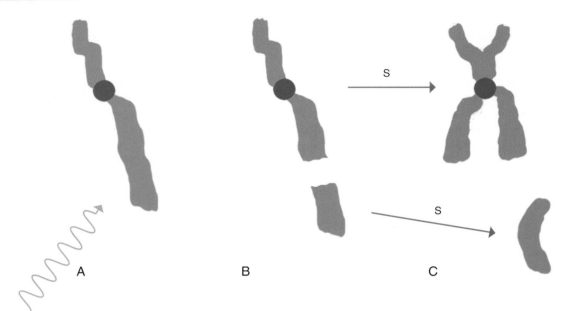

FIG 7.12 The process of deletion, in which part of a chromosome is lost at the next cell division, thus creating an acentric fragment. (A) The chromatid or single-strand chromosome break results from a photon interaction. (B) The fragment is fully separated from the rest of the chromatid. (C) After the next DNA synthesis phase of the cell cycle (labeled S), the remainder of the single-strand chromosome has been replicated normally but with fragments missing from the two arms of the metaphase chromosome. The replicated fragment is acentric, a section of genetic material without a centromere.

an aberration known as an *acentric fragment* (Fig. 7.12). This results in a cell mutation.

3. *Broken-end rearrangement,* whereby a grossly misshapen chromosome may be produced. Ring chromatids, dicentric chromosomes, and anaphase bridges are examples of such distorted chromosomes and chromatids (Fig. 7.13). This results in a cell mutation.

4. *Broken-end rearrangement without visible damage to the chromatids,* whereby the chromatid's genetic material has been rearranged even though the chromatid appears normal. Translocations are examples of such rearrangements (Fig. 7.14). This results in a cell mutation.

Changes such as those outlined in items 2, 3, and 4 inevitably result in mutation because the positions of the genes on the chromatids have been rearranged, thus altering the heritable characteristics of the cell.

Target Theory

The biologic effects of exposure to radiation stem primarily from the ionizations occurring at sensitive cellular points secondary to energy transfers from that radiation. These affected locations in a cell or, more specifically, on a vital molecule within the cell are known as *targets.* Whether or not such locations are struck by radiation is a random process. From all existing evidence, it appears that producing a serious effect usually requires more than one radiation "hit" on a specific target. The damage from a single hit normally is not conclusive because of repair mechanisms. This concept of radiation damage resulting from discrete and random events is known as target theory.

Amid the many different types of molecules that lie within the cell, a master, or key, molecule that maintains normal cell function is believed to be present (Fig. 7.15). This master molecule is necessary for the survival of the cell. Because this molecule is unique in any given cell, no similar molecules in the cell are available to replace it; if a critical location on the master molecule is a target receiving multiple hits from ionizing radiation, the master molecule may well be inactivated. Normal cell function will then cease, and the cell will die

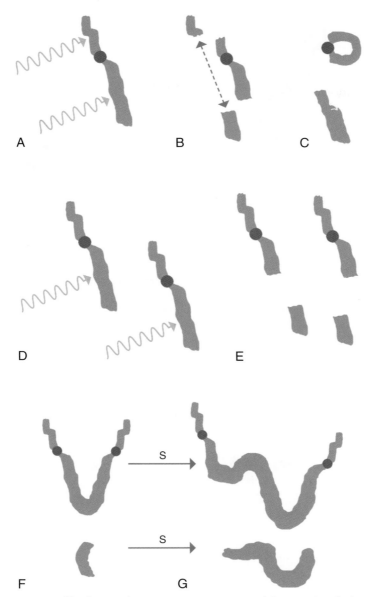

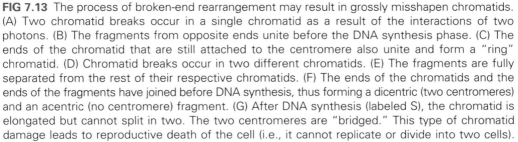

FIG 7.13 The process of broken-end rearrangement may result in grossly misshapen chromatids. (A) Two chromatid breaks occur in a single chromatid as a result of the interactions of two photons. (B) The fragments from opposite ends unite before the DNA synthesis phase. (C) The ends of the chromatid that are still attached to the centromere also unite and form a "ring" chromatid. (D) Chromatid breaks occur in two different chromatids. (E) The fragments are fully separated from the rest of their respective chromatids. (F) The ends of the chromatids and the ends of the fragments have joined before DNA synthesis, thus forming a dicentric (two centromeres) and an acentric (no centromere) fragment. (G) After DNA synthesis (labeled S), the chromatid is elongated but cannot split in two. The two centromeres are "bridged." This type of chromatid damage leads to reproductive death of the cell (i.e., it cannot replicate or divide into two cells).

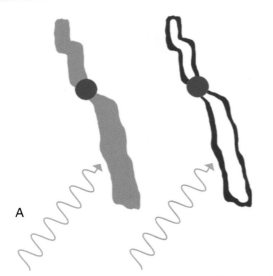
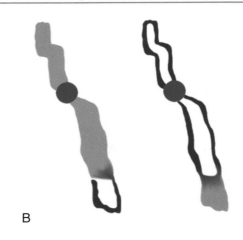

A

B

FIG 7.14 If radiation breaks off parts of two different chromatids that are near each other (A) then the broken parts may reattach to the wrong chromatids (B) resulting in no visible damage. However, this rearrangement of genetic material may drastically alter a cell's function and lead to cell death or failure to replicate. This same type of damage could occur to a chromosome if S phase had already occurred. In this case, the cell may divide, but the genetic material in the daughter cells is compromised and those cells may not function properly.

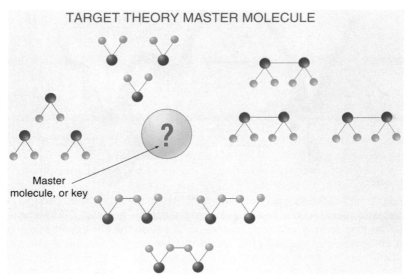

TARGET THEORY MASTER MOLECULE

Master
molecule, or key

FIG 7.15 A master, or key, molecule that maintains normal cell function is believed to be present in every cell. This molecule is vital to the survival of the cell and is presumed to be DNA. (From *Radiobiology and Radiation Protection: Mosby's Radiographic Instructional Series,* St. Louis, 1999, Mosby.)

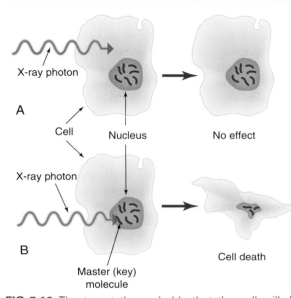

FIG 7.16 The target theory holds that the cell will die after exposure to ionizing radiation only if the master, or key, molecule (DNA) is inactivated in the process. (A) An x-ray photon passes through the cell without interacting with the master molecule, which is located in the cell's nucleus; no measurable effect results. (B) An x-ray photon enters the nucleus and interacts with and inactivates the master molecule; the cell dies as a result.

(Fig. 7.16). If, conversely, it receives only a single hit, then the master molecule most likely will still be operational. Experimental data strongly support this concept and indicate that DNA, as one might suspect, is the irreplaceable master, or key, molecule that serves as the preeminent vital target. Destruction of some other important large-scale molecules that are present in the cell does not normally result in cell death. The reason for this is simply that cells have a redundancy of similar molecules to take over and perform necessary functions in the event of the destruction of one or more of them. Consequently, if only a few non-DNA cell molecules are made dysfunctional by radiation exposure, the cell will probably not show any evidence of injury after irradiation.

In its passage through the molecular structure of living systems, radiation does not preferentially seek out master molecules in cells to destroy them; it interacts with these key molecules only by chance. The target theory concept then is useful for explaining cell death and nonfatal cell abnormalities caused by exposure to radiation.

Interactions between ionizing radiation and molecular targets such as DNA occur through both direct and indirect action. However, discerning which of the two types of effects or actions has been at work in any given case of cell death is virtually impossible.

EFFECTS OF IRRADIATION ON THE ENTIRE CELL

For the cell as a whole, damage to the cell's nucleus reveals itself in one of the following ways:
1. Instant death
2. Reproductive death
3. Apoptosis, or programmed cell death (interphase death)
4. Mitotic, or genetic, death
5. Mitotic delay
6. Interference with function

Instant Death

Instant death of large numbers of cells occurs when a volume is irradiated with an x-ray or gamma ray dose of approximately 1000 Gy_t in a period of seconds or a few minutes. This large influx of energy causes gross disruption of cellular form and structure and severe changes in chemical machinery. As a result of receiving such a massive dose of ionizing radiation, the cell's DNA macromolecule breaks up and cellular proteins coagulate. Radiation doses high enough to cause this type of damage are vastly greater than those used for diagnostic examinations or even standard therapeutic treatments.

Reproductive Death

Reproductive death generally results from exposure of cells to doses of ionizing radiation in the range of 1 to 10 Gy_t. Although the cell does not die when reproductive death occurs, it permanently loses its ability to procreate but continues to metabolize and to synthesize nucleic acids and proteins. The termination of the cell's reproductive abilities does, however, prevent the transmission of damage to future generations of cells.

Apoptosis

A nonmitotic, or nondivision, form of cell death that occurs when cells die without attempting division during the interphase portion of the cell life cycle is termed **apoptosis**, or programmed cell death. This was formerly called *interphase death*. Apoptosis occurs spontaneously in both normal tissue and in tumors. It can occur in human beings and other vertebrate animals and amphibians, both in the embryo and in the adult. An example of this process is the sequence of events during embryonic development whereby tadpoles lose their tails.

Certain types of *programmed cell death* are integral to the development and maintenance of organisms. Many types of cells are destined to die for the good of the organism. For example, human beings lose webbing between their digits during embryonic development, and all through life human skin cells die, are replenished, and maintain the protective outer coating we usually refer to as *skin*. In apoptosis the cell shrinks and produces tiny membrane-enclosed structures called *blebs*. The cell nucleus breaks up and then the cell itself breaks up, and its fragments are usually ingested by neighboring cells.

Researchers believe that apoptosis may be instigated by radiation under some circumstances. The mechanisms of apoptosis and its relationship with radiosensitivity are areas of active research in radiobiology. It appears that radiosensitivity of the individual cell governs the dose required to induce apoptosis; the more radiosensitive the cell is, the smaller the dose required to cause apoptotic death during interphase. For example, a few hundred centigray (cGy_t) can initiate apoptosis in very sensitive cells such as lymphocytes or spermatogonia, but for less radiosensitive cells, such as those in bone, it seems that apoptosis may require radiation doses of several thousand cGy_t. A new type of radiation therapy seeks to involve activation of the genes that regulate apoptosis so that the occurrence becomes much more likely after irradiation in a tumor. It should also be noted that the phenomenon of apoptosis is considered by many to be integrally related to the "ageing process."

Mitotic Death

Ionizing radiation can adversely affect cell division. It may retard the mitotic process or permanently inhibit it; cell death follows permanent inhibition. *Mitotic*, or *genetic*, *death* occurs when a cell dies after one or more divisions. Even relatively small doses of radiation have a possibility of causing this type of cell death. The radiation dose required to produce mitotic death is less than the dose needed to produce apoptosis in slowly dividing cells or nondividing cells.

Mitotic Delay

Exposing a cell to as little as 0.01 Gy_t of ionizing radiation just before it begins dividing can cause *mitotic delay*, the failure of the cell to start dividing on time. After this delay the cell may resume its normal mitotic function. The underlying cause of this phenomenon is not known. Possible reasons for the delay are as follows:
1. Alteration of a chemical involved in mitosis
2. Proteins required for cell division not being synthesized
3. A change in the rate of DNA synthesis after irradiation

Interference With Function

Permanent or temporary interference with cellular function independent of the cell's ability to divide can be brought about by exposure to ionizing radiation. If repair enzymes are able to fix the damage, the cell can recover and continue to properly function. Otherwise, the cell will be unable to reproduce or will die.

SURVIVAL CURVES FOR MAMMALIAN CELLS

Cells vary in their radiosensitivity. This fact is particularly important in determining the types of cancer cells that will respond to radiation therapy. A classic method of displaying the sensitivity of a particular type of cell to radiation is the **cell survival curve**.[5] A cell survival curve is constructed from data obtained by a series of experiments. First, the cells are made to grow "in culture," meaning in a laboratory environment such as a Petri dish. Then the cells are exposed to a specified dose of radiation. After radiation exposure, the ability of the cells to divide, or form new "colonies" of cells, is measured. The fraction of cells that are able to form new colonies through cell division is then reported as the fraction of cells that have survived irradiation. The process is repeated for a range of radiation doses, and the results are graphed with the logarithm* of the surviving fraction on the vertical axis and the dose on the horizontal axis.

Fig. 7.17 shows two cell survival curves, one for high-LET radiation and one for low-LET radiation. The curve for low-LET radiation shows very little change in survival at low doses, followed by a linear portion in which survival decreases in regular proportions at higher doses. This indicates that at low doses the cell is able to find and

---

*In the ordinary decimal counting system, the logarithm (log) of a number N is, by definition, the power to which 10 must be raised to give N (e.g., log 1000 = 3 because 10^3 = 1000). So using logarithm values as one axis of an x-y graph permits a convenient display of very wide-ranging (orders of magnitude) data values.

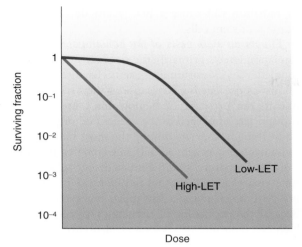

FIG 7.17 Cell survival curves for the same cell line irradiated with both low- and high-linear energy transfer (LET) radiation. With low-LET radiation, a "shoulder" to the curve at lower doses indicates the cell's ability to repair some damage at low doses. High-LET radiation typically has no shoulder, thus indicating that little or no repair takes place.

repair some of the damage. At higher doses the repair mechanism is overwhelmed. For the high-LET curve, no survival shoulder exists. If damage occurs, it is usually so extensive that it is irreparable.

CELL RADIOSENSITIVITY

Cell Maturity and Specialization

The human body is composed of different types of cells and tissues, which vary in their degree of radiosensitivity. Immature cells are nonspecialized (undifferentiated) and undergo rapid cell division, whereas more mature cells are specialized in their function (highly differentiated) and divide at a slower rate or do not divide. These factors affect the cells' degree of radiosensitivity. Examples of radiosensitive and radioinsensitive cells are listed in Box 7.4. Because combinations of both immature and mature cells in various ratios form the different body tissues and organs, radiosensitivity varies from one tissue and organ to another.

Oxygen Enhancement Effects

If oxygen is present when a tissue is irradiated, more free radicals will be formed in the tissue; this increases the indirect damage potential of the radiation.

During imaging procedures, fully oxygenated human tissues are exposed to x-radiation or gamma radiation. However, both radiographic and nuclear medicine procedures employ low doses of radiation that are also low LET. Consequently, very few cells are killed by the types of radiation used in these procedures.

In radiotherapy, the presence of oxygen plays a significant role in radiosensitivity and thereby treatment efficacy. When megavoltage x-radiation is used to treat certain types of cancerous tumors that are known to be oxygen depleted, high-pressure (hyperbaric) oxygen has sometimes been employed in conjunction with the radiation to increase tumor radiosensitivity. Cancerous tumors often contain both hypoxic cells, which lack an adequate amount of oxygen, and normally aerated cells. The poorly oxygenated cells severely inhibit the indirect mechanism of radiation interaction with cells and therefore are radioresistant (particularly to low-LET radiation); hence hypoxic cells are more difficult to destroy than normally oxygenated cells. However, when oxygen tensions in capillaries are increased by hyperbaric oxygenation, hypoxic cells may reoxygenate and become sensitive to radiation; consequently, the chances of their being destroyed by therapeutic radiation increase. Radiosensitization has also been accomplished with chemical-enhancing agents such as misonidazole.[3]

Law of Bergonié and Tribondeau

In 1906 Jean A. Bergonié, a French radiologist, and Louis F. A. Tribondeau, a French physician, observed the effects of ionizing radiation on testicular germ cells of rabbits they had exposed to x-rays. These researchers established that radiosensitivity was a function of the metabolic state of the cell receiving the exposure. Their findings eventually became known as the law of Bergonié and Tribondeau. It states that the radiosensitivity of cells is directly proportional to their reproductive activity and inversely proportional to their degree of differentiation. Thus the most pronounced radiation effects occur in cells with the least maturity and specialization or differentiation, the greatest reproductive activity, and the longest mitotic phases.[6] Although the law was originally applied only to germ cells, it is actually true for all types of cells in the human body. Consequently, within the realm of diagnostic imaging, the embryo-fetus, which contains a large number of immature, nonspecialized cells, is much more susceptible to radiation damage than is an adult or even a child. All imaging professionals should be ever mindful of this.

Effects of Ionizing Radiation on Human Cells and Tissues

As we have seen, the more mature and specialized in performing functions a cell is, the less sensitive it is to radiation. In the following sections, the radiation response of some of the most important cell groups is examined in detail.

Blood Cells

Hematologic depression. Ionizing radiation adversely affects blood cells by depressing the number of cells in the peripheral circulation. A whole-body dose of 0.25 Gy_t delivered within a few days produces a measurable hematologic depression. This dose by far exceeds normal doses sustained by the working population of the radiation industry. Therefore the use of blood count tests for purposes of dosimetry is not valid.

Depletion of immature blood cells. Most blood cells are manufactured in bone marrow. Radiation causes a decrease in the number of immature blood cells (stem or precursor) produced in bone marrow and hence a reduction, ultimately, in the number of mature blood cells in the bloodstream. The higher the radiation dose received by the bone marrow, the greater will be the severity of the resulting cell depletion.

Repopulation after a period of recovery. If the bone marrow cells have not been destroyed by exposure to ionizing radiation, they can repopulate after a period of recovery. The time necessary for recovery depends on the magnitude of the radiation dose received. If a relatively low dose (less than 1 Gy_t) of radiation is received, bone marrow repopulation occurs within weeks after irradiation. Moderate (1 to 10 Gy_t) to high (10 or more Gy_t) doses, which severely deplete the number of bone marrow cells, require a longer recovery period. Very high doses

of radiation can cause a permanent decrease in the number of stem cells.

Effects on stem cells of the hematopoietic system. Radiation affects primarily the stem cells of the hematopoietic (blood-forming) system. Erythrocytes, also known as *red blood cells* because of their reddish color due to the presence of hemoglobin*, are the main transporters of oxygen to the tissues and organs of the body. Initially, they are among the most radiosensitive of human cells. As with all cells, however, that transform from an immature, undifferentiated state to a mature, functional state, the mature red blood cells, which do not have a cell nucleus, are much less radiosensitive. Because the population of circulating red blood cells is high and their life span is long, depletion of red cells is not usually the cause of death in high-dose irradiation (i.e., several Gy_t delivered to the whole body). Death, if it occurs, is more typically caused by infection that cannot be overcome by the immune system because of the destruction of *myeloblasts* (an immature cell of bone marrow that is the most basic precursor of granulocyte** white blood cells) and internal hemorrhage resulting from destruction of megakaryoblasts (cells that are the ancestors of platelets***).

Whole-body doses in excess of 5 Gy_t. Human beings who receive whole-body doses in excess of 5 Gy_t may die within 30 to 60 days because of effects related to initial depletion of the stem cells of the hematopoietic system. The use of antibiotics or isolation from pathogens in the environment (e.g., placing the patient in a sterile environment, feeding only sterilized food) has been shown to

---

*Hemoglobin is the main functional component of the red blood cell. It serves as an oxygen-carrying protein. Iron is present within its molecular structure. Because an iron atom has a free valence electron, it can readily bind chemically with a molecule of oxygen. Thus the hemoglobin protein has an affinity for oxygen, which when achieved is expressed by the formation of an iron oxide combination. This creates the red color for which the cell is known.

**Granulocytes are cells that are so called because they have visible small grains called *granules* inside the cell. Granulocytes are a category of white blood cells that are essential in fighting infections.

***Platelets, also known as *thrombocytes*, are small cell fragments that originate in the bone marrow as pieces broken off from large cells. They circulate within our blood and when they recognize damaged blood vessels, clump together in large numbers at the damaged site, as a result causing a plug or blood clot.

TABLE 7.1 LD 50/30 Values for Various Species	
	LD 50/30
Species	**Gy$_t$**
Human being	3.0–4.0*
Monkey	4.0–4.75
Dog	3.0
Hamster	7.0
Rabbit	7.25
Rat	9.0
Turtle	15.0
Newt	30.0

*Depending on the source of the radiation exposure, LD 50/30 (dose that produces death in 50% of the subjects within 30 days) varies. LD 50/30 may be higher if medical intervention is available. For humans, LD 50/60 may be more realistic because humans are more likely to survive longer than 30 days after an acute whole-body exposure, especially if medical treatment is provided.

mitigate these effects in animals and humans. Humans, however, recover more slowly than do laboratory animals. The lethal dose in animals is usually specified as LD 50/30 (dose that produces death in 50% of the subjects within 30 days). The lethal dose in human beings is usually given as LD 50/60 because a human's recovery is slower than that of the laboratory animals, and death may still occur at a later time after a substantial whole-body exposure. Whether survival lasts for 30 days or 60 days, the lethal whole-body dose for humans is generally estimated to be 3.0 to 4.0 Gy$_t$ without treatment and higher if medical intervention is available. Table 7.1 presents an overview of LD 50/30 for various species.

Effects of ionizing radiation on lymphocytes. White blood cells are collectively called *leukocytes.* They include cells with and without the small grains known as *granules.* Lymphocytes belong to the granule-free category and are of major importance in defending the body against foreign objects (antigens) by producing protective proteins (antibodies) to combat disease. Lymphocytes, which live for only approximately 24 hours, have the shortest life span of all the blood cells. They are manufactured in bone marrow and are the most radiosensitive blood cells in the human body. A radiation dose as low as 0.25 Gy$_t$ is sufficient to noticeably depress the number of such cells present in the circulating blood. When significant numbers of lymphocytes are damaged by radiation exposure, the body loses its natural ability to combat

infection and becomes very susceptible to bacterial and viral antigens.

The normal white blood cell count for an adult ranges from 5000 to 10,000/mm^3 of blood. At this dose level of 0.25 Gy$_t$ or less, complete blood cell recovery occurs shortly after irradiation. However, when a higher dose range of whole-body radiation (0.5 to 1 Gy$_t$) is received, the lymphocyte count decreases to zero within a few days. Full recovery generally requires a period of several months after this level of exposure. During that period the body is highly susceptible to antigens.

Effects of ionizing radiation on neutrophils. Neutrophils, another kind of white blood cell but belonging to the granule-containing category, also play an important role in fighting infection. A dose of 0.5 Gy$_t$ of ionizing radiation will noticeably reduce the number of neutrophils present in the circulating blood, making a person susceptible to infection. When larger doses of radiation (2 to 5 Gy$_t$), however, are received, these cells decrease in number to 10% or less within a few weeks of irradiation with a consequently high potential for serious infection. In this latter situation, it will require several months after the exposure until the number of neutrophils present in the blood returns to its original value.

Effects of ionizing radiation on thrombocytes (platelets). Thrombocytes, or platelets, initiate blood clotting and prevent hemorrhage. They have a life span of approximately 30 days. The normal platelet count in the human adult ranges from 150,000 to 350,000/mm^3 of blood. A dose of radiation greater than 0.5 Gy$_t$ lessens the number of platelets in the circulating blood, but when exposed to radiation in the range of 1 to 10 Gy$_t$, these cells may become significantly depleted and begin to regain their original numbers only approximately 2 months after being irradiated. During this period wound clotting will be highly compromised.

Radiation exposure during diagnostic imaging procedures. Neither the blood nor the blood-forming organs of patients should undergo appreciable damage from radiation exposure received during diagnostic imaging procedures. However, numerous studies indicate some chromosome aberrations in circulating lymphocytes that have received radiation doses within the diagnostic radiology range. Prime candidates for developing such aberrations are patients either for whom high-level fluoroscopy was employed or for whom very long fluoroscopic exposure times occurred (e.g., cardiac catheterization and other specialized invasive procedures).

Monitoring of patients undergoing radiation therapy treatment. A therapeutic dose of ionizing radiation, especially doses delivered to locations that include blood-forming organs, decreases the blood count. Consequently, patients who are undergoing radiation therapy treatment are monitored frequently (in the form of weekly or biweekly complete blood counts, also known as *CBCs*) to determine whether all of their blood constituent counts are adequate.

Occupational radiation exposure monitoring. As previously discussed, a periodic blood count is not recommended as a method for monitoring occupational radiation exposure because biologic damage has already been sustained when an irregularity is seen in the blood count. In addition, a blood count is a relatively insensitive test that is unable to indicate doses of less than 10 cGy$_t$. State-of-the-art optically stimulated luminescence (OSL) dosimeters detect effective radiation doses in the microsievert range and therefore may be used to reveal potentially hazardous working conditions before actual harm occurs.

Epithelial Tissue. Epithelial tissue lines and covers body tissue. The cells of these tissues lie close together, with few or no substances between them. Epithelial tissue is devoid of blood vessels, and it regenerates through the process of mitosis. The cells are found in the lining of the intestines, the mucous lining of the respiratory tract, the pulmonary alveoli, and the lining of blood and lymphatic vessels. Because the body constantly regenerates epithelial tissue, the cells that comprise this tissue are highly radiosensitive.

Muscle Tissue. Muscle tissue contains fibers that affect movement of an organ or part of the body. Since muscle tissue cells are highly specialized and do not divide, they are relatively insensitive to radiation.

Nervous Tissue. Nervous tissue (conductive tissue) is found in the brain and spinal cord. A nerve cell (neuron) (Fig. 7.18) consists of a cell body, which contains its nucleus, and two kinds of stringlike tissue segments, called *processes,* that extend outward from the cell body, namely *dendrites* (fine tentacle-like extensions that carry impulses toward the cell) and the *axon* (a broad, long, tentacle that carries impulses away from it). Nerve cells relay messages to and from the brain. A message enters the nerve cell through the dendrites. It passes through the

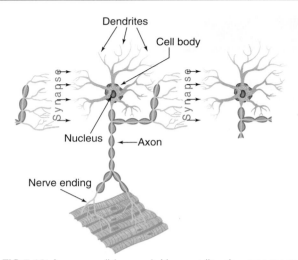

FIG 7.18 A nerve cell (neuron). Nerve cells relay messages to and from the brain. A message enters a nerve cell through its dendrites, passes through the cell body, and exits the cell through the axon, which transmits the message across a synapse, the communication area leading to the next nerve cell in the chain.

cell body and exits the cell through the axon, which transmits the message across a *synapse*, the communicating area leading to the next nerve cell in the chain.

Nerve tissue in the human adult. In the adult, nerve cells are highly specialized. They perform specific functions for the body and, similar to muscle cells, do not divide. Nerve cells contain a nucleus. If the nucleus of one of these cells is destroyed, the cell dies and is never restored. If the cell nucleus has been damaged but not destroyed by exposure to radiation, the damaged nerve cell may still be able to function but in an impaired fashion. Radiation also can produce temporary or permanent damage in a nerve's processes (dendrites and axon). When this occurs, communication with and control of some areas of the body may be disrupted. Whole-body exposure to very high doses of radiation causes severe damage to the central nervous system (CNS). A single exposure amounting to a dose in excess of 50 Gy$_t$ of ionizing radiation may lead to death within a few hours or days.

Nerve tissue in the embryo-fetus. Developing nerve cells in the embryo-fetus are more radiosensitive than are the mature nerve cells of the adult. Irradiation of the embryo can lead to CNS anomalies, microcephaly (small head circumference), and intellectual disability. Study of the Japanese atomic bomb survivors provides strong evidence of a "window of maximal sensitivity" extending from 8 to 15 weeks after gestation. This time span covers the end of *neuron organogenesis* (a period of development and change of the nerve cells) into the beginning of the fetal period. After this a lower level of elevated risk remains until week 25, at which time the risk is not found to be significantly different from that of young adults. During the window of maximal sensitivity, a 0.1-Sv fetal EqD is associated with as much as a 4% chance of intellectual disability. This level is considered significant compared with risks during a normal pregnancy. Therefore special consideration is given to the irradiation of the abdomen or pelvis of a pregnant patient, particularly during the period of greatest sensitivity. The fetal EqD associated with abdominal fluoroscopy, however, is generally about 0.05 Sv. Thus if the referring physician and radiologist believe that the diagnostic imaging procedure is vital to the medical management of the mother or embryo-fetus, the risk associated with the needed radiation exposure may be justified. For such a situation a genetic study might be recommended afterwards.

Reproductive Cells

Spermatogonia. Human reproductive cells (germ cells) are relatively radiosensitive, although the exact responses of male and female germ cells to ionizing radiation vary because their processes of development from immature to mature status differ. The male testes contain both mature and immature spermatogonia. Because the developed spermatogonia are specialized and do not divide, they are relatively insensitive to ionizing radiation. The "young" spermatogonia, however, are unspecialized and divide rapidly, and therefore these germ cells are extremely radiosensitive. A radiation dose of 2 Gy_t may cause temporary sterility for as long as 12 months, and a dose of 5 or 6 Gy_t can cause permanent sterility. Even small doses of ionizing radiation (doses as low as 0.1 Gy_t) could depress the male sperm population. Male reproductive cells that have been exposed to a radiation dose of 0.1 Gy_t or more may cause genetic mutations in future generations. To prevent mutations from being passed on to children, male patients receiving this level of testicular radiation dose should refrain from unprotected sex for a few months after such an exposure. By that time, cells that were irradiated during their most sensitive stages will have matured and disappeared. It is

highly unlikely that germ cells of patients undergoing diagnostic imaging procedures would ever receive doses of 0.1 Gy_t, and radiographers working under normal occupational conditions would never receive a gonadal dose of this level.

Ova. The ova, the mature female germ cells, do not divide constantly. After puberty, one of the two ovaries expels a mature ovum approximately every 28 to 36 days (the exact number of days varies among women). During the reproductive life of a woman (from approximately 12 to 50 years old), 400 to 500 mature ova are produced. Radiosensitivity of ova varies considerably throughout the lifetime of the germ cell. Immature ova are very radiosensitive, whereas more mature ova have little radiosensitivity. After irradiation, a mature ovum can still unite with a male germ cell during conception. However, these irradiated cells may contain damaged chromosomes. If fertilization of an ovum with damaged chromosomes occurs, hereditary damage can be passed on to the child, potentially resulting in congenital abnormalities. In general, whenever chromosomes in male or female germ cells are damaged by exposure to ionizing radiation, it is possible for mutations to be passed on to succeeding generations. Even low doses received from diagnostic imaging procedures could cause some chromosomal damage. For this reason, the reproductive organs should be shielded whenever possible.

Exposure to ionizing radiation also may cause female sterility. The dose necessary to produce this depends partly on the age of the patient. Sterility occurs when radiation exposure destroys new and/or mature ova. The ovaries of the female fetus and those of a young child are very radiosensitive because they contain a large number of stem cells (oogonia) and immature cells (oocytes). As the female child matures from birth to puberty, the number of immature cells (oocytes) decreases. Therefore the ovaries become less radiosensitive. This decrease continues up to the age of 30 years; women between the ages of 20 and 30 years exhibit the lowest level of sensitivity. After a woman reaches age 30 years, the overall sensitivity of the ovaries increases constantly until menopause because the new ova being destroyed are not replenished.[7-9] Because the ovaries of a younger woman are less sensitive overall than the ovaries of an older woman, a higher dose of radiation is required to cause sterility in the younger woman.

Temporary sterility usually results from a single radiation dose of 2 Gy_t to the ovaries. If the radiation dose is fractionated (i.e., given as a combination of smaller doses with time between doses) over a period of several weeks, thus permitting the cells to repair some of the damage, doses as high as 20 Gy$_t$ may be tolerated.[10,11] A single dose of 5 Gy$_t$ generally causes permanent sterility in mature women. Even small doses of ionizing radiation (doses as low as 0.1 Gy$_t$) could cause menstrual irregularities such as delay or suppression of menstruation. Although some evidence suggests that immature ova are capable of repairing radiation damage, women who have received 0.1 Gy$_t$ or more are sometimes advised to postpone attempting conception for 30 days or more to allow the damaged immature ova to be expelled. Because all the ova a woman will ever possess are present from birth until the time they are fertilized or expelled, the best solution is to avoid substantial exposures in the first place.

SUMMARY

- Linear energy transfer (LET)
  - LET is the average energy deposited per unit length of track by ionizing radiation as it passes through and interacts with a medium along its path.
    - It is described in units of keV per micron (1 micron [μm] =10^{-6} m).
  - The LET value of the radiation involved is a very important factor in assessing potential tissue and organ damage from exposure to that type of ionizing radiation.
  - Because of a property known as *wave-particle duality,* x-rays and gamma rays can also be referred to as a stream of particles called *photons.*
  - Low-LET radiation (x-rays and gamma rays) doses that are not excessive mainly cause indirect damage to biologic tissues that usually can be reversed by repair enzymes.
  - High-LET radiation (alpha particles, ions of heavy nuclei, and low-energy neutrons) can produce irreparable damage to DNA because of inducing multiple-strand breaks that cannot be undone by repair enzymes.
- Relative biologic effectiveness (RBE)
  - RBE of the type of radiation being used is the ratio of the dose of a reference radiation (conventionally 250-kVp x-rays) to the dose of radiation of the type in question that is necessary to produce the same biologic reaction in a given experiment.

The reaction is what is produced by a dose of test radiation delivered under the same conditions.
  - As the LET of radiation increases, so do biologic effects; RBE quantitatively describes this relative effect.
  - RBE describes the relative capabilities of radiation with differing LETs to produce a particular biologic reaction.
  - The concept of RBE is not practical for specifying radiation protection dose levels in humans. Therefore to overcome this limitation, a radiation weighting factor (W$_R$) is used to calculate the equivalent dose (EqD) to determine the ability of a dose of any kind of ionizing radiation to cause biologic damage.
- Oxygen enhancement ratio (OER)
  - OER is a comparative measure used to obtain the amount of cellular injury for a species of ionizing radiation. It is the ratio of the radiation dose required to cause a particular biologic response of cells or organisms in an oxygen-deprived environment to the radiation dose required to cause an identical response under normal oxygenated conditions.
- Radiation-induced biologic damage in living systems is observed on molecular, cellular, and organic systems levels.
- Radiation action on the cell is either direct or indirect, depending on the site of interaction.
  - If sufficient quantities of somatic cells are affected by exposure to ionizing radiation, entire body processes can be disrupted. Conversely, if radiation damages the germ cells, the damage may be passed on to future generations in the form of genetic mutations.
  - Action is direct when biologic damage occurs as a result of the ionization of atoms on essential molecules (e.g., DNA, RNA, proteins, enzymes) produced by straight interaction with the incident radiation.
  - Action is indirect when effects are produced by reactive free radicals created by the interaction of radiation with water molecules; these unstable, highly reactive molecules can cause substantial disruption to molecules such as DNA and result in cell death.
  - High-LET radiation is more likely to cause biologic damage through direct action than is low-LET radiation.

- Because the human body is 80% water and less than 1% DNA, essentially all effects of low-LET irradiation in living cells result from indirect action.
- Point lesions commonly occur with low-LET radiation and are often reversible through the action of repair enzymes.
- Double-strand breaks of DNA happen more commonly with densely ionizing (high-LET) radiation and often are associated with the loss of one or more nitrogenous bases. Chance of repair from this type of damage is very low; the possibility of a lethal alteration of nitrogenous bases within the genetic sequence is far greater.
- When two interactions, one on each of the two sugar–phosphate chains, occur within the same rung of the DNA ladder-like configuration, the result is a cleaved or broken chromosome, with each new portion containing an unequal amount of genetic material. If this damaged chromosome divides, each new daughter cell will receive an incorrect amount of genetic material, resulting in either death or impaired functioning of the new daughter cell.
- Because the genetic information to be passed on to future generations is contained in the strict sequence of nitrogenous bases, the loss or change of a base in the DNA chain represents a mutation.
- Chromosome aberrations and chromatid aberrations are two types of chromosome anomalies that have been observed at metaphase.
- Consequences to the cell from structural changes within the nucleus can result in restitution, deletion, broken-end rearrangement, or broken-end rearrangement without visible damage to the chromatids. The last three types of consequences result in mutation because the position of the genes on the chromatids have been rearranged, thus altering the heritable characteristics of the cell.
- Target theory states that when cell DNA is directly or indirectly inactivated by exposure to radiation, the cell will die.
- When a cell nucleus is significantly damaged by exposure to ionizing radiation, the cell can die or experience reproductive death, apoptosis, mitotic death, mitotic delay, or interference with function.
- The cell survival curve is used to display the radiosensitivity of a particular type of cell, which helps determine the types of cancer cells that will respond to radiation therapy.
- The human body is composed of different types of cells and tissues, which vary in their degree of radiosensitivity.
- The law of Bergonié and Tribondeau states that the most pronounced radiation effects occur in cells with the least maturity and specialization or differentiation, the greatest reproductive activity, and the longest mitotic phases.
- The embryo-fetus is very susceptible to radiation damage, which can cause CNS anomalies, microcephaly, and intellectual disability.
- Lymphocytes are the most radiosensitive blood cells, and when they are damaged the body loses its natural ability to combat infection and becomes more susceptible to bacterial and viral antigens.
- Neither the blood nor the blood-forming organs of patients should undergo appreciable damage from radiation exposure received during diagnostic imaging procedures, but several studies have indicated some chromosome aberrations in circulating lymphocytes that have received radiation doses within the diagnostic radiology range. X-ray procedures responsible for these aberrations include high-level fluoroscopy or fluoroscopy with long exposure time such as cardiac catheterization and other specialized invasive procedures.
- Because the body constantly regenerates epithelial tissue, the cells comprising this tissue are highly radiosensitive.
- Muscle tissue is relatively insensitive to radiation.
- Nerve cells in the adult are highly specialized. If the cell nucleus has been damaged but not destroyed by exposure to radiation, the damaged nerve cell may still be able to function but in an impaired fashion. Radiation can cause temporary or permanent damage to a nerve's processes, thus disrupting communication with and control of some body areas.
- Developing nerve cells in the embryo-fetus are more radiosensitive than are the mature nerve cells of the adult. Studies indicate that the eighth to the fifteenth week after gestation is the time frame of maximal radiosensitivity. A lower but still significant level of risk remains until the twenty-fifth week after gestation.
- Human germ cells are relatively radiosensitive, although the exact responses of male and female

germ cells to ionizing radiation differ because their courses of development from immature to mature status differ. For both males and females, temporary sterilization occurs at 2 Gy_t, and permanent sterilization occurs at 5 to 6 Gy_t.

REFERENCES

1. Bushong SC: *Radiologic science for technologists: physics, biology and protection*, ed 10, St. Louis, 2013, Elsevier.
2. Forshier S: *Essentials of radiation biology and protection*, Albany, NY, 2002, Delmar.
3. Hall EJ: *Radiobiology for the radiologist*, ed 5, Philadelphia, 2000, Lippincott Williams & Wilkins.
4. Travis EL: *Primer of medical radiobiology*, ed 2, Chicago, 1989, Year Book.
5. Puck TT, Marcus PI: Action of x-rays on mammalian cells. *J Exp Med* 103:653, 1956.
6. Bergonié J, Tribondeau L: De quelques résultats de la radiothérapie et assai de fixation d'une technique rationelle. *CR Acad Sci (Paris)* 143:983, 1906.
7. United Nations Scientific Committee on the Effects of Atomic Radiation (UNSCEAR): Ionizing radiation sources and biologic effects, Report E.82.IX.8. New York, 1992, United Nations.
8. International Commission on Radiological Protection (ICRP): Non-stochastic effects of ionizing radiation, ICRP Publication No. 41. Oxford, 1984, Pergamon.
9. Upton AR: Cancer induction and non-stochastic effects. *Br J Radiol* 60:1, 1987.
10. Lushbaugh CC, Ricks RC: Some cytokinetic and histopathologic consideration of irradiated male and female gonadal tissue. In Vath JM, editor: *Frontiers of radiation therapy and oncology* (vol 6). Basel, 1972, Karger.
11. Lushbaugh CC, Casarett GW: The effects of gonadal irradiation in clinical radiation therapy: a review. *Cancer* 37:1111, 1976.

GENERAL DISCUSSION QUESTIONS

1. Why is it necessary for persons who administer radiation to humans for medical purposes to have a basic understanding of cell structure, composition, and function, as well as the adverse effects of ionizing radiation on these entities?
2. What will an ionized atom of biologic tissue not be able to do?
3. Why is the LET value of the radiation involved a very important factor in assessing potential tissue and organ damage from exposure to that type of ionizing radiation?
4. Why is high-LET radiation more destructive to biologic matter than low-LET radiation?
5. Why is the concept of relative biologic effectiveness (RBE) alone not practical for specifying radiation protection dose levels in humans?
6. Why does the presence of oxygen in biologic tissue make the damage produced in that tissue by free radicals nonrestorable?
7. What consequences can occur if ionizing radiation damages germ (reproductive) cells?
8. How can ionizing radiation interact with a DNA macromolecule and create a point lesion?
9. Why is the embryo-fetus more susceptible to radiation damage than either the child or the adult?
10. Why is LD 50/60 a more accurate way to assess lethal dose for humans than LD 50/30?
11. Why is a periodic blood count test not recommended for monitoring radiation exposure?
12. Why can x-rays and gamma rays also be referred to as a stream of particles called *photons*?

REVIEW QUESTIONS

1. For radiation protection, high-LET radiation is of *greatest* concern when internal contamination is possible, that is, when a radionuclide has been implanted, ingested, injected, or inhaled because:
   A. Only single-strand breaks in DNA are possible
   B. Then the potential exists for reparable damage of single-strand breaks in DNA
   C. Then the potential exists for irreparable damage because multiple-strand breaks in DNA are possible.
   D. Then the potential exists for reparable damage in DNA resulting from multiple-strand breaks
2. Free radicals behave as an extremely reactive single entity as a result of the presence of:
   A. Paired valence electrons
   B. Unpaired valence electrons
   C. Paired neutrons and protons
   D. Unpaired neutrons and protons
3. Which of the following are classified as high-LET radiation?

  1. Alpha particles
  2. Gamma rays
  3. X-rays
  A. 1 only
  B. 2 only
  C. 3 only
  D. 1, 2, and 3

4. A biologic reaction is produced by 3 Gy_t of a test radiation. It takes 12 Gy_t of 250-kVp x-radiation to produce the same biologic reaction. What is the relative biologic effectiveness (RBE) of the test radiation?
  A. 2.5
  B. 3
  C. 4
  D. 8

5. Which action of ionizing radiation is *most* harmful to the human body?
  A. Direct action
  B. Indirect action
  C. Epidemiologic action
  D. Linear-quadratic action

6. Which molecules in the human body are most commonly directly acted on by ionizing radiation to produce molecular damage through an indirect action?
  A. Protein
  B. Carbohydrate
  C. Fat
  D. Water

7. When does ionizing radiation cause complete chromosome breakage?
  A. When a single strand of the sugar–phosphate chain sustains a direct hit
  B. When two direct hits occur in the same rung of the DNA macromolecule
  C. When two direct hits occur in different rungs of the DNA macromolecule
  D. When two direct hits are sustained at opposite ends of the DNA macromolecule

8. When significant numbers of lymphocytes are damaged by exposure from ionizing radiation, the body:
  1. Loses its natural ability to combat infection
  2. Becomes more susceptible to bacteria
  3. Becomes more susceptible to viral antigens
  A. 1 and 2 only
  B. 1 and 3 only
  C. 2 and 3 only
  D. 1, 2, and 3

9. With respect to the law of Bergonié and Tribondeau, which of the following would *best* complete this statement? "The most pronounced radiation effects occur in cells with the _____."
  A. Least reproductive activity, shortest mitotic phases, and most maturity and specialization or differentiation
  B. Greatest reproductive activity, shortest mitotic phases, and most maturity and specialization or differentiation
  C. Greatest reproductive activity, longest mitotic phases, and least maturity and specialization or differentiation
  D. Least reproductive activity, shortest mitotic phases, and least maturity and specialization or differentiation

10. What do basal cells of the skin, intestinal crypt cells, and reproductive cells have in common?
  A. All cells are hypoxic.
  B. All cells are premalignant.
  C. All cells are radioinsensitive.
  D. All cells are radiosensitive.

8

Early Tissue Reactions and Their Effects on Organ Systems

OBJECTIVES

After completing this chapter, the reader will be able to perform the following:

- Define all key terms.
- Identify what early tissue reactions depend upon and the time frames in which these reactions appear.
- List and describe several possible high-dose consequences of ionizing radiation on living systems.
- Describe acute radiation syndrome (ARS), and list three separate dose-related syndromes that occur as part of this total-body condition.
- Identify and describe the four major response stages of ARS.
- Explain why cells that are exposed to sublethal doses of ionizing radiation recover after irradiation, and discuss the cumulative effect that exists after repeated radiation injuries.
- Describe local tissue damage that occurs when any part of the human body receives high radiation exposure.
- List three factors on which organ and tissue responses to radiation exposure depend.
- Describe radiation-induced skin damage from a historical perspective.
- Differentiate among the three layers of human skin, and identify other related accessory structures.

- State the single absorbed dose of ionizing radiation that can cause radiation-induced skin erythema within 24 to 48 hours after irradiation, and describe how this dose first manifests.
- Explain the difference between moderate and large radiation doses with regard to epilation.
- State the energy range of grenz rays, and give a historical example of their use in treating disease.
- Discuss the concept of orthovoltage radiation therapy treatment, and identify how this radiation energy range affects human skin.
- Discuss the impact on human skin when high-level fluoroscopy is used for extended periods of time during cardiovascular or therapeutic interventional procedures.
- Define cytogenetics, and explain how cytogenetic analysis of chromosomes may be accomplished.
- Explain the process of karyotyping, and identify the phase of cell division in which chromosome damage caused by radiation exposure can be evaluated.
- List two types of chromosomal aberrations that can be caused by exposure to ionizing radiation, and explain what determines the rate of production of these aberrations.

CHAPTER OUTLINE

Somatic and Genetic Effects
Somatic Effects
    Early Tissue Reactions
    Lethal Dose
    Repair and Recovery

Local Tissue Damage
Effects on the Skin
Effects on the Reproductive
    System

Hematologic Effects
Cytogenetic Effects
Summary

KEY TERMS

acute radiation syndrome (ARS)	genetic mutations	prodromal stage
biologic dosimetry	grenz rays	radiodermatitis
cytogenetics	karyotype	recovery
desquamation	latent period	somatic effects
early tissue reactions	manifest illness	somatic tissue reactions
epilation	metaphase	
genetic effects	pluripotential stem cell	

When biologic effects of radiation occur relatively soon after humans receive high doses of ionizing radiation, the biologic responses demonstrated are called *early effects.* Numerous laboratory animal studies and data from observation of some irradiated human populations provide substantial evidence of the consequences of such responses. Although early tissue reactions are not common in diagnostic imaging, they are discussed in this chapter to provide the reader with a broader and more complete understanding of the impact of high radiation exposure on the human body.

SOMATIC AND GENETIC EFFECTS

The term *somatic* comes from the Greek "soma" meaning "body." So, somatic effects are effects upon the body that was irradiated. Genetic effects are effects upon future generations due to irradiation of germ cells in previous generations.

SOMATIC EFFECTS

Depending on the length of time from the moment of irradiation to the first appearance of symptoms of radiation damage, somatic effects are classified as either:

1. Early
2. Late

This chapter discusses *early* somatic radiation effects on organ systems. If the consequences include cell killing and are directly related to the dose received, they are termed somatic tissue reactions. As the radiation dose increases, the severity of early somatic tissue reactions also increases. These results have a threshold, a point at which they begin to appear and below which they are absent (Fig. 8.1). The amount of biologic damage depends on the actual absorbed dose of ionizing radiation.

Early Tissue Reactions

Early tissue reactions vary depending on the duration of time after exposure to ionizing radiation. Subject to their nature, they may appear within:

- Minutes
- Hours
- Days
- Weeks

A substantial dose of ionizing radiation is required to produce biologic changes very soon after irradiation, and the severity of these changes is dose related. Early tissue reactions are precipitated by cell death.

With the exception of certain lengthy high–dose-rate fluoroscopic procedures, diagnostic imaging examinations do not normally impose radiation doses sufficient to cause early tissue reactions. Therefore they are of little concern in this modality. It should be noted, however, that prolonged exposure to x-rays in the diagnostic energy range results in a high radiation dose to the skin, whereas underlying tissues receive a substantially lower dose. Therefore unacceptably high x-ray exposures in radiology result primarily in skin effects, which are discussed later in this chapter. For completeness of knowledge of radiobiology, radiographers are also expected to understand the consequences of large doses to the whole body as would result from exposure to types of radiation other than x-rays.

Possible high radiation dose consequences include:

- Nausea
- Fatigue
- Erythema (diffuse redness over an area of skin after irradiation) (Fig. 8.2)
- Epilation (loss of hair)
- Blood disorders
- Intestinal disorders
- Fever

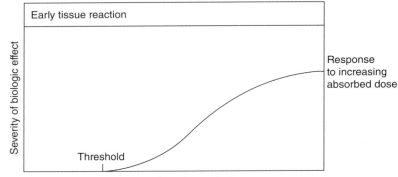

FIG 8.1 This graph demonstrates the existence of a threshold whereby early tissue reactions of an absorbed dose of ionizing radiation begin and increase in severity as the dose of radiation received increases.

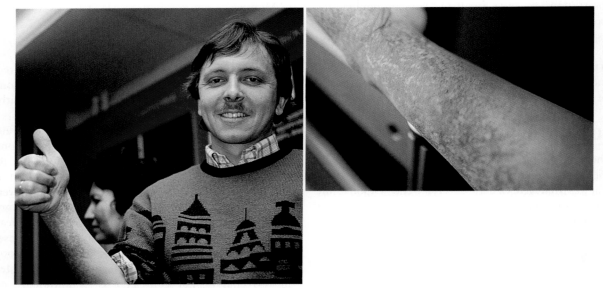

FIG 8.2 Radiation burn or erythema on the arm of a former worker who was present at the Chernobyl nuclear power plant during the 1986 radiation accident. (From Ken Graham Photography.)

- Dry and moist desquamation (shedding of the outer layer of skin) (Fig. 8.3)
- Depressed sperm count in the male
- Temporary or permanent sterility in the male and female
- Injury to the central nervous system (at extremely high radiation doses)

The various types of organic damage may be related to the cellular effects discussed in Chapter 7. For example, intestinal disorders are caused by damage to the sensitive epithelial tissue lining the intestines (Fig. 8.4). When the whole body is exposed to a dose of 6 Gy_t of ionizing radiation, many of these manifestations of organic damage occur soon thereafter and in succession. These early tissue reactions are called acute radiation syndrome (ARS).

Acute Radiation Syndrome (ARS). ARS, or radiation sickness, occurs in humans after whole-body reception of large doses of ionizing radiation delivered over a short period (from several hours to a few days). Data from epidemiologic studies of human populations exposed to

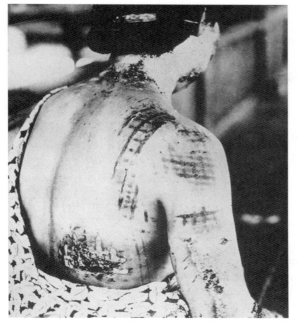

FIG 8.3 Dry and moist desquamation. The back of this female Japanese atomic bomb survivor demonstrates the pattern of the kimono she was wearing at the time of the bombing. Radiation burns resulting in the shedding of the outer layer of skin are visible. (From PhotoAssist, Inc.)

doses of ionizing radiation sufficient to cause this syndrome have been obtained from:

- Atomic bomb survivors of Hiroshima and Nagasaki
- Marshall Islanders who were inadvertently subjected to high levels of fallout during an atomic bomb test in 1954
- Nuclear radiation accident victims, such as those injured in the 1986 Chernobyl disaster
- Patients who have undergone radiation therapy

Symptoms of acute radiation syndrome. Syndrome is the medical term that defines a collection of symptoms. Thus ARS is a collection of symptoms associated with high-level radiation exposure. Three separate dose-related syndromes or conditions occur as part of the total-body syndrome:

- Hematopoietic syndrome
- Gastrointestinal syndrome
- Cerebrovascular syndrome

Hematopoietic syndrome. The hematopoietic form of ARS, or "bone marrow syndrome," occurs when people receive whole-body doses of ionizing radiation ranging from 1 to 10 Gy_t (Fig. 8.5). The hematopoietic system manufactures the corpuscular elements of the blood and is the most radiosensitive vital organ system in humans. Radiation exposure causes the number of red blood cells, white blood cells, and platelets in the circulating blood to decrease. Dose levels that produce this syndrome also may damage cells in other organ systems and cause the affected organ or organ system to fail.

For persons with hematopoietic syndrome, survival time shortens as the radiation dose increases. Because additional bone marrow cells are being destroyed, the body becomes more susceptible to infection (mostly from its own intestinal bacteria) and more prone to hemorrhage. When death occurs, it is because of excessive bone marrow destruction causing anemia and little or no resistance to severe infection.

Death may occur 6 to 8 weeks after irradiation in some very sensitive human subjects who receive a whole-body dose just exceeding 2 Gy_t. But as the whole-body dose increases from 2 to 10 Gy_t, all irradiated individuals will die and in a shorter period. If the radiation exposure is, however, in the range of 1 to 2 Gy_t, bone marrow cells will eventually repopulate to a level adequate to support life in most individuals. Many of these people recover 3 weeks to 6 months after irradiation. The irradiated person's general state of health at the time of irradiation strongly influences the possibility of recovery.

Survival probability of patients with hematopoietic syndrome is enhanced by intense supportive care and special hematologic procedures. As an illustration, victims who received doses in excess of 5 Gy_t, such as those of the nuclear power station accident in Chernobyl, benefited from bone marrow transplants from appropriate histocompatible donors. During the operation, hematopoietic stem cells are transplanted to facilitate bone marrow recovery. This operation, however, is not an absolute cure for patients with hematopoietic syndrome because many individuals undergoing bone marrow transplant die of burns or other radiation-induced damage they sustained before the transplanted stem cells have had a chance to support recovery.

Gastrointestinal syndrome. In humans, the gastrointestinal (GI) form of ARS appears at a threshold dose of approximately 6 Gy_t and peaks after a dose of 10 Gy_t. Without medical support to sustain life, exposed persons receiving doses of 6 to 10 Gy_t may die 3 to 10 days after being exposed. Even if medical support is provided, the exposed person will live only a few days longer. Survival time does not change with dose in this syndrome.

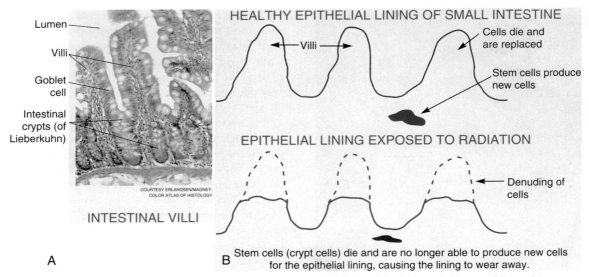

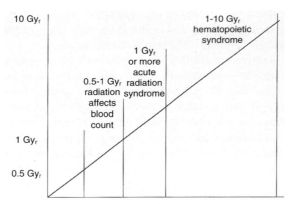

FIG 8.4 (A) Intestinal villi. (B) The top drawing depicts the healthy lining of the small intestine. The bottom drawing shows the epithelial lining of the small intestine after it has been exposed to radiation. Stem cells (crypt cells) die and are no longer able to produce new cells for the epithelial lining, thus causing the lining to wear away. (From *Radiobiology and Radiation Protection: Mosby's Radiographic Instructional Series*, St. Louis, 1999, Mosby.)

FIG 8.5 The prodromal stage of acute radiation syndrome occurs within hours after a whole-body absorbed dose of 1 Gy_t or more is received. Doses ranging from 1 to 10 Gy_t are responsible for causing the hematopoietic form of acute radiation syndrome. (From *Radiobiology and Radiation Protection: Mosby's Radiographic Instructional Series*, St. Louis, 1999, Mosby.)

A few hours after the dose required to cause the GI syndrome has been received, the *prodromal, or beginning, stage* occurs. Severe nausea, vomiting, and diarrhea persist for as long as 24 hours. This is followed by a latent period, which lasts as long as 5 days. During this time, the outward symptoms disappear. The *manifest illness stage* follows this period of false calm. Again, the human subject experiences:

- Severe nausea
- Vomiting
- Diarrhea
  Other signs and symptoms that may occur include:
- Fever (as in hematopoietic syndrome)
- Fatigue
- Loss of appetite
- Lethargy
- Anemia
- Leukopenia (decrease in the number of white blood cells)
- Hemorrhage (GI tract bleeding because the body loses its blood-clotting ability)
- Infection
- Electrolyte imbalance
- Emaciation

Fatality occurs primarily because of catastrophic damage to the epithelial cells that line the gastrointestinal tract. This results in the death of the exposed person within 3 to 5 days from a combination of infection, fluid loss, and electrolytic imbalance. Although expiration from GI syndrome is primarily from damage to the bowel, it also can be induced by destruction of the bone marrow.

The small intestine is the most severely affected part of the GI tract. Because epithelial cells function as an essential biologic barrier, their breakdown leaves the body vulnerable to:

- Infection (mostly from its own intestinal bacteria)
- Dehydration
- Severe diarrhea

Some epithelial cells regenerate in the period before death occurs. However, because of the large number of epithelial cells damaged by the radiation, death may occur before sufficient cell regeneration is accomplished. The workers and firefighters at Chernobyl are examples of humans who died as a result of GI syndrome.

Cerebrovascular syndrome. The cerebrovascular form of ARS results when the central nervous system and cardiovascular system receive doses of 50 Gy_t or more of ionizing radiation. A dose of this magnitude can cause death within a few hours to 2 or 3 days after exposure. After irradiation, the prodromal stage begins. Signs and symptoms include:

- Excessive nervousness
- Confusion
- Severe nausea
- Vomiting
- Diarrhea
- Loss of vision
- Burning sensation of the skin
- Loss of consciousness

A latent period lasting up to 12 hours follows. During this time, symptoms lessen or disappear. After the latent period, the manifest illness stage occurs. During this period, the prodromal syndrome recurs with increased severity, and other symptoms appear, including:

- Disorientation and shock
- Periods of agitation alternating with stupor
- Ataxia (confusion and lack of muscular coordination)
- Edema in the cranial vault
- Loss of equilibrium
- Fatigue
- Lethargy
- Convulsive seizures
- Electrolytic imbalance
- Meningitis
- Prostration
- Respiratory distress
- Vasculitis
- Coma

Injured blood vessels and capillaries permit fluid to leak into the brain. This creates an increase in intracranial pressure, which causes tissue damage. The final result of this damage is failure of the central nervous and cardiovascular systems, which brings death in a matter of minutes. Because the gastrointestinal and hematopoietic systems are more radiosensitive than the central nervous system, they fail to function after a dose of this magnitude. However, because death occurs quickly, the consequences of the failure of these two systems are not demonstrated.

An overview of acute radiation lethality is presented in Table 8.1. The radiation dose required to cause a particular syndrome and the average survival time are

TABLE 8.1	**Overview of Acute Radiation Lethality**		
Stage	**Dose (Gy_t)**	**Average Survival Time**	**Symptoms**
Prodromal	1	—	Nausea, vomiting, diarrhea, fatigue, leukopenia
Latent	1–100	—	None
Hematopoietic	1–10	6–8 wk (doses over 2 Gy_t)	Nausea; vomiting; diarrhea; decrease in number of red blood cells, white blood cells, and platelets in the circulating blood; hemorrhage; infection
Gastrointestinal	6–10	3–10 days	Severe nausea, vomiting, diarrhea, fever, fatigue, loss of appetite, lethargy, anemia, leukopenia, hemorrhage, infection, electrolytic imbalance, and emaciation
Cerebrovascular	50 and above	Several hours to 2–3 days	Same as hematopoietic and gastrointestinal, plus excessive nervousness, confusion, lack of coordination, loss of vision, burning sensation of the skin, loss of consciousness, disorientation, shock, periods of agitation alternating with stupor, edema, loss of equilibrium, meningitis, prostration, respiratory distress, vasculitis, coma

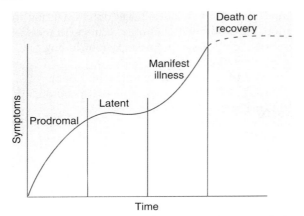

FIG 8.6 The graph depicts the stages of acute radiation syndrome following whole-body reception of large doses of ionizing radiation delivered over a short period. The length of time involved for the syndrome to run its course and the final outcome of the syndrome depend on the dose received. (From *Radiobiology and Radiation Protection: Mosby's Radiographic Instructional Series*, St. Louis, 1999, Mosby.)

the most important measures used to quantify human radiation lethality. The progression of each syndrome, the length of time required for the consequential chain of events to occur, and the final outcome depend on the effective dose received.

Major response stages of acute radiation syndrome. ARS presents in four major response stages:
- Prodromal
- Latent period
- Manifest illness
- Recovery or death (Fig. 8.6)

The **prodromal stage,** also called *prodromal syndrome,* occurs within hours after a whole-body absorbed dose of 1 Gy_t or more (see Fig. 8.6).

The severity of its symptoms is dose related; the higher the dose, the more severe the symptoms. The length of time involved for this stage to run its course may be hours or a few days. After the prodromal stage, a **latent period** of approximately 1 week follows during which no visible signs occur. Actually, it is during this period that either recovery or lethal effects begin. Toward the end of the first week, the next stage commences. This stage is called **manifest illness** because it is the period when signs and symptoms involving the hematopoietic, GI, and cerebrovascular systems become visible. These signs and symptoms can include:

- Apathy and confusion
- Fluid loss and dehydration
- Epilation
- Headaches and exhaustion
- Vomiting and severe diarrhea
- Fever and infection
- Decreased numbers of red and white blood cells and platelets in the circulating blood
- Hemorrhage
- Cardiovascular collapse

If, after receiving a whole-body near-lethal dose such as 2 to 3 Gy_t, exposed persons pass through the first three stages but display less severe symptoms than those seen with highly lethal doses of 6 to 10 Gy_t, **recovery** may occur in approximately 3 months. However, such persons may show some signs of permanent radiation damage and experience late effects.

Acute radiation syndrome as a consequence of the Chernobyl nuclear power plant accident. The massive explosion that blew apart the unit 4 reactor at the nuclear power station in Chernobyl in the Soviet Union on April 26, 1986, provides an example of humans developing ARS. During the explosion, several tons of burning graphite, uranium dioxide fuel, and other contaminants such as cesium-137, iodine-131, and plutonium-239 were ejected upward into the atmosphere in a 3-mile-high radioactive plume of intense heat. Of 444 people working at the power plant at the time of the explosion, 2 died instantly, and 29 died within 3 months of the accident as a consequence of thermal trauma and severe injuries caused by whole-body doses of ionizing radiation of approximately 6 Gy_t or more.[1-3]

Without effective physical monitoring devices, biologic criteria such as the occurrence of nausea and excessive vomiting played an important role in the identification of radiation casualties during the first 2 days after the nuclear disaster. Acute radiation syndrome caused the hospitalization of at least 203 people.[3,4] A determination of the lapse of time from the incidental exposure of the victims to the onset of nausea and vomiting completed the biologic criteria. Dose assessment was determined from serial measurements of levels of lymphocytes and granulocytes in the blood and a quantitative analysis of the frequency of dicentric chromosomes (altered chromosomes with two centromeres) present in blood and hematopoietic cells, coming from bone marrow. The data were compared with doses and effects from earlier radiation mishaps.[2,3] An analysis such as this in which damage to tissues is used to estimate radiation dose is referred to as biologic dosimetry.

Acute radiation syndrome as a consequence of the atomic bombing of Hiroshima and Nagasaki. The Japanese atomic bomb survivors of Hiroshima and Nagasaki are examples of a human population affected by ARS as a consequence of war. Follow-up studies of the survivors who did not rapidly die of this syndrome demonstrated late tissue reactions (e.g., cataracts) and stochastic effects of ionizing radiation such as induction of leukemia. The atomic bombing of Japan and the nuclear accident at Chernobyl made the medical community recognize the need for a thorough understanding of ARS and appropriate medical support of persons affected.

Lethal Dose

LD 50/30. The term *LD 50/30* signifies the whole-body dose of radiation that can be lethal to 50% of the exposed population within 30 days. As mentioned previously, the LD 50/30 for adult humans is estimated to be 3.0 to 4.0 Gy_t without medical support (Fig. 8.7). For x-rays and gamma rays, this is equal to an equivalent dose of 3.0 to 4.0 Sv. Whole-body doses greater than 6 Gy_t will cause the death of the entire population in 30 days without medical support. With medical support, some human beings have survived doses as high as 8.5 Gy_t.[5]

LD 10/30, LD 50/60, and LD 100/60. Other measures of lethality also are quoted, such as *LD 10/30, LD 50/60,* and *LD 100/60.* All these measures refer to the percentage of subjects who die after a certain number of days. The values reported in the literature vary widely because most lethal dose data represent an estimate of the role played by radiation in fatalities in which other factors (e.g., fire at Chernobyl, physical effects of a large explosion at Hiroshima and Nagasaki, chemical contamination in some nuclear accidents) were present. Specifications of lethal effects are further complicated by the medical treatment that the patient may receive during the prodromal and latent stages, before many of the symptoms of ARS appear. When medical treatment is given promptly, the patient is supported through initial symptoms, and so, answering the question of long-term survival may simply be delayed. For this reason, LD 50/60 for humans is probably a more accurate measure for human survival than any shorter period. Table 8.2 gives estimates of lethal doses, including the treatment

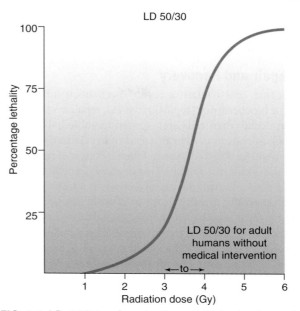

FIG 8.7 LD 50/30 refers to the whole-body dose of radiation that can be lethal to 50% of the exposed population within 30 days. As can be seen in the graph, no deaths are expected below 1 Gy_t. In this particular graph, which represents the human response to radiation exposure, LD 50/30 is reached at 3.5 Gy_t, a dose that falls between 3.0 and 4.0 Gy_t. This is the point at which half of those exposed to 3.5 Gy_t of ionizing radiation would die. The graph also demonstrates that at a dose of 6 Gy_t no one is expected to survive. In reality, survival is possible with extensive medical intervention.

TABLE 8.2 Lethal Dose Values for Healthy Adults Who Receive the Specified Medical Treatment After Exposure to Low–Linear Energy Transfer Radiation at Dose Rates of More Than 100 mGya/Min

Effect	Treatment	Dose (Gy_a)
LD 50/60	Minimal	3.2–4.5
LD 50/60	Optimal supportive	4.8–5.4
LD 50/60	Autologous bone marrow transplantation	11

From Fry RJM: Acute radiation effects. In Wagner LK Fabrikant JI, Fry RJM, editors: *Radiation Bioeffects and Management: Test and Syllabus,* Reston, VA, 1991, American College of Radiology.

given in populations studied. Regardless of treatment, whole-body equivalent doses of greater than 12 Gy$_t$ are considered fatal.[6]

Repair and Recovery

Because cells contain a repair mechanism inherent in their biochemistry (repair enzymes), repair and recovery can occur when cells are exposed to sublethal doses of ionizing radiation. After this level of irradiation, surviving cells will be able to divide and thereby begin to repopulate in the irradiated region. This process permits an organ that has sustained functional damage as a result of radiation exposure to regain some or most of its useful ability. In the repair of sublethal damage, cells that are oxygenated, which as a result receive more nutrients, have a better prospect for recovery than do hypoxic, or poorly oxygenated, cells that consequently receive fewer nutrients. When both cell categories are exposed to a comparable dose of low-LET radiation, the oxygenated cells are more severely damaged, but those that survive can repair themselves and recover from the injury. Even though they are less severely damaged, the hypoxic cells do not repair and recover as efficiently.

Research has shown that repeated radiation injuries have a cumulative effect. Hence a percentage (approximately 10%) of the radiation-induced damage will be irreparable, whereas the remaining 90% may be repaired over time.

Local Tissue Damage

A destructive response in biologic tissue will likely occur when any part of the human body receives a high radiation dose. Significant cell death usually results, leading to the shrinkage of organs and tissues, a process referred to as *atrophy*. Atrophied organs and tissues can lose their ability to function, or they may possibly recover. If recovery does occur, it might be partial or complete, depending on the types of cells involved and the dose of radiation received. Should this not happen, then necrosis, or death, of the irradiated biologic structure results.

Organ and tissue response to radiation exposure depend on factors such as:
- Radiosensitivity
- Reproductive characteristics
- Growth rate

Some local tissues suffer immediate consequences from high radiation doses. Examples of such tissues include the following:

- Skin
- Male and female reproductive organs
- Bone marrow

Effects on the Skin

From the experiences of early pioneers, radiation accident victims, atomic bomb survivors, and patients who have received radiation therapy or unusually high doses during prolonged fluoroscopy in certain areas, a considerable amount of information is available on radiation-induced skin damage. Recall that many early radiologists and dentists developed radiodermatitis, a significant reddening of the skin caused by excessive exposure to relatively low-energy ionizing radiation that eventually led to cancerous lesions on the hands and fingers. In 1898 after personally suffering severe burns, which he eventually attributed to accumulated radiation exposures, William Herbert Rollins, a Boston dentist, began investigating the potential hazards of radiation exposure. This led to his becoming the first known determined advocate for radiation protection. Rollins performed experiments on guinea pigs that led to "three important safety practices for radiographers: wear radiopaque glasses; enclose the x-ray tube in protective housing; and irradiate only areas of interest on the patient, covering adjacent areas with radiopaque materials."[7] Unfortunately, at the time Rollins made these insightful recommendations, they were not given much attention. The misfortune of ignoring his suggestions led to continuing radiation-induced injuries. Eventually, however, our pioneers did learn from their misfortunes, and these recommendations became universally accepted.

The skin consists of three layers (Fig. 8.8):
- Epidermis, or outer, layer
- Dermis, or middle, layer composed of connective tissue
- Hypodermis, a subcutaneous layer of fat and connective tissue

Accessory structures include hair follicles, sensory receptors, sebaceous glands, and sweat glands. All the layers of the skin, as well as its accessory structures, are actively involved in the response of the tissue to radiation exposure.

Because the skin functions as an ongoing regeneration system, it is relatively radiosensitive. Approximately 2% of the body's surface skin cells are replaced daily by stem cells from an underlying basal layer. The characteristics of these stem cells are actually responsible for the radiosensitivity of the skin. A single absorbed dose of 2 Gy$_t$

THICK SKIN   THIN SKIN

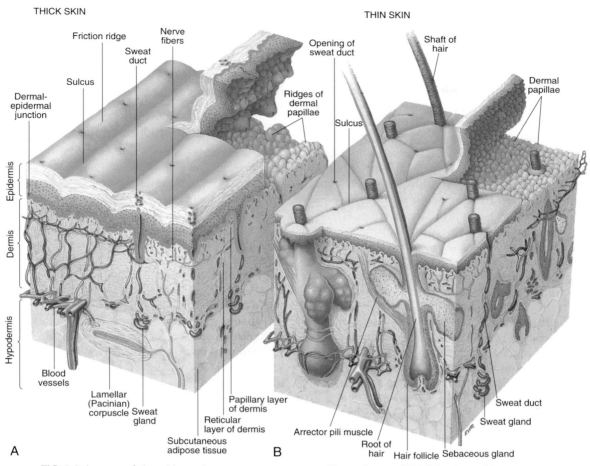

FIG 8.8 Layers of the skin and accessory structures. (From Patton KT, Thibodeau GA: *Anatomy and Physiology*, ed 9, St. Louis, 2016, Elsevier.)

can cause radiation-induced skin erythema within 24 to 48 hours after irradiation. As time progresses, over the next week or two, the erythema becomes much greater until it reaches its maximal intensity. **Desquamation,** or shedding of the outer layer of skin, occurs at higher radiation doses. It generally manifests first as moist desquamation, and then dry desquamation may develop (see Fig. 8.3).

Epilation, or hair loss (also called *alopecia*), can be caused from exposure to radiation because hair follicles are growing tissue. Moderate doses of radiation generally produce temporary hair loss, whereas large radiation doses can result in permanent hair loss.

Historically, skin diseases, such as ringworm, were treated and successfully cured by irradiating the affected area with **grenz rays** (x-rays in the energy range of 10 to 20 kVp).[5] These very low energy photons were adequate to cure the disease. However, if the ringworm was located on the scalp, the local irradiation of that area also caused the hair to fall out for a period of time. This would normally be followed by regrowth, provided the radiation dose delivered to the patient was not sufficient to cause permanent hair loss.

Significant evidence of skin damage as a consequence of exposure to orthovoltage radiation therapy (x-rays in the range of 200 to 300 kVp) comes from oncology patients who underwent such treatments in earlier years for deep-seated tumors. With orthovoltage irradiation used for this purpose, the ability of an individual person's skin to tolerate this exposure actually determined the total amount of treatment radiation the individual could receive, especially when only one radiation entrance surface portal was employed. Modern radiation therapy uses much higher energy photons (ranging from 6 to 18 MeV) produced by linear accelerators* and with multiple skin entrance locations. The combination of the two effectively spares the shallow body tissues from what would now be considered unacceptable exposure levels while precisely delivering cell-killing doses to solid tumors at any depth and location within the body. High energy gamma-emitting isotopes such as cobalt 60 (gamma ray energy of 1.25 MeV) have also historically been much utilized to bring about skin sparing while successfully treating nonsuperficial cancers.

The overall goal of the therapeutic treatment was to deposit the radiant energy at a planned location within a specified treatment volume enclosing the tumor while sparing as much healthy surrounding tissue as possible. Single-portal orthovoltage radiation treatments caused the patient's skin to receive a considerably higher radiation dose than the dose received by the tumor volume because radiation in this energy range was substantially absorbed while traversing the skin and other intervening tissue layers before it reached the tumor. Thus to deliver a specific dose to the tumor, the superficial, or skin dose, would unavoidably have to be significantly greater than the tumor dose. This often resulted in an area of diffuse redness, or erythema, of the skin at the treatment entrance site. If that radiation dose was high enough, moist desquamation of the irradiated skin would occur, followed by dry desquamation of the skin. Eventually, before the advent of modern, much higher energy treatment machines, some multiportal orthovoltage treatment plans were devised leading to lesser entrance skin doses per irradiated area and resultant improved skin sparing.

During cardiovascular or other therapeutic interventional procedures that use high-level fluoroscopy for

extended periods, the effects of ionizing radiation on the skin are significant. Patient exposure rates have been estimated to range from 100 to 200 mGy$_a$/min and sometimes even greater. As a result of numerous reported injuries to patients that were associated with the use of high-level fluoroscopy, imposing strict controls on its use is essential.

Effects on the Reproductive System

Some of the early tissue reactions from ionizing radiation have been discussed in Chapter 7.

Human germ cells are relatively radiosensitive. Doses as low as 0.1 Gy$_t$ can depress the male sperm population, and this same dose has the potential to cause genetic mutations in future generations. In girls and women, a gonadal dose of 0.1 Gy$_t$ may delay or suppress menstruation.

Animal experiments and data from irradiated human populations have provided significant information on gonadal response to radiation exposure. Irradiated human populations include:
- Patients who have undergone radiation therapy
- Radiation accident victims
- Volunteer convicts[8,9]

The testes of the male and the ovaries of the female do not respond in the same way to irradiation because of the difference in the way in which these cells are produced and progress from elementary stem cells to mature cells. The spermatogonia, the stem cells of the testes, constantly reproduce. They mature and become spermatocytes. The latter cells then multiply and develop into spermatids that eventually differentiate and become spermatozoa, or sperm, which are the functionally mature germ cells (Fig. 8.9). The development of the male stem cell into a functionally mature germ cell takes 3 to 5 weeks.[5]

*A linear accelerator is essentially a highly evacuated straight-line device that, by virtue of superimposed oscillating electrical potentials, accelerates electrons injected into it from a heated filament into a megavoltage energy beam. This beam is then directed by a magnetic field onto a high atomic number target (e.g., tungsten and/or lead). The resulting interactions generate highly energetic x-rays (megavoltage range), which themselves are formed into a useful beam that can be employed to effectively treat deep-seated tumors while sparing superficial tissues.

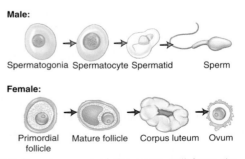

FIG 8.9 Development of the germ cell from the stem cell phase to the mature cell.

In the female, the oogonia, the ovarian stem cells, multiply to millions of cells only during fetal development, before birth, and then they steadily decline in number throughout life. During the later part of fetal development, the oogonia become encapsulated by numerous primordial (primary) follicles that actually grow around them (see Fig. 8.9). The oogonia in due course become oocytes, which contain follicles that are nests of cells, some of which eventually mature during the reproductive life of a woman. Before these primary oocyte-containing follicles grow into mature follicles, they actually remain dormant until puberty. Then, just before puberty, the oocytes are reduced in number to only several hundred thousand. Some of the cells of the primary follicles proliferate in response to stimulation by hormones from the pituitary gland, and these cells begin to mature. At the same time, the ovum contained within each of the follicles undergoes meiosis. As puberty begins, the developed ova, or mature female germ cells*, within the follicles are ejected when the follicles themselves rupture. Usually, only one follicle will fully mature and move toward the surface of the ovary to be expelled, and the others disintegrate. This process occurs at regular time intervals of approximately 28 days. Of the mature ova that are actually enclosed within the follicles, only 400 to 500 are produced, matured, and made available for fertilization during a woman's reproductive life.

Follicles range in size from small to large. Of these, the intermediate-size follicles are the most radiosensitive, and the small follicles are the least radiosensitive. Large mature follicles possess only a moderate degree of radiosensitivity.[10] During the female menstrual cycle, a mature follicle releases an ovum during the period of ovulation, when a ripe ovum is expelled from an ovary into the pelvic cavity. If that ovum is not fertilized by a waiting male sperm in the uterus, it will be lost during menstruation and not replaced.

Hematologic Effects

As a brief review, recall that during the 1920s and 1930s, periodic blood counts were the only means of radiation exposure monitoring for radiation workers engaged in radiologic practices. The use of personnel dosimeters for monitoring of occupational exposure made

*Mature female germ cells or eggs are those that have entered stage M2 of meiosis. The end result of meiosis is the halving of the number of chromosomes and genetic material.

the former practice obsolete. Through the years when such predosimeter monitoring was employed, a whole-body dose as low as 0.25 Gy_t would produce measurable hematologic depression. This dose could cause enough of a decrease in the number of lymphocytes in the blood to leave the body vulnerable to infection by foreign invaders. This method therefore was totally unfounded with respect to modern principles of radiation protection.

Hematopoietic System. The hematopoietic system consists of:

- Bone marrow
- Circulating blood
- Lymphoid organs (lymph nodes, spleen, and thymus gland)

Cells of this system all develop from a single precursor cell, the **pluripotential stem cell**. The following are other types of cells that originate from this one type of elementary cell: lymphocytes, granulocytes, thrombocytes or platelets, and erythrocytes. Fig. 8.10 demonstrates the progressive development of these cells from a single pluripotential stem cell. Most of these blood cells are manufactured in bone marrow at different intervals, and when they mature, they enter the blood capillaries and the peripheral circulation. Even though blood cells are constantly being produced, the life span of each individual type of blood cell differs, varying, on average, from only a few hours (e.g., lymphocytes) to almost 120 days (e.g., erythrocytes).

The human body may experience health-related consequences throughout life if there is a decrease in the numbers of these various cells. Some of these consequences will be increased susceptibility to aggressive infectious organisms, greater risk of hemorrhage, and anemia.

Radiation doses resulting from diagnostic imaging procedures during which appropriate radiation protection methods have been employed for patients and all personnel result in negligible damage to the blood and the blood-forming organs. However, in this dose range, some chromosomal changes in circulating lymphocytes have been observed.

Cytogenetic Effects

In simple terms, **cytogenetics** may be defined as the study of cell genetics with an emphasis on cell chromosomes. The techniques used to study and observe the chromosomes of each human cell have greatly contributed to

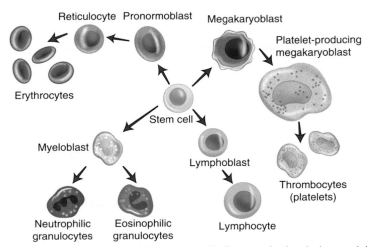

FIG 8.10 Progressive development of various cells from a single pluripotential stem cell.

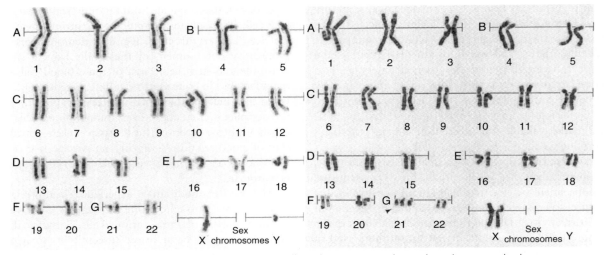

FIG 8.11 A photomicrograph of the human cell nucleus at metaphase that shows each chromosome individually demonstrated. The karyotype is constructed by cutting out the individual chromosomes and pairing them with their sister chromosomes. These chromosome pairs are usually aligned by size, beginning with the largest pair and ending with the smallest pair. The left karyotype is male, and the right is female. (From Carolyn Caskey Goodner, Identigene, Inc.)

advancing genetic analysis and the understanding of the influence of radiation on genetics.

A cytogenetic analysis of chromosomes may be accomplished through the use of a chromosome map called a **karyotype**. This map consists of a photograph, or *photomicrograph*, that is taken of the human cell nucleus during metaphase, when each chromosome can be individually demonstrated. The karyotype is constructed by cutting out the individual chromosomes and pairing them on the map with their sister chromosomes. These chromosome pairs are usually aligned by size, beginning with the largest pair and ending with the smallest pair (Fig. 8.11).

Metaphase is the phase of cell division in which chromosome damage caused by radiation exposure can be evaluated. *Chromosome aberrations* (deviation from normal development or growth) and *chromatid aberrations* have been observed at metaphase.

Both low and high radiation doses can cause chromosomal damage that may not be apparent immediately. Most chromosomal damage results from the process of indirect action of ionizing radiation on vital biologic macromolecules.

Almost every type of chromosome aberration can be brought about by exposure to ionizing radiation. However, some aberrations can "only" be produced by radiation exposure.[5] The total radiation dose given to a somatic or genetic cell and the period of time in which that dose was delivered determine the rate of production of chromosome aberrations.

Attempts have been made to measure chromosome aberrations after diagnostic x-ray imaging procedures, but successful results have not been achieved in these studies. For some imaging procedures that involve much higher radiation dose rates, studies demonstrated that radiation-induced chromosome imperfections were observed shortly after the imaging procedure was completed.

Increased frequency of chromosome translocations is an established radiation biomarker and may also suggest increased cancer risk.[11] An occupational epidemiologic study of 146,000 US radiologic technologists began in 1982 and is still in progress. This study is a collaborative effort of the University of Minnesota School of Public Health, the National Cancer Institute, and the American Registry of Radiologic Technologists.[12,13] The purpose of the research is "to determine whether their personal cumulative exposure to diagnostic x-rays was associated with increased frequencies of chromosome translocations"[11] and possible associated cancer risk. Included in the study were mail surveys, telephone interviews, and a collection of 150 blood samples for testing purposes. Results of the blood tests indicated increased chromosome damage as a consequence of cumulative work-related exposure from routine x-ray procedures.[11] For patients, increased computed tomography (CT) and nuclear medicine procedures can contribute substantially to higher radiation exposure. "Some studies have found increased chromosome abnormalities immediately after radiation exposure from CT scanning"[11,14] or in patients with unusually high numbers of diagnostic procedures.[11,15]

SUMMARY

- Biologic effects that occur relatively soon after humans receive high doses of ionizing radiation are general referred to as *early effects*.

- Early tissue reactions are not common in diagnostic radiology.
- Somatic effects are effects upon the body that was irradiated.
- Genetic effects are effects upon future generations due to irradiation of germ cells in previous generations.
- Somatic tissue reactions include cell killing and are directly related to the dose of radiation received. As dose increases, so does the severity of these early tissue reactions.
  - Early tissue reactions vary depending on the duration of time after exposure to ionizing radiation. Subject to their nature, they may appear within minutes, hours, days, or weeks after receiving a high dose of ionizing radiation.
  - Possible high radiation dose consequences generally include nausea and fever, extreme fatigue, erythema, epilation, and blood and intestinal disorders. In addition, temporary or permanent sterility in the male and female and injury to the central nervous system (at extremely high radiation doses) can occur.
- Acute radiation syndrome (ARS) occurs in humans after whole-body reception of large doses of ionizing radiation delivered over a short period.
  - ARS can manifest as hematopoietic syndrome, syndrome, and cerebrovascular syndrome.
  - ARS presents in four major response stages: prodromal, latent period, manifest illness, and recovery or death.
- LD (lethal dose) 50/30 signifies the whole-body dose of ionizing radiation that can be lethal to 50% of an exposed population within 30 days.
  - LD 50/30 for adult humans is estimated to be 3 to 4 Gy_t without medical support.
  - When cells are exposed to sublethal doses of ionizing radiation, repair and recovery are possible.
  - After receiving a sublethal dose of radiation, surviving cells will be able to divide and thereby begin to repopulate in the irradiated region.
  - Approximately 90% of radiation-induced damage may be repaired over time; 10% is irreparable.
- High radiation doses to any part of the human body can result in local tissue damage.
- Significant cell death usually results after a substantial radiation exposure, leading to potential atrophy of involved organs and tissues.
- Depending on the types of cells included and the dose of radiation received, recovery may be partial or

complete, or it may fail to occur, resulting in death of the irradiated biologic structure.

- Factors such as radiosensitivity, reproductive characteristics, and growth rate govern organ and tissue response to radiation exposure.
- Many early radiologists and dentists developed radiodermatitis as a consequence of radiation exposure to the skin that eventually led to the development of cancerous lesions.
  - Human skin consists of three layers and several accessory structures, all of which are actively involved in the response of tissue to radiation exposure.
  - A single absorbed dose of 2 Gy_t can cause radiation-induced skin erythema within 24 to 48 hours after irradiation.
  - High radiation doses to the skin can cause moist and then dry desquamation.
  - Moderate radiation doses to the scalp can cause temporary hair loss, and large radiation doses can result in permanent hair loss.
  - Significant evidence of skin damage as a consequence of exposure to orthovoltage radiation therapy comes from oncology patients who underwent such treatments in earlier years for deep-seated tumors.
  - The use of high-level fluoroscopy for extended periods can result in radiation-induced skin injuries for patients.
- Human germ cells are relatively radiosensitive.
  - In males, a radiation dose of 0.1 Gy_t can depress the sperm population and possibly cause genetic mutations in future generations.
  - In females, a gonadal dose of 0.1 Gy_t may delay or suppress menstruation.
- Periodic blood counts have been replaced by personnel dosimeters as a means to monitor occupational radiation exposure.
  - Through the years, when predosimeter monitoring was employed, a whole-body dose of radiation as low as 0.25 Gy_t would produce measurable hematologic depression.
- Mapping of chromosomes is called *karyotyping*.
  - Karyotyping is done during metaphase, when each chromosome can be individually demonstrated and radiation-induced chromosome and chromatid aberrations can be observed.
  - Chromosomal damage can be caused by both low and high radiation doses.
  - Chromosome aberrations have been observed in individuals after completion of some imaging

procedures in which very high radiation dose rates were administered.

REFERENCES

1. Finch SC: Acute radiation syndrome. *JAMA* 258:666, 1987.
2. Gale RP: Immediate medical consequences of nuclear accidents: lessons from Chernobyl. *JAMA* 258:625, 1987.
3. Perry AR, Iglar AF: The accident at Chernobyl: radiation doses and effects. *Radiol Technol* 61:290, 1990.
4. Linnemann RE: Soviet medical response to Chernobyl nuclear accident. *JAMA* 258:639, 1987.
5. Bushong SC: *Radiologic science for technologists: physics, biology and protection*, ed 10, St. Louis, 2013, Mosby.
6. Fry RJM: Acute radiation effects. In Wagner LK, Fabrikant JI, Fry RJM, editors: *Radiation bioeffects and management: test and syllabus*, Reston, VA, 1991, American College of Radiology.
7. Hidden giants. *ASRT Scanner* 41:1, 2008.
8. George Washington University: Staff memo: experiments on prisoners. Available at: http://www.gwu.edu/~nsarchiv/radiation/dir/mstreet/commeet/meet1/brief1/br1n.txt.
9. Advisory Committee on Human Radiation Experiments (ACHRE) report: Chapter 9: The Oregon and Washington experiments. Available at: http://www.hss.energy.gov/healthsafety/ohre/roadmap/achre/chap9_2.html.
10. Forshier S: *Essentials of radiation biology and protection*, Albany, NY, 2002, Delmar.
11. Sigurdson AJ, et al: Routine diagnostic x-ray examinations and increased frequency of chromosome translocations among U.S. radiologic technologists. Available at: http://www.ncbi.nlm.nih.gov/pubmed/18974125.
12. University of Minnesota, Health Science Section: *U.S. Radiologic Technologists Study*, (vol 2). Minneapolis, 2004, University of Minnesota.
13. University of Minnesota, Health Studies Section: U.S. Radiologic Technologists Study. Available at: www.radtechstudy.org.
14. M'kacher R, Violot D, et al: Premature chromosome condensation associated with fluorescence in situ hybridization detects cytogenic abnormalities after a CT scan: evaluation of the low-dose effect. *Radiat Prot Dosimetry* 103:35, 2003.
15. Weber J, Scheid W, Traut H: Biological dosimetry after extensive diagnostic exposure. *Health Phys* 68:266, 1995.

GENERAL DISCUSSION QUESTIONS

1. Although early tissue reactions are not common in diagnostic radiology, what type of diagnostic imaging procedure could possibly produce a radiation dose sufficient to cause such a reaction?
2. In what do unacceptable high x-ray exposures in radiology primarily result?
3. How can a cytogenetic analysis of chromosomes be accomplished?
4. What are genetic effects?
5. How have scientists become aware of radiation-induced skin damage in early pioneers?
6. What are the three separate dose-related syndromes that occur as part of acute radiation syndrome, and what are the four major response stages?
7. What is radiodermatitis?
8. After the reception of a single absorbed dose of 2 Gy$_t$ of radiation, approximately how long will it take to cause radiation-induced skin erythema?
9. How has information on the gonadal response to radiation exposure been acquired?
10. How significant is the chance of causing sterility in imaging personnel who perform routine procedures?
11. What are the somatic effects of radiation exposure?
12. From where does the term *somatic* originate?

REVIEW QUESTIONS

1. The total radiation dose given to a somatic or genetic cell and the period of time in which that dose was delivered determine the rate of production of:
   A. Cell division
   B. Chromosome aberrations
   C. Genetic analysis
   D. Karyotyping
2. Acute radiation syndrome presents in four major response stages. In what order do these stages occur?
   A. Latent period, prodromal, manifest illness, recovery or death
   B. Manifest illness, prodromal, latent period, recovery or death
   C. Prodromal, latent period, manifest illness, recovery or death
   D. Manifest illness, latent period, prodromal, recovery or death

3. Which of the following systems is the *most* radiosensitive vital organ system in human beings?
   A. Cerebrovascular
   B. Gastrointestinal
   C. Hematopoietic
   D. Skeletal
4. When cells are exposed to sublethal doses of ionizing radiation, approximately _____ of radiation-induced damage may be repaired over time and about _____ is irreparable.
   A. 25%, 75%
   B. 50%, 50%
   C. 75%, 25%
   D. 90%, 10%
5. As radiation dose increases, the severity of early tissue reactions:
   A. Also increases
   B. Gradually decreases
   C. Increases sharply and then gradually decreases
   D. Remains constant
6. Prolonged exposure to x-rays in the diagnostic energy range results in high radiation dose to the skin while underlying tissues receive:
   A. A much greater dose
   B. A slightly greater dose
   C. No dose
   D. A substantially less dose
7. In 1898 after personally developing burns attributed to radiation exposure, this Boston dentist began investigating the hazards of radiation exposure and became the first advocate of radiation protection. Who is this person?
   A. William Herbert Rollins
   B. Wilhelm Conrad Roentgen
   C. Thomas Alva Edison
   D. Clarence Madison Dally
8. In the female, the ovarian stem cells:
   A. Begin as a single cell during fetal development, before birth, and then gradually increase in number throughout life
   B. Multiply to a few hundred cells during fetal life, before birth, and then gradually increase in number throughout life
   C. Multiply to millions of cells only during fetal development, before birth, and then steadily decline in number throughout life
   D. Multiply to millions of cells only during fetal development, before birth, and then steadily continue to increase in number throughout life

9. Which of the following types of cells develop from single precursor cell, the pluripotential stem cell?
    1. Lymphocytes and granulocytes
    2. Thrombocytes and erythrocytes
    3. Platelets
   A. 1 only
   B. 2 only
   C. 3 only
   D. 1, 2, and 3

10. With regard to radiation exposure, which part of the gastrointestinal tract is *most* severely affected?
    A. Esophagus
    B. Stomach
    C. Small intestine
    D. Large intestine

9

Stochastic Effects and Late Tissue Reactions of Radiation in Organ Systems

OBJECTIVES

After completing this chapter, the reader will be able to perform the following:
- Define all key terms.
- Explain how scientists use epidemiologic studies to predict the risk of cancer in human populations exposed to low doses of ionizing radiation.
- Explain the purpose of a radiation dose–response curve.
- Draw diagrams demonstrating various dose–response relationships.
- Explain why regulatory agencies continue to use the linear dose–response model for establishing radiation protection standards.
- Differentiate between threshold and nonthreshold relationships.

- List and describe the various late tissue reactions and stochastic effects of ionizing radiation on living systems.
- Describe the concept of risk for radiation-induced malignancies, and explain the models that are used to give risk estimates.
- Identify ionizing radiation-exposed human populations or groups that prove radiation induces cancer.
- Explain how spontaneous mutations occur.
- Discuss the concept and processes of radiation-induced genetic effects.
- Differentiate between dominant and recessive gene mutations.
- Explain the doubling dose concept, and give an example of how the number of mutations increases as dose increases.

CHAPTER OUTLINE

KEY TERMS

absolute risk	late somatic effects	radiation dose–response
carcinogenesis	late tissue reaction	relationship
cataractogenesis	linear nonthreshold curve	relative risk
doubling dose	linear-quadratic nonthreshold	sigmoid, or S-shaped (nonlinear),
embryologic effects (birth	curve	threshold curve
defects)	nonthreshold	stochastic effects
epidemiology	organogenesis	threshold
genetic, or hereditary, effects		

Radiation-induced damage at the cellular level may lead to measurable somatic and hereditary damage in the living organism as a whole further on in life. These *late effects* are the long-term results of radiation exposure. Some examples of measurable delayed biologic damage are:

- Cataracts
- Leukemia
- Genetic mutations

Cataracts are considered to be a **late tissue reaction** that is non-random, whereas leukemia and genetic mutations are viewed as stochastic or random consequences that, if they appear, do not do so for extended periods. This chapter focuses on organic system–level damage from ionizing radiation that occurs months or years after radiation exposure.

EPIDEMIOLOGY

Epidemiology is defined as a "science that deals with the incidence, distribution, and control of disease in a population."[1] Epidemiologic studies consist of observations and statistical analysis of data, such as the incidence of disease within groups of people. The latter studies include the risk of radiation-induced cancer. The incident rates at which these irradiation-related malignancies occur are determined by comparing the natural incidence of cancer occurring in a human population with the incidence of cancer occurring in an irradiated population. Risk factors are then determined for the general human population.

Epidemiologic studies are of significant value to radiobiologists who use the information from these studies to formulate *dose–response estimates* for making predictions of the risk of cancer in human populations exposed to low doses of ionizing radiation.

RADIATION DOSE–RESPONSE RELATIONSHIP

Dose–Response Curves

The **radiation dose–response relationship** is demonstrated graphically through a curve (the DR curve) that maps the observed effects of radiation exposure in relation to the dose of radiation received. The "effect" in question may be the incidence of a disease (e.g., cases of cancer per million in a population or fatalities due to cancer per million in a population), or it may be the severity of an effect, such as the severity of cataracts as dose increases. The DR curve is either linear (straight line) or nonlinear (curved to some degree), and it depicts either a threshold dose or a nonthreshold dose (Fig. 9.1).

Threshold and Nonthreshold Relationships

The term **threshold** may be defined as a point or level at which a response or reaction to an increasing stimulation first occurs. With reference to ionizing radiation, this means that below a certain absorbed radiation dose, no biologic effects are observed. The latter begin to occur only when the threshold dose is reached. A **nonthreshold** relationship, on the other hand, indicates that a radiation absorbed dose of any magnitude has the capability of producing a biologic effect. Therefore if the DR curve is as shown in Fig. 9.2, biologic effect responses will be caused by ionizing radiation in living organisms in a directly proportional manner all the way down to dose levels approaching zero. This behavior is referred to as a *linear nonthreshold (LNT) relationship*. It proclaims that no radiation dose can be considered absolutely "safe," with the severity of the biologic effects increasing directly with the magnitude of the absorbed dose.

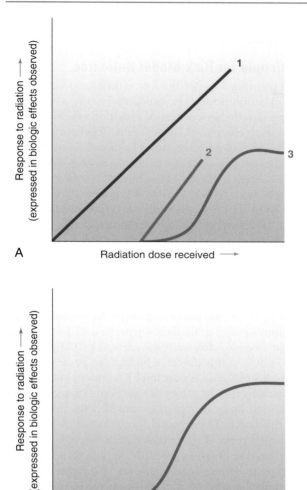

A

Radiation dose received ⟶

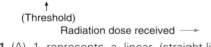

(Threshold)

B   Radiation dose received ⟶

FIG 9.1 (A) 1 represents a linear (straight-line) non-threshold curve of radiation dose–response relationship; 2 represents a linear threshold curve of radiation dose–response relationship; 3 represents a nonlinear threshold curve of radiation dose–response relationship. (B) Sigmoid (S-shaped, hence nonlinear) threshold curve of radiation dose–response relationship generally employed in radiation therapy to demonstrate high-dose cellular response.

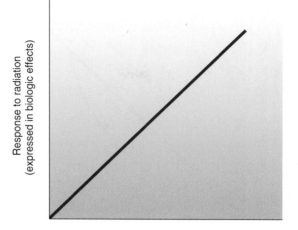

Radiation dose

FIG 9.2 Linear nonthreshold curve of radiation dose–response relationship. The straight-line curve passing through the origin in this graph indicates both that the response to radiation (in terms of biologic effects) is directly proportional to the dose of radiation and that no known level of radiation dose exists below which the chance of sustaining biologic damage is zero. In contrast to a cell-survival curve, as seen in Chapter 7, both the vertical and horizontal axes of a dose–response curve are ordinary linear scales.

Risk Models Used to Predict Cancer Risk and Heritable Damage in Human Populations

In a 1980 report, the Committee on the Biological Effects of Ionizing Radiation (BEIR), under the auspices of the National Academy of Sciences, looking at atomic bomb survivors concluded that most stochastic effects (e.g., cancer) and hereditary effects at low-dose levels from low LET radiation, such as the type of radiation used in diagnostic radiology, appear to follow a linear-quadratic nonthreshold dose–response curve (LQNT DR) (Fig. 9.3). The term *linear-quadratic* implies that the equation that best fits the data has components that depend on dose to the first power (linear or straight-line behavior) and also on dose squared (quadratic or curved behavior). Since the 1980 report, newer risk models and updated dosimetry techniques have provided a better follow-up study of Hiroshima and Nagasaki atomic bomb survivors. In 1990 the BEIR Committee's revised risk estimates indicated that the risk from radiation exposure was about three to four times greater than previously projected.

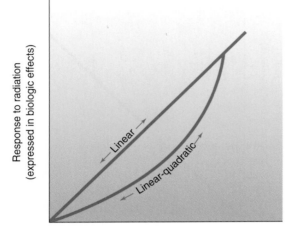

FIG 9.3 Linear-quadratic nonthreshold dose–response relationship. The curve estimates the risk associated with low-dose levels from low LET radiation.

Currently, the committee recommends the use of the **linear nonthreshold curve** of radiation dose–response (LNT DR) for most types of cancers. With the LNT DR curve, if the absorbed dose is doubled, the biologic response probability, and therefore its actual occurrence in a large population sample, is also doubled (see Fig. 9.2).

Risk Models Used to Predict Leukemia, Breast Cancer, and Heritable Damage

Currently, advocates of LNT theorize that because all radiation exposure levels possess the potential to cause biologic damage, radiographers must never fail to employ aggressive radiation safety measures whenever humans are exposed to radiation during diagnostic imaging procedures. As we have seen, another nonthreshold risk estimate curve is the **LQNT DR** curve (see Fig. 9.3). It displays a *more conservative dose–response outcome for low-level radiation*. The 1990 BEIR Committee considered the LQNT relationship to be an improved reflection of stochastic and genetic effects at low-dose levels from low-LET radiation. The following health concerns are presumed to follow this DR curve:
- Leukemia
- Breast cancer
- Heritable damage

For leukemia, the LQNT hypothesis appears to be supported by an analysis of the leukemia occurrences in Nagasaki and Hiroshima that used a more recent reevaluation of the radiation dose distribution in these two cities.[2,3]

Rationale for Risk Model Selection

The continued use of the linear dose–response model for radiation protection standards has the potential to exaggerate the seriousness of radiation effects at lower dose levels from low-LET radiation. Regulatory agencies such as the Nuclear Regulatory Commission continue to review scientific literature to determine if evidence supports changes in the use of this model for setting radiation protection standards. In establishing such standards, the regulatory agencies have chosen to be conservative—that is, to use a model that may overestimate risk at low doses but is not expected to underestimate risk.

Risk Model Used to Predict High-Dose Cellular Response

Acute reactions from significant radiation exposure such as skin erythema and hematologic depression may be demonstrated graphically through the use of a radiation *linear threshold dose–response curve* (LT DR) as shown in Fig. 9.4. In this model, a biologic response does not occur below a specific dose level. Laboratory experiments on animals and data from human populations observed after high doses of radiation provided the foundation for this curve. The **sigmoid, or S-shaped (nonlinear), threshold curve** of the radiation dose–response relationship (see Fig. 9.1B) is generally employed in radiation therapy to demonstrate high-dose cellular response to the radiation absorbed doses within specific tissues such as skin, lens of the eye, and various types of blood cells. Different effects require different minimal doses. The tail of the curve indicates that limited recovery occurs at lower radiation doses. At the highest radiation doses, the curve gradually levels off and then veers downward because the affected living specimen or tissue dies before the observable effect appears.

SOMATIC EFFECTS

When living organisms that have been exposed to radiation sustain biologic damage, the effects of this exposure are classified as *somatic effects*, from the Greek *sōmatikos*, meaning "of the body." The classification of somatic effects may be subdivided into:
- Stochastic effects
- Tissue reactions

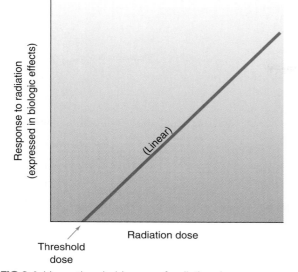

FIG 9.4 Linear threshold curve of radiation dose–response. This depicts those cases for which a biologic response does not occur below a specific radiation dose.

In stochastic effects, the probability that the effect happens depends upon the received dose, but the severity of the effect does not. The occurrence of a cancer is an instance of a stochastic somatic effect. In tissue reactions, however, both the probability and the severity of the effect depend upon the dose.

A *non-somatic* effect is an effect in offspring of the individual who was irradiated. An example of a nonsomatic effect is irradiation of an individual's genetic material (sperm or eggs) leading to a genetic malformation in offspring.

Late Somatic Effects

Late somatic effects are consequences of radiation exposure that appear months or years afterwards. Late effects may be either stochastic or tissue reactions. Stochastic effects, such as the incidence of cancers in a population, usually require years to be noticeable in a population. Tissue reactions, such as skin effects, may be noticeable sooner in individuals, although months or more may be required for their full expression. Tissue reactions are the result of slowly developing changes to body tissues that may be modified by other factors, such as medical intervention, after the exposure. Stochastic effects, such as the incidence of cancer, are generally determined at the time of irradiation.

BOX 9.1   Late Effects of Radiation

Late Tissue Reactions
Cataract formation
Fibrosis
Organ atrophy
Loss of parenchymal cells
Reduced fertility
Sterility

Teratogenic Effects
(i.e., effects of radiation on the embryo-fetus in utero that depend on the fetal stage of development and the radiation dose received)
Embryonic, fetal, or neonatal death
Congenital malformations
Decreased birth weight
Disturbances in growth and/or development
Increased stillbirths
Infant mortality
Childhood malignancy
Childhood mortality

Stochastic Effects
Cancer
Genetic (hereditary) effects

Examples of both classes of late effects are listed in Box 9.1.

Risk Estimate for Contracting Cancer From Low-Level Radiation Exposure

Low-level doses are a consideration for patients and personnel exposed to ionizing radiation as a result of diagnostic imaging procedures. The risk estimate for humans contracting cancer from low-level radiation exposure is still controversial. No conclusive proof currently exists that low-LET ionizing radiation absorbed doses below 0.1 Gy cause a significant increase in the risk of malignancy. The risk, in fact, may be negligible or even nonexistent. Sources of such low-level radiation include the following:

- X-rays and radioactive materials used for diagnostic purposes
- Employment-related exposures in medicine and industry
- Natural background exposure

In general, low-level low LET radiation dosage has been defined as "an absorbed dose of 0.1 Sv or less delivered over a short period of time" and as "a larger dose delivered over a long period of time—for instance, 0.5 Sv in 10 years."[4] The effective dose of a typical routine two-view chest radiograph is approximately 0.06 mSv (note: this can be somewhat greater or lesser, depending on the patient's body size), so this is far below what is considered a low-level exposure.[5] Numerous laboratory experiments on animals and studies on human populations that had been exposed to *high doses* of ionizing radiation from various causes were conducted to catalog the occurrence and degree of adverse health effects. Using all data available on high radiation exposure, members of the scientific and medical communities have concluded that three categories of harmful health consequences also require study at *low dose levels*:

- Cancer induction
- Damage to the unborn from irradiation in utero
- Genetic effects

Low-Level Effects Summary

Cells that survive the initial irradiation may have incurred some form of damage. Theoretically, radiation damage to just one or a few cells of an individual could actually produce a stochastic effect such as a malignancy or a hereditary disorder many years after radiation exposure. Tissue reactions such as skin reactions do not usually demonstrate a late onset. Extreme reactions associated with high skin doses may persist for some time but will usually occur in weeks or months after the exposure.

Major Types of Late Effects

To summarize, the three major types of late effects are:

- **Carcinogenesis**
- **Cataractogenesis**
- **Embryologic effects (birth defects)**

Of these, carcinogenesis and embryologic effects are considered stochastic events, and cataractogenesis is regarded as a late tissue reaction.

Risk Estimates for Cancer

Exposure to ionizing radiation may cause cancer as a stochastic effect. At high doses, for groups such as the atomic bomb survivors, the risk is measurable in human populations. At low equivalent doses, that is, below 0.1 Sv, which includes groups such as occupationally exposed individuals and virtually all patients in diagnostic radiology, this risk is not directly measurable in population studies. Either the risk is overshadowed by other causes (e.g., environmental exposures, genetic predisposition,

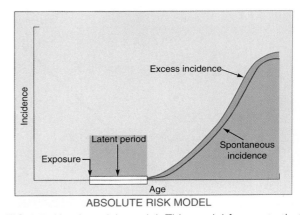

FIG 9.5 Absolute risk model. This model forecasts that a specific number of malignancies will occur as a result of exposure. (From *Radiobiology and Radiation Protection: Mosby's Radiographic Instructional Series*, St. Louis, 1999, Mosby.)

lifestyle factors such as smoking) of cancer in humans, or the risk is zero. Current conservative radiation protection philosophy, namely the LNT model, assumes that risk still exists and may be determined by extrapolating from high-dose data, in which risk has been directly observed, down to low doses, in which it has not been observed. This remains a very controversial concept.

Absolute Risk and Relative Risk Models. Risk estimates to predict cancer incidence may be given in terms of absolute risk or relative risk caused by a specific exposure to ionizing radiation (over and above background exposure). Both models forecast the number of excess cancers or cancers that would not have occurred in the population in question without the exposure to ionizing radiation. The absolute risk model forecasts that a specific number of malignancies will occur as a result of exposure (Fig. 9.5). The relative risk model predicts that the number of excess cancers will increase as the natural incidence of cancer increases with advancing age in a population (Fig. 9.6). It is relative in the sense that it predicts a percentage increase in incidence rather than a specific number of cases. More recent studies of atomic bomb survivors tend to support the relative risk model over the absolute risk model.

Epidemiologic Studies for Determining the Risk of Cancer. Epidemiologic studies suggest that although the radiation doses encountered in diagnostic radiology

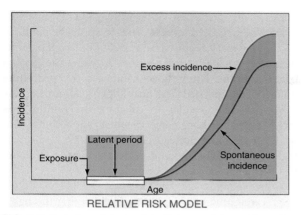

FIG 9.6 Relative risk model. This model predicts that the number of excess cancers will increase as the natural incidence of cancer increases with advancing age in a population. (From *Radiobiology and Radiation Protection: Mosby's Radiographic Instructional Series*, St. Louis, 1999, Mosby.)

should be considered, the benefit to the patient of the information gained from an imaging procedure greatly exceeds the minimal theoretical risk to the patient for developing cancer as a late stochastic response to radiation exposure. Even at the relatively high doses encountered by the Japanese atomic bomb survivors, the probability of causation of an excess fatal cancer is surprisingly low—approximately 5% per sievert.[6]

Models for Extrapolation of Cancer Risk From High-Dose to Low-Dose Data. Researchers commonly use two models for extrapolation of risk from high-dose to low-dose data. As discussed previously, these are linear and linear-quadratic models. In the linear model (Fig. 9.7A) as we have seen, the risk per centigray is constant; the occurrence of cancer follows a straight-line or dose-proportional progression throughout the entire dose range. Although this model appears to fit the high-dose data, it may substantially overestimate the risk at low doses. The linear-quadratic model (see Fig. 9.7B) includes additional mathematical terms that produce a deviation from straight-line behavior at low doses so that the risk per additional centigray at low doses is projected to be less than at high doses. The 1989 BEIR V report supported the linear-quadratic model for leukemia only. For all other cancers, the BEIR V Committee recommended adoption of the linear model to fit the available data.[7]

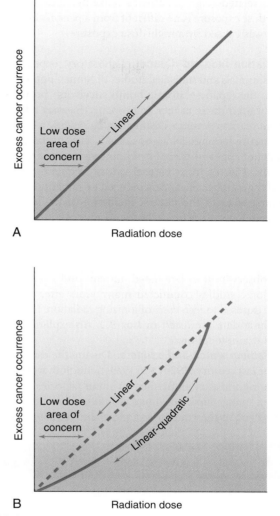

FIG 9.7 (A) Linear model used to extrapolate the occurrence of cancer from high-dose information to low doses. This model suits current high-dose information satisfactorily but exaggerates the actual risk at low doses and dose rates. (B) Linear-quadratic model used to extrapolate the occurrence of cancer from high-dose information to low doses. This model suits current high-dose information satisfactorily, but risk at low doses may be underestimated.

Carcinogenesis

Cancer is the most important late stochastic effect caused by exposure to ionizing radiation. Recall that this effect is a random occurrence that does not seem to have a threshold and for which the severity of the disease is not dose related (e.g., a patient's leukemia induced by a low-dose exposure is no different from a person's leukemia that was caused by a high-dose exposure).

Radiation-Induced Cancer. Laboratory experiments with animals and statistical studies of human populations (e.g., the Japanese atomic bomb survivors) prove that radiation induces cancer. In humans, this may take 5 or more years to develop. Distinguishing radiation-induced cancer by its physical appearance is difficult because it does not appear different from cancers initiated by other agents. Cancer from natural causes frequently occurs, and the number of cancers induced by radiation is small compared with the natural incidence of malignancies even at doses many times those encountered in diagnostic radiology. Therefore, cancer caused by low-level radiation is extremely difficult to identify. In general, evidence of radiation-induced carcinogenesis in humans comes from the observation of irradiated humans and from epidemiologic studies conducted many years after subjects were exposed to *high doses* of ionizing radiation. Examples of these data are listed in Box 9.2. An explanation of each example follows.

Radium watch-dial painters. During the early years of the last century (1920s and 1930s), a radium watch-dial painting industry flourished in some factories in New Jersey. Young, unprotected, and ill-informed young women employed in these factories hand-painted the luminous

---

BOX 9.2 Human Evidence for Radiation Carcinogenesis

1. Radium watch-dial painters (1920s and 1930s)
2. Uranium miners (early years, and Navajo people of Arizona and New Mexico during the 1950s and 1960s)
3. Early medical radiation workers (radiologists, dentists, technologists) (1896 to 1910)
4. Patients injected with the contrast agent Thorotrast (1925 to 1945)
5. Infants treated with x-radiation to reduce an enlarged thymus gland (1940s and 1950s)
6. Children of the Marshall Islanders inadvertently subjected to high levels of fallout during an atomic bomb test in 1954
7. Japanese atomic bomb survivors (1945)
8. Patients with benign postpartum mastitis who were given radiation therapy treatments (mid 1900s)
9. Evacuees from the Chernobyl nuclear power station disaster in 1986

---

numerals on watches and clocks with a radium-containing paint. The girls used sable brushes to apply the paint. To do the fine work required, some would place the paint-saturated brush tip on their lips to draw the bristles to a fine point. The girls who followed this procedure unfortunately ingested large quantities of radium. Because it is chemically similar to calcium, the radium was incorporated into bone tissue. Eventually the accumulation of this toxic substance caused:

- Development of osteoporosis (decalcification of bone)
- Osteogenic sarcoma (bone cancer)
- Other malignancies such as
  - carcinoma of the epithelial cells lining the nasopharynx and paranasal sinuses

The bones most frequently affected by cancer included the pelvis, femur, and mandible. Doses of 5 Gy_t or more are assumed to have induced the aforementioned malignancies. The number of head carcinomas attributed to the radium watch-dial painting industry, although small, is statistically significant. Of 1474 women in the industry, 61 were diagnosed with cancer of the paranasal sinuses and 21 with cancer of the mastoid air cells. Studies attributed the death of at least 18 of the radium watch-dial painters to radium poisoning.

Uranium miners. During the early years of the last century, people worked in European mines to extract pitchblende, a uranium ore. Uranium ($^{238}U_{92}$) is a radioactive element with a very long half-life of 4.5 billion years. It decays through a series of radioactive nuclides by emitting alpha, beta, and gamma radiation. One of the most important members of its decay family is radon*, which decays to the radioactive gas, radon. Because of its gaseous nature, radon was able to seep through tiny gaps in rocks within the mines and created an ever-present insidious airborne hazard to miners. Consequently, throughout many years of employment, some miners inevitably inhaled significant amounts of radon, leading to about 50% of the miners eventually succumbing to lung cancer.

During the 1950s and 1960s, at the height of the Cold War between the United States and the Soviet Union, the US government needed fuel for nuclear weapons and power plants. The Navajo people of Arizona and New Mexico mined uranium to meet this need. Because the

---

*Radium (atomic number Z = 88) has an unstable nucleus and decays with a half-life of 1622 years by alpha particle emission to the radioactive element radon (Z = 86).

government did not regulate working conditions in the mines to ensure safety from exposure—despite an awareness of risk—some 15,000 Navajo and other workers in the uranium mines received substantial doses of ionizing radiation by breathing radioactive dust and drinking radioactive water. Researchers have estimated that each miner unknowingly got an approximate equivalent dose of 10 Sv or more.[8] The families of the miners also were affected because the clothing worn by the miners was contaminated by radioactive material.

Early medical radiation workers. Many of the first generation of radiation workers (radiologists, dentists, and technologists) were exposed to large amounts of ionizing radiation without realizing the dangers of this exposure. This resulted in a large number of severe radiation injuries to these individuals. An example of that was the development of cancerous skin lesions on the hands of radiologists and dentists (Fig. 9.8). When compared with their nonradiologist counterparts, a significant number of these early radiation workers also had a higher incidence of blood disorders such as:

- Aplastic anemia
- Leukemia

Because all worked without the benefit of protective devices, which led to some receiving doses estimated at more than 1 Gy/year, the occurrence of these radiation-induced injuries is very understandable. Today, as a result of programs stressing radiation safety education, appropriate usage of protective devices, and safety improvements in x-ray imaging equipment, radiation workers employed in medical imaging need not experience any adverse health effects as a consequence of their work. Detailed studies of radiographers and physicians who began their careers in radiology after the 1940s have demonstrated that these radiation workers had no increase in adverse health effects as a result of their occupational exposure. This finding is attributed to increased knowledge and use of proper protective measures and improved safety devices.[9]

Patients injected with the contrast agent Thorotrast. Between 1925 and 1945, Thorotrast was used as a contrast agent for diagnostic angiography. This medium contained a radioactive colloidal suspension that was approximately 25% thorium dioxide (ThO_2) by weight.[10] When administered by intravascular injection, the radioactive material emitted alpha particles that were deposited in the patient's reticuloendothelial system. The liver and spleen became the primary recipients of this substance. After a period of 15 to 20 years, the cumulative destruction wrought by the alpha particle–emitting contrast agent resulted in many cases of:

- Liver cancer
- Spleen cancer
- Angiosarcomas
- Biliary duct carcinomas

When the contrast agent was administered by extravascular injection, the tissue surrounding the injection site itself eventually became cancerous.

Infants treated for an enlarged thymus gland. The thymus is a gland located adjacent to the thyroid in the mediastinal cavity. The thymus gland plays a crucial role in the body's defenses against infection. During the 1940s and early 1950s, physicians diagnosed thymus gland enlargement in many infants with respiratory distress. To reduce the size of the gland, physicians treated the infants with therapeutic doses (1.2 to 60 Gy_t) of x-radiation. Because the thyroid is so close to the thymus, the thyroid gland also received a substantial radiation dose. This resulted in the development, some 20 years later, of thyroid nodules and carcinomas in many of these treated infants.

Incidence of breast cancer in radiation treatment of benign postpartum mastitis. Studies showed that postpartum patients treated with ionizing radiation for relief

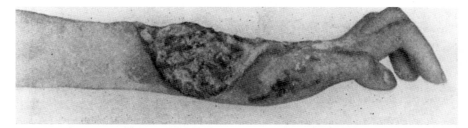

FIG 9.8 Carcinoma of the distal arm and hand developing after an x-ray burn (in 1904). (From Allen CW: *Radiotherapy and Phototherapy Including Radium and High Frequency Currents,* New York, 1904, Lea Brothers.)

of mastitis are another group of individuals in whom the results of radiation exposure to healthy breast tissue via scattered radiation indicate that radiation can cause breast cancer. In a particular study of 531 women who received a mean dose of 247 cGy$_t$, "breast cancer incidence doubled from 3.2% expected to 6.3% actual."[11] Because there is ongoing concern that mammography performed for either screening or diagnostic purposes could possibly cause the development of breast cancer, epidemiologic studies that provide such statistical information continue to be a high priority.

Children of the Marshall Islanders. Thyroid cancer also occurred in the children of the Marshall Islanders who were inadvertently subjected to high levels of fallout during an atomic bomb test (code name Bravo) on March 1, 1954. During the detonation of a 15-megaton thermonuclear device on Bikini Atoll, the wind shifted and carried the fallout over the neighboring islands. As a consequence of this exposure, the children received substantial absorbed doses to the thyroid from both external exposure and internal ingestion of radioiodine. It has been estimated that inhabitants of Rongelap Atoll received a mean dose of radiation to the thyroid gland of 21 Gy$_t$, and the inhabitants of Utrik Atoll received 2.80 Gy$_t$.[12,13] Hence a dose of 12 Gy$_t$ is considered to be representative of a population average dose for these two areas combined.

Japanese atomic bomb survivors

Atomic bomb detonation on Hiroshima and Nagasaki. On August 6, 1945, the United States dropped the first atomic bomb on the Japanese city of Hiroshima, thus marking the pivotal moment in the latter stages of World War II. Three days later, on August 9, 1945, a second bomb was dropped on the city of Nagasaki. Of the 300,000 people living in these two cities at the time of these bombings, approximately 88,000 people were killed and at least 70,000 more were injured. Many of those who died were killed by the heat and the blast (Fig. 9.9). Many of those who survived became victims of radiation injuries. These individuals have been observed since that time for signs of stochastic effects of radiation.

Data obtained from epidemiologic studies. Epidemiologic studies of approximately 100,000 Japanese survivors of the atomic bombings at Hiroshima and Nagasaki indicate that ionizing radiation causes leukemia (proliferation of the white blood cells). "Studies of the atomic bomb survivors in both Hiroshima and Nagasaki show a statistically significant increase in leukemia incidence in the exposed population compared with the

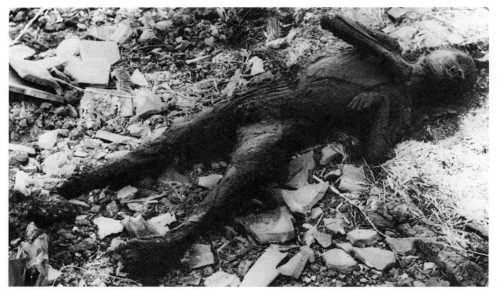

FIG 9.9 Charred human remains found in the epicenter of Nagasaki after the detonation of the atomic bomb on August 9, 1945. (From Magnum Photos.)

non-exposed population. In the period 1950 to 1956, 117 new cases of leukemia were reported in the Japanese survivors; approximately 64 of these can be attributed to radiation exposure."[1]

Incidence of leukemia rate of other radiation-induced malignancies. Among the atomic bomb survivors, the number of leukemia victims has slowly declined since the late 1940s and early 1950s. However, the occurrence rates of other radiation-induced malignancies have continued to escalate since the late 1950s and early 1960s. Among these are a variety of solid tumors such as:

- Thyroid cancer
- Breast cancer
- Lung cancer
- Bone cancers

Fig. 9.10 demonstrates the nominal risk of malignancy, as identified by Warren K. Sinclair, from a dose of 0.01 Gy_t of uniform whole-body radiation.[14] The graph indicates that leukemia occurs approximately 2 years after the initial exposure, rises to its highest level of incidence between 7 and 10 years, and then declines to almost zero at about 30 years. Unlike leukemia, solid tumors take approximately 10 years to develop and generally increase in occurrence at the same rate that cancer increases as people age. Whether the risk for solid tumors continues to rise beyond

40 years or declines, as with leukemia, is still unknown. Follow-up studies of the atomic bomb survivors may eventually provide the answer.

Incidence of breast cancer in Japanese women. In general, Japanese women have a lower natural incidence of breast cancer than US and Canadian women.[15] Studies of the female Japanese atomic bomb survivors provide strong evidence that ionizing radiation can induce breast cancer. The incidence of breast cancer in these women rises with radiation dose. It follows a linear nonthreshold curve. Numerous studies of female survivors indicate a relative risk for breast cancer ranging from 4:1 to as high as 10:1.

Effectiveness of ionizing radiation as a cancer-causing agent. Although studies from Hiroshima and Nagasaki confirm that high doses of ionizing radiation cause cancer, radiation is not a highly effective cancer-causing agent. For example, follow-up studies of approximately 82,000 atomic bomb survivors from 1950 to 1978 reveal an excess of only 250 cancer deaths attributed to radiation exposure. Instead of the expected 4500 cancer deaths, 4750 actually occurred. This indicates that of about every 300 atomic bomb survivors, 1 died of a malignancy attributed to an average whole-body radiation dose of approximately 0.14 Sv.

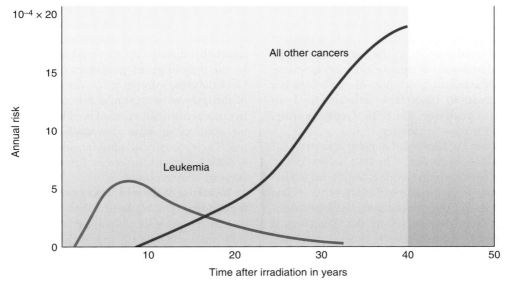

FIG 9.10 Nominal risk of malignancy from a dose of 0.01 Gy_t of uniform whole-body radiation. (From Sinclair WK: Radiation protection recommendations on dose limits: the role of the NCRP and the ICRP and future developments, *J Radiat Oncol Biol Phys* 131:387, 1995.)

Radiation dose and radiation-induced leukemia. Epidemiologic data about the Hiroshima atomic bomb survivors also indicate that a linear relationship exists between radiation dose and radiation-induced leukemia. In other words, the chance of contracting leukemia as a result of exposure to radiation is directly proportional to the magnitude of the radiation exposure. Available information of the kind necessary to establish the existence of a threshold dose–response relationship (i.e., whether a harmless dose exists) is inconclusive. Hence radiation-induced leukemia is assumed to follow a linear non-threshold dose–response relationship compared with leukemia in a population that has not been exposed to ionizing radiation.[10] More recent reevaluations of the quantity and type of radiation that was released in the cities of Hiroshima and Nagasaki provide a better foundation for radiation dose and damage assessment. Originally, neutrons were credited with the damage in Hiroshima. However, when more recent studies revealed that the uranium-fueled bomb dropped on Hiroshima provided more gamma radiation exposure and less neutron exposure than previously believed, data on the survivors were updated to reflect this more accurate information. As a result, researchers have established that gamma radiation and neutrons each provided about 50% of the radiation dose inflicted on the population of Hiroshima. Conversely, the inhabitants of Nagasaki, who were exposed to a plutonium bomb, received only 10% of their exposure from neutrons and 90% from gamma radiation. Based on the revised atomic bomb data, radiation-induced leukemias and solid tumors in the survivors may be attributed predominantly to gamma radiation exposure. The impact of the atomic bomb dosimetry revision is a significant increase in cancer risk estimates for both gamma and x-ray irradiation. The BEIR V report provides a summary of the newer estimates.

Evacuees from the Chernobyl nuclear disaster

Need for follow-up studies. The 1986 nuclear power station accident at Chernobyl requires long-term follow-up studies to assess the magnitude and severity of late effects on the exposed population. Detailed observations investigating potential increases in the incidence of leukemia, thyroid problems, breast cancer, and other possible radiation-induced malignancies will continue.

Evacuation of people within 36 hours after the accident. Within 36 hours of the nuclear catastrophe, 49,360 people residing at Pripyat, a city 2 miles from the plant, were evacuated. An additional 85,640 people, most of whom were living within a 10-mile (30-km) radial zone about Chernobyl, were also evacuated over a period of 14 days after the disaster. In general, the 135,000 evacuees received an average equivalent dose of 0.12 Sv per person. Of the 135,000, approximately 24,000 people received an equivalent dose of about 0.45 Sv. The remaining 111,000 people received from 0.03 to 0.06 Sv.[16,17] If the evacuees are monitored for at least 30 years, important estimates of radiation-induced leukemias, thyroid cancers, and other malignancies may be obtained.

Worldwide effects of the accident. The possibility of late effects occurring from the Chernobyl power station disaster is still a source of concern worldwide. Because winds carried the radioactive plume in several different directions during the 10 days after the accident, more than 20 countries were affected by fallout, with approximately 400,000 people receiving some degree of radiation exposure. In February 1989, Dr. Richard Wilson, professor of physics at Harvard University in Cambridge, Massachusetts, estimated "that about 20,000 people throughout the world" will develop a radiation-induced malignancy from the Chernobyl accident.[18]

Attempts by physicians to prevent thyroid cancer in children. Iodine-131 ($^{131}I_{53}$) is one of the radioactive materials that became airborne in the radioactive plume.[131] I concentrates in the thyroid gland and may cause cancer many years after the initial exposure. In an attempt to prevent thyroid cancer resulting from the accidental overdose of ^{131}I, physicians administered potassium iodide to children in Poland and other countries after the Chernobyl disaster. By offering a substitute for take-up by the thyroid gland, potassium iodide is intended to block the gland's uptake of ^{131}I. The degree of effectiveness of this preventive treatment remains to be determined. In other accidentally exposed populations, thyroid cancer has occurred in some individuals at doses of 1 Gy_t or less. The approximate time for the appearance of such radiation-induced thyroid malignancies is usually 10 to 20 years after exposure.

Incidence of thyroid cancer and breast cancer since the accident. During the first 10 years after the Chernobyl disaster, the incidence of thyroid cancer increased dramatically among children living in the regions of Belarus, Ukraine, and Russia (Fig. 9.11), where the heaviest radioactive iodine contamination occurred. Thyroid cancer has been the "most pronounced health effect" of the radiation accident.[19] As of April 1996, more than 700 cases of thyroid cancer were diagnosed in children residing

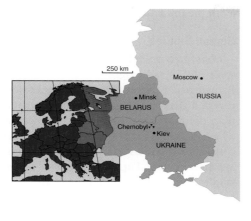
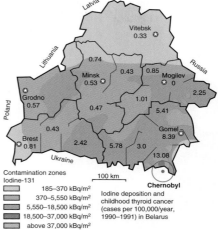

FIG 9.11 In the first 10 years after the Chernobyl nuclear accident, a dramatic increase in thyroid cancer was seen among children living in the regions of Belarus, Ukraine, and Russia, where the heaviest contamination occurred. (From Abelin T, Egger M, Ruchti C: Fallout from Chernobyl. Belarus increase was probably caused by Chernobyl, *BMJ* 12:1298, 1994.)

in these areas. The number of new thyroid cancer cases identified since the Chernobyl incident is significantly higher than anticipated, and by 1998 a total of 1700 cases had been diagnosed.[20] Radiation scientists from the Western and Eastern Hemispheres are collaborating to determine the reason for this increase. Some possible explanations for the higher-than-expected number of thyroid cancers are as follows:

1. Chronic iodine deficiency during the years preceding the accident in the children living in the regions contaminated
2. Genetic predisposition to developing thyroid malignancy after radiation exposure in some subgroups of the exposed population[19]

If the first theory is valid, the thyroid glands of these individuals would have preferentially assimilated isotopes of the radioactive material inhaled from a cloud or ingested from contaminated milk supplies. If the second theory is valid, some of the exposed individuals may have a disorder that prevents the mechanism normally used by healthy cells to initiate repair and mend the genetic damage.

Why early studies did not demonstrate a significant increase in the incidence of leukemia after the accident. From the earlier discussion of the Japanese atomic bomb survivors, we have learned that radiation causes leukemia and that the disease is assumed to follow a linear nonthreshold dose–response curve. However, early studies of the Chernobyl victims did not demonstrate a significant increase in the incidence of leukemia, possibly because the radioactive iodine and cesium expelled into the environment during the accident may produce damaging health effects in different ways.[21] For example, ^{131}I has a relatively short half-life (about 8 days) and is assimilated by the body and quickly distributed to the thyroid gland, thereby delivering an abrupt, acute dose to that organ. Radioactive cesium, conversely, has a much longer life (e.g., for $_{55}$Cs^{137}, $T_{1/2} = 30$ years). It causes whole-body irradiation over a lengthy time span through its long-term presence in the environment and food supply lines. This probably increases the incidence of childhood leukemia (Fig. 9.12). However, this increase is difficult to detect without very sensitive and reliable monitoring procedures.

Subsequent findings. Later studies began to demonstrate some of the expected effects. Reports indicated an approximately 50% increase in leukemia cases in children and adults in the Gomel region since the Chernobyl disaster.[22,23] Although the World Health Organization (WHO) reported that it found no increase in leukemia in the populations hit hardest by fallout from Chernobyl by 1993,[24] in 1995 the WHO reported that nearly 700 cases of thyroid cancer among children and adolescents had been linked to the Chernobyl accident.[25] In addition, in June 2001 at the Third International Conference, held

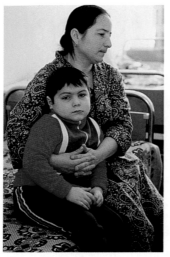

FIG 9.12 Mother with son who has radiation-induced leukemia. The child is a victim of the 1986 nuclear power plant explosion at Chernobyl. (From Ken Graham Photography.)

in Kiev, a statistically significant rise in the number of leukemia cases was reported in the Russian cleanup workers who worked during 1986 and 1987 at the Chernobyl power station complex.[26] Since the time of the Chernobyl accident, there has also been an increase in the incidence of breast cancer directly attributed to the radiation exposure.[27] If these findings continue to be substantiated, it will take many more years of observation and analysis before all the adverse health effects can be understood. Further investigation is indeed necessary.

Given that the actual levels of risk from the accident are still unknown, because of the limited data provided by the Russians, the risk for development of radiation-induced malignancies is difficult to determine.

Life Span Shortening
Animal Studies

Laboratory experiments on small animals have shown that the life span of animals that were exposed to nonlethal doses of ionizing radiation was shortened as a consequence of the exposure. When compared with a control group of unexposed small animals, the exposed animals died sooner. Radiation was then believed to have accelerated all causes of death. This reduction in the life cycle was termed *nonspecific life span shortening*. It was also believed that radiation accelerated the aging process, thus making the animals more susceptible to several diseases. In

actuality, early demise of the experimental animals resulted from the induction of cancer.

Human Studies

American radiologists. In humans, studies of the life span of US radiologists that were conducted by the Radiological Society of North America from 1945 to 1954 revealed that radiologists did have a shorter life span than nonradiologist physicians.[10] However, the process of evaluation of the information has been subject to considerable criticism, and the conclusions of the study are questionable. Further analysis of the epidemiologic studies showed that shortening of the life span in both animals and humans was the result of cancer and leukemia and not other "nonspecific" causes or accelerated aging.

American radiologic technologists. Initiated in 1982 and currently still in progress, an extensive study of approximately 146,000 US radiologic technologists (USRT) is continuing to evaluate potential radiation-related adverse health effects resulting from long-term, repeated exposures to low-dose ionizing radiation. These responses include cancer incidence and other work-related conditions. This occupational epidemiologic study is a collaborative effort among the University of Minnesota School of Public Health, the National Cancer Institute, and the American Registry of Radiologic Technologists. The study involves a series of mail surveys to all participating technologists and telephone interviews with approximately 1200 retired technologists who were in the field before 1950. The interviews provide important information about work practices that were common in the early years before personnel monitoring devices were routinely used.[28,29]

As reported in the Volume 2, Spring 2004 edition of the USRT Newsletter, among the 90,305 technologists who completed the first survey in the mid-1980s, there were 1283 deaths from cancer. A comparison was made between technologists who started working in the 1960s or later and those who began working before 1940. A slightly higher risk of dying from any type of cancer was found in technologists working before 1940. Technologists who began working after 1940 did not demonstrate any elevated risk. However, technologists entering the medical radiation industry before 1950 demonstrated a somewhat higher risk of dying from leukemia compared with individuals entering the workforce in 1950 or later. The risk of dying from breast cancer has also been studied in technologists working in the field before 1940, in those working between 1940 and 1950, and in those entering the field in 1960 or later. Technologists who began working before 1940 had the greatest risk of dying of breast cancer, followed by those who worked up to 1950. When the risk of dying of breast cancer in women who began their careers in the 1950s is compared with that in women employed from 1960 or later, the risk is only slightly higher for the women first employed in the 1950s. Improvements in radiologic technology, medical imaging equipment, and radiation safety are factors in cancer risk reduction. Readers interested in obtaining more information about this ongoing study can visit the website at www.radtechstudy.org, or they can write to US Radiologic Technologist Study, University of Minnesota, Health Science Section, MMC 807, 420 Delaware Street S.E., Minneapolis, MN 55455. "Studies are ongoing by other well-known experts in the field such as researchers of the National Cancer Institute's Radiation Epidemiology Branch. Their more recent work has focused on interventional technologists who are exposed to higher doses of radiation than the general population of technologists."[30]

Cataractogenesis

The lens of the eye contains transparent fibers that transmit light. The lens focuses light on the retina so that as the image forms, it may be transmitted through the optic nerve (Fig. 9.13B). The probability that a single dose of ionizing radiation of approximately 2 Gy_t will induce the formation of cataracts (opacity of the eye lens) (see Fig. 9.13A) is high. Cataracts result in partial or complete loss of vision. Laboratory experiments with mice show that cataracts may be induced with doses as low as 0.1 Gy_t. Highly ionizing neutron radiation is extremely efficient in inducing cataracts. A neutron dose as low as 0.01 Gy_t has been known to cause cataracts in mice. Radiation-induced cataracts in humans follow a threshold nonlinear dose–response relationship. Evidence of human radiation cataractogenesis comes from the observation of small groups of people who accidentally received substantial doses to the eyes. These groups include:

- Japanese atomic bomb survivors
- Nuclear physicists working with cyclotrons (units that produce beams of high-energy particles such as 150-MeV proton beams) between 1932 and 1960
- Patients undergoing radiation therapy who received significant exposures to the eyes during treatment

Recent data tend to show that the threshold for cataract induction is lower than was previously thought.[31] The

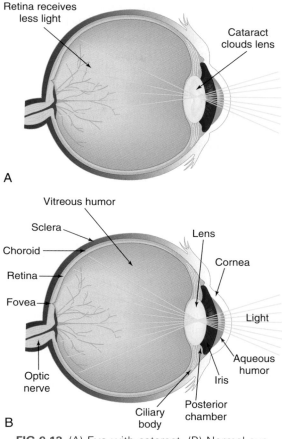

FIG 9.13 (A) Eye with cataract. (B) Normal eye.

threshold for single exposures is therefore now considered to be 0.5 Gy (50 cGy).[32] Even with this lower value, the chance of radiation-induced cataracts to radiographers occurring from general diagnostic imaging procedures is very remote. However, in the realm of diagnostic radiology, some very lengthy fluoroscopic procedures can result in not insignificant radiation exposure to the lens of the eye from cumulative scatter radiation. Occupational dose to this sensitive area can be substantially reduced when radiologists and radiographers wear protective eyewear while participating in the examination. In patients, exposure to the lens of the eye, and subsequent dose, can be decreased by also having them wear protective eye shields, provided the use of such shields does not compromise the diagnostic value of the fluoroscopic examination.

Embryologic Effects (Birth Defects)

Stages of Gestation in Humans. All life forms seem to be most vulnerable to radiation during the embryonic stage of development. The period of gestation during which the embryo-fetus is exposed to radiation governs the effects (death or congenital abnormality) of the radiation. Gestation in humans is divided into three stages:

1. Preimplantation, which corresponds to 0 to 9 days after conception
2. Organogenesis, which lasts approximately from 10 days postconception to 12 weeks after conception
3. The fetal stage, which extends from the twelfth week to term (Fig. 9.14)

Embryonic Cell Radiosensitivity During the First Trimester of Pregnancy. Because embryonic cells begin dividing and differentiating after conception, they are extremely radiosensitive and hence may easily be damaged by exposure to ionizing radiation. Thus the first trimester of pregnancy is the most crucial period with respect to harmful consequences from irradiation because the developing central nervous system and related sensory organs of the embryo-fetus contain a large number of stem cells during this period of gestation.

When a high dose of radiation is received by the embryo within approximately 2 weeks of fertilization (before the start of organogenesis), prenatal death is the most obvious adverse consequence of such an exposure. This usually manifests as a spontaneous abortion. If this does not occur, the pregnancy will simply continue to term without any negative effect.[10] Irradiation of the embryo-fetus during the first 12 weeks of development to equivalent doses in excess of 200 mSv frequently may result in death or in severe congenital abnormalities.

During the preimplantation stage, the fertilized ovum divides and forms a ball-like structure containing undifferentiated cells. If this structure is irradiated with a dose in the range of 0.05 to 0.15 Gy_t, embryonic death will occur. Malformations resulting from radiation exposure do not occur at this stage. Because organogenesis occurs at approximately 10 days to 12 weeks after conception, the developing fetus is most susceptible to radiation-induced congenital abnormalities during this period. This is actually the time when the undifferentiated cells are beginning to differentiate into organs. Abnormalities occurring as a consequence of irradiation during the period of organogenesis may include:

- Growth inhibition
- Intellectual disability
- Microcephaly
- Genital deformities
- Sensory organ damage

During the late stages of organogenesis, the presence of nonminor abnormalities in the fetus will cause neonatal death (death at birth). Skeletal damage from radiation exposure occurs most frequently during the period from week 3 to week 20 of development. Cancer and functional disorders during childhood are other possible effects of irradiation during the fetal stage (a growth period).

Embryonic Cell Radiosensitivity During the Second and Third Trimesters of Pregnancy. Fetal radiosensitivity decreases as gestation progresses. Hence, during the second and third trimesters of pregnancy when lesser numbers

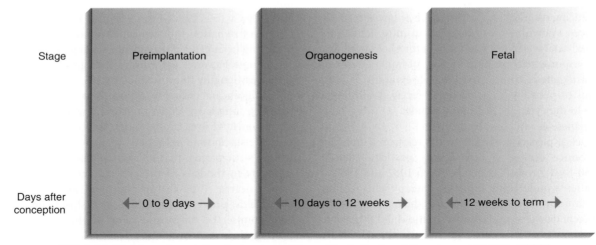

| Stage | Preimplantation | Organogenesis | Fetal |

| Days after conception | ← 0 to 9 days → | ← 10 days to 12 weeks → | ← 12 weeks to term → |

FIG 9.14 Division of gestation in humans. (From Riegh R: *Am J Roentgenol* 89:182, 1963.)

of cells are differentiating, the developing fetus is less susceptible to ionizing radiation exposure. However, even in these later trimesters, congenital abnormalities and functional disorders such as sterility may be caused by radiation exposure.

Much of the evidence for radiation-induced congenital abnormalities in humans comes from more than four decades of follow-up studies of children exposed in utero during the atomic bomb detonations in Hiroshima and Nagasaki. Although the risk of radiation-induced leukemia is greater when the embryo-fetus is irradiated during the first trimester, leukemia also may be brought on by exposure to radiation during the second and third trimesters. Studies of the latter, however, have not demonstrated any significant rates of cancer and leukemia deaths.[33]

Embryonic Effects Resulting From the Chernobyl Nuclear Power Plant Accident.

Of the 135,000 evacuees from the 18-mile (30-km) radial zone of the Chernobyl nuclear power plant, approximately 2000 were pregnant women. Each received an average total-body equivalent dose of 0.43 Sv. No obvious abnormalities were observed in the 300 live babies born by August 1987. However, from after 1987 through 1990, the Ministry of Health in the Ukraine recorded an increased number of miscarriages, premature births, and stillbirths.[22,23] Also recorded by the ministry was an increase to three times the normal rate of deformities and developmental abnormalities in newborns.[22,23]

Review of Fetal Effects by UNSCEAR.

Fetal effects such as mortality, malformations, intellectual disability, and childhood cancer were reviewed by the United Nations Scientific Committee on the Effects of Atomic Radiation (UNSCEAR).[34] This group proposed an upper-limit *increased combined radiation risk* for the aforementioned fetal effects of "3 chances per 1000 children (0.3%) for each rem of fetal dose."[35] Without radiation, these fetal effects have an estimated *normal total risk* of "60 chances per 1000 children (6%)."[35] Thus the radiation was shown to produce an increased risk of 3 per 1000 children over the existing risk of 60 per 1000, leading to a total risk of 63 per 1000.

International Chernobyl Project.

In 1990 the International Chernobyl Project was initiated in response to a request for assistance from the former Soviet Union. The director of the Radiation Effects Research Foundation in Hiroshima, Japan, led this project. The study compared seven contaminated Russian villages with six uncontaminated villages. By 1990 no significant increases in fetal and genetic abnormalities were seen in this population.[36] However, because of the relatively long latency period for radiogenic cancer, particularly solid tumors, researchers expect that more time will be required before the ultimate impact on the population of Russia is known. Estimates of as many as 500 excess cancers in the former Soviet Union during the next 50 to 60 years have been made.[37]

Effects of Low-Level Ionizing Radiation on the Embryo-Fetus.

The effects of low-level ionizing radiation on the embryo-fetus can only be poorly estimated. Documentation of the effects of low-level radiation on the unborn irradiated in utero is insufficient because some types of abnormalities occur in a small percentage (approximately 4%) of all live births in the United States. However, if the exposure occurs during a period of major organogenesis, the abnormality and its occurrence may be more pronounced. Precise assessment of radiation-induced birth abnormalities from low-level exposure can be very difficult because human genes vary naturally, and the expression of the traits they encode is affected by the environment.

Because the embryo-fetus is extra sensitive to radiation, radiation workers should exercise caution and employ appropriate safety measures when performing radiographic procedures on pregnant patients. Medical physicists are able to make fetal dose estimates for specific patients based upon characteristics such as patient size and the actual technical parameters used in the studies in cases where there are concerns about medical management.

GENETIC (HEREDITARY) EFFECTS

Cause of Genetic Mutations

Biologic effects of ionizing radiation on future generations are termed genetic, or hereditary, effects. They can occur as a result of radiation-induced damage to the DNA molecule in the sperm or ova of an adult, leading to germ cell mutations. These cause faulty genetic information to be transmitted to the offspring. This altered hereditary information may manifest as various diseases or malformations.

Natural Spontaneous Mutations

Some mutations in genetic material occur spontaneously, without a known cause. Such randomly occurring mutations in genes and DNA are called *spontaneous mutations*.

These mutations can be transmitted from one generation to the next and can cause a wide variety of disorders or diseases, including:

- Hemophilia
- Huntington's chorea
- Down syndrome (mongolism)
- Duchenne's muscular dystrophy
- Sickle cell anemia
- Cystic fibrosis
- Hydrocephalus

Hereditary disorders are common in any animal population. In humans, a hereditary disorder is present in approximately 10% of all live births in the United States.

Mutagens Capable of Inducing Genetic Mutations

Certain agents can increase the frequency of mutations. Some of these include:

- Ionizing radiation
- Viruses
- Specific chemicals

These agents are called *mutagens,* and ionizing radiation is one of the more effective mutagens known. Any nonlethal radiation dose received by the germ cells can cause chromosome mutations that may be transmitted to successive generations.

Radiation Interaction With DNA Macromolecules

When radiation interacts with DNA macromolecules, it can modify the structure of these molecules by causing breaks in the chromosomes or by causing a deletion or an alteration in the sequence of nitrogen bases. Such modifications change the cell's hereditary information. A mutation of this type could eventually lead to genetic disease in subsequent generations.

Incapacities of Mutant Genes

Mutant genes cannot properly govern the cell's normal chemical reactions or properly control the sequence of amino acids in the formation of specific proteins. These incapacities result in various genetic diseases. For example, sickle cell anemia arises from the defective synthesis of the protein hemoglobin. About 300 amino acids combine to form the hemoglobin molecule. Sickle cell anemia is caused by the omission of only a single vital amino acid.

Dominant or Recessive Point Mutations

Point mutations (genetic mutations at the molecular level) may be either *dominant* (probably expressed in the offspring) or *recessive* (probably not expressed for several generations). Radiation is thought to cause primarily recessive mutations. For a recessive mutation to appear in the offspring, both parents must have the same genetic defect. This means that the defect must be located on the same part of a specific DNA base sequence in each parent. Because this rarely occurs, the effects of recessive mutations are not likely to appear in a population. However, an increase in the number of individuals who receive radiation exposure raises the likelihood that two individuals with the same type of mutation will have children. Therefore it is important to limit the radiation exposure of the entire population. Damage from recessive mutations sometimes manifests more subtly and may play a role in many commonly encountered disorders related to metabolism or the immune system.

Ionizing Radiation as a Possible Cause of Genetic (Hereditary) Effects

The only concrete evidence showing that ionizing radiation causes genetic effects comes from extensive experimentation with fruit flies and mice at high radiation doses. The data on mice have been extrapolated to low doses and then applied to humans. The information obtained from the fruit fly experiments suggests that *hereditary effects do not have a threshold dose.* Because this means that even the smallest radiation dose could cause some hereditary damage, there is, according to these data, no such thing as a "100% safe" gonadal radiation dose.

Existing data on radiation-induced genetic effects in humans, however, are both contradictory and inconclusive. Some of the data accumulated come from observation of test groups of children conceived after one or both parents had been exposed to radiation as a result of the atomic bomb detonation in Hiroshima or Nagasaki. As of the third generation, no radiation-induced genetic effects are known. However, this does not mean that they will not be seen in subsequent generations. J. F. Crow, a geneticist who spent many years experimenting with fruit flies, stated the following: "The most frequent mutations in man are not those leading to freaks or obvious hereditary diseases, but those causing minor impairments leading to higher embryonic death rates, lower life expectancy, increase in disease, or decreased fertility."[38] The position of the scientific community to date remains unresolved.

In 2001 an UNSCEAR study on the hereditary effects of radiation concluded that no radiation-induced genetic diseases had so far been demonstrated in human populations exposed to ionizing radiation. However, some counterexamples are thought to be found in the scientific literature.[23]

Currently, evidence of radiation-induced hereditary effects has not been observed in persons employed in diagnostic imaging or in patients undergoing radiologic examinations. Even with this information, it is still recommended that gonadal shielding be effectively used and all radiation exposure be maintained as low as reasonably achievable (ALARA).

Doubling Dose Concept

Animal studies of radiation-induced hereditary changes led to the development of the doubling dose concept. This dose measures the effectiveness of ionizing radiation in causing mutations. Doubling dose is the radiation dose that causes the number of spontaneous mutations occurring in a given generation to increase to two times their original number. For example, if 7% of the offspring in each generation are born with mutations in the absence of radiation other than background levels, the administration of the doubling dose to all members of the population would eventually increase the number of mutations to 14% (Box 9.3). The radiation doubling equivalent dose for humans, as determined from studies of the children of the atomic bomb survivors of Hiroshima and Nagasaki, is estimated to have a mean value of 1.56 Sv based on the hereditary indicators of untoward pregnancy outcome (e.g., stillbirths, major congenital abnormalities, death

during the first postnatal week), childhood mortality, and sex chromosome aneuploidy (possession of an abnormal number of chromosomes).

■ SUMMARY

- Scientists use the information from epidemiologic studies to formulate dose–response graphical relationships to predict the risk of cancer in human populations exposed to low doses of ionizing radiation.
  - Curves that demonstrate radiation dose–response relationships can be either linear or nonlinear and depict either a threshold or a nonthreshold dose.
  - An LNT curve currently is used for most types of cancers.
  - Risk associated with low-level radiation other than cancer is usually estimated with the LQNT curve.
  - Late tissue reactions may be demonstrated graphically through the use of an LT curve of radiation dose–response.
  - High-dose cellular response may be demonstrated through the use of a sigmoid threshold curve.
- Late effects include carcinogenesis, cataractogenesis, and embryologic (birth) defects.
- Effects that have no threshold, that occur arbitrarily, that have a severity that does not depend on dose, and that occur months or years after exposure are called *stochastic effects.*
- Cancer is the most important stochastic somatic effect caused by exposure to ionizing radiation.
- Risk estimates are given in terms of absolute risk or relative risk.
  - The absolute risk model forecasts that a specific number of malignancies will occur as a result of radiation exposure.
  - The relative risk model predicts that the number of excess cancers rises as the natural incidence of cancer increases with advancing age in a population.
  - Linear and linear-quadratic models are used for extrapolation of risk from high-dose to low-dose data.
- The first trimester of pregnancy is the most critical period for radiation exposure of the embryo-fetus.
  - Radiation-induced congenital abnormalities can occur approximately 10 days to 12 weeks after conception.
  - Skeletal abnormalities most frequently occur from weeks 3 to 20.

BOX 9.3	Doubling Dose Concept	
Percentage (%) of offspring born in each generation with mutations in the absence of radiation other than background	Estimated radiation dose in sieverts (Sv) received	Percentage (%) of offspring born with mutation after receiving a doubling equivalent dose
7%	1.56 Sv	14%

- Radiation exposure even in the second and third trimesters can potentially cause congenital abnormalities, functional disorders, and a predisposition to the development of childhood cancer.
- Genetic effects of ionizing radiation are biologic effects on generations yet unborn.
  - Radiation-induced abnormalities are caused by unrepaired damage to DNA molecules in the sperm or ova of an adult.
  - There is no 100% safe gonadal radiation dose; even the smallest radiation dose could cause some hereditary damage.
  - Doubling dose measures the effectiveness of ionizing radiation in causing mutations; it is the radiation dose that causes the number of spontaneous mutations in a given generation to increase to two times their original number.
  - For humans, the doubling dose is estimated to have a mean value of 1.56 Sv.

REFERENCES

1. Travis EL: *Primer of medical rradiobiology*, ed 2, Chicago, 1989, Year Book.
2. Straume T, Dobson RL: Implications of new Hiroshima and Nagasaki dose estimates: cancer risks and neutron RBE. *Health Phys* 41:666, 1981.
3. Webster EW: Critical issues in setting radiation dose limits, Proceedings No. 3, Washington, DC, 1982, National Council on Radiation Protection and Measurements (NCRP).
4. Hendee WR, editor: *Health effects of low-level radiation*, Norwalk, CT, 1984, Appleton-Century-Crofts.
5. Doses from medical x-ray procedures. Available at: http://hps.org/physicians/documents/Doses_from_Medical_X-Ray_Procedures.pdf.
6. International Commission on Radiological Protection (ICRP): Recommendations of the International Commission on Radiological Protection, ICRP publication No. 60. *Ann ICRP* 21:1–3, 1991.
7. National Research Council, Commission of Life Sciences, Committee on Biological Effects on Ionizing Radiation (BEIR V), Board on Radiation Effects Research: Health effects of exposure to low levels of ionizing radiations, Washington, DC, 1989, National Academies Press.
8. Tilke B: Navajo miners battle long-term effects of radiation. *Adv Radiol Technol* 3:3, 1990.
9. Berrington de Gonzalez A, et al: Long-term mortality in 43763 U.S. radiologists compared with 64990 U.S. psychiatrists. *Radiology* 2016. doi:10.1148/radiol.2016152472. posted online 19 July.
10. Bushong SC: *Radiologic science for technologists: physics, biology and protection*, ed 10, St. Louis, 2013, Elsevier/Mosby.
11. Dowd SB, Tilson ER: *Practical radiation protection and applied radiobiology*, ed 2, Philadelphia, 1999, Saunders.
12. Hamilton TE, et al: Thyroid neoplasia in Marshall Islanders exposed to nuclear fallout. *JAMA* 258:629, 1987.
13. Lessard E, et al: Thyroid absorbed dose for people at Rongelap, Utrik, and Sifo on March 1, 1954, U.S. Department of Energy publication (BNL) 51-882, Upton, NY, 1985, Brookhaven National Laboratory.
14. Sinclair WK: Radiation protection recommendations on dose limits: the role of the NCRP and the ICRP and future developments. *Int J Radiat Oncol Biol Phys* 131:387–392, 1995.
15. Hall EJ: *Radiobiology for the radiologist*, ed 5, Philadelphia, 2000, Lippincott Williams & Wilkins.
16. Gale RP: Immediate medical consequences of nuclear accidents: lessons from Chernobyl. *JAMA* 258:625, 1987.
17. Perry AR, Iglar AF: The accident at Chernobyl: radiation doses and effects. *Radiol Technol* 61:290, 1990.
18. WGBH Transcript: Back to Chernobyl, Nova No. 1604, Boston, 1989 (television program originally broadcast on PBS on February 14, 1989).
19. Balter M: Children become the first victims of fallout. *Science* 272:357, 1996.
20. United Nations Scientific Committee on the Effects of Atomic Radiation (UNSCEAR): 2000 report to the General Assembly, with Scientific Annexes, UNSCEAR 2000: sources and effects of ionizing radiation, New York, 2000, United Nations.
21. Williams N: Leukemia studies continue to draw a blank. *Science* 272:358, 1996.
22. Otto Hug Strahleninstit: Information, Ausgabe 9/2001 K 2001.
23. Chernobyl: the facts—what you need to know almost 20 years after the disaster. Available at: http://www.chernobyl-international.org/documents/chernobylfacts2.pdf.
24. Walker SJ: *Permissible dose: a history of radiation protection in the twentieth century*, Berkeley, 2000, University of California Press.
25. Chernobyl accident. Available at: http://www.martinfrost.ws/htmlfiles/chernobyl1.html.
26. Conclusions of 3rd International Conference: Health effects of the Chernobyl accident. *Int J Radiat Med* 3:3–4, 2001.
27. Fifteen years after the Chernobyl accident: lessons learned, International Conference Executive Summary, Kiev, 2001.

28. University of Minnesota, Health Studies Section: U.S. Radiologic Technologists Study, vol 2, Minneapolis, 2004.

29. University of Minnesota, Health Studies Section: U.S. Radiologic Technologists Study. Available at: www .radtechstudy.org.

30. Rajaraman, et al: Cancer risks in the U.S. radiologic technologists working with fluoroscopic guided interventional procedures, 1994-2008. *AJR Am J Roentgenol* 1–9, 2016.

31. Bouffler S, et al: Radiation-induced cataracts: the Health Protection Agency's response to the ICRP statement on tissue reactions and recommendation on the dose limit for the eye lens. *J Radiol Prot* 32(4):479–488, 2012. doi:10.1088/0952-4746/32/4/479. [Epub 2012 Nov 27].

32. International Commission on Radiological Protection, Statement on Tissue Reactions, ICRP ref. 4825-3093-1464, April 21, 2011.

33. Stewart A, et al: A survey of childhood malignancies. *Br Med J* 1:1495, 1958.

34. United Nations Scientific Committee on the Effects of Atomic Radiation (UNSCEAR): Biological effects of pre-natal irradiation, 35th Session of UNSCEAR, Vienna, April 1986, New York, 1986, United Nations.

35. Webster EW, the Biological Effects Committee of the American Association of Physicists in Medicine (AAPM): A primer on low-level ionizing radiation and its biological effects, AAPM Report No. 18, New York, 1986, American Institute of Physics (published for the American Association of Physicists in Medicine).

36. Eijgenraam F: Chernobyl's cloud: a lighter shade of gray. *Science* 252:1245, 1991.

37. Goss LB: International team examines health in zones contaminated by Chernobyl. *Phys Today* 40:20, 1991.

38. Crow JF: Genetic effects of radiation. *Bull At Sci* 14:19, 1958.

GENERAL DISCUSSION QUESTIONS

1. How can the information obtained from a radiation dose–response curve be used?
2. What did the BEIR Committee's 1990 revised risk estimates for the atomic bomb survivors of Hiroshima and Nagasaki indicate?
3. What rationale is used when regulatory agencies establish radiation protection standards?
4. What is the difference between late tissue reaction and stochastic effects of ionizing radiation?
5. What is the difference between the absolute risk model and the relative risk model used for estimating risk caused by a specific exposure to ionizing radiation?

6. Name five groups of humans exposed to high doses of ionizing radiation that demonstrate proof that radiation induces cancer, and explain the circumstances that led to the exposure received by each group.
7. What is organogenesis, and what are the consequences to the developing fetus if irradiated during this period?
8. Describe the concept of doubling dose.
9. Describe the importance of epidemiologic studies as they related to radiation-induced cancer.
10. Name two groups of individuals who have demonstrated an increase in the incidence of breast cancer after radiation exposure.
11. Where is the thymus gland located?
12. Where is a sigmoid threshold curve of radiation dose–response relationship generally employed, and what is the curve used for?

REVIEW QUESTIONS

1. Cancer and genetic defects are examples of:
   A. Stochastic effects
   B. Early tissue reactions
   C. Birth effects
   D. Late tissue reactions
2. Some examples of measurable late biologic damage are:
   1. Cataracts
   2. Leukemia
   3. Nausea and vomiting
   4. Genetic mutations
   A. 1 and 2 only
   B. 2 and 3 only
   C. 1, 2, and 3 only
   D. 1, 2, and 4 only
3. Which of the following provide the foundation for the sigmoid, or S-shaped, threshold curve of radiation dose response?
   1. Data from human populations observed after acute high doses of radiation
   2. Data from human populations observed after chronic low doses of radiation
   3. Laboratory experiments on animals
   A. 1 only
   B. 2 only
   C. 3 only
   D. 1, 2, and 3

4. The linear nonthreshold curve implies that biologic response is:
   A. Directly proportional to the dose
   B. Inversely proportional to the dose
   C. Insignificant in relation to dose
   D. Not able to be plotted on a dose–response curve

5. Reevaluation of the quantity and type of radiation that was released in the atomic bombing of the cities of Hiroshima and Nagasaki has led to revised atomic bomb data in which radiation-induced leukemia and solid tumors may now be attributed predominantly to:
   A. Alpha radiation exposure
   B. Gamma radiation exposure
   C. Neutron radiation exposure
   D. X-radiation exposure

6. The radiation dose–response relationship is demonstrated graphically through the use of a curve that maps the observed effects of radiation exposure in relation to the dose of radiation received. Which of the following curves expresses a linear-quadratic nonthreshold dose response?
   A. ∠
   B. ∠
   C. ∠
   D. ∠

7. During the 10 years immediately after the 1986 Chernobyl nuclear power station accident, which of the following was the *most pronounced* health effect observed?
   1. Dramatic increase in the incidence of childhood leukemia

2. Dramatic increase in thyroid cancer in children living in the regions where the heaviest radioactive contamination occurred
   3. Major increase in the number of solid tumors in the general population of the former Soviet Union
   A. 1, 2, and 3
   B. 1 only
   C. 2 only
   D. 3 only

8. The early demise of experimental animals exposed to nonlethal doses of ionizing radiation actually resulted from:
   A. Accelerated aging
   B. Hemorrhage
   C. Induction of cancer
   D. Respiratory distress

9. According to data from studies performed on US radiologic technologists, individuals who began working before 1950 had a somewhat higher risk of dying of _____ when compared with technologists who started working in 1950 and later.
   A. Darkroom disease
   B. Leukemia
   C. Pancreatic cancer
   D. Thyroid cancer

10. Most diagnostic procedures result in equivalent doses:
    A. Above 0.1 Sv but less than 1.56 Sv
    B. Less than 0.1 Sv
    C. Between 1.56 Sv and 1.75 Sv
    D. Above 1.75 Sv

Dose Limits for Exposure to Ionizing Radiation

OBJECTIVES

After completing this chapter, the reader will be able to perform the following:

- Define all key terms.
- List and describe the function of the four major organizations that share the responsibility for evaluating the relationship between radiation equivalent dose and induced biologic effects and five US regulatory agencies responsible for enforcing established radiation effective dose limiting standards.
- Explain the function of the radiation safety committee (RSC) in a medical facility, and describe the role of the radiation safety officer (RSO) by listing the various responsibilities he or she must fulfill.
- Explain the purpose of the Radiation Control for Health and Safety Act of 1968 and the Consumer Patient Health and Safety Act of 1981.
- List the important provisions of the code of standards for diagnostic x-ray equipment that began on August 1, 1974.
- Explain the ALARA concept.
- Discuss current radiation protection philosophy.
- Identify radiation-induced responses that warrant serious concern for radiation protection.
- Explain the concept of risk as it relates to the medical imaging industry.
- Describe the effective dose limit and the effective dose limiting system.
- Identify the risk from exposure to ionizing radiation at low absorbed doses.
- Discuss current National Council on Radiation Protection and Measurements recommendations.

- Calculate the cumulative effective dose for the whole body for a radiation worker.
- Discuss the significance of action limits in health care facilities.
- Explain the concept of radiation hormesis.
- State the following in terms of International System (SI) units:
  - Annual occupational effective dose limit and cumulative effective dose (CumEfD) limit for whole-body exposure excluding medical and natural background exposure, which are based on stochastic effects
  - Annual occupational equivalent dose limits for tissues and organs such as lens of the eye, skin, hands, and feet, which are based on tissue reactions
  - Annual effective dose limits for continuous (or frequent) exposure and for infrequent exposure of the general public from manmade sources other than medical and natural background, which are based on stochastic effects
  - Annual equivalent dose limits for tissues and organs such as lens of the eye, skin, hands, and feet of members of the general public, which are based on tissue reactions
  - Annual effective dose limit for an occupationally exposed student under the age of 18 years (excluding medical and natural background radiation exposure)
  - Occupational monthly equivalent dose limit to the embryo-fetus (excluding medical and natural background radiation) once the pregnancy is known

KEY TERMS

action limits
agreement states
ALARA concept
annual occupational effective
dose limit
cumulative effective dose
(CumEfD) limit
effective dose (EfD)
effective dose (EfD) limiting system
effective dose limit (EDL)

equivalent dose (EqD)
International Commission on
Radiological Protection (ICRP)
lifetime effective dose
National Council on Radiation
Protection and Measurements
(NCRP)
negligible individual dose (NID)
Nuclear Regulatory Commission
(NRC)

optimization
radiation hormesis
radiation-induced malignancy
radiation safety committee (RSC)
radiation safety officer (RSO)
stochastic effects
tissue reactions
tissue weighting factor (W_T)

Exposure of the general public, patients, and radiation workers to ionizing radiation must be limited to minimize the risk of harmful biologic effects. To this end, scientists have developed occupational and nonoccupational *effective dose (EfD)* limits and *equivalent dose (EqD)* limits for tissues and organs such as the lens of the eye, skin, hands, and feet. An *effective dose (EfD) limiting system* (i.e., a set of numeric dose limits that are based on calculations of the various risks of cancer and genetic [hereditary] effects to tissues or organs exposed to radiation) has been incorporated into Title 10 of the Code of Federal Regulations, Part 20, a document prepared and distributed by the US Office of the Federal Register. The rules and regulations of the Nuclear Regulatory Commission (NRC) and fundamental radiation protection standards governing occupational radiation exposure are included in this document.

BASIS OF EFFECTIVE DOSE LIMITING SYSTEM

The concept of radiation exposure and of the associated risk of *radiation-induced malignancy* is the basis of the effective dose limiting system. Information contained in Report No. 116 of the National Council on Radiation Protection and Measurement (NCRP) and Publication No. 60 of the International Commission on Radiological Protection (ICRP) serves as a resource for the revised recommendations. Future radiation protection standards are expected to continue to be based on *risk*.

Because medical imaging professionals share the responsibility for patient safety from radiation exposure and are subject themselves to such exposure in the performance of their duties, they must be familiar with previous, existing, and new guidelines. By keeping informed, they will be more conscious of good radiation safety practices. A radiographer may obtain the required knowledge by becoming familiar with the functions of the various advisory groups and regulatory agencies discussed in this chapter (Fig. 10.1).

RADIATION PROTECTION STANDARDS ORGANIZATIONS

The discussion that follows concerns the four major organizations responsible for evaluating the relationship between radiation EqD and induced biologic effects. In addition, the following organizations are concerned with

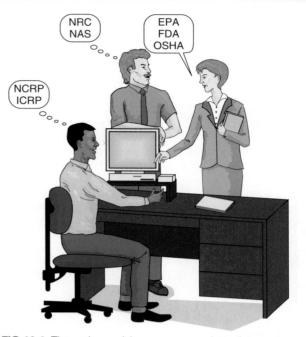

FIG 10.1 The various advisory groups and regulatory agencies, usually referred to by abbreviations and acronyms, may be extremely confusing.

formulating risk estimates of somatic and genetic effects of irradiation:

1. International Commission on Radiological Protection (ICRP)
2. National Council on Radiation Protection and Measurements (NCRP)
3. United Nations Scientific Committee on the Effects of Atomic Radiation (UNSCEAR)
4. National Academy of Sciences/National Research Council Committee on the Biological Effects of Ionizing Radiation (NAS/NRC-BEIR)

A summary of radiation standards organizations is presented in Table 10.1.

International Commission on Radiological Protection

The **International Commission on Radiological Protection (ICRP)** is considered the international authority on the safe use of sources of ionizing radiation. It is composed of a main commission with 12 active members, a chairman, and four standing committees, which include committees on radiation effects, radiation exposure, protection in medicine, and the application of ICRP

TABLE 10.1 Summary of Radiation Protection Standards Organizations

Organization	Function
International Commission on Radiological Protection (ICRP)	Evaluates information on biologic effects of radiation and provides radiation protection guidance through general recommendations on occupational and public dose limits
National Council on Radiation Protection and Measurements (NCRP)	Reviews regulations formulated by the ICRP and decides ways to include those recommendations in US radiation protection criteria
United Nations Scientific Committee on the Effects of Atomic Radiation (UNSCEAR)	Evaluates human and environmental ionizing radiation exposure and derives radiation risk assessments from epidemiologic data and research conclusions; provides information to organizations such as the ICRP for evaluation
National Academy of Sciences/National Research Council Committee on the Biological Effects of Ionizing Radiation (NAS/NRC-BEIR)	Reviews studies of biologic effects of ionizing radiation and risk assessment and provides the information to organizations such as the ICRP for evaluation

recommendations.[1] Since its inception in 1928, the ICRP has been the leading international organization responsible for providing clear and consistent radiation protection guidance through its recommendations for:

- Occupational dose limits
- Public dose limits

Originally, these recommendations were published as reports in selected scholarly journals. Since 1959 the ICRP has had its own series of publications, and from 1977 onward the scientific journal *Annals of the ICRP* has published ICRP information. The information that serves as a basis for the recommendations is supplied by scientific articles published in scholarly journals and by organizations such as UNSCEAR and NAS/NRC-BEIR, which are discussed later in this chapter. The ICRP only makes recommendations; it does not function as an enforcement agency. Each nation must develop and enforce its own specific regulations.

National Council on Radiation Protection and Measurements

In the United States a nongovernmental, nonprofit, private corporation known as the National Council on Radiation Protection and Measurements (NCRP), chartered by Congress in 1964, reviews the recommendations formulated by the ICRP. The NCRP determines the way ICRP recommendations are incorporated into US radiation protection criteria. The council implements this task by:

- Formulating general recommendations
- Publishing their recommendations in the form of various NCRP reports

These reports may be purchased from NCRP Publications in Bethesda, Maryland. A listing of current NCRP reports available for purchase at cost may be found at www.ncrp.com.

Because the NCRP is not an enforcement agency, enactment of its recommendations lies with federal and state agencies that have the power to enforce such standards after they have been established. To facilitate understanding of the function of the NCRP, the council's objectives are identified in Box 10.1. Governmental organizations (e.g., the NRC, the Environmental Protection Agency [EPA], and state governments) use the recommendations of the NCRP as the scientific basis for their radiation protection activities.[2] Nongovernmental groups desiring to improve their radiation safety practices and their promotion and disbursement of pertinent radiation protection materials look to this public service organization for direction.

United Nations Scientific Committee on the Effects of Atomic Radiation (UNSCEAR)

UNSCEAR, which was established in 1955, is another group that plays a prominent role in the formulation of radiation protection guidelines. This group evaluates human and environmental ionizing radiation exposures from a variety of sources, including:

- Radioactive materials
- Radiation-producing machines
- Radiation accidents

UNSCEAR uses epidemiologic data (e.g., information from follow-up studies of Japanese atomic bomb survivors), information acquired from the Radiation Effects Research Foundation (a group run by the government of Japan primarily for the purpose of studying the survivors), and research conclusions to derive radiation risk assessments for radiation-induced cancer and for genetic (hereditary) effects.

National Academy of Sciences/National Research Council Committee on the Biological Effects of Ionizing Radiation (NAS/NRC-BEIR)

NAS/NRC-BEIR is another advisory group that reviews studies of biologic effects of ionizing radiation and risk assessment. This group formulated the 1990 BEIR V Report,

Health Effects of Exposure to Low Levels of Ionizing Radiation. BEIR V supersedes four earlier BEIR reports that listed studies of biologic effects and the associated risk of groups of people who were either routinely or accidentally exposed to ionizing radiation. Such groups include:
- Early radiation workers
- Atomic bomb victims of Hiroshima and Nagasaki
- Evacuees from the Chernobyl nuclear power station disaster

As previously noted, recommendations for EfD limits and EqD limits are made by the ICRP, NCRP, UNSCEAR, and NAS/NRC-BEIR. Based on these recommendations, limits on radiation exposure are established by congressional act or state mandates. National and state agencies are charged with the responsibility of enforcing standards after they have been established.

US REGULATORY AGENCIES

After radiation protection standards have been determined, responsible agencies must enforce them for the protection of the general public, patients, and occupationally exposed personnel.

Regulatory agencies include the following:
1. Nuclear Regulatory Commission (NRC)
2. Agreement states
3. Environmental Protection Agency (EPA)
4. US Food and Drug Administration (FDA)
5. Occupational Safety and Health Administration (OSHA)

A summary of the US regulatory agencies is presented in Table 10.2.

Nuclear Regulatory Commission

The **Nuclear Regulatory Commission (NRC)**, formerly known as the *Atomic Energy Commission,* is a federal agency that has the authority to control the possession, use, and production of atomic energy in the interest of national security. This agency also has the power to enforce radiation protection standards. However, the NRC does not regulate or inspect x-ray imaging facilities. The main function of the NRC is to oversee the nuclear energy industry. This agency supervises the:
- Design and working mechanics of nuclear power stations
- Production of nuclear fuel
- Handling of expended fuel
- Supervision of hazardous radioactive waste material

TABLE 10.2   Summary of US Regulatory Agencies

Agency	Function
Nuclear Regulatory Commission (NRC)	Oversees the nuclear energy industry, enforces radiation protection standards, publishes its rules and regulations in Title 10 of the US Code of Federal Regulations, and enters into written agreements with state governments that permit the state to license and regulate the use of radioisotopes and certain other material within that state
Agreement states	Enforce radiation protection regulations through their respective health departments
Environmental Protection Agency (EPA)	Facilitates the development and enforcement of regulations pertaining to the control of radiation in the environment
US Food and Drug Administration (FDA)	Conducts an ongoing product radiation control program, regulating the design and manufacture of electronic products, including x-ray equipment
Occupational Safety and Health Administration (OSHA)	Functions as a monitoring agency in places of employment, predominantly in industry

In addition, the NRC controls the manufacture and use of radioactive substances formed in nuclear reactors and used in:

- Research
- Industry
- Nuclear medicine imaging procedures
- Therapeutic treatments

The NRC also licenses users of such radioactive materials and periodically makes unannounced inspections to determine whether these users are in compliance with the provisions of their licenses. Up until 2008 the NRC did not regulate the use of radioactive substances that either are naturally occurring, like radium, or are produced outside of a reactor by high-energy particle accelerators, such as cyclotrons. These materials are given the word designation *NARM*. It stands for "naturally occurring and/or accelerator produced materials." Two common examples of cyclotron-produced radioisotopes are:

- Thallium-201 (^{201}Tl) used in nuclear medicine for heart stress tests
- Palladium-103 (^{103}Pd) used for therapeutic prostate seed implants

NARM materials were formerly solely regulated by state bureaus of radiation protection. In 2008 the NRC expanded its definition of by-product substances to include NARM materials. This meant that by a certain specified date, all facilities in nonagreement states (i.e., those states that have decided to maintain their own designed independent radiation protection program for radioactive materials), in order to be in compliance, would have to amend their NRC radioactive materials licenses to include all NARM materials that they are currently using.

The NRC writes rules and regulations. The US Office of the Federal Register prepares and distributes these rules in Title 10 of the US Code of Federal Regulations. Radiation protection standards governing occupational radiation exposure may be found in Part 20 of Title 10. For the latter the abbreviation 10 CFR 20 is used.

Agreement States

The NRC has the authority to enter into written contracts with state governments. These agreements permit the contracting state to undertake the responsibility of licensing and regulating the use of radioisotopes and certain other radioactive materials within that state.

Most states in the United States have entered into such "agreements" with the NRC, thereby also assuming responsibility for enforcing radiation protection regulations through their respective health departments. These states are known as **agreement states**. In *nonagreement states*, both the state and the NRC jointly enforce radiation protection regulations by sending agents to health care facilities. Hospitals are evaluated to determine whether they are in compliance with existing radiation safety regulations. Individual states also may legislate their own regulations regarding radiation safety. Inspection of nuclear reactors and assurance of adherence to federal radiation safety regulations in agreement or nonagreement states fall solely under the jurisdiction of the NRC.

Environmental Protection Agency (EPA)

The EPA was established on December 2, 1970. It was created through the reorganization plan of former US president Richard M. Nixon. The agency was created to bring several departments under one organization that would be responsible for protecting the health of humans and for safeguarding the natural environment.

The EPA, as part of its general overseer responsibilities, facilitates the development and enforcement of regulations pertaining to the control of radiation in the environment. Specifically it:

- Directs federal agencies
- Oversees the general area of environmental monitoring
- Has oversight authority for specific areas such as determining the action level for radon

US Food and Drug Administration (FDA)

Under Public Law 90-602, the Radiation Control for Health and Safety Act of 1968, the FDA conducts an ongoing product radiation control program, regulating the design and manufacturing of electronic products, including diagnostic x-ray equipment.

A more detailed explanation of the Radiation Control for Health and Safety Act of 1968 is given later in this chapter.

To determine the level of compliance with standards in a given x-ray facility, the FDA conducts on-site inspections of x-ray equipment, especially mammography units. Compliance with FDA standards ensures the protection of occupationally and nonoccupationally exposed persons from faulty manufacturing.

Occupational Safety and Health Administration (OSHA)

OSHA functions as a monitoring agency in places of employment, predominantly in industry. OSHA regulates occupational exposure to radiation through Part 1910 of Title 29 of the US Code of Federal Regulations (29 CFR 1910). It is responsible for regulations concerning an employee's "right to know" with regard to hazards that may be present in the workplace. A series of statutes passed by the individual states requires that employees be made aware of these hazards in the workplace. The act covers:

- Hazardous substances
- Infectious agents
- Ionizing radiation
- Nonionizing radiation (e.g., ultraviolet, microwaves, etc.)

The act requires employers to evaluate their workplaces for hazardous agents and to provide training and written information to their employees. OSHA also regulates training programs in the workplace.

RADIATION SAFETY PROGRAM

Requirement

Facilities providing imaging services shall have an effective and detailed radiation safety program to ensure adequate safety of patients and radiation workers. The implementation of an effective program begins with the administration of the facility. Individuals in executive positions must provide the resources necessary for creating and maintaining this program. They can:

- Delegate operational funds in the budget
- Oversee the development of policies and procedures
- Provide the equipment necessary for starting and for continuing the program

Radiation Safety Committee and Radiation Safety Officer

The NRC mandates that a radiation safety committee (RSC) be established for the facility. This committee provides guidance for the program and facilitates its ongoing operation. A radiation safety officer (RSO) should also be selected to:

- Oversee the program's daily operation
- Provide for formal review of the program each year

An RSO is normally a medical physicist, health physicist, radiologist, or other individual qualified through adequate training and experience. This person has been designated by a health care facility and approved by the NRC and the state.

Responsibilities of the Radiation Safety Officer. The RSO is specifically responsible for developing an appropriate radiation safety program for the facility that follows internationally accepted guidelines for radiation protection. He or she is charged with ensuring that the facility's operational radiation practices are such that all persons, especially those who are or could be pregnant, are adequately protected from unnecessary exposure. To fulfill this responsibility, management of the facility must grant the RSO the authority necessary to implement and enforce the policies of the radiation safety program.

The RSO also must review and maintain radiation-monitoring records for all personnel and be available to provide counseling for individuals (e.g., those who receive monitor readings in excess of allowable limits).

Required Training and Experience for a Radiation Safety Officer. The necessary training and experience for an RSO are described in Part 35.50 and Part 35.900 of Title 10 of the Code of Federal Regulations. The NRC publishes regulatory guides to accompany its rules. Although on a legal level health care facilities do not need to comply with the guide, they frequently choose to do so to facilitate the chances of a successful outcome of an NRC inspection or approval of license changes. The guide is actually the NRC's interpretation of how to implement its own rules.

The training and experience requirements for the RSO allow for three training pathways. These pathways are identified in Box 10.2.

Authority of the Radiation Safety Officer. 10 CFR 35.24 requires that the licensee provide the RSO:
• Sufficient authority
• Organizational freedom
• Management prerogative to perform certain duties
These tasks are identified in Box 10.3. The licensee must establish, in writing, the authority, functions, and responsibilities of the RSO. Because the RSO is responsible for the day-to-day supervision of the facility's radiation

safety program, he or she must have independent authority to stop operations that are considered unsafe. In addition, this individual must be given adequate time and resources and have a sufficient commitment from management to ensure that radioactive materials are used in a safe manner. The NRC requires the name of the RSO on the facility's radioactive materials license to ensure that licensee management has always identified a responsible, qualified person who can directly interact with the NRC during inspections and also concerning any inquiries about the facility's safety program. Usually, the RSO is a full-time employee of the licensed facility; however, the NRC has authorized individuals who are not employed by the licensee (e.g., a consultant) to fill the role of an RSO or to provide support to the facility's RSO. Training for this role is covered in 10 CFR 35. A list of these requirements may also be found in Appendix H.

RADIATION CONTROL FOR HEALTH AND SAFETY ACT OF 1968

In 1968 the US Congress passed the Radiation Control for Health and Safety Act (Public Law 90-602) to protect the public from the hazards of unnecessary radiation exposure resulting from electronic products such as microwave ovens and color televisions. Diagnostic x-ray equipment also was included. The act permitted the establishment of the Center for Devices and Radiological Health (CDRH). Until 1982 this organization was known as the *Bureau of Radiological Health*. The CDRH falls under the jurisdiction of the FDA. Essentially, it is responsible for conducting an ongoing electronic product radiation control program. This includes setting up standards for the manufacture, installation, assembly, and maintenance of machines for radiologic procedures. Further responsibilities include:
• Assessing the biologic effects of ionizing radiation
• Evaluating radiation emissions from electronic products in general
• Conducting research to reduce radiation exposure

Code of Standards for Diagnostic X-Ray Equipment

The code of standards for diagnostic x-ray equipment (Public Law 90-602) went into effect on August 1, 1974. This code applies to complete systems and major components manufactured after that date. Equipment in use before August 1, 1974, does not need to be modified or

BOX 10.2 Allowable Pathways for a Radiation Safety Officer to Meet Training and Experience Requirements as Described in 10 CFR 35.50 and 10 CFR 35.900

1. Certification by one of the professional boards approved by the Nuclear Regulatory Commission (NRC)
2. Didactic and work experience as described in detail in the regulations
3. Identification as an authorized user, authorized medical physicist, or authorized health physicist on the license, with experience in the types of uses for which the individual has radiation safety officer (RSO) responsibilities

BOX 10.3 Duties That 10 CFR 35.24 Requires the Licensee to Freely Provide the Radiation Safety Officer to Perform

1. Identify radiation safety problems.
2. Initiate, recommend, or provide corrective action.
3. Stop unsafe operations involving by-product material.
4. Verify implementation of corrective actions.

BOX 10.4 Provisions Included in the Standards for Diagnostic X-Ray Equipment

1. Automatic limitation of the radiographic beam to the image receptor regardless of image receptor size, a condition known as *positive beam limitation.*
2. Appropriate minimal permanent filtration of the x-ray beam to ensure an acceptable level of beam quality. Filtration provides significant reduction in the intensity of very "soft" x-rays that contribute only to the added patient-absorbed dose.
3. Ability of x-ray units to duplicate certain radiation exposures for any given combination of kilovolts at peak value (kVp), milliamperes (mA), and time to ensure both exposure reproducibility and linearity. *Reproducibility* is defined as consistency in output in radiation intensity for identical generator settings from one individual exposure to subsequent exposures.* A variance of 5% or less is acceptable. *Exposure linearity* is defined as consistency in output radiation intensity at a selected kVp setting when changing from one milliamperage and time combination (mAs = mA × exposure time) to another. *Linearity,* which is defined as the ratio of the difference in mR/mAs values between two successive generator stations to the sum of those mR/mAs values, must be less than 0.1.
4. Inclusion of beam limitation devices for spot films taken during fluoroscopy. Such devices should be located between the x-ray source and the patient.
5. Presence of "beam on" indicators to give visible warnings when x-ray exposures are in progress and both visual and audible signals when exposure has terminated.
6. Inclusion of manual backup timers for automatic (photo-timed) exposure control to ensure the termination of the exposure if the automatic timer fails.

*Mathematically, reproducibility is described by the coefficient of variation C, which is equal to the standard deviation of at least five successive output measurements employing the same technique factors divided by the average, or mean value, of those measurements. The regulation requires that C must not exceed 0.05.

discarded. Some important provisions of the standards for diagnostic x-ray equipment are listed in Box 10.4.

Public Law 90-602 does not regulate the diagnostic x-ray user. It is strictly an equipment performance standard.

ALARA CONCEPT

In 1954 the National Committee on Radiation Protection (later known as the *National Council on Radiation Protection and Measurements*) put forth the principle that radiation exposures should be kept "as low as reasonably achievable" (ALARA) with consideration for economic and societal factors. According to NCRP Report No. 160, "The protection from radiation exposure is as low as reasonably achievable when the expenditure of further resources would be unwarranted by the reduction in exposure that would be achieved."[3]

The ALARA concept is accepted by all regulatory agencies. In 1987 the NCRP described it as "the continuation of good radiation protection programs and practices which traditionally have been effective in keeping the average and individual exposures for monitored workers well below the limit."[4] It also may be referred to as optimization in accordance with ICRP Publication No. 37 and Publication No. 55. Medical imaging personnel and radiologists share the responsibility to keep occupational and nonoccupational dose limits ALARA.

In practice this translates into EfDs and EqDs well below maximum allowable levels. This goal can usually be simply achieved through the employment of proper safety procedures performed by qualified personnel. Such procedures should be clearly described in a facility's radiation safety program. To define ALARA, health care facilities usually adopt *investigation levels,* defined as level I and level II. In the United States, these levels are traditionally one-tenth to three-tenths the applicable regulatory limits.

Model for the ALARA Concept

The ALARA concept adopts an extremely conservative model with respect to the relationship between ionizing radiation and potential risk. The relationship is the linear nonthreshold model discussed in Chapter 9 (reproduced in Fig. 10.2). The central principle of radiation protection is that in the interest of safety, risk of injury should be overestimated rather than underestimated.

FOOD AND DRUG ADMINISTRATION WHITE PAPER

The US Food and Drug Administration supports the premise that "each patient should get the right imaging examination, at the right time, with the right radiation dose."[5] This declaration is clearly stated in the FDA document known as *the White Paper,* published in February 2010, in which they announced "the launch of a cooperative *Initiative to Reduce Unnecessary Radiation*

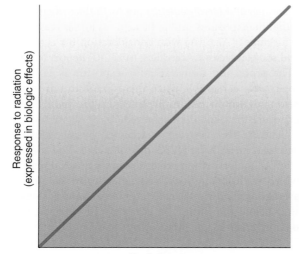

FIG 10.2 Dose–response curve. Hypothetical linear (straight-line) nonthreshold curve for radiation dose–response relationship. The straight-line curve passing through the origin in this graph indicates both that the response to radiation (in terms of biologic effects) is directly proportional to the dose of radiation and that no known level of radiation dose exists below which absolutely no chance of sustaining biologic damage is evident.

Exposure from Medical Imaging.[5] Working in conjunction with their partners, the FDA intends to take action to:
1. "Promote safe use of medical imaging devices"[5]
2. "Support informed clinical decision"[5]
3. "Increase patient awareness"[5]

By coordinating these efforts, the FDA will be able to "optimize patient exposure to radiation from certain types of medical exams, and thereby reduce related risks while maximizing the benefits of these studies."[5] For those desiring more information about this document, a link to the website is provided in Reference 5 at the end of this chapter.

CONSUMER-PATIENT RADIATION HEALTH AND SAFETY ACT OF 1981

The Consumer-Patient Radiation Health and Safety Act of 1981 (Title IX of Public Law 97-35) (see Appendix I) provides federal legislation requiring the establishment of minimal standards for the accreditation of education programs for persons who perform radiologic procedures and the certification of such persons. The purpose of

this federal act, which is under the directorship of the secretary of Health and Human Services, is to ensure that standard medical and dental radiologic practices adhere to rigorous safety precautions and standards. Individual states are encouraged to enact similar statutes and administer certification and accreditation programs based on the standards established therein. Because no legal penalty exists for noncompliance, many states, unfortunately, have not responded with appropriate legislation.

RADIATION-INDUCED RESPONSES OF CONCERN IN RADIATION PROTECTION

Categories for Radiation-Induced Responses

At the present time, the two main categories of radiation-induced responses of serious concern in radiation protection programs are:
1. Tissue responses
2. Stochastic (probabilistic) effects

Recent Changes in Terminology

Many texts and source materials continue to use a number of terms to refer to the categories of effects of radiation. These terms include *stochastic, nonstochastic, deterministic,* and *tissue reactions.* Modern terminology, as defined by the ICRP and the NCRP, has settled upon the two terms *stochastic* and *tissue reactions.* Following is a brief explanation.

In the 1970s[6] radiation effects were divided into two broad categories: stochastic and nonstochastic. Stochastic effects are those effects whose severity does not depend on the radiation dose, but the probability of occurrence is dose dependent. The only examples are cancer and hereditary effects. Stochastic effects occur as a result of injury to a single cell or a small number of cells. Effects that occurred as a result of injury to a large number of cells were therefore referred to as nonstochastic. By the 1990s[7] it was decided that effects that were previously called nonstochastic were produced by stochastic effects in a large number of cells. So the term *nonstochastic* was no longer considered appropriate. Effects involving injury or death of many cells were referred to as *deterministic* because the severity of the effects was determined by the dose. By the early 2000s[8–10] it was acknowledged that the effects that had been referred to as deterministic were not actually determined at the time of irradiation but could be altered by the use of various biologic response

BOX 10.5 Recent Changes in the Terminology Used to Describe Radiation Effects for the Purpose of Radiation Protection Guidelines

Approximate Year of Adoption	Terminology
1977–1991	stochastic vs. nonstochastic
1991–2012	stochastic vs. deterministic
2012–present	stochastic vs. tissue reactions (early or late)

modifiers (e.g., chemical agents such as radioprotectors and radiosensitizers) and by medical intervention after the irradiation. The term *tissue reactions* was then adopted and has replaced the older terms *nonstochastic* and *deterministic*. Both early and late tissue reactions are recognized. This development in terminology is summarized in Box 10.5.

Tissue Reactions. As described in the preceding chapters, tissue reactions are biologic somatic effects of ionizing radiation that can be directly related to the dose received. They exhibit a threshold dose below which the response does not normally occur and above which the severity of the biologic damage increases as the dose increases. For example, if a certain dose of radiation produces a skin burn, a higher dose of radiation will cause the skin burn to be more severe; however, a dose below the threshold level for skin burn will not demonstrate the effect. When radiation-induced biologic damage escalates, it does so because greater numbers of cells interact with the increased number of x-ray photons that are present at higher radiation exposures. As mentioned in Chapter 9, in general, tissue reactions typically occur only after large doses of radiation. However, they could also result from long-term individual low doses of radiation sustained over several years. In either instance the cumulative amounts of such radiation doses are usually much greater than those typically encountered by a patient in diagnostic radiology.*

---

*A significant exception to this is high–dose-rate fluoroscopic procedures. For these studies, entrance dose rates as great as 200 mGy_a/min are possible. A fluoroscopic exposure of 15 minutes at this level would result in a patient entrance dose of approximately 3 Gy_a.

Early and late tissue reactions. Tissue effects may be early, such as:
- Diffuse redness over an area of skin after irradiation (erythema)
- A decrease in the white blood cell count
- Epilation, or loss of hair

As we discussed in Chapter 8, other, and far more serious, early consequences of radiation sickness can also arise, such as:
- Hematopoietic syndrome
- Gastrointestinal syndrome
- Cerebrovascular syndrome

Recall that these effects usually occur within a few hours or days after a very high-level radiation exposure to a significant portion of the body. Some late tissue reactions due to high-level radiation exposure, though, occur months or more afterward. They include:
- Cataract formation
- Fibrosis
- Organ atrophy
- Loss of parenchymal cells
- Reduced fertility
- Sterility caused by a decrease in reproductive cells

Early tissue reactions such as erythema and late tissue reactions such as cataract formation have a high probability of occurring when entrance radiation doses exceed 2 Gy_t. The frequency of occurrence of high-dose tissue reactions is not linear with respect to dose but rather follows a nonlinear threshold curve that is sigmoidal (S-shaped) with a threshold (see Fig. 9.1B).

Stochastic Effects. We have seen that stochastic effects are nonthreshold, randomly occurring biologic somatic changes. Their chances of occurrence increase with each radiation exposure. Examples of stochastic effects are:
- Cancer
- Genetic alterations

Stochastic responses may be demonstrated with the use of both the linear (see Fig. 9.2) and the linear-quadratic dose–response curves (see Fig. 9.3). Because a stochastic event is an all-or-none, random effect, ionizing radiation could induce cancers within a general large population, but determining beforehand which members of that population will develop cancer is not possible. Injury may result from exposure of a single cell or from damage in a sensitive substructure, such as a gene. The assumption is that no minimal safe dose exists. The frequency of an occurrence in a population, however, does increase

BOX 10.6 Summary of Serious Radiation-Induced Responses of Concern

Tissue Reactions	Stochastic (Probabilistic)
Early Reactions	Effects
Erythema (diffuse redness over an area of skin after irradiation)	Cancer
Blood changes (decrease of lymphocytes and platelets)	**Genetic (Hereditary) Effects**
Epilation (loss of hair)	Mutagenesis (irradiation of DNA of somatic cells leading to abnormalities in new cells as they divide in that individual)
Acute radiation syndrome	
Hematopoietic syndrome	
Gastrointestinal syndrome	
Cerebrovascular syndrome	
Late Reactions	
Cataract formation	
Fibrosis	
Organ atrophy	
Loss of parenchymal cells	
Reduced fertility	
Sterility	

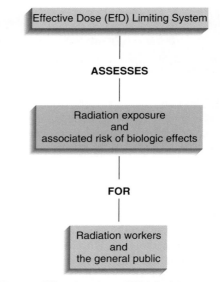

FIG 10.3 Effective dose (EfD) limiting system.

in proportion to the magnitude of the absorbed dose of ionizing radiation delivered to the entire population. Therefore the net effect on the population group depends not only on the number of individuals irradiated but also on the mean dose that each individual receives.

A summary of both early and late tissue reactions and stochastic (probabilistic) effects is presented in Box 10.6.

CURRENT RADIATION PROTECTION PHILOSOPHY

Both genetic and somatic responses to ionizing radiation were considered in developing the present EfD limiting recommendations. Current radiation protection philosophy is based on the assumption that a linear nonthreshold relationship exists between radiation dose and biologic response. Thus even the most minuscule dose of radiation has a nonzero potential to cause some harm. The current philosophy also acknowledges that ionizing radiation possesses a beneficial potential. It proposes that, when employed the potential benefits of exposing the patient to ionizing radiation must far outweigh any potential risk.

Effective Dose Limiting System

The EfD limiting system is the current method for controlling risk of biologic damage to radiation workers and the general public from radiation exposure (Fig. 10.3). The effective dose limit (EDL) is the upper boundary dose of ionizing radiation that results in a negligible risk of:
- Bodily injury
- Hereditary damage

EDLs may be specified for whole-body exposure, partial-body exposure, and exposure of individual organs. Separate limits are set for occupationally exposed individuals and for the general public. The sum of both the external and internal whole-body exposures is considered when effective dose limits are established. Their values are such as to minimize the risk to humans in terms of early and late tissue reactions and stochastic effects, and they do not include natural background and medical exposure.

Upper boundary radiation exposure limits for occupationally exposed persons are associated with risks that are similar to those encountered by employees in other industries that are generally considered to be reasonably safe. These industries include:
- Manufacturing
- Trade
- Government

Quantitative values for radiation risks are derived from the complete injury caused by radiation exposure. The potential for terminal cancer, hereditary imperfections induced by reproductive cell mutations, shortening of life span because of the induction of cancer, or other abnormalities and the overall poorer quality of life are collectively taken into account.

Revised Concepts of Radiation Exposure and Risk

Revised concepts of radiation exposure and risk have brought about more recent changes in NCRP recommendations for limits on exposure to ionizing radiation. Because many conflicting views exist on assessing the risk of cancer induction from low-level radiation exposure, the trend has been to create more rigorous radiation protection standards.

The adoption of the EfD limiting system is a direct consequence of this conservatism.

Occupational Risk

The risk to a radiographer from radiation exposure may be equated with occupational risk in other industries that are generally considered reasonably safe. That risk is generally estimated to be a 2.5% chance of fatal accident over an entire career. The lifetime fatal risk in hazardous occupations is many times greater. Examples of such occupations include:

- Logging
- Deep sea fishing

To ensure that the hazard to radiation workers is no greater than the hazard to the general working public, the NCRP proposes that radiation protection programs for radiation workers be designed to prevent individual workers from having a total external plus internal cumulative EfD in excess of their age in years times 10 mSv.[4] Consider the following situation: A worker at age 40 years has been employed at a nuclear power plant for 10 years. He had previously been employed as a radiation worker in another industry, during the course of which he received a cumulative EfD of 100 mSv. Therefore the radiation protection program for his current position should have ensured that he has not accumulated a total EfD greater than 300 mSv during his 10 years of employment.

Vulnerability of the Embryo-Fetus to Radiation Exposure

We have already seen that the embryo-fetus in utero is particularly sensitive to radiation exposure. Epidemiologic studies of atomic bomb survivors exposed in utero provided conclusive evidence of a dose-dependent increase in the incidence of severe intellectual disability for fetal doses greater than approximately 0.4 Sv. The greatest risk for radiation-induced intellectual disability occurred when the embryo-fetus was exposed 8 to 15 weeks after conception.

BASIS FOR THE EFFECTIVE DOSE LIMITING SYSTEM

Concept Underlying Radiation Protection

The essential concept underlying radiation protection is that any organ in the human body is vulnerable to damage from exposure to ionizing radiation. Even though some organs are known to be more sensitive to radiation than others, every organ is at some risk because of the assumed random nature of somatic or hereditary radiation-induced effects.

The EfD limiting system includes, for the determination of EqD for tissues and organs, all radiation-vulnerable human organs that can contribute to potential risk, rather than only those human organs considered critical. In earlier recommendations such as NCRP Report No. 39 (released in 1971), only critical organs such as the gonads, blood-forming organs, and lung tissue were identified.[11]

Tissue Weighting Factor

Although this factor has already been discussed, a brief description follows to reinforce greater understanding of its importance as it relates to the EfD limiting system. The EfD limiting system is an attempt to equate the various risks of cancer and hereditary effects to the tissues or organs that were exposed to radiation. Because various tissues and organs do not have the same degree of sensitivity to these effects, the system employed must compensate for the differences in risk from one organ to another. Therefore a **tissue weighting factor** (W_T) is used. This factor "indicates the ratio of the risk of stochastic effects attributable to irradiation of a given organ or tissue (T) to the total risk when the whole body is uniformly irradiated."[12] Organ or tissue weighting factors (W_T) recommended by the ICRP in Report No. 60, released in 1991, and adopted by the NCRP in Report No. 116, released in 1993, are reproduced in Box 10.7.

*The remainder takes into account the following additional tissues and organs: adrenals, brain, small intestine, large intestine, kidney, muscle, pancreas, spleen, thymus, and uterus.

†In extraordinary circumstances in which one of the remainder tissues or organs receives an equivalent dose in excess of the highest dose in any of the 12 organs for which a weighting factor (W_T) is specified, a W_T of 0.025 should be applied to that tissue or organ and a W_T of 0.025 to the average dose in the other remainder tissues or organs. From National Council on Radiation Protection and Measurements (NCRP): *Limitation of exposure to ionizing radiation, Report No. 116*, Bethesda, MD, 1993, NCRP. Reprinted with permission of the National Council on Radiation Protection and Measurements, http://NCRPonline .org.

CURRENT NATIONAL COUNCIL ON RADIATION PROTECTION AND MEASUREMENTS RECOMMENDATIONS

National Council on Radiation Protection and Measurements Reports

The NCRP periodically reiterates and updates its position on radiation protection standards and publishes recommendations on these standards in the form of reports. Recommendations contained in NCRP Report No. 116 now supersede those contained in NCRP Reports No. 91 and No. 39. A summary of some important issues and changes follows.

Cumulative Effective Dose (CumEfD) Limit. A radiation worker's lifetime effective dose must be limited to his or her age in years times 10 mSv. This is called the cumulative effective dose (CumEfD) limit and pertains to the whole body. Adhering to this limit ensures that

the lifetime risk for these workers remains acceptable. CumEfD limits, however, do not include:
- Radiation exposure from natural background radiation
- Exposure acquired as a consequence of a worker's undergoing medical imaging procedures
The limits do include the possibility of both:
- Internal exposure
- External exposure

The cumulative effective dose is therefore the sum or total of both the internal and external EqDs. The example in Box 10.8 demonstrates the application of the CumEfD limit for the whole body.

Medical imaging personnel hardly ever receive EqDs that are close to the annual occupational effective dose limit. If a radiation safety program is well structured and properly maintained, occupational exposure will not remotely approach 50 mSv in any given year.

International Commission on Radiological Protection Recommendation for Downward Revision of the Annual Effective Dose Limit. In 1991 the ICRP recommended that the annual EfD limit for occupationally exposed persons be reduced from 50 mSv to 20 mSv as a result of newer information obtained regarding the Japanese atomic bomb survivors in whom the risk of radiation from the atomic bomb detonations was estimated to be approximately three to four times greater (more damaging) than previously estimated.[13] The NCRP has not acted yet but very well might recommend lower limits on exposure because of the:
1. Revised risk estimates derived from the more recent reevaluations of dosimetric studies on the atomic bomb survivors of Hiroshima and Nagasaki[11]

2. Appearance, as a result of longer follow-up time, of increased numbers of solid tumors in the survivor population

Therefore, in the future, the annual whole-body EfD limit for occupationally exposed persons in the United States may be limited to 10 to 20 mSv per year. Of course, such a change will necessitate further evaluation of actual risk for persons employed in radiation industries. In the United States, lowering of the current limits is the responsibility of the NRC, individual states, and the FDA.

Limits for Nonoccupationally Exposed Individuals. In addition to limits for occupationally exposed individuals, the NCRP sets limits for nonoccupationally exposed individuals who are not undergoing medical imaging procedures. An example would be a person accompanying a patient to the imaging department such as a:

- Spouse
- Parent
- Guardian

A limit also has been set for individual members of the general public not occupationally exposed. The NCRP-recommended annual EDL is 1 mSv for continuous or frequent exposures from artificial sources other than medical irradiation and natural background and a limit of 5 mSv annually for infrequent exposure.[4] The annual EfD nonoccupational limit set for individual members of the general public is designed to limit that exposure "to reasonable levels of risk comparable with risks from other common sources, i.e., about 10^{-4} to 10^{-6} annually."[4] The 5-mSv annual limit for infrequent exposure is made because "annual exposures in excess of the 1 mSv recommendation, usually to a small number of people, need not be regarded as especially significant to the group as a whole provided it does not occur often to the same groups and that the average exposure to individuals in these groups does not exceed an average annual EfD of about 1 mSv."[4]

Limits for Pregnant Radiation Workers. To reduce exposure for pregnant radiation workers and control the exposure to the unborn during potentially sensitive periods of gestation, the NCRP now "recommends" a monthly EqD limit not exceeding 0.5 mSv per month to the embryo-fetus and a limit during the entire pregnancy not to exceed 5.0 mSv after declaration of the pregnancy. The recommended monthly limit is more stringent. Nevertheless, both limits are proposed to reflect the fact that not all pregnant workers are monitored monthly and that personnel dosimetry does not result in exact measures of EqD, just approximations based on the personnel dosimeter readings. This 9-month EqD value excludes both medical and natural background radiation. It is designed to restrict significantly the total lifetime risk of leukemia and other malignancies in persons exposed in utero.[4] The occurrence of tissue reactions is expected to be statistically negligible if the EqD remains at or below the recommended limit. These reactions include:

- Small head size
- Intellectual disability

Limits for Education and Training Purposes. For education and training purposes, the same dose limits should apply to students of radiography in general and to those individuals under 18 years of age. The dose limit is the same for kindergarten through twelfth-grade students attending science demonstrations involving ionizing radiation as it is for student radiologic technologists who begin their education before they are 18 years old. The limit for any education and training exposures of individuals under the age of 18 years is an EfD of 1 mSv annually. Occasional exposure for the purpose of education and training is permitted, provided special care is taken to ensure that the annual EfD limit of 1 mSv is not exceeded.

Limits for Tissues and Organs Exposed Selectively or Together With Other Organs. Annual occupational dose limits for tissue reactions, for tissues and organs exposed selectively, or together with other organs have been set to prevent excessive doses to those organs and tissues. They include 150 mSv to the crystalline lens of the eyes and 500 mSv for localized areas of the skin, the hands, and the feet.[4] Even though the established annual dose limit for localized areas of skin provides adequate protection for that organ against stochastic effects, it will actually be necessary to specify an additional limit to prevent tissue reactions.

Negligible Individual Dose. To provide a low-exposure cutoff level so that regulatory agencies may consider a level of effective dose as being of negligible risk, an annual negligible individual dose (NID) of 0.01 mSv/year per source or practice has been set. This means that at this EfD level, a reduction of individual exposure is unnecessary.

ACTION LIMITS

Health care institutions go to great lengths to avoid having personnel even approach EfD limits. In a well-designed and well-run facility, radiologic technologists' personnel dosimeter readings should be significantly below a tenth of the maximum EfD limits, even for those technologists who receive the most exposure. Hospitals normally establish their own internal action limits. These limits are usually set at levels far below the actual limits, typically a tenth of the limit, but at levels that are still not routinely exceeded by personnel. The purpose of these action limits is to trigger an investigation when they are exceeded that should uncover the reason for any abnormal exposure. A prime reason for an unusual reading can result from a personnel dosimeter accidently remaining in an x-ray room while exposures were being made because it had unknowingly fallen off the uniform of a technologist. Sometimes work habits, such as where the technologist stands during interventional radiography, can lead to personnel readings that exceed the action limit. Corrective actions can then be initiated by the RSO. In general, the RSO must be an active participant along with the imaging department manager in an ongoing program that is designed to prevent personnel from receiving anywhere near the maximum allowed exposures.

RADIATION HORMESIS

The concept of radiation hormesis is that there exists a beneficial aspect or result to groups of individuals from continuing exposure to small amounts of radiation. This essentially contradicts the concept that repetitive low doses of radiation will generate an accumulation of mutations that inevitably will result in transforming a normal cell into one that continues to divide without end, ultimately leading to cancer.

In Report No. 5 of the National Academy of Science on the Biological Effects of Ionizing Radiation (BEIR V), conclusions regarding the adverse effects on health of low levels of ionizing radiation are based on extrapolations from radiation EqDs greater than 0.5 Sv. Such radiation levels are more than a factor of 1000 greater than ordinary background radiation levels (3.3 mSv/year). BEIR V espouses the conservative linear "no threshold" view of the Japanese atomic bomb lifetime survival study (LSS) data. However, studies from the Radiation Effects Research Council in Hiroshima have indicated an apparent threshold dosage in the atomic bomb LSS data that is approximately 0.2 to 0.5 Sv. This lower value corresponds to the amount of natural radiation that average US residents receive *in their lifetimes*. What is curious is that the lifetime survival data possibly appear to indicate that Japanese atomic bomb survivors with moderate radiation exposure of 5 mSv to 50 mSv, the equivalent of 1.5 to 15 years of natural radiation, have a reduced cancer death rate compared with a normally exposed control population. Additional recent reanalysis of the atomic bomb survivor data has shown that effects on survivors are more consistent with a threshold model than the LNT model.[14] All of this contradicts the predictions of the BEIR V report and, if substantiated, seems to cast doubt on the BEIR V conclusion that any amount of radiation is potentially harmful. The reverse could actually be true, at least for very moderate amounts of radiation exposure. More specifically, in seven Western states with background radiation levels higher than other states by approximately 1 mSv per year, residents experience approximately 15% fewer cancer deaths per 1000 individuals than the US average. There is also much evidence from animal studies that supports the view that low doses of radiation actually reduce the chances of both cancer and nonmalignant disease occurrence.[15]

A study was conducted in China from 1972 to 1975 of two stable populations of approximately 70,000 persons, each of whose annual background radiation levels differed by approximately 2 mSv. This study disclosed a cancer rate in the more exposed population of only approximately 50% of that of the other group. Other intriguing studies exist, such as annex B of the UNSCEAR 1994 Report, which actually discusses the beneficial aspects of low-dose radiation.[16] All of these suggest a potential *radiation hormesis effect,* which is a positive consequence of radiation for populations continuously exposed to moderately higher levels of radiation than ordinary background levels. During the course of human evolution over millions of years, advantageous genetic mutations caused by radiation exposure may have occurred, resembling those that allow lower animals today to demonstrate radiation hormesis. Therefore, to assume risk from very small amounts of radiation exposure (two or three or four times normal background levels) may be incorrect.

As we have seen in earlier chapters, the risk from low-level, low-LET radiation exposure is mainly an indirect process involving the production of highly reactive free radicals. It is these chemical agents that have the capacity of damaging cellular DNA. But the human body has an elaborate system of antioxidants that can neutralize many of these reactants. When the immune system is subjected over a period of time to low doses of radiation, it initiates adaptive protection responses[17] that can lessen the potential DNA damage and consequently the malignant transformation of cells.

However, until the radiation hormesis theory is proven, the medical radiation industry will continue to follow a rigid principle of ALARA and the no-threshold concept for radiation protection purposes.

OCCUPATIONAL AND NONOCCUPATIONAL DOSE LIMITS

Effective Dose Limits for Radiation Workers and the Population as a Whole

For the protection of radiation workers and the population as a whole, EfD limits have been established as guidelines (Table 10.3). All medical imaging personnel should be familiar with current NCRP recommendations. For this group the most important item is the 50 mSv/year whole-body occupational dose limit.

TABLE 10.3 Summary of the National Council on Radiation Protection and Measurements (NCRP) Recommendations*† (NCRP Report No. 116)

A. Occupational exposures‡	
1. Effective dose limits	
a. Annual	50 mSv
b. Cumulative	10 mSv × age
2. Equivalent dose annual limits for tissues and organs	
a. Lens of eye	150 mSv
b. Localized areas of the skin, hands, and feet	500 mSv
B. Guidance for emergency occupational exposure‡ (see Section 14, NCRP No. 116)	
C. Public exposures (annual)	
1. Effective dose limit, continuous or frequent exposure‡	1 mSv
2. Effective dose limit, infrequent exposure‡	5 mSv
3. Equivalent dose limits for tissues and organs‡	
a. Lens of eye	15 mSv
b. Localized areas of the skin, hands, and feet	50 mSv
4. Remedial action for natural sources	
a. Effective dose (excluding radon)	>5 mSv
b. Exposure to radon and its decay products§	>26 $(J/s)m^{-3}$¶
D. Education and training exposures (annual)‡	
1. Effective dose limit	1 mSv
2. Equivalent dose limit for tissues and organs	
a. Lens of eye	15 mSv
b. Localized areas of the skin, hands, and feet	50 mSv
E. Embryo and fetus exposures‡	
1. Equivalent dose limit	
a. Monthly	0.5 mSv
b. Entire gestation	5.0 mSv
F. Negligible individual dose (annual)‡	0.01 mSv

*Excluding medical exposures.
†See Tables 4.2 and 5.1 in NCRP Report No. 116 for recommendations on radiation weighting factors and tissue weighting factors, respectively.
‡Sum of external and internal exposures, excluding doses from natural sources.
§WLM stands for working level month and refers to a cumulative exposure for a working month (170 hours). As applied to radon and its daughter products, 1 WLM represents the cumulative exposure experienced in a 170-hour period resulting from a radon concentration of 100 pCi/L. The occupational limit for miners is 4 WLM per year, which results in an equivalent dose of approximately 0.15 Sv per year.
¶A measure of the rate of release of energy (joules per second) by radon and its decay products per unit volume of air (cubic meters).

This annual upper boundary is designed to limit the stochastic (probabilistic) effects of radiation. It takes into account the EqD in all radiation-sensitive organs found in the body.

Special Limits for Selected Areas

Because the tissue weighting factors (see Box 10.7) used for calculating EfD are so small for some organs, an organ that is associated with a low weighting factor may receive an unreasonably large dose, whereas the EfD remains within the allowable total limit. Therefore, special limits are set for the crystalline lens of the eye and localized areas of the skin, hands, and feet to prevent tissue reactions. These special limits may be found in Table 10.3.

At the present time, international radiation protection advisory groups such as the ICRP and most governmental regulatory agencies in other countries limit exposure of the lens of the eye to less than 20 mSv per year, in view of recent data that show a lower threshold for cataracts than was originally thought. In the United States, the NCRP is continuing to study the matter but is unlikely to change its guidance in the near future.[18] Although this seems to be a very large discrepancy, the NCRP, in addition to its special limit for the lens of the eye, maintains a cumulative limit of 10 mSv times the worker's age, which indicates a de facto lower limit to the lens.

▌ SUMMARY

- Effective Dose Limiting System.
  - Adherence to occupational and nonoccupational EfD limits helps prevent harmful biologic effects of radiation exposure.
  - The concept of radiation exposure and the associated risk of radiation-induced malignancy is the basis of the EfD limiting system.
  - The sum of both external and internal whole-body exposures is considered when establishing the CumEfD limit.
  - Accounting for tissue weighting factors is important because various tissues and organs do not have the same degree of sensitivity.
  - Different biologic threats posed by different types of ionizing radiation must be taken into consideration even when the absorbed dose is the same.
  - Radiation hormesis is the hypothesis that a positive effect exists for certain populations that are continuously exposed to moderately higher levels of radiation.

- Major organizations involved in regulating radiation exposure include the following:
  - The United Nations Scientific Committee on the Effects of Atomic Radiation (UNSCEAR) and the National Academy of Sciences/National Research Council Committee on the Biological Effects of Ionizing Radiation (NAS/NRC-BEIR) supply information to the International Commission on Radiological Protection (ICRP).
  - The ICRP makes recommendations on occupational and public dose limits.
  - The National Council on Radiation Protection and Measurements (NCRP) reviews ICRP recommendations and may adopt them into recommendations for US radiation protection policy.
  - The Nuclear Regulatory Commission (NRC) is the watchdog of the nuclear energy industry; it controls the manufacture and use of radioactive substances.
  - The Environmental Protection Agency (EPA) develops and enforces regulations pertaining to the control of environmental radiation.
  - The US Food and Drug Administration (FDA) regulates the design and manufacture of products used in the radiation industry.
  - The Occupational Safety and Health Administration (OSHA) monitors the workplace and regulates occupational exposure to radiation.
- Individual health care facilities establish a radiation safety committee (RSC) and designate a radiation safety officer (RSO).
- The RSO is responsible for developing a radiation safety program for the health care facility; he or she maintains personnel radiation-monitoring records and provides counseling in radiation safety.
- The ALARA concept (optimization) states that radiation exposure should be kept "as low as reasonably achievable."
- Serious radiation-induced responses may be classified as having either tissue reactions or stochastic effects.
  - Tissue reactions are those biologic somatic effects of ionizing radiation that exhibit a threshold dose below which the effect does not normally occur and above which the severity of the biologic damage increases as the dose increases.
  - Stochastic effects are nonthreshold, randomly occurring biologic somatic changes in which the chance of occurrence of the effect rather than the severity of the effect is proportional to the dose of ionizing radiation.

- EfD limits for occupationally exposed personnel include the following:
  - The NCRP has established an annual occupational EfD limit of 50 mSv and a lifetime EfD that does not exceed 10 times the occupationally exposed person's age in years.
  - Internal action limits are established by health care facilities to trigger an investigation to uncover the reasons for any unusual high exposures received by individual staff members.

REFERENCES

1. International Commission on Radiological Protection (ICRP): *ICRP: structure and organization.* Available at: http://www.icrp.org/.
2. National Council on Radiation Protection and Measurements (NCRP): *Background information.* Available at: www.ncrp.com/info.html.
3. National Council on Radiation Protection and Measurements (NCRP): *Ionizing radiation exposure of the population of the United States, Report No. 160,* Bethesda, MD, 2009, NCRP.
4. National Council on Radiation Protection and Measurements (NCRP): *Limitation of exposure to ionizing radiation, Report No. 116,* Bethesda, MD, 1993, NCRP.
5. FDA White Paper: *Initiative to reduce unnecessary radiation exposure from medical imaging.* 2010, Center for Devices and Radiological Health, U.S. Food and Drug Administration. Available at: http://www.fda.gov/Radiation-EmittingProducts/RadiationSafety/RadiationDoseReduction/ucm199994.htm.
6. *Recommendations of the International Commission on Radiological Protection.* ICRP Publication 26, http://www.icrp.org, Ann. ICRP 1977.
7. *1990 Recommendations of the International Commission on Radiological Protection.* ICRP Publication 60, http://www.icrp.org, Ann. ICRP 1991.
8. *ICRP 118 – ICRP Statement on Tissue Reactions / Early and Late Effects of Radiation in Normal Tissues and Organs – Threshold Doses for Tissue Reactions in a Radiation Protection Context ICRP Publication 118 Ann.* ICRP 41 (1/2), 2012.
9. *NCRP 168 – Radiation Dose Management for Fluoroscopically-Guided Interventional Procedures,* NCRP Report No. 168, 2010, 325 pp., National Council on Radiation Protection and Measurements, 7910 Woodmont Avenue, Suite 400, Bethesda, MD 20814-3095; www.ncrponline.org.
10. *NCRP Statement 11 – Outline of Administrative Policies for Quality Assurance and Peer Review of Tissue Reactions Associated with Fluoroscopically-Guided Interventions,* *NCRP Statement No. 11,* Dec. 31, 2014, National Council on Radiation Protection and Measurements, 7910 Woodmont Avenue, Suite 400, Bethesda, MD 20814-3095; www.ncrppublications.org.
11. National Council on Radiation Protection and Measurements (NCRP): *Basic radiation protection criteria, Report No. 39,* Washington, DC, 1971, NCRP.
12. National Council on Radiation Protection and Measurements (NCRP): *Recommendations on limits for exposure to ionizing radiation, Report No. 91,* Bethesda, MD, 1987, NCRP.
13. *Committee on Biological Effects of Ionizing Radiation, National Research Council, Commission of Life Sciences, Board of Radiation Research: Health effects of exposure to low levels of ionizing radiation (BEIR V Report),* Washington, DC, 1989, National Academies Press.
14. Doss M: Linear no-threshold model vs. radiation hormesis. *Dose Response* 11:480–497, 2013.
15. Doss M: Shifting the paradigm in radiation safety. *Dose Response* 10:562–583, 2012.
16. See References 14 and 15.
17. Feinendegen LE, et al: Hormesis by low dose radiation effects: low dose cancer risk modelling must recognize up-regulation of protection. In Baum RP, editor: *Therapeutic nuclear medicine,* Berlin, 2013, Springer.
18. Boice J: *Health Physics Society News,* May 2014. http:ncrponline.org/wp-content/themes/ncrp/PDFs/BOICE-HPnews/24_The_Eyes_Have_It_May2014.pdf.

GENERAL DISCUSSION QUESTIONS

1. Why must radiation exposure of the general public, patients, and radiation workers be limited?
2. What is the basis of the effective dose limiting system?
3. Why must health care facilities have an effective and detailed radiation safety program?
4. Describe the responsibilities of a radiation safety officer.
5. What authority must a radiation safety officer have?
6. What responsibilities does the Center for Devices and Radiological Health (CDRH) fulfill?
7. What was the former name of the Nuclear Regulatory Commission?
8. What is the difference between the late tissue reactions and stochastic effects of ionizing radiation?
9. Describe the effective dose limiting system.

10. Describe current NCRP dose limiting recommendations.
11. What is a radiation hormesis effect?
12. What is the purpose of action limits for radiation exposure of personnel in a health care facility?

REVIEW QUESTIONS

1. Which of the following agencies is responsible for enforcing radiation safety standards?
   A. ICRP
   B. NRC
   C. NCRP
   D. UNSCEAR
2. Determine the cumulative effective dose (CumEfD) to the whole body of an occupationally exposed person who is 27 years old.
   A. 2700 mSv
   B. 270 mSv
   C. 27 mSv
   D. 2.7 mSv
3. Biologic effects such as cataracts that result from exposure to ionizing radiation appear to have which of the following?
   A. Exponential dose–response threshold relationship
   B. Linear nonthreshold dose pattern
   C. Sigmoid threshold dose–response curve
   D. Sigmoid nonthreshold dose–response relationship
4. For radiation workers, such as medical imaging personnel, occupational risk may be equated with occupational risk in which of the following?
   A. Other industries that are generally considered reasonably safe
   B. Somewhat hazardous industries
   C. Hazardous industries
   D. Extremely hazardous industries
5. Revised estimates derived from more recent reevaluations of dosimetric studies on the atomic bomb survivors of Hiroshima and Nagasaki indicate which of the following?
   A. A decrease in the number of solid tumors in the survivor population
   B. An increase in the number of solid tumors in the survivor population
   C. That low-level radiation causes cancer
   D. That the risk of radiation-induced cancer is nonexistent

6. When exposed to radiation as part of their educational experience, 18-year-old students should *not* exceed an effective dose limit of _____ annually.
   A. 0.5 mSv
   B. 1 mSv
   C. 5 mSv
   D. 50 mSv
7. Which of the following groups has provided sufficient evidence of the induction of stochastic effects in humans resulting from high radiation absorbed doses?
   A. Japanese atomic bomb survivors
   B. General population of the United States
   C. Population of occupationally exposed radiographers in the United States
   D. The 2 million people living within 50 miles of the Three Mile Island nuclear power plant after the accident on March 28, 1979
8. Responsibilities of a medical facility's radiation safety officer (RSO) include which of the following?
   1. Developing an appropriate radiation safety program
   2. Maintaining radiation-monitoring records for all personnel
   3. Repairing all broken or defective imaging equipment
   A. 1 and 2 only
   B. 1 and 3 only
   C. 2 and 3 only
   D. 1, 2, and 3
9. To reduce exposure for pregnant imaging professionals and to control the exposure of the unborn during potentially sensitive periods of gestation, the NCRP now recommends a monthly equivalent dose limit not exceeding _____ per month to the embryo-fetus and a limit during the entire pregnancy not to exceed _____ after declaration of a pregnancy.
   A. 0.5 mSv, 5.0 mSv
   B. 5 mSv, 7.0 mSv
   C. 150 mSv, 300 mSv
   D. 250 mSv, 500 mSv
10. Which of the following is the annual occupational effective dose that applies to radiographers during routine operations?
    A. 5 mSv
    B. 50 mSv
    C. 250 mSv
    D. 750 mSv

11

Equipment Design for Radiation Protection

OBJECTIVES

After completing this chapter, the reader will be able to perform the following:

- Define all key terms.
- Explain the requirements for a diagnostic-type protective tube housing, x-ray control panel, radiographic examination table, and source-to-image distance indicator, and discuss their purpose.
- List the various x-ray beam limiting devices, and describe each.
- Explain the importance of luminance of the collimator light source, state the requirements for good coincidence between the radiographic beam and the localizing light beam, and explain the function of the collimator's positive beam limitation (PBL) feature.
- Explain the function of x-ray beam filtration in diagnostic radiology, list two types of filtration used to filter the beam adequately, describe half-value layer (HVL), and give examples of HVLs required for selected peak kilovoltages.
- Explain the function of a compensating filter in radiography, and list two types of such filters.

- Explain the significance of exposure reproducibility and exposure linearity.
- Explain how radiographic grids increase patient dose.
- Identify the minimal source-skin distance (SSD) that must be used for mobile radiography to ensure patient safety, and state the reason for this minimal SSD requirement.
- Explain the process of digital radiography and computed radiography, and discuss why care must be taken that patients undergoing digital imaging procedures not be overexposed initially.
- Explain how patient exposure may be reduced during routine fluoroscopic procedures, C-arm fluoroscopic procedures, digital fluoroscopic procedures, and high-dose (high level control [HLC]) fluoroscopy interventional procedures.
- Discuss the use of fluoroscopic equipment by nonradiologist physicians who perform interventional procedures or other potentially lengthy tasks, and identify the responsibilities of the radiographer during such procedures.

CHAPTER OUTLINE

Radiation Safety Features of Radiographic Equipment, Devices, and Accessories
  Diagnostic-Type Protective Tube Housing
  Control Panel, or Console
  Radiographic Examination Table
  Source-to-image Receptor Distance Indicator
  X-Ray Beam Limitation Devices
  Filtration
  Compensating Filters

  Exposure Reproducibility
  Exposure Linearity
  Usage of Screen-Film as an Image Receptor and Recording Medium
  Radiographic Grids
  Mobile Radiography
General Information and Radiation Safety Features of Digital Imaging Equipment, Devices, and Accessories
  Digital Imaging

KEY TERMS

brightness
computed radiography (CR)
control panel, or console
cumulative timer
diagnostic-type protective tube housing
digital fluoroscopy (DF)
digital radiography (DR)
entrance skin exposure rates
exposure linearity

exposure reproducibility
filtration
half-value layer (HVL)
high level control fluoroscopy (HLCF)
image matrix
light-localizing variable-aperture rectangular collimator
off-focus radiation
positive beam limitation (PBL)

primary protective barrier
pulsed progressive systems
radiographic examination table
radiographic grid
scattered radiation
source-to-image receptor distance (SID)
source-to-skin distance (SSD)
useful, or primary, beam
x-ray beam limitation device

State-of-the-art diagnostic radiographic and fluoroscopic equipment is designed with many devices that radiologists and technologists can use to optimize the quality of the image while at the same time reducing radiation exposure to patients. Multiple features have been built into new x-ray–producing machines by the manufacturers to ensure radiation safety, and some extra characteristics have also been included to meet enhanced federal regulations. In addition, various accessories are available to further lower radiation doses. Lastly, in the newest systems, all dimensions for patient setup are now given in metric units. Table 11.1 provides an overview of standard English system dimensions with their corresponding metric unit replacements.

In summary, this chapter provides an overview of equipment components and accessories that imaging professionals can use to minimize exposure of patients.

RADIATION SAFETY FEATURES OF RADIOGRAPHIC EQUIPMENT, DEVICES, AND ACCESSORIES

All necessary measures must be taken to ensure that radiographic equipment operates safely. Every diagnostic imaging system must have a protective tube housing and a correctly functioning control panel, or console. The radiographic examination table and other devices and accessories also are required to be constructed so as to reduce the patient's radiation dose.

Diagnostic-Type Protective Tube Housing

A diagnostic-type protective tube housing (Fig. 11.1) is required to safeguard the patient and imaging personnel

TABLE 11.1 **Conversion of English Units of Measure to Effective Metric Equivalent Units**	
English Unit Effective	**Metric Equivalent Unit**
40 inches	100 cm
48 inches	120 cm
72 inches	180 cm
10 inches × 10 inches	25 cm × 25 cm

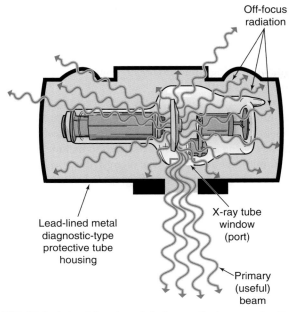

Off-focus radiation

Lead-lined metal diagnostic-type protective tube housing

X-ray tube window (port)

Primary (useful) beam

FIG 11.1 A lead-lined metal diagnostic-type protective tube housing protects patients and imaging personnel from off-focus, or leakage, radiation by restricting x-ray emission to the area of the primary (useful) beam.

from off-focus, or leakage, radiation by restricting the emission of x-rays to the area of the useful, or primary, beam (those x-rays emitted through the x-ray port or tube window).

X-Ray Tube Housing Construction and Functions. The housing enclosing the x-ray tube must be constructed with lead lining so that radiation leakage through any portion of the housing away from the useful beam, measured at a distance of 1 m from the x-ray source, does not exceed 1 mGy$_a$/hr (100 mR/hr) when the tube is operated at its highest voltage at the highest current that allows continuous operation. The protective tube housing also serves as a shield against the high voltage entering the x-ray tube, thereby preventing electric shock while also facilitating cooling of the x-ray tube. Because the x-ray tube and housing assembly are relatively heavy, the overall structure is robustly built to give needed mechanical support and minimize the potential for damage of the x-ray tube in the event that rough handling occurs.

Control Panel, or Console

The control panel, or console, is where technical exposure factors such as milliamperes (mA), peak kilovoltage (kVp), and exposure duration (mS) are selected and visually displayed. It must be located behind a suitable protective barrier that has a radiation-absorbent window that permits observation of the patient during any procedure. It is mandatory that this panel display the conditions of exposure and provide a positive indication when the x-ray tube is energized.[1] For some state-of-the-art operating consoles, digital controls for kVp and mAs are available on a *touch* screen. Generally, when an x-ray exposure begins, a tone is emitted and a radiation sign illuminates. When the exposure terminates, the sound stops and the light goes out.

Radiographic Examination Table

The radiographic examination table must be strong enough to adequately support patients whose weight is in excess of 300 pounds. Frequently, this piece of equipment has a floating tabletop that makes it easier to maneuver the patient during an imaging procedure. The thickness of the tabletop must be uniform, and for under-table x-ray tubes as used in fluoroscopy, the patient support surface should be as radiolucent as possible, thereby reducing the patient's radiation dose. A carbon fiber material is commonly used in the tabletop to meet this requirement.

Source-to-image Receptor Distance Indicator

When x-ray imaging a patient, radiographers must have a means to measure the distance from the anode focal spot to the image receptor to ensure that the recommended* source-to-image receptor distance (SID) is maintained. To meet this need, radiographic equipment comes with an indicator that will perform this function. Frequently, a simple device such as a tape measure is

*For most ordinary x-ray imaging examinations, a standard distance of 100 to 120 cm (40 to 48 inches) is now used in many radiography facilities. For chest radiography of patients who can assume an upright position, a 180 cm (72 inch) distance is traditional. However, an SID as great as 300 cm (120 inches), is sometimes employed. The benefits of increased SID are reduced magnification of the anatomic part being imaged, increased spatial resolution, and an approximate 10% reduction in radiation dose for the patient.[2]

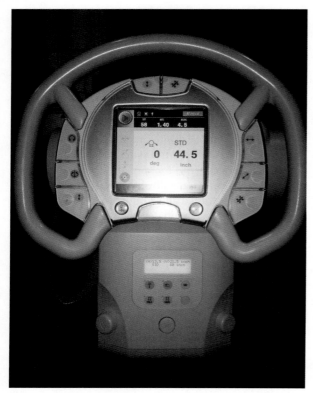

FIG 11.2 Light-localizing variable-aperture rectangular collimator.

attached to the collimator or tube housing so that the radiographer can manually measure the SID. Lasers are also sometimes used to accomplish the same task. SID accuracy is essential. "Distance and centering indicators must be accurate to within 2% and 1% of the source-to-image receptor distance (SID), respectively."[1]

X-Ray Beam Limitation Devices

The primary x-ray beam shall be adequately collimated so that it is no larger than the size of the image receptor being used for the examination. With modern equipment, this is accomplished by providing the unit with a light-localizing variable-aperture rectangular collimator to adjust the size and shape of the x-ray beam either automatically or manually (Fig. 11.2). The collimator is currently the predominant x-ray beam limitation device in use.

Additional Types of X-Ray Beam Limitation Devices.
Some earlier x-ray beam limitation devices included:
- Cones
- Cylinders

These devices confine the useful, or primary, beam before it enters the area of clinical interest and thereby limits the surface area of body tissue irradiated. This also reduces the amount of scattered radiation in the tissue, thus preventing unnecessary exposure to anatomy not under examination.

Scattered radiation is all the radiation that arises from the interaction of an x-ray beam with the atoms of a patient or any other object in the path of the beam. When the size of the x-ray field is restricted to include only the anatomic structures of clinical interest, this also improves the overall quality of the radiographic image.

Light-Localizing Variable-Aperture Rectangular Collimators

Construction. As stated earlier, the collimator is the most versatile device for defining the size and shape of the radiographic beam. The light-localizing variable-aperture rectangular collimator is the type of collimator used with multipurpose x-ray units. It is box shaped and contains the radiographic beam–defining system (Fig. 11.3). This system consists of:
- Two sets of adjustable lead shutters mounted within the device at different levels
- A light source to illuminate the x-ray field and permit it to be centered over the area of clinical interest
- A mirror to deflect the light beam toward the patient to be radiographed

The first set of shutters, the upper shutters, are mounted as close as possible to the tube window to reduce the amount of x-rays emitted from parts of the tube other than the focal spot, coming from the primary beam and exiting at various angles from the x-ray tube window. This off-focus radiation can never be completely eliminated because the metal shutters cannot be placed immediately beneath the actual focal spot of the x-ray tube. However, by placing the first set, or upper, shutters as close as possible to the tube window, this off-focus radiation can be reduced significantly, thereby decreasing the patient's exposure.

The second set of collimator shutters, the lower shutters, are mounted below the level of the light source and mirror and function to further confine the radiographic beam to the area of clinical interest (see Fig. 11.3; Fig. 11.4). This set of shutters consists of two pairs of lead plates oriented at right angles to each other. Each set may be adjusted independently so that an extensive variety of rectangular shapes can be selected. In this way, the field is not limited to the circular or fixed square shapes

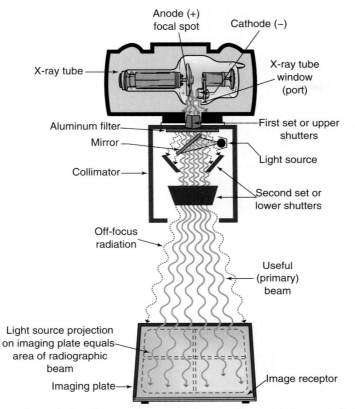

FIG 11.3 Diagram of a typical collimator demonstrating a radiographic beam-defining system: *1,* anode focal spot; *2,* x-ray tube window; *3,* first set of shutters, or upper shutters; *4,* aluminum filter; *5,* mirror; *6,* light source; *7,* second set of shutters, or lower shutters. The metal shutters collimate the radiographic beam so that it is no larger than the image receptor.

that sometimes cause areas of the patient not requiring imaging to receive radiation.

Skin sparing. To minimize skin exposure to electrons produced by photon interaction with the collimator, the patient's skin surface should be at least 15 cm below the collimator. Some collimator housings contain "spacer bars," which project down from the housing to prevent the collimators from being closer than 15 cm to the patient.

Luminance. Luminance is a scientific term referring to the brightness of a surface. Specifically, luminance quantifies the intensity of a light source (i.e., the amount of light per unit area coming from its surface). Luminance is determined by measuring the concentration of light over a particular field of view. This may be understood by examining the units used to describe luminance. The primary unit is the candela per square meter, known

more simply as the *nit*. One candela corresponds to 3.8 million billion photons per second being emitted from a light source through a cone-like field of view. A good analogy is the sound intensity emerging from a drill sergeant with a megaphone held to his lips. With appropriate dimensions, the megaphone's larger opening corresponds to the conelike field of view associated with the candela. The luminance of the collimator light source must be sufficient to permit the localizing light beam to outline the margins of the radiographic beam adequately on the patient's anatomy. Because the light field and the x-ray field are designed to coincide, then if the light field were not sufficiently bright, a radiographer could improperly position the x-ray field on a patient or, at the very least, have great difficulty accurately centering the x-ray beam. With insufficient brightness, the x-ray

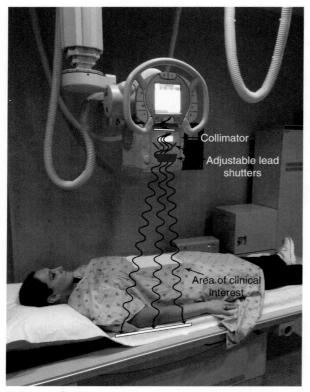

FIG 11.4 Collimator containing the radiographic beam-defining system, which establishes the parameters (margins) of the beam. Adjustable lead shutters limit the cross-sectional area of the beam and confine it to the area of clinical interest.

unit may fail a state inspection. According to standard regulation criteria, luminance must be high enough so that a calibrated light meter reading taken at a distance of 100 cm will be at least 15 foot-candles when averaged over the four quadrants of a 25 × 25-cm field size. A foot-candle is approximately equivalent to 10.76 nit (the unit of luminance). Therefore a reading of 15 foot-candles corresponds to a collimator light source with a luminance of approximately 161 nit, or 161 candela per square meter.

In summary, if the luminance of the collimator light source is adequate, the localizing light beam will satisfactorily outline the margins of the radiographic beam on the area of clinical interest on *all* patients.

Coincidence between the radiographic beam and the localizing light beam. When a light-localizing variable-aperture rectangular collimator is used, good coincidence

(i.e., both physical size and alignment) between the radiographic beam and the localizing light beam is essential to eliminate collimator cutoff of the body structures being irradiated. The sum of the cross-table and along-the-table alignment differences between the x-ray and light beams must not exceed 2% of the SID. This condition is also imposed on the relative "sizing" differences between the x-ray and light beams. These coincidence requirements are collectively known as:

• Alignment
• Congruence

As an example, 100 cm (or 40-inch) is a commonly used SID in radiography. For this the maximum allowable total difference in length and width alignments of the projected light field with the radiographic beam at the level of the image receptor must be no more than 2% of 100 cm (approximately 40-inch), which equals 2 cm (0.8 inch). Acceptable congruence at a 100-cm (40-inch) SID requires that the sum of the dimensions of the x-ray field should also differ from the length and width span of the light field by no more than 2 cm (0.8 inch).

The SID used in radiography actually depends on the individual radiographic projection. For example, a 180-cm (or 72-inch) SID is normally used for routine chest x-ray examinations performed on ambulatory patients. In some imaging departments, the use of 120-cm (or 48-inch) SID for many projections has become standard instead of using 100-cm (40-inch) SID because increasing the SID causes less geometric divergence of the x-ray beam within the patient's body. This will improve the sharpness, or spatial resolution, of the radiographic image. The extended SID can also decrease the patient's dose.[1-4]

Positive beam limitation. In some earlier collimation systems the radiographer could inadvertently use an image receptor size much smaller than the size of the radiation field. Thus areas of the patient would be irradiated that would not be recorded on the image receptor. Either the radiation field size should be smaller (if the additional anatomy is not of diagnostic interest) or the image receptor should be larger (if the anatomy is indeed of diagnostic interest). To prevent such a mismatch, radiographic collimators that are part of fixed radiographic equipment manufactured in the United States generally include a feature called **positive beam limitation (PBL)**. The PBL feature consists of electronic sensors in an image receptor holder that sends signals to the collimator housing. When PBL is activated, the collimators are automatically adjusted so that the radiation field matches the size of the image receptor. If special conditions require the radiographer to have complete control of the system, with the turn of a key, the PBL feature may be deactivated. However, in such a circumstance a warning light is automatically lit to indicate that the PBL system has been deactivated.

The PBL system illustrates an important principle of patient protection during radiographic procedures. The radiographer must ensure that collimation is adequate by adjusting the radiographic beam so that it is no larger than the image receptor (Fig. 11.5). State requirements for agreement of the PBL setting with the actual

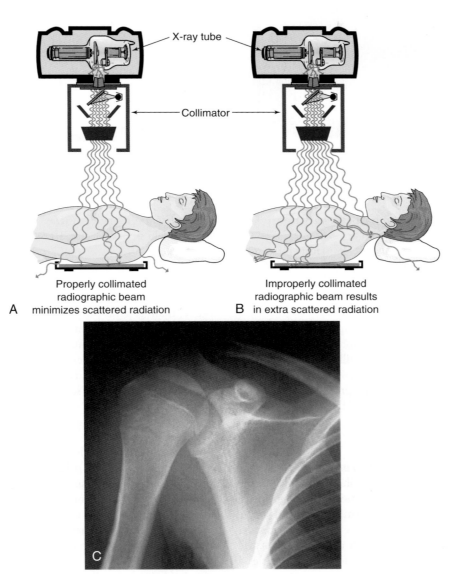

FIG 11.5 Collimate the radiographic beam so that it is no larger than the image receptor. Limiting the beam to the area of clinical interest decreases the amount of tissue irradiated and minimizes patient exposure by reducing the amount of scattered and absorbed radiation. (A) Good collimation. (B) Poor collimation. (C) Anteroposterior radiograph of the shoulder demonstrating good collimation.

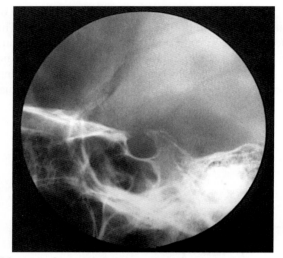

FIG 11.6 Coned-down lateral projection of the sella turcica. (From Ballinger PW, Frank ED: *Merrill's Atlas of Radiographic Positioning and Procedures,* ed 10, St. Louis, 2003, Elsevier.)

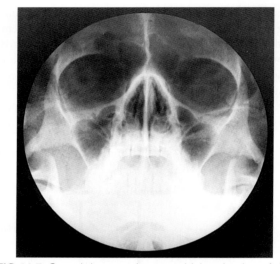

FIG 11.7 Coned-down parietoacanthial projection of the maxillary sinuses. (From Long BW, Rollins JH, Smith BS: *Merrill's Atlas of Radiographic Positioning and Procedures,* ed 13, St. Louis, 2016, Elsevier.)

dimensions of the radiographic beam vary from 2% to 3% of the SID.

Alignment of the x-ray beam. It is imperative that the x-ray beam and the image receptor be correctly aligned with each other. Every radiographic tube must have a device in place to ensure accurate beam alignment.

Cones. Light-localizing variable-aperture rectangular collimators have replaced cones for most radiographic examinations. However, cones are still sometimes used for radiographic examinations of specific areas such as the:
- Head (e.g., coned-down lateral projection of the sella turcica [Fig. 11.6], projections of the paranasal sinuses [Fig. 11.7])
- Vertebral column
- Chest

Flared metal tubes and straight cylinders. Radiographic cones are circular metal tubes that attach to the x-ray tube housing or variable rectangular collimator to limit the x-ray beam to a predetermined size and shape. The design of this collimating device is simple, consisting of either a flared metal tube with the diameter of the upper end smaller than the diameter of the lower end or a straight cylinder with the diameter the same at both the upper and lower ends (Fig. 11.8). Although the length and diameter of the cones vary, it is primarily the lower rim of the cone that governs beam limitation. Sharper

size restriction is achieved when the cone or cylinder is longer. Field size at selected SIDs should be indicated on the cone.

Beam-defining cones used in dental radiography. Beam-defining cones are widely used in dental radiography. Because dental x-ray equipment is usually less bulky than general-purpose equipment, a one-piece beam limitation device, such as a cone made of plastic, is convenient. Some dental cones are lined with lead. By using lead-lined cones instead of the conventional plastic cones, dentists reduce the patient's exposure by eliminating the source of secondary radiation (the plastic cone itself).[5]

Filtration

Purpose of Radiographic Beam Filtration. Filtration of the radiographic beam reduces exposure to the patient's skin and superficial tissue by absorbing most of the lower-energy photons (long wavelength, or soft x-rays) from the heterogeneous beam (Fig. 11.9). This increases the mean energy, or "quality," of the x-ray beam. This change is also referred to as "hardening" the beam.

Effect of Filtration on the Absorbed Dose to the Patient. Because filtration absorbs some of the photons in a radiographic beam, it decreases the overall intensity (quantity, or amount) of incident radiation. The remaining photons,

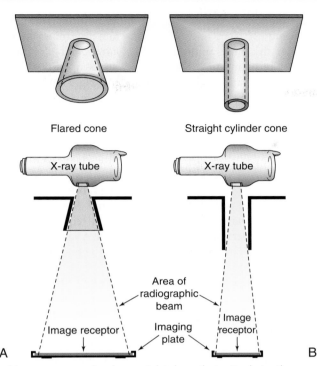

FIG 11.8 Radiographic cones are circular metal tubes that attach to the x-ray tube housing or variable rectangular collimator to limit the radiographic beam to a predetermined size and shape. (A) Cone fashioned in the form of a flared metal tube. (B) Cone fashioned in the form of a straight cylinder.

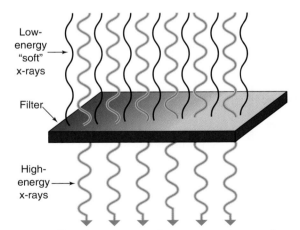

FIG 11.9 Filtration removes low-energy photons (long-wavelength or "soft" x-rays) from the beam by absorbing them and permits higher-energy photons to pass through. This reduces the amount of radiation that the patient receives.

however, are, as a whole, more penetrating and therefore less likely to be absorbed in body tissue. Hence, the absorbed dose to the patient decreases when the correct amount and type of filtration are placed in the path of the radiographic beam. If adequate filtration were not present, very low-energy photons (20 keV or lower) would enter the patient and be almost totally absorbed in the body, thus increasing the patient's radiation dose, especially near or at the surface, but contributing nothing to the image process. The low-energy photons should be removed from the radiographic beam through filtration. Filter material used for this purpose includes elements that are built in or added to the x-ray tube.

Types of Filtration. The following two types of filtration are available:
- Inherent filtration
- Added filtration
  Inherent filtration includes the:
- Glass envelope encasing the x-ray tube

- Insulating oil surrounding the tube
- Glass window in the tube housing

This intrinsic material provides the same amount of filtration as a 0.5 mm thickness of aluminum. The light-localizing collimator mirror provides an additional attenuation of almost 1 mm aluminum equivalent. Taken all together then, there is always a minimum of about 1.5 millimeters of equivalent aluminum filtration imposed on the x-ray beam prior to it exiting from the collimator.

Added filtration usually consists of:

- Sheets of aluminum (or the equivalent) of appropriate thickness

This extra filtration is generally located outside the glass window of the tube housing above the collimator shutters. It is readily accessible to service personnel and may be changed as the x-ray tube ages. The inherent filtration and added filtration combine to equal the required amount necessary to filter the useful beam adequately (Box 11.1).

BOX 11.1   Total Filtration

Total filtration = Inherent filtration plus added filtration

Requirement for Total Filtration. The kVp of a given x-ray unit determines the amount of attenuation required. *Total filtration* of 2.5 mm aluminum equivalent for fixed x-ray units operating above 70 kVp is the regulatory standard (Fig. 11.10).[6] Therefore the manufacturer needs only to place an additional 1 mm aluminum equivalent filter between the tube housing and collimator to meet the minimum regulatory requirement.

Stationary (fixed) radiographic equipment requires total filtration of 1.5 mm aluminum equivalent for x-ray units operating at 50 to 70 kVp, whereas fixed units operating at below 50 kVp require only 0.5 mm aluminum equivalent.[6] Mobile diagnostic units and fluoroscopic equipment require a minimum of 2.5 mm aluminum equivalent. A summary of required minimum total filtration may be found in Box 11.2.

Filtration for General Diagnostic Radiology. In general diagnostic radiology, aluminum (Z = 13) is the metal most widely selected as a filter material because it effectively removes low energy (soft) x-rays from a polyenergetic (heterogeneous) x-ray beam without severely decreasing the x-ray beam intensity. In addition, aluminum is:

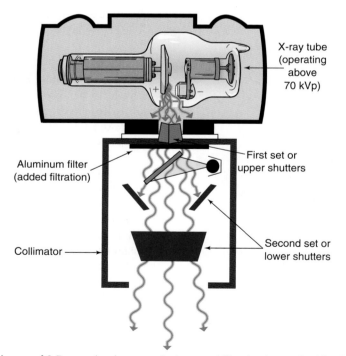

FIG 11.10 A minimum of 2.5 mm aluminum equivalent total filtration is required for fixed radiographic units operating at above 70 kVp.

BOX 11.2 **Summary of Required Minimum Total Filtration**

Stationary (Fixed) Radiographic Equipment

Tube Potential Minimum Total Filtration Required (kVp)	Minimum Total Filtration Required (Specified in mm Al Eq)*
Above 70	2.5
50–70	1.5
Below 50	0.5

Mobile Diagnostic Units and Fluoroscopic Equipment

Mobile diagnostic units and fluoroscopic equipment require a minimum of 2.5 mm Al Eq total permanent filtration.

Al Eq, Aluminum equivalent.
*Modified from National Council on Radiation Protection and Measurements (NCRP): *Medical x-ray, electron beam and gamma-ray protection for energies up to 50 MeV (equipment design, performance, and use), Report No. 102,* Bethesda, MD, 1989, NCRP.

TABLE 11.2 **Half-Value Layer Required by the Radiation Control for Health and Safety Act of 1968 and Detailed by the Bureau of Radiological Health* in 1980**

Peak Kilovoltage	Minimum Required HVL in Millimeters of Aluminum
30	0.3
40	0.4
50	1.2
60	1.3
70	1.5
80	2.3
90	2.5
100	2.7
110	3.0
120	3.2

HVL, Half-value layer.
*The Bureau of Radiological Health changed its name to the Center for Devices and Radiological Health in 1982.

- Lightweight
- Sturdy
- Relatively inexpensive
- Readily available

In compliance with the Radiation Control for Health and Safety Act of 1968, a diagnostic x-ray beam must always be adequately filtered. This means that a sufficient quantity of low-energy photons has been removed from a beam produced at a given kVp. The half-value layer (HVL) of the beam must be measured to verify this. HVL is defined as the thickness of a designated absorber required to decrease the intensity of the primary beam by 50% of its initial value. A radiologic physicist should obtain this measurement at least once a year and also after an x-ray tube is replaced or repairs have been made on the diagnostic x-ray tube housing or collimation system. For diagnostic x-ray beams, the HVL is expressed in millimeters of aluminum. Because it is a measure of beam quality, or effective energy of the x-ray beam, a certain minimal HVL is required at a given kVp. Examples of required HVLs for selected kVp values are listed in Table 11.2.

Compensating Filters

Dose reduction and uniform radiographic imaging of body parts that vary considerably in thickness or tissue composition may be accomplished by use of compensating filters constructed of:

- Aluminum
- Lead-acrylic
- Other suitable materials

These devices are shaped so as to partially attenuate x-rays that are directed toward the thinner, or less dense, anatomic areas while permitting more x-radiation to strike the thicker, or denser, areas to be imaged. For example, the *wedge filter* (Fig. 11.11) is used to provide uniform density when the foot is undergoing radiography in the dorsoplantar projection. For this examination, the wedge is attached to the lower rim of the collimator and positioned with its thickest part toward the toes and thinnest part toward the heel.

The *trough,* or *bilateral, wedge filter,* which is used in some dedicated chest radiographic units, is another example of a compensating filter. This filter is thin in the center to permit adequate x-ray penetration of the mediastinum and thick laterally to reduce exposure of the aerated lungs. With this device, a radiographic image with uniform average density is obtained. Some modern digital systems correct for such nonuniformities of exposure with digital image processing rather than by using physical filters.

Exposure Reproducibility

Exposure reproducibility has been previously defined as consistency in radiation output intensity for identical

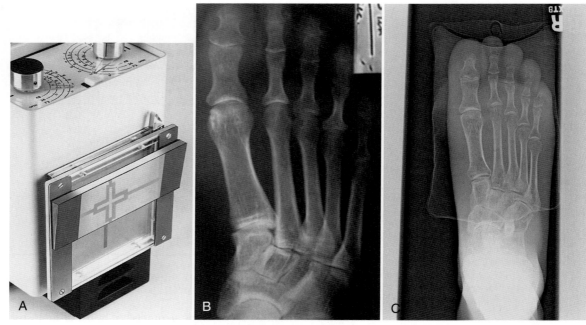

FIG 11.11 (A) Wedged-shaped lead-acrylic compensating filter used to provide uniform density for (B) a dorsoplantar projection of the foot without a compensating filter. (C) A dorsoplantar projection of the foot with a wedge-shaped lead-acrylic compensating filter.

generator settings from one individual exposure to subsequent exposures. This means that the x-ray unit must be able to duplicate certain radiographic exposures for any given combination of kilovolts at peak (kVp), milliamperes (mA), and time settings. A variance of 5% or less is acceptable. Reproducibility may be verified by using the same technical exposure factors to make a series of repeated radiation exposures and then, observing with a calibrated ion chamber, how radiation intensity typically varies.

Exposure Linearity

Exposure linearity, also previously described, refers to a *consistency* in output radiation intensity at any selected kVp when generator settings are changed from one milliamperage and time combination (mAs = mA × exposure time) to another. *Linearity (L)* has been mathematically defined as the ratio of the difference in mSv/mAs or mR/mAs values between two successive generator stations to the sum of those mSv/mAs or mR/mAs values. It must be less than 0.1 (i.e., L cannot exceed 10%).

Usage of Screen-Film as an Image Receptor and Recording Medium

In the past, radiographic images were acquired and saved on film. Devices called *intensifying screens* received x-ray photons and converted their energy to enhanced visible light, which exposed the film, creating a durable image. With advances in technology, most health care facilities now use digital image receptors that include digital radiography (DR) and computed radiography (CR) modalities and are discussed later in this chapter. Radiographers should be aware of screen-film systems because older films still exist as part of some patients' history. But radiographers are not expected to have detailed knowledge of this technology. The use of screen-film systems has largely been abandoned in modern medicine.

Radiographic Grids

Construction, Purpose, Technical Value, and Impact of Radiographic Grid on Patient Dose. A radiographic grid (Fig. 11.12) is a device made of parallel radiopaque strips alternately separated with low-attenuation strips of:

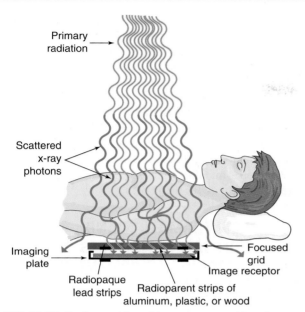

FIG 11.12 Radiographic grids remove scattered x-ray photons that emerge from the patient being radiographed before this scattered radiation reaches the image receptor and decreases radiographic quality.

- Aluminum
- Plastic fiber
- Wood

It is placed between the patient and the radiographic image receptor to remove scattered x-ray photons that emerge from the patient before they reach the image receptor. This significantly improves:

- Radiographic contrast
- Visibility of detail

Generally, this device is used when the thickness of the body part to be radiographed is 10 cm (about 4 inches) or greater. Although the use of a grid increases patient dose, the benefit obtained in terms of the improved quality of the recorded image, making available a greater quantity of diagnostic information, is a fair compromise. Because several different types of grids and grids with different ratios are available, care must be taken to ensure that the correct type and grid ratio* are used for a particular examination, or else a repeat examination may be necessary, which would additionally increase patient dose.

Grid ratio is defined as the ratio of the height of the lead strips in the grid to the distance between them. High-ratio grids reduce scatter radiation more effectively than do low-ratio grids. However, high-ratio grids require more radiation exposure.

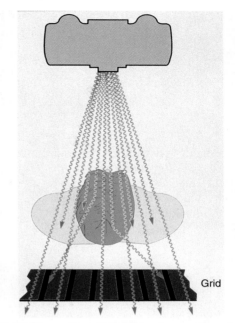

FIG 11.13 The radiographic grid acts as a sieve to block the passage of photons that have been scattered at some angle from their original path. (From *Radiobiology and Radiation Protection: Mosby's Radiographic Instructional Series,* St. Louis, 1999, Elsevier.)

Summarizing the Function of a Radiographic Grid. To summarize, when x-rays pass through an object, some of the photons are scattered away from their original path as a result of coherent and Compton scattering processes. Radiographic quality is highest when these scattered photons are not recorded on the image. If scattered photons are recorded, a general darkening of the image occurs, which detracts from the viewer's ability to distinguish among the different structures of the object being radiographed. Ideally, only those photons that have passed through matter with no deviation from their original geometric path should be recorded. To minimize the influence of scattered photons, a grid is inserted between the patient and the image receptor. It is designed to act as a sieve to block the passage of photons that have been scattered beyond some maximum angle from their original path (Fig. 11.13).

Grid Ratio and Patient Dose. As previously noted, grids are made of parallel radiopaque lead strips alternately separated by low-attenuation strips of aluminum, plastic fiber, or wood. Therefore because some fraction of the

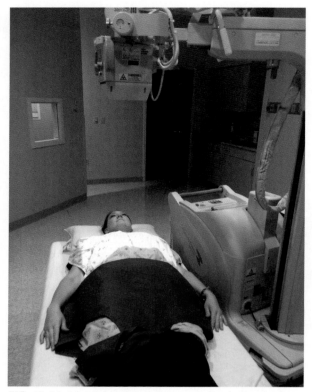

FIG 11.14 Mobile radiographic examinations require a minimal source-skin distance of 30 cm (12 inches). The 30 cm distance limits the effects of inverse square falloff of radiation intensity with distance.

image receptor is covered with lead, more mAs must be used to compensate. Thus patient dose increases whenever a grid is inserted, and because extra lead is contained in higher-ratio grids (e.g., 16:1), patient dose increases as grid ratio increases.

Mobile Radiography

Requirement. Mobile radiographic units require special precautions to ensure patient safety. When operating the unit, the radiographer must use a source-skin distance (SSD) of at least 30 cm (12 inches) (Fig. 11.14). The 30-cm (12-inch) distance limits the effects of the inverse square falloff of radiation intensity with distance. This falloff is more pronounced the shorter the SSD. In practice, much longer distances (e.g., 100 cm [40 inches] from the x-ray source to image receptor or even 120 cm [48 inches]) are generally used.

Use of Mobile Units. Mobile (portable) units should be used to perform radiographic procedures only on patients who cannot be transported to a fixed radiographic installation (an x-ray room). Mobile units are not designed to replace specially designated imaging rooms.

Effect of Source-Skin Distance on Patient Entrance Exposure. For all types of x-ray units, when the SSD is small, the patient's entrance exposure is significantly greater than the exit exposure. By increasing SSD, the radiographer maintains a more uniform distribution of exposure throughout the patient.

GENERAL INFORMATION AND RADIATION SAFETY FEATURES OF DIGITAL IMAGING EQUIPMENT, DEVICES, AND ACCESSORIES

Digital Imaging

Modern computers are capable of rapidly processing vast amounts of independent groups of information. Since the 1970s, the use of computers has virtually revolutionized the medical industry. In particular, computers have had a major impact on imaging. They are now used extensively in almost all imaging modalities. The primary examples of this are:
- Computed tomography (CT)
- Computed radiography (CR)
- Digital radiography (DR)
- Digital fluoroscopy (DF)
- Digital mammography (DM)
- Nuclear medicine (NM) imaging
- Magnetic resonance imaging (MRI)
- Ultrasound (US)

Conventional Radiography: Analog Image. Historically, in conventional radiography, after x-rays passed through an anatomic area of clinical interest, they formed an invisible, or latent, image of that area on radiographic film. This temporary image then had to be chemically processed to make the unseen image visible. The finished radiograph that resulted from this process is an "analog image." Conventional radiography permitted the production of optimal-quality images that made possible adequate visualization and demonstration of various anatomic structures. However, the use of this technology has some disadvantages in addition to the waiting time it took for the chemical processing of these film-based images. Radiographic film needed to be physically handled by authorized personnel and then stored in a centralized file. Manually retrieving radiographs was often time consuming and required adequate personnel power. As a consequence of human error, film jackets containing patients' radiographs were sometimes misfiled or misplaced, thus making these records unavailable at a time when a physician needed them for patient care.

Digital Radiography. The information contained in a conventional image on radiographic film consisted of various shades of gray that represent the amount of x-ray penetration through various biologic tissues. With **digital radiography (DR)**, the latent image, formed by x-ray photons on a radiation detector, is actually an electronic latent image.[7] Because this anatomic information is subsequently collected by a computer and shown on its display, it is called a *digital image*.[8] The familiar radiographic densities then appear as levels of brightness associated with shades of gray. "**Brightness** is defined as the amount of luminance (light emission) of a display monitor. The shades of gray that are displayed constitute the contrast in the image. The number of different shades of gray that can be stored in memory and displayed on a computer monitor is termed grayscale. Digital images are composed of numerical data that can be easily manipulated by a computer."[9]

The numeric values of the digital image are aligned in a fixed number of rows and columns (an array) that form many individual miniature square boxes, each of which corresponds to a particular place in the image. These individual boxes collectively constitute the **image matrix**. Each miniature square box in this matrix is called a *picture element,* or *pixel.* The pixels collectively produce a two-dimensional representation of the information contained in a volume of tissue.[10] The size of the pixels determines the sharpness of the image. Resolution is sharper when pixels are smaller. Common matrix sizes are 512 pixels high by 512 pixels wide or simply 512 × 512 and similarly 1024 × 1024. The latter corresponds to a much higher resolution because it has four times as many elements distributed over the same area. The pixels are therefore smaller, which leads to improved image detail.

When compared with an optimal quality image produced on radiographic film, the resolution of the digital image is actually somewhat lower. However, the digital image is still diagnostic, permitting adequate visualization of anatomic structures because it has better image contrast. This is so, because unlike in a developed film, the contrast in the digital image can be enhanced by computer manipulation.

The image receptors used in DR convert the energy of x-rays into electrical signals. The image receptor is divided into small detector elements that make up the picture elements, or pixels, of the digital image. There are various types of DR image receptors. Some use a *scintillator,* such as amorphous silicon,* to convert the x-ray energy into visible light. The visible light is then transformed into electrical signals by an assortment of transistors or an array of charge-coupled devices (CCDs), such as those found in video cameras. Other systems use a *photoconductor,* such as amorphous selenium, to convert the x-ray energy directly into electrical signals that are then read by an ordered grouping of transistors. In all these systems, the number and size of small transistors or CCDs determine the number and size of pixels in the digital image. Advances in materials technology have resulted in pixel sizes as small as 50 micrometers, which approaches the resolution of screen-film imaging systems (Fig. 11.15).

DR images can be accessed at several workstations at the same time, thus making image viewing very convenient for physicians providing patient care. Patient information and reports can be included in the patient's DR imaging file, along with records from other imaging modalities.[11]

Repeat Rates in Digital Radiography. Because the image contrast and overall brightness may be manipulated after image acquisition, DR eliminates the need for almost all retakes required as a result of improper technique selection (Fig. 11.16). However, repeat rates for reasons of poor positioning are not lowered. Because the image receptor is part of the imaging equipment and does not need to be removed for processing, the technologist can simply view the image on a monitor in the room. This raises a concern about knowing the number of repeats required because of mispositioning. There is no direct "penalty" to a technologist repeating images because of unacceptable technique, so the examination and resultant radiation exposure could be delivered multiple times, instead of

---

*A noncrystalline grouping of silicon atoms in which, rather than in a regular geometric pattern, the silicon atoms are distributed in a continuous random fashion.

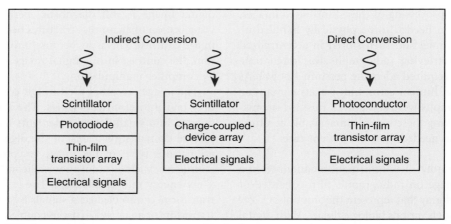

FIG 11.15 Some large area detectors provide indirect conversion of x-ray energy to electrical charge through intermediate steps involving photodiodes or charge-coupled devices. Other area detectors provide direct conversion of x-ray energy to electrical charge through the use of a photoconductor. (From Hendee WR, Ritenour ER: *Medical Imaging Physics*, ed 4, Chicago, 2002, John Wiley & Sons.)

just once, without the knowledge of supervisors. Therefore either each image should be monitored by an independent quality control technologist at a separate monitor or a quality control system should be devised whereby for each technologist the number of images per examination is compared with the number ordered.

Computed Radiography. Computed radiography (CR) involves the use of conventional radiographic equipment, traditional patient positioning performed by a radiographer, and the selection and use of standard technical exposure factors. The unseen radiographic image is actually produced in a rectangular, closed cassette containing a photostimulable phosphor (europium-activated barium fluorohalide is the most commonly employed phosphor[1]) imaging plate as the image receptor. This reusable device is inserted in place of radiographic film into a light-tight, closed cassette that resembles that found in conventional radiography.

When the enclosed phosphor is exposed to x-rays, it becomes energized. An image reading unit is used to scan the photostimulable phosphor imaging plate with a helium–neon laser beam. This results in the emission of violet light that is changed into an electronic signal by a device called a *photomultiplier tube.*

A computer then converts the electronic signal into a digitized image of the anatomic area or part and stores the digital image for visual display on a monitor. If desired, the image can be printed on a laser film when hard copy is needed. While the digital image is displayed on a monitor, the radiographer, by manipulating the computer mouse[2] (Fig. 11.17), can adjust it to the correct:

- Size
- Brightness
- Contrast

After adjustments have been completed, the image can be electronically sent for reading.

Avoiding overexposure of the patient. Although the radiographer can manipulate the CR image of the patient's anatomy of interest to adjust image size, brightness, and contrast, this technologic flexibility does not excuse overexposing the patient. Even with sophisticated digital technology, it is still the radiographer's responsibility to determine and use correct technical exposure factors the first time a patient is x-rayed to minimize radiation exposure. If patients are overexposed by radiographers who claim the rationale that computerized images can be manipulated later on to produce a diagnostic-quality image, patients are actually receiving higher radiation doses than are necessary to produce those initial images. This type of practice leads to a phenomenon known in many facilities as *dose creep.* Therefore the routine practice of overexposing patients to avoid possible repeat radiographic exposures is unethical and unacceptable.

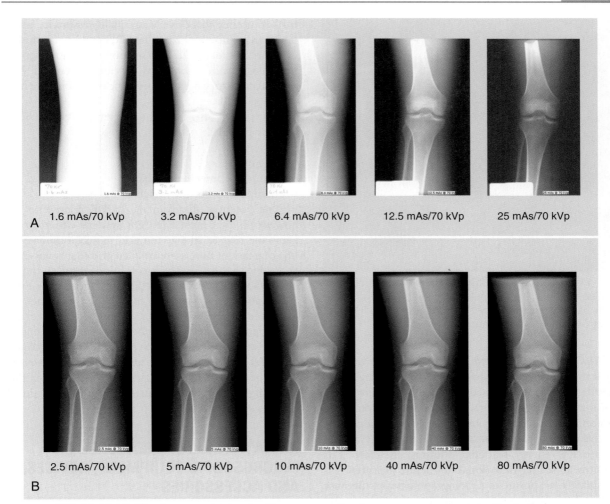

FIG 11.16 (A) The images obtained with a screen-film image receptor system illustrate how changing technical exposure factors greatly affects film image quality. (B) Computed radiography (CR) images obtained through the same technique ranges as those used for (A) have much less effect on image quality because "CR image contrast is constant, regardless of radiation exposure." (From Betsy Shields, Presbyterian Hospital, Charlotte, North Carolina. In Bushong SC: *Radiologic Science for Technologists: Physics, Biology and Protection,* ed 11, St. Louis, 2017, Elsevier.)

To conform with ALARA protection guidelines, radiographers must exercise good judgment in selecting correct technical exposure factors the first time.

Kilovoltage. As in conventional radiography, kilovoltage controls radiographic contrast. However, CR imaging has greater kilovoltage flexibility than does conventional screen-film radiography. Therefore a radiographer can select an appropriate kVp setting from a broader range of settings than have been traditionally suitable for a particular radiographic projection.[2] An acceptable range of kVp that is adequate for penetration of the anatomy of interest should, however, always be used. Kilovoltage above or below this acceptable range should not be used. Technique charts indicating optimal kVp values for all CR projections must be available in the x-ray room near the operating console for the radiographer.

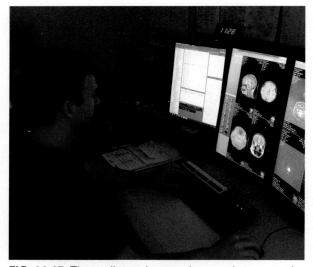

FIG 11.17 The radiographer at the monitor uses the mouse to adjust the computed radiography image of the body part to the proper size, density, and contrast before electronically sending the image for reading.

X-ray beam collimation. For the computer to form a CR image correctly, the body area or part being radiographed must be positioned in or near the center of the CR image receptor. In practical application, only one projection per image is taken on a CR imaging plate.

Use of radiographic grids. The CR imaging plate can absorb low energy scattered photons; therefore it is sensitive to scatter radiation, both before and after it is sensitized by exposure to a radiographic beam.[3] Because of this increased sensitivity, a radiographic grid should be used more frequently. For chest radiography, Carlton and Adler advocated the use of a grid for optimum images when chest measurements exceed 24 to 26 cm.[3] Some CR imaging manufacturers recommend the use of a grid for certain radiographic projections that require relatively high-kVp settings. Grid selection depends on several factors: size of the anatomic features to be radiographed, kVp selected, amount of scatter removal preferred, and grid frequency (lines per centimeter or inch), for example.[3]

It is customary and, for the best image quality, necessary to use a grid for anatomy sections more than 10 cm thick or for techniques that exceed 70 kVp. This need remains true with both CR and DR. The problem one faces with CR in general is that the mAs required and, consequently, the patient dose received are significantly higher than for non-CR. The addition of a grid will only further increase that dose. Many quality assurance teams, however, are now realizing that CR, because of its higher exposure latitude, makes grid use on the pediatric population less necessary than was previously believed. As a result, satisfactory nongrid pediatric protocols have been developed and used.

DR systems offer several advantages over CR. Some of these include:
- Lower dose
- Ease of use
- Immediate imaging results
- Manipulation of the image

One potential disadvantage of DR relative to CR, however, is that most fixed DR systems either do not allow the user to change the grid to accommodate the imaging task or have a preinstalled grid that is not easily accessible to the user. These conditions result in the use of grids for pediatric imaging, thereby unnecessarily giving these patients a higher dose of radiation. Facilities will now need to work with their radiation safety officer and physics group more than ever before to ensure the highest quality imaging for the smallest patients. As a technologist, one must find out whether grids are truly not removable from the digital imaging equipment or whether they are being used merely because it is the manufacturer's recommendation.

RADIATION SAFETY FEATURES OF FLUOROSCOPIC EQUIPMENT, DEVICES, AND ACCESSORIES

Fluoroscopic Procedures and Patient Radiation Exposure Rate

Fluoroscopy is the process in which an x-ray examination is performed that demonstrates dynamic, or active, motion of selected anatomic structures (e.g., a stomach filled with barium sulfate and air during an upper gastrointestinal series) by producing a real-time image of those structures on a television monitor that works in conjunction with an image intensification system. Fluoroscopic procedures (Fig. 11.18) yield the greatest patient radiation exposure rate in diagnostic radiology. Therefore the referring physician should carefully evaluate the need for a fluoroscopic examination to ascertain whether the potential benefit to the patient, in terms of information gained, outweighs any adverse somatic or genetic effects of the examination. If the fluoroscopic procedure is necessary,

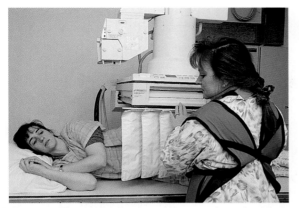

FIG 11.18 Fluoroscopic procedures produce the largest patient radiation exposure rate in diagnostic radiology.

every precaution must be taken to minimize patient exposure time.

Fluoroscopic Imaging Systems

Traditionally, fluoroscopic imaging systems have the x-ray tube positioned under the x-ray examination table and the image intensifier and a spot film system mounted on a linked C-arm–like structure that is centered and suspended over the x-ray examination table. The C-arm design keeps the x-ray tube and the image receptor in constant alignment. Other equipment configurations are possible; for example, the unit can be arranged so that the x-ray tube can be placed over the x-ray examination table while the image receptor lies beneath the x-ray examination table. A fluoroscopic imaging system can also be set up as a remote control facility, thus permitting the equipment operator to remain outside the fluoroscopic room. In the interest of patient and personnel safety, radiologists and assisting radiologic technologists have a responsibility to become fully knowledgeable regarding the safe operation of the equipment they use.

Image Intensification Fluoroscopy

Benefits. Modern fluoroscopy (Fig. 11.19) involves the use of a signal amplification device called an *image intensifier tube* (Fig. 11.20) to greatly increase the brightness of the real-time image produced on a screen during fluoroscopy. It, or a digital device that performs the same function, is used in virtually all state-of-the-art fluoroscopic equipment. Image intensification fluoroscopy has three significant benefits, which are listed in Box 11.3.

> **BOX 11.3 Benefits of Image Intensification Fluoroscopy**
>
> 1. Increased image brightness
> 2. Saving of time for the radiologist
> 3. Patient dose reduction

Brightness of the Fluoroscopic Image. The x-ray image intensification system converts the x-ray image pattern into a corresponding amplified visible light pattern. The overall brightness of the fluoroscopic image increases to roughly 10,000 times the brightness of the image on the long since discontinued non–image intensifier fluoroscopy systems* operating under the same conditions. This dramatic increase in brightness has greatly improved the radiologist's perception of the fluoroscopic image.

Milliamperage Required and Effect on Patient Dose. Because an image intensification system greatly increases brightness, image intensification fluoroscopy requires less milliamperage than does old-fashioned fluoroscopy (approximately 1.5 to 2 mA is used for many procedures with image intensification systems, whereas 3 to 5 mA was usually required prior to image intensification fluoroscopy). The consequent decrease in exposure rate can result in a sizable dose reduction for the patient.

Multifield, or Magnification, Image Intensifier Tubes. An image intensifier tube is basically an "electronic device that receives the image-forming x-ray beam and converts it into a visible-light picture of high intensity."[1] A simple diagram of this tube with components labeled may be found in Fig. 11.20. Multifield, or magnification, image intensifier tubes are found in the majority of image intensifiers. They are also found in digital fluoroscopy (DF) units (see the discussion on DF presented later in this chapter). Depending on their manufacturer and geographic location, multifield image intensification tubes

---

*A pre–image intensification fluoroscopic operating system consisted of the fluoroscopic tube, mounted beneath the radiographic table as with most modern fluoroscopic systems, producing x-rays that passed through the tabletop and the patient before striking a zinc-cadmium sulfide (ZnCdS) screen. The latter then phosphoresced and produced an image of the anatomy of interest, which was very dim, thus yielding a poor visibility of detail of those structures for the radiologist.

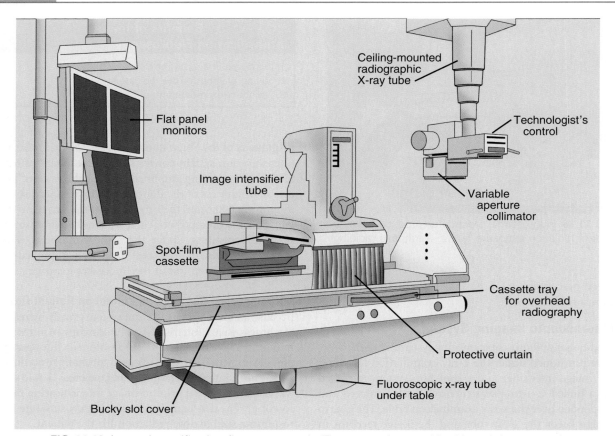

FIG 11.19 Image intensification fluoroscopy unit. The x-ray tube used in this unit is mounted beneath the unit's radiographic table, which supports the patient. The image intensifier and other image detection devices are then drawn forward and placed over the patient on the table to perform the examination. Other fluoroscopic equipment arrangements are possible. (From Bushong SC: *Radiologic Science for Technologists: Physics, Biology and Protection,* ed 10, St. Louis, 2013, Elsevier.)

vary in size, but the 30/25/20-cm (12/10/8-inch) diameter trifield model is typical for general-purpose fluoroscopic units. However, other sizes and magnification modes are available. When the normal viewing mode of 30 cm (12 inches) is used, photoelectrons from the entire surface of a cesium iodide (CsI) phosphor (i.e., the input surface when the x-ray photons passing through the patient first strike the image intensifier assembly) are accelerated to a zinc–cadmium sulfide output phosphor. However, when magnification in the fluoroscopic image is needed and the viewing mode is changed to the 25-cm mode (10 inches) or even less (e.g., 20 cm or 8 inches in many new systems), the voltage on the electrostatic focusing lenses increases, thereby causing the focal point of the electrons

to move to a greater distance away from the output phosphor.[1] As a result, only electrons from the central 25-cm diameter portion of the input phosphor actually reach the output phosphor of the image intensifier. This added distance from the focal point location of the electrons to the output phosphor surface, however, creates a larger image but with a decreased field of view (Fig. 11.21). The quality of the magnified image, if there are no other changes, as viewed on a monitor, is somewhat degraded. This decrease in image clarity occurs because of a reduction in minification gain (i.e., increase in brightness resulting from minification of the image) caused when fewer photoelectrons are available to strike the output phosphor on the image intensifier. Therefore

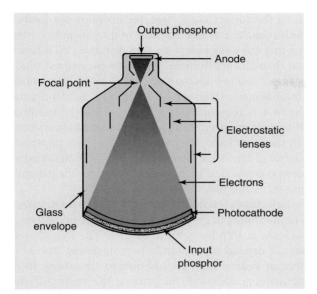

FIG 11.20 Basic components of an image intensifier tube. (From Bushong SC: *Radiologic Science for Technologists: Physics, Biology and Protection*, ed 10, St. Louis, 2013, Elsevier.)

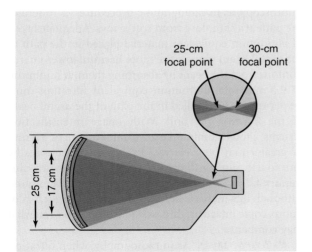

FIG 11.21 A 30/25/20 image intensifier tube produces a magnified image in 25-cm mode, whereas the 20-cm mode produces an image that is even more highly magnified. (From Bushong SC: *Radiologic Science for Technologists: Physics, Biology and Protection*, ed 10, St. Louis, 2013, Elsevier.)

the resultant image is dimmer. Because it is necessary and desirable to maintain a constant level of brightness on the monitor, fluoroscopic mA increases automatically to counter this. The overall quality of the image will now be at least as good as the larger-diameter modes because a greater number of x-ray photons will be used to form the magnified image. This image will have a more even appearance (less noise), and it will be possible to distinguish among similar tissues in an easier manner because of improved contrast. However, the increase in tube mA raises the dose to the patient.

Multifield or Magnification with Digital Detectors. In digital systems, changing the image size may simply mean that the system just displays a different subset of pixels. Thus a "digital zoom" of the image may not involve a change in patient exposure. For some adjustments of image size the manufacturer might adjust patient exposure, but without the analog image intensifier, the change does not depend upon the area of the input phosphor. Therefore to know whether changing the field size changes patient dose, the medical physicist or the manufacturer must be consulted. Similarly, with digital systems, changing the collimation may not significantly alter the patient exposure at any point, although "collimating in" will decrease the volume of the patient irradiated and therefore will decrease scattered radiation.

Pulsed and Interrupted Fluoroscopy

Effect on Patient Dose. Intermittent, or pulsed, fluoroscopy involves manual or automatic periodic activation of the fluoroscopic tube by the fluoroscopist, rather than continuous activation. This practice:

- Significantly decreases patient dose, especially in long procedures
- Helps extend the life of the tube

In pulsed (discontinuous) mode the system software automatically turns the radiation beam on and off at an operator selected repetition rate. The most common rates are 30, 15, and 7.5 pulses per second, with each radiation pulse lasting no more than 10 milliseconds. Shorter pulse durations improve the sharpness of the image but decrease the signal-to-noise ratio because of the smaller number of x-rays involved. A 30 p/s rate would normally be used for imaging studies involving very rapid anatomic or process motion (e.g., interventional catheter procedures) to achieve acceptable temporal resolution. Barium swallow studies, on the other hand, could make use of 7.5 p/s.

Many systems include a last image hold feature that allows the fluoroscopist to see the most recent image without exposing the patient to another pulse of radiation (i.e., to momentarily halt the radiation). Frequently making use of last image hold through lengthy procedures will significantly reduce patient dose.

Limiting Fluoroscopic Field Size

Benefit of fluoroscopic field size limitation. The radiologist must limit the size of the fluoroscopic field to include only the area of clinical interest. This involves visually moving the shutters placed between the fluoroscopic tube and the patient to define the desired x-ray field of view. When fluoroscopic field size is limited, patient area or integral dose decreases substantially. It is also possible, for lengthy procedures, to spread out the patient entrance dose area and thereby minimize the potential for skin effects while maintaining the same anatomic field of view by moving or rotating the patient so that the radiation enters multiple portions of the patient surface during the procedure.

Fluoroscopic beam length and width limitation. Primary beam length and width must be confined within the image receptor boundary. Regardless of the distance from the x-ray source to the image receptor, the useful beam should not extend outside the image receptor. Ideally, visible borders should appear on the image monitor. If this is not so, a patient could receive substantial irradiation in certain procedures to sensitive areas adjacent to the study area. Thus this conformity between the x-ray field and the input phosphor of the image intensifier is an important item of regulatory concern.

Technical Exposure Factors

Selection of technical exposure factors for adult patients. The fluoroscopist must select technical exposure factors that will minimize patient dose during manual fluoroscopic procedures. Increases in kVp and filtration reduce the patient radiation exposure rate. Most fluoroscopic examinations performed with image intensification systems employ a range of 75 to 110 kVp for adult patients, depending on the body area being examined. This kVp range produces the correct level of fluoroscopic image brightness. Lower kVp, when used for greater diameter regions, increases patient dose because use of a lesser penetrating x-ray beam necessitates the use of a higher milliamperage (a larger quantity of x-ray photons in the beam) to obtain adequate image brightness. Besides

using the correct kilovoltage, the operator can further limit excessive entrance exposure of the patient by ensuring that the x-ray source-to-skin distance (SSD) is not less than 38 cm (15 inches) for stationary (fixed) fluoroscopes and not less than 30 cm (12 inches) for mobile (fluoroscopes) (C-arms). A 30-cm (12-inch) minimal distance is required, but a 38-cm (15-inch) minimal distance is preferred for all image intensification systems. On the other hand, the position of the input phosphor surface of the image intensifier should be maintained as close as is practical to the patient to reduce the patient's entrance exposure rate as well.

Selection of technical exposure factors for children. Safe fluoroscopic procedures for children necessitate a decrease in kVp by as much as 25%. The kVp chosen should depend on anatomic part thickness, just as it does in radiography. In addition to decreasing kVp, maintaining SSD and minimizing the height of the image intensifier entrance surface above the patient will further limit excessive entrance exposure of the pediatric patient.

Filtration

Purpose and requirements. The function of a filter in fluoroscopy, as in radiographic procedures, is to reduce the patient's skin dose from soft x-rays. Adequate layers of aluminum equivalent material placed in the path of the useful beam remove the more harmful lower-energy photons from the beam by absorbing them. A minimum of 2.5 mm total aluminum equivalent filtration must be permanently installed in the path of the useful beam of the fluoroscopic unit. With image intensification systems, a total aluminum equivalent filtration of 3.0 mm or greater may be preferred. Patient dose decreases by one-fourth during fluoroscopic procedures when aluminum filtration increases from 1 to 3 mm aluminum. Although this increase in filtration causes a slight loss of fluoroscopic image brightness, increasing kVp somewhat may compensate.

Half-value layer. As in radiography, when filtration of the x-ray beam is questionable, the HVL of the beam must be measured. In *standard* image intensification fluoroscopy, an x-ray beam HVL of 3 to 4.5 mm aluminum is considered acceptable when kVp ranges from 80 to 100.

Cumulative Timing Device

A cumulative timer must be provided and used with each fluoroscopic unit. This resettable device measures the x-ray beam-on time and sounds an audible alarm or in some cases temporarily interrupts the exposure after the fluoroscope has been activated for 5 minutes. It serves to make the radiologist aware of how long the patient has been receiving x-ray exposure for each fluoroscopic examination. When the fluoroscope is activated for shorter periods, the patient, radiologist, and radiographer will all receive less exposure. Total fluoroscopic beam-on time should be documented for every fluoroscopic procedure.

Exposure Rate Limitations. Current federal standards limit entrance skin exposure rates of general-purpose intensified fluoroscopic units with maximum technique factors engaged to a maximum of 100 mGy$_a$ per minute (10 R/min), as measured at tabletop, with the image intensifier entrance surface at a prescribed 30 cm (12 inches) above the tabletop. This limit for ordinary fluoroscopic systems has been imposed to give protection against patients accidentally receiving skin-damaging entrance dose levels in short periods. Special fluoroscopic units equipped with *high level control (HLC),* however, may produce a skin entrance exposure rate as great as 200 mGy$_a$ per minute (20 R/min). Because special fluoroscopic procedures can result in the largest patient doses in diagnostic x-ray imaging, sometimes reaching the level of therapeutic doses, a concerted effort must be made to keep fluoroscopic exposure rates and cumulative exposure times within established limits.

Primary Protective Barrier. A primary protective barrier of 2 mm lead equivalent is required for a fluoroscopic unit. The image intensifier assembly or a digital detector provides this barrier to direct radiation. The assembly must be physically joined with the x-ray tube and interlocked so that the fluoroscopic x-ray tube cannot be activated when the image intensifier is in the parked position.

Fluoroscopic Exposure Control Switch. The fluoroscopic exposure control switch (e.g., the foot pedal) must be of the dead-man type (i.e., only continuous pressure applied by the operator [usually a radiologist] can keep the switch activated and the fluoroscopic tube emitting x-radiation). This means that the exposure automatically terminates if the person operating the switch becomes incapacitated (e.g., has a medical emergency) or for any reason removes his or her foot from the pedal.

RADIATION SAFETY FEATURES OF MOBILE C-ARM FLUOROSCOPY EQUIPMENT, DEVICES, AND ACCESSORIES

Mobile C-Arm Fluoroscopy

A mobile C-arm fluoroscopic unit is a portable x-ray unit that is C-shaped. It has an x-ray tube attached to one end of its curved arm and an image intensifier attached to the other end. C-arm fluoroscopes (Fig. 11.22) are frequently used in the operating room for orthopedic procedures (e.g., pinning of a fractured hip). They are also used for:

- Cardiac imaging
- Interventional procedures

The use of C-arm fluoroscopy in procedures such as these carries the potential for a relatively large patient radiation dose. C-arm fluoroscope operators, if standing close to the patient, could also receive a significant increase in occupational exposure from patient scatter radiation during such cases. For this reason, equipment operators, including attending physicians, must have appropriate education and training to ensure that they will be able

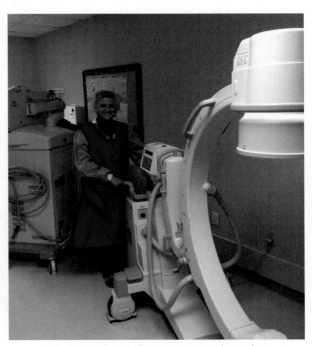

FIG 11.22 C-arm fluoroscope and monitor.

to follow guidelines for safe C-arm operation and also meet radiation safety protocols essential to patient and personnel safety. An essential component of this is the wearing of wrap-around lead aprons and thyroid shields by all involved personnel throughout each procedure.

Mobile fluoroscopic units are required to have a minimal source-to-end of collimator assembly distance of 30 cm (12 inches). Some type of spacer, or collimator, extension is usually installed to prevent any part of the patient from coming closer than 30 cm (12 inches) to

the tube target. During C-arm fluoroscopic procedures, the patient–image intensifier distance should be as short as possible (Fig. 11.23). This reduces patient entrance dose. In addition, for dose-reduction purposes it is preferable to position the C-arm so that the x-ray tube is under the patient. With the x-ray tube in this position, scatter radiation is less intense (Fig. 11.24). When the x-ray tube is positioned over the patient, scatter radiation becomes more intense, and radiation exposure of personnel increases correspondingly.

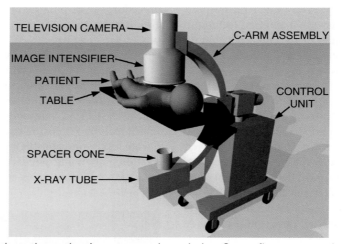

FIG 11.23 To reduce the patient's entrance dose during C-arm fluoroscopy, the patient–image intensifier distance should be as short as possible. (Courtesy Mark Rzeszotarski.)

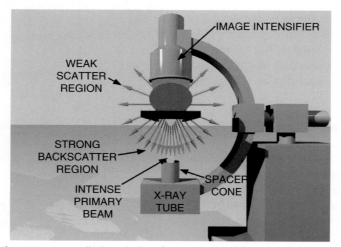

FIG 11.24 To reduce scatter radiation during C-arm fluoroscopy, position the C-arm so that the x-ray tube is under the patient whenever possible. (Courtesy Mark Rzeszotarski.)

RADIATION SAFETY FEATURES OF DIGITAL FLUOROSCOPIC EQUIPMENT, DEVICES, AND ACCESSORIES

Digital Fluoroscopy

Use of Pulsed Progressive Systems for Dose Reduction.
Various methods are used to obtain digital images in some fluoroscopic equipment. The electrical signal from the video camera attached to the output phosphor may be digitized. Alternatively, the TV camera may be replaced by a digital device such as a CCD camera or other digital detector. However the digital image is acquired, the use of digital technology offers the possibility of some methods of dose reduction. One such method makes use of the fact that a brief high-intensity pulse of radiation can create an entire image on the output phosphor. The lines composing the image are progressively scanned (i.e., the image on the camera, namely the TV lines, is scanned or painted in a natural sequence, from left to right followed by right to left and so on in a manner referred to as *raster scanning* from top to bottom) to provide the picture that appears on a monitor during a brief period (one-sixtieth of a second). The x-ray beam is turned off while the image is being scanned, thereby decreasing patient dose, and then pulsed back on for the next image. These systems are known as pulsed progressive systems and are commonly used to lower patient dose.

Use of Last Image Hold Feature for Dose Reduction.
Another dose-reduction technique that is particularly effective in DF systems is last image hold. In "last image hold" the image formed when the x-ray tube was last energized remains on the monitor so that no further radiation exposure is needed to regenerate it. In a digital system, using embedded processing software, this image could be composed of several frames of information that have been added together to reduce the effect of quantum or random noise that would be particularly apparent in a single frame.

RADIATION SAFETY FOR HIGH LEVEL CONTROL INTERVENTIONAL PROCEDURES

High Level Control Interventional Procedures

Justification for Use of High Level Control Interventional Procedures.
Interventional procedures are invasive procedures performed by a physician with the aid of fluoroscopic imaging. The interventional physician, usually a radiologist or cardiologist, inserts catheters into vessels or directly into patient tissues for the purpose of:
- Drainage
- Biopsy
- Alteration of vascular occlusions or malformations

For these procedures, high level control fluoroscopy (HLCF) is often employed. HLCF is an operating mode for state-of-the-art fluoroscopic equipment in which exposure rates are substantially higher than those normally allowed in routine procedures. The higher exposure rate allows visualization of smaller and lower-contrast objects that do not usually appear during standard fluoroscopy. HLCF therefore is used for interventional procedures in which visualization of fine catheters or not easily seen structures is crucial. An audible signal constantly reminds personnel that the high level control is engaged. *It is strongly recommended that pulsed mode and frequent last image hold be the standard methods of operation for such units.*

Public Health Advisory About the Dangers of Overexposure of Patients and Exposure Rate Limits.
More than a few fluoroscopically guided therapeutic interventional procedures have the potential for substantial patient exposure. On September 30, 1974, the Food and Drug Administration (FDA) issued a public health advisory to alert health care workers to the dangers of overexposure of patients through the use of high-level fluoroscopy. The FDA x-ray equipment standards, issued in 1994, limited the tabletop exposure rate of fluoroscopic equipment for routine procedures to 100 mGy_a/min (10 R/min) unless a high level control was present, in which case routine fluoroscopy was limited to 50 mGy_a/min (5 R/min) when the system was not in HLC mode and unlimited when it was in HLC mode.[12] The authors of the standards believed that the high-level capability was necessary for certain vital situations involving therapeutic interventional procedures in which the potential risks to the patient of increased radiation exposure would be subordinate to a successful medical outcome of an intervention. Although HLC allowed unlimited exposure rate levels, it required manual continuous, positive pressure on a special high-level foot pedal, as well as a continuous audible signal to remind personnel that the high-level fluoroscopic mode was in use. For this method of operation, patient exposure rates have been estimated to range from 200 to a very concerning 1200 mGy_a/min (20 to 120 R/min). When the rule was issued, total patient

exposure was limited by the heat-loading capabilities of the x-ray tube. Amazingly, the thinking was that the tube would reach its heat limit before any detectable early tissue reactions could occur. By the early 1990s, however, advances in x-ray tube technology and the development of vascular interventional procedures that require long fluoroscopy times (Box 11.4) had created a situation in which serious skin reactions had been reported in some patients. Radiogenic skin injuries such as erythema (diffuse reddening) and desquamation (sloughing off of skin cells) are early tissue reactions in which the severity of the disorder increases with radiation dose. As the data in Table 11.3 show, a half hour of total beam-on time at one location on a patient's skin is sufficient to produce erythema. The effect does not appear for approximately 10 days. Because manifestations of skin injury are delayed, a radiologist would not usually be the first person to observe the onset of the symptoms. Therefore patient monitoring, radiation dosimetry, and accurate record keeping are important for the future medical management of adverse reactions. The FDA has recommended that a notation be placed in the patient's record if a skin dose in the range of 1 to 2 Gy_t is received. The location of the area of the patient's skin that received the absorbed dose should also be noted using:

- A diagram
- Annotated photograph
- Narrative description

Since 2000, however, alarmed state regulatory agencies have imposed a restriction on high-level radiation exposure

---

BOX 11.4 Procedures Involving Extended Fluoroscopic Time

- Percutaneous transluminal angioplasty
- Radiofrequency cardiac catheter ablation
- Vascular embolization
- Stent and filter placement
- Thrombolytic and fibrinolytic procedures
- Percutaneous transhepatic cholangiography
- Endoscopic retrograde cholangiopancreatography
- Transjugular intrahepatic portosystemic shunt
- Percutaneous nephrostomy
- Biliary drainage
- Urinary or biliary stone removal

From the US Food and Drug Administration (FDA): *Public health advisory: avoidance of serious x-ray-induced skin injuries to patients during fluoroscopically guided procedures*, Rockville, MD, September 30, 1994, FDA.

TABLE 11.3 Radiation-Induced Skin Injuries

		HOURS OF FLUOROSCOPIC "ON TIME" TO REACH THRESHOLD*		
Effect	Typical Threshold Absorbed Dose $(Gy_t)^\dagger$	Usual Fluoroscopic Dose Rate of 0.02 Gy_a/min	High-Level Dose Rate of 0.2 Gy_a/min	Time to Onset of Effect‡
Early transient erythema	2	1.7	0.17	Hours
Temporary epilation	3	2.5	0.25	3 weeks
Main erythema	6	5.0	0.50	10 days
Permanent epilation	7	5.8	0.58	3 weeks
Dry desquamation	10	8.3	0.83	4 weeks
Dermal atrophy	11	9.2	0.92	0.14 weeks
Telangiectasias	12	10.0	1.00	0.52 weeks
Moist desquamation	15	12.5	1.25	4 weeks
Late erythema	15	12.5	1.25	6–10 weeks
Dermal necrosis	18	15.0	1.50	0.10 weeks
Secondary ulceration	20	16.7	1.67	0.6 weeks

*Time required to deliver the typical threshold dose at the specified dose rate.
†The unit for absorbed dose is the gray (Gy_t) in the International System of Units.
‡Time after single irradiation to observation of effect.
Modified from Wagner LK, Eifel PJ, Geise RA: Potential biological effects following high x-ray dose interventional procedures, *J Vasc Interv Radiol* 5:71, 1994.

rates. With the image intensifier at a distance of 30 cm (12 inches) above the tabletop, the maximum *continuous* fluoroscopic entrance exposure rate permitted is 200 mGy$_a$/min (20 R/min). This is not true, though, for pulsed mode for which the instantaneous exposure rates can be very much higher.

Use of Fluoroscopic Equipment by Nonradiologist Physicians. Fluoroscopic devices are capable of subjecting the patient, the equipment operator, and other personnel near the fluoroscopic equipment to substantial doses of ionizing radiation. These devices include:
- C-arm fluoroscopes
- Fluoroscopes on stationary equipment with HLC mode used for interventional procedures
- Biplane interventional fluoroscopic systems

Ongoing education and training in the safe use of fluoroscopic equipment should be mandatory for nonradiologist physicians and equipment operators. Many institutions have therefore set up through their RSOs radiation safety accreditation programs that must be taken and passed before nonradiologist physicians are permitted to use such devices.

Some of the causes of high radiation exposures to personnel during interventional procedures include:
- Operation of the fluoroscopic tube for longer periods in continuous mode in place of pulsed mode

- Failure to use the protective curtain or floating shields on the stationary fluoroscopic equipment's image intensifier as a means of protection

Monitoring and documenting procedural fluoroscopic time are essential. The responsibility for this documentation generally belongs to the radiographer assisting with the procedure. With newer systems the computer software automatically produces a record of both accumulated continuous and pulsed radiation time, as well as estimates of delivered dose and dose area product. In addition, if a physician loses track of how long a procedure is taking and how much radiation is being delivered to a localized area of the patient's body, it becomes the radiographer's ethical responsibility to call this to his or her attention in the interest of the safety of all concerned. In the event of a critical situation in which there is significantly excessive fluoroscopic operation time, the radiographer is responsible for notifying an appropriate supervisor, who should then follow the imaging facility's established protocol.

The National Cancer Institute and the Society of Interventional Radiology have conjointly designed some guidelines to assist physicians in developing strategies that will enable them to fulfill their interventional clinical objectives while controlling patient radiation dose and minimizing exposure to occupationally exposed personnel and any other assisting personnel. These strategies are listed in Box 11.5.

BOX 11.5 Strategies to Manage Radiation Dose to Patients, Operators, and Staff During Interventional Fluoroscopy

Immediate	Long-Term
Optimize Dose to Patient Use proper radiologic technique: • Maximize distance between x-ray tube and patient • Minimize distance between patient and image receptor • Limit use of electronic magnification Control fluoroscopic time: • Limit use to necessary evaluation of moving structures • Employ last image hold function to review findings Control images: • Limit acquisition to essential diagnostic and documentation purposes Reduce dose: • Reduce field size (collimate) and minimize field overlap • Use pulsed fluoroscopy and low frame rate	Include medical physicist in decisions: • Machine selection and maintenance Incorporate dose-reduction technologies and dose-measurement devices in equipment Establish a facility quality improvement program that includes an appropriate x-ray equipment quality assurance program, overseen by a medical physicist, which includes equipment evaluation/inspection at appropriate intervals

Continued

SUMMARY

- A diagnostic-type tube housing protects the patient and imaging personnel from off-focus, or leakage, radiation by restricting the emission of x-rays to the area of the useful, or primary, beam.
  - Leakage radiation from the tube housing measured at 1 m from the x-ray source must not exceed 1 Gy_a/hr (100 mR/hr) when the tube is operated at its highest voltage at the highest current that allows continuous operation.
- The control panel, or console, must be located behind a suitable protective barrier that has a radiation-absorbent window that permits observation of the patient during any procedure.
  - This panel must indicate the conditions of exposure and provide a positive indication when the x-ray tube is energized.[1]
- The radiographic examination tabletop must be of uniform thickness, and for under-table tubes as used in fluoroscopy, the patient support surface also should be as radiolucent as possible so that it will absorb only a minimal amount of radiation, thereby reducing the patient's radiation dose.
  - The tabletop is frequently made of a carbon fiber material.
- Radiographic equipment must have an SID indicator.

- X-ray beam limitation devices must be used to confine the useful beam before it enters the anatomic area of clinical interest.
  - The light-localizing variable-aperture rectangular collimator, cones, and extension cylinders are the beam limitation devices used.
  - The patient's skin surface should always be at least 15 cm below the collimator to minimize exposure to the epidermis.
  - Good coincidence between the x-ray beam and the light-localizing beam of the collimator is necessary; both alignment and length and width dimensions of the two beams must correspond to within 2% of the SID.
  - States vary in their exact requirements for agreement of PBL setting and radiation field, varying from 2% to 3% of SID.
- Exposure to the patient's skin may be reduced through proper filtration of the radiographic beam.
  - Inherent filtration amounting to 0.5 mm aluminum equivalent is always present in the x-ray beam reaching the collimator.
  - Together, the inherent filtration and added filtration comprise the total filtration. Stationary x-ray units operating at above 70 kVp are required to have a total filtration on emerging x-rays of 2.5 mm aluminum equivalent.

- The HVL of the beam is measured to determine whether an x-ray beam is adequately filtered.
- Compensating filters are used in radiography to provide uniform imaging of body parts when considerable variation in thickness or tissue composition exists.
- Diagnostic x-ray units must have consistent exposure reproducibility, that is, the ability to duplicate certain radiographic exposures for any given combination of kVp, mA, and time.
- Exposure linearity is essential. When a change is made from one mA station to a neighboring mA station, the most linearity can vary is 10%.
- Radiographic grids increase patient dose in radiography. Their use for examination of thicker body parts is a fair compromise because they remove scattered radiation emanating from the patient that would otherwise degrade the recorded image.
  - Because of increased sensitivity of photostimulable phosphor to scatter radiation before and after exposure to a radiographic beam, a grid may be used more frequently during CR imaging. The use of a grid does increase patient dose but significantly improves radiographic contrast and visibility of detail.
- To limit the effects of inverse square falloff of radiation intensity with distance during a mobile radiographic examination, an x-ray SSD of at least 30 cm (12 inches) must be used.
- With digital radiography, the latent image formed by x-ray photons on a radiation detector is actually an electronic latent image. It is called a *digital image* because it is produced by computer representation of anatomic information. The image receptor is divided into small detector elements that make up the two-dimensional picture elements, or pixels, of the digital image.
- Radiographers must select correct technical exposure factors the first time to avoid overexposing patients when digital images are obtained.
- CR results when the invisible, or latent, image generated in conventional radiography is produced in a digital format using computer technology.
- The digital image can be displayed on a monitor for viewing, and it can be printed on a laser film when hard copy is needed.
- Fluoroscopic procedures produce the largest patient radiation exposure rate in diagnostic radiology.
  - Minimize patient exposure time whenever possible.

- Limit the size of the fluoroscopic field to include only the area of anatomy that is of clinical interest.
- Employ the practice of interrupted and pulsed fluoroscopy to reduce the overall length of exposure.
- Select the correct technical exposure factors to help minimize the amount of radiation received by a patient.
- Ensure that the SSD is no less than 38 cm (15 inches) for stationary (fixed) fluoroscopes and no less than 30 cm (12 inches) for mobile fluoroscopes.
- During C-arm fluoroscopic procedures, the patient–image intensifier distance should be as short as possible.
  - Reduce patient dose by using intermittent activation of the fluoroscope to locate the catheter, limiting the time of the digital run, and using the last image hold feature to view the most recent image.
- During digital fluoroscopy the use of pulsed progressive systems lowers patient dose.
  - Use of the last image hold feature is another effective dose-reduction technique in DF.
- HLCF is used for interventional procedures and uses exposure rates that are substantially higher than those allowed for routine fluoroscopic procedures.
  - If skin dose is received in the range of 1 to 2 Gy_t the FDA requires that a notation be placed in the patient's record.
  - The radiographer generally has the responsibility for monitoring and documenting procedural fluoroscopic time when fluoroscopic equipment is used by nonradiologist physicians.

REFERENCES

1. Bushong SC: *Radiologic science for technologists: physics, biology and protection*, ed 10, St. Louis, 2013, Elsevier/Mosby.
2. Long BW, Rollins JH, Smith BJ: *Merrill's atlas of radiographic positioning & procedures*, (vol 1). ed 13, St. Louis, 2016, Elsevier/Mosby.
3. Carlton RR, Adler AM: *Principles of radiographic imaging: an art and a science*, ed 5, Albany, NY, 2013, Delmar Cengage Learning.
4. Kebart RC, James CD: Benefits of increasing focal film distance. *Radiol Technol* 62:434, 1991.
5. Edwards C, Statkiewicz-Sherer MA, Ritenour ER: *Radiation protection for dental radiographers*, Denver, 1984, Multi-Media.

6. National Council on Radiation Protection and Measurements (NCRP): *Medical x-ray, electron beam and gamma ray protection for energies up to 50 MeV: equipment design, performance, and use*, Report No. 102, Bethesda, Md, 1989, NCRP.
7. Bushong SC: *Radiologic science for technologists: physics, biology and protection*, ed 8, St. Louis, 2004, Mosby.
8. Roberts TD: *The Effect of Computers in Imaging and Radiation Safety*. Available at: http://e-edcredits.com/xraycredits/article.asp?testID=17.
9. Johnston JN, Fauber TL: *Essentials of radiographic physics and imaging*, ed 2, St. Louis, 2016, Elsevier Inc.
10. Seeram E: Digital image processing. *Radiol Technol* 75:6, 2004.
11. Cullinan AM, Cullinan JE: *Producing quality radiographs*, ed 2, Philadelphia, 1994, Lippincott.
12. Office of the Federal Register: *Federal register* August 15, 1972 (37 FR 16461), Washington, DC, 1972, U.S. Government Printing Office.

GENERAL DISCUSSION QUESTIONS

1. What are the x-ray tube housing construction requirements when a tube is operated at its highest voltage at the highest current that allows continuous operation?
2. What must the control panel, or console, indicate?
3. How do light-localizing variable-aperture rectangular collimators and cones and cylinders reduce the amount of scattered radiation being produced during a radiographic examination?
4. How does filtration of the radiographic beam reduce exposure to the patient's skin and superficial tissues?
5. When should the half-value layer of a diagnostic x-ray tube be measured?
6. When should a radiologic physicist measure the half-value layer of a diagnostic x-ray beam?
7. What is exposure linearity?
8. What is the effective metric equivalent unit for the English unit 48 inches?
9. Why is the use of a radiographic grid a fair compromise if its use increases patient dose?
10. What can a radiographer do to avoid overexposing the patient when a computed radiographic system is used?
11. What effect does the use of interrupted, or pulsed, fluoroscopy have on patient dose?
12. Why is there concern over the use of mobile C-arm fluoroscopes during surgical, vascular, interventional, and other potentially lengthy procedures?
13. To what does the scientific term *luminance* refer?
14. What strategies can physicians use during interventional fluoroscopic procedures to control patient radiation dose and minimize exposure of occupationally exposed personnel and any other assisting personnel?
15. During digital fluoroscopy, how does the use of a pulsed progressive system lower patient dose?

REVIEW QUESTIONS

1. The radiographic beam should be collimated so that it is which of the following?
   A. Slightly larger than the image receptor
   B. No larger than the image receptor
   C. Twice as large as the image receptor
   D. Four times as large as the image receptor
2. Both alignment and length and width dimensions of the radiographic and light beams must correspond to within:
   A. 1% of the SID
   B. 2% of the SID
   C. 5% of the SID
   D. 10% of the SID
3. What is the function of a filter in diagnostic radiology?
   A. To permit only alpha rays to reach the patient's skin
   B. To permit only beta particles to interact with the atoms of the patient's body
   C. To decrease the x-radiation dose to the patient's skin and superficial tissue
   D. To remove gamma radiation from the useful beam
4. HVL may be defined as the thickness of a designated absorber required to do which of the following?
   A. Increase the intensity of the primary beam by 50% of its initial value
   B. Increase the intensity of the primary beam by 25% of its initial value
   C. Decrease the intensity of the primary beam by 50% of its initial value
   D. Decrease the intensity of the primary beam by 25% of its initial value
5. The photostimulable phosphor in the computed radiography imaging plate is more sensitive to scatter

radiation before and after it is sensitized through exposure to a radiographic beam. Because of this increased sensitivity, which of the following is true?
1. Five millimeters of added aluminum equivalent filtration must always be used during routine CR imaging.
2. A radiographic grid may be used more frequently during CR imaging.
3. Any source-to-image receptor distance can be used during CR imaging without adjustment in technical exposure factors.
A. 1 only
B. 2 only
C. 3 only
D. 1, 2, and 3

6. To minimize skin exposure to electrons produced by photon interaction with the collimator, how far below the collimator should the patient's skin surface be?
A. At least 1 cm below
B. At least 5 cm below
C. At least 10 cm below
D. At least 15 cm below

7. Which of the following aluminum equivalents for total permanent filtration meets the minimum requirement for mobile diagnostic and fluoroscopic equipment?
A. 0.5 mm aluminum equivalent
B. 1.0 mm aluminum equivalent
C. 2.0 mm aluminum equivalent
D. 2.5 mm aluminum equivalent

8. The trough, or bilateral wedge, filter, which is used in some dedicated chest radiographic units, is an example of which of the following?
A. Compensating filter
B. Filter used in all digital imaging systems
C. Filter used in all dedicated mammographic units
D. Filter used in all computed tomography systems

9. To *decrease* patient exposure during fluoroscopic procedures, the fluoroscopist can:
1. Limit the size of the fluoroscopic field to include only the area of anatomy that is of clinical interest
2. Employ the practice of pulsed fluoroscopy to reduce the overall length of exposure
3. Choose to use a conventional fluoroscope instead of an image intensification fluoroscope
A. 1 and 2 only
B. 1 and 3 only
C. 2 and 3 only
D. 1, 2, and 3

10. A diagnostic-type protective tube housing must be constructed so that leakage radiation measured at a distance of 1 m from the x-ray source does *not* exceed _____ when the tube is operated at its highest voltage at the highest current that allows continuous operation.
A. 5 Gy_a/hr
B. 3 Gy_a/hr
C. 1 Gy_a/hr
D. 0.1 Gy_a/hr

12

Management of Patient Radiation Dose During Diagnostic X-Ray Procedures

OBJECTIVES

After completing this chapter, the reader will be able to perform the following:

- Define all key terms.
- Explain the meaning of a holistic approach to patient care, and recognize the need for effective communication between imaging department personnel and the patient.
- Discuss how voluntary motion can be eliminated or at least minimized and how involuntary motion can be compensated for during a diagnostic radiographic procedure.
- Give reasons for the use of protective shielding during diagnostic imaging procedures, state the rationale for employing gonadal shielding or other specific area shielding, and compare the various types of shields available.
- Discuss the need to use the appropriate radiographic technical exposure factors for all radiologic procedures, and show how these factors may be adjusted to reduce patient dose.
- Explain how a radiographer can achieve a balance in radiographic exposure factors to ensure the presence of adequate information in the recorded image while minimizing patient dose.
- Clarify how adequate immobilization and correct image postprocessing techniques reduce radiographic exposure for the patient.

- Compare the use of an air gap technique for certain examinations with the use of a midratio grid (8:1).
- State the reasons for repeat analysis programs, and describe their benefits.
- List six nonessential radiologic examinations, and explain why each is considered unnecessary.
- List four ways to indicate the amount of radiation received by a patient from diagnostic imaging procedures, and give details for each.
- Discuss the concept of fluoroscopically guided positioning, and clarify why this is an unacceptable practice.
- Define the term *genetically significant dose (GSD)*.
- Describe special precautions employed in radiography to protect the pregnant or potentially pregnant patient during an x-ray examination.
- Discuss the protocol to be followed when irradiation of an unknown pregnancy occurs, and explain how the absorbed dose to the patient's embryo-fetus is determined.
- Explain the reason children require special radiation protection when they undergo conventional diagnostic imaging procedures.
- Pledge to Image Gently and Image Wisely.

CHAPTER OUTLINE

Effective Communication
Verbal Messages and Body Language
Importance of Clear, Concise Instructions
Appropriate Communication for Procedures That Will Cause Pain or Discomfort
Repeat Radiographic Exposures That Result From Poor Communication

Immobilization
Need for Patient Immobilization
Types of Patient Motion
Protective Shielding
Need for Protective Shielding
Gonadal Shielding
Specific Area Shielding

KEY TERMS

air gap technique
Alliance for Radiation Safety in
    Pediatric Imaging
bone marrow dose
effective communication
entrance skin exposure (ESE)

fluoroscopically guided
    positioning (FGP)
genetically significant dose (GSD)
gonadal dose
Image Gently Campaign
Image Wisely Campaign

repeat image
scattered radiation
skin dose
thermoluminescent dosimeters
    (TLDs)

During a diagnostic x-ray procedure, a holistic approach to patient care is essential. This means treating the whole person rather than just the area of concern. Holistic patient care must begin with effective communication between the radiographer and the patient. Effective communication is "an interaction that produces a satisfying result through an exchange of information."[1] This can be accomplished through verbal messages, body language, and clear and concise instructions. This type of dialog alleviates the patient's uneasiness and increases the likelihood for cooperation and successful completion of the procedure. To take care of all patients appropriately,

the radiographer should develop easily understandable communication skills.

Radiographers must limit the patient's exposure to ionizing radiation by:

- Employing appropriate radiation reduction techniques
- Using protective devices that minimize radiation exposure

Patient exposure can be substantially reduced by:

- Use of proper body or body part immobilization
- Motion reduction techniques
- Appropriate beam limitation devices
- Adequate filtration of the x-ray beam

- Use of gonadal or other specific area shielding
- Selection of suitable technical exposure factors used in conjunction with computer-generated digital images
- Use of appropriate digital image processing
- Elimination of repeat radiographic exposures

This chapter provides an overview of methods and techniques that radiographers can use to minimize the patient's exposure to radiation during radiologic examinations.

EFFECTIVE COMMUNICATION

Verbal Messages and Body Language

When verbal messages and body language, or nonverbal messages, are understood as intended, communication between the radiographer and the patient is effective. Good communication:

- Encourages reduction in anxiety and emotional stress
- Enhances the professional image of the radiographer as a person who cares about the patient's well-being
- Increases the chance for successful completion of the x-ray examination, thereby reducing the potential of repeat exposures resulting from poor communication

Everyone within the imaging department should always behave as a compassionate professional. Words and actions must demonstrate understanding and respect for human dignity and individuality.

Importance of Clear, Concise Instructions

Patient protection during a diagnostic x-ray procedure should begin with clear, concise instructions (Fig. 12.1). When health care professionals do not thoroughly explain procedures, patients fear the unknown and become anxious, especially during lengthy examinations. To alleviate the problem, the radiographer must take adequate time to explain the procedure in simple terms that the patient can understand. Patients should also be given the opportunity to ask questions. The radiographer must listen attentively to these questions and answer them truthfully in an appropriate tone of voice and in accordance with ethical guidelines. This creates a sense of trust between the patient and the radiographer and encourages further communication.

Appropriate Communication for Procedures That Will Cause Pain or Discomfort

If the radiographic procedure (e.g., angiocatheterization or another study requiring an injection of a contrast

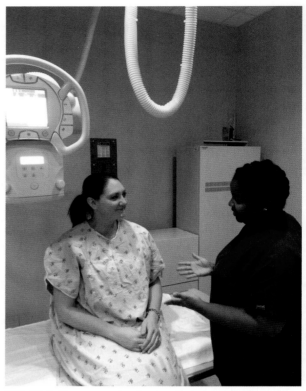

FIG 12.1 Clear, concise instructions promote effective communication between the radiographer and the patient.

medium, such as an intravenous urogram) will cause pain, discomfort, or any strange sensations, the patient must be informed before the procedure begins (Fig. 12.2). However, to prevent the patient from imagining more pain or discomfort than the procedure will actually cause, the radiographer should try not to overemphasize this aspect of the examination.

Repeat Radiographic Exposures That Result From Poor Communication

Repeat radiographic exposures can sometimes be attributed to poor communication between the radiographer and the patient. Inadequate or misinterpreted instructions may prevent the patient from being able to cooperate as needed. For example, during an interventional radiographic examination that creates some uncomfortable warmth, patients could move abruptly because they are surprised or want to inform the technologist or physician that something seems to be wrong. Such physical movement usually results in a repeat exposure. Effective

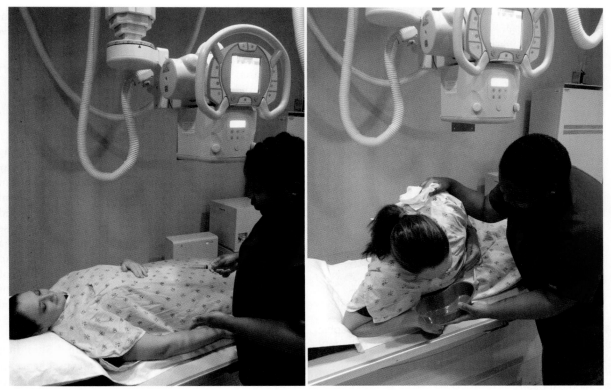

FIG 12.2 Before the procedure begins, inform the patient of any pain, discomfort, or strange sensations that he or she will experience during the procedure.

communication between the radiographer and patient will prevent this problem from occurring.

IMMOBILIZATION

Need for Patient Immobilization

If a patient moves during a radiographic exposure, the radiographic image will be blurred. Because blurred images have little or no diagnostic value, a repeat examination is necessary, even though it results in additional radiation exposure for the patient. Proper body or body part immobilization and the use of motion reduction techniques can eliminate or at least minimize patient motion.

Types of Patient Motion

Two types of patient motion exist:
- Voluntary
- Involuntary

Motion controlled by will is classified as *voluntary motion.* Lack of such control may be attributed to:

- The patient's age
- Breathing patterns or problems
- General anxiety
- Physical discomfort
- Excitability
- Fear of the examination
- Fear of unfavorable prognosis
- Mental instability

To eliminate voluntary patient movement during radiography, the radiographer must gain the cooperation of the patient or adequately immobilize that individual during the radiographic exposure (Fig. 12.3). Various suitable restraining devices are available to immobilize either the whole body or the individual body part to be radiographed. These aids should be used whenever necessary.

Involuntary motion, caused by muscle groups such as those associated with the digestive organs or the heart, cannot be willfully controlled. Other clinical manifestations also cause involuntary motion. These include:

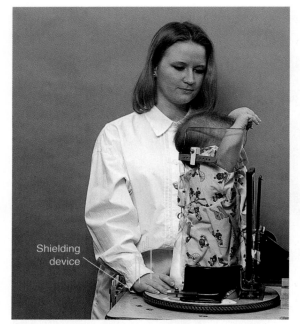

FIG 12.3 Adequate immobilization during radiographic examinations eliminates or at least minimizes voluntary motion. This restraint has a shield *(left)* that may be adjusted to protect the child's reproductive organs from radiation exposure.

- Chills
- Tremors such as those experienced by patients with Parkinson's disease
- Muscle spasms
- Pain
- Active withdrawal

Shortening the length of exposure time with an appropriate increase in milliamperes (mA) to maintain sufficient milliampere-seconds (mAs) for useful radiographic brightness (lightness or darkness of an image on a display monitor) and using very-high-speed imaging receptors can compensate for this type of motion.

PROTECTIVE SHIELDING

Need for Protective Shielding

The potential for radiation exposure to the radiosensitive body organs or tissues of a patient requires the use of intelligent patient positioning and/or personal shielding (i.e., a device made of lead or lead-impregnated materials that will adequately attenuate ionizing radiation) to reduce or eliminate a radiation dose that would otherwise

result in biologic damage. Areas of the body that should be shielded from the useful beam whenever possible are the:
- Lens of the eye
- Breasts
- Thyroid gland
- Reproductive organs

Gonadal Shielding

Use of Gonadal Shielding Devices. Gonadal shielding devices are used on patients during diagnostic x-ray procedures to protect the reproductive organs from exposure to the useful beam when these organs are in or within approximately 5 cm of a properly collimated beam. Gonadal shielding is used unless it will compromise the diagnostic value of the examination. It should be a secondary protective measure, not a substitute for an adequately collimated beam. Adequate collimation of the radiographic beam, to include only the anatomy of interest (Fig. 12.4), must always be the first step in gonadal protection.

Dose Reduction From the Use of Gonadal Shielding for Female and Male Patients. As a consequence of their anatomic location, the female reproductive organs receive about three times more exposure during a given radiographic procedure involving the pelvic region than do the male reproductive organs. Gonadal exposure, however, for both male and female patients can be greatly reduced through the application of appropriate shielding. For female patients, the use of a flat contact shield placed over the reproductive organs reduces exposure by approximately 50% (Fig. 12.5A). Primary beam exposure for male patients may be reduced as much as 90% to 95% when the gonads are also covered with a contact shield (Fig. 12.5B). Gonadal shielding ought to always be used whenever it will not obscure necessary clinical information. Every imaging department should establish a written shielding protocol for each of its radiologic procedures. Ultimately, this practice reduces the cumulative population gonad dose.

Placement of Gonadal Shielding Devices. When a gonadal shield is employed, it must be positioned directly over the patient's reproductive organs, as shown in Fig. 12.5. External anatomic landmarks on the patient can be used to guide placement of a testicular or ovarian shield. For example, when a male patient is in the supine

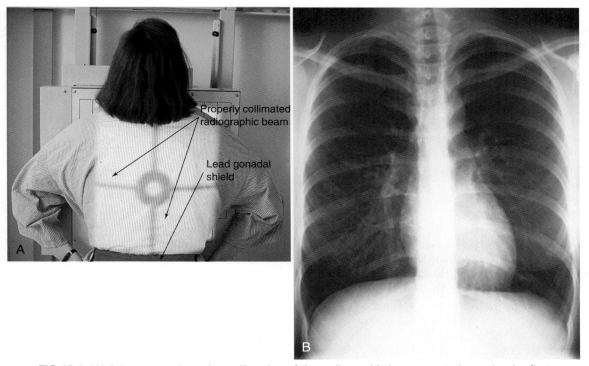

FIG 12.4 (A) Adequate and precise collimation of the radiographic beam must always be the first step in gonadal protection. (B) When the gonads are not in the area of clinical interest, precise collimation of the radiographic beam reduces gonadal exposure.

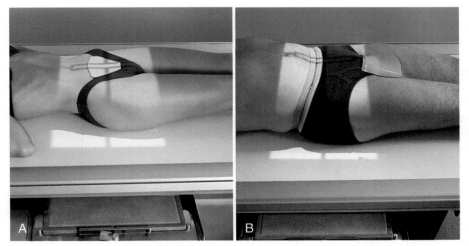

FIG 12.5 (A) Contact shield correctly placed over the reproductive organs of a female patient. (B) Contact shield correctly placed over the reproductive organs of a male patient. (From Frank ED, Long BW, Smith BS: *Merrill's Atlas of Radiographic Positioning & Procedures,* ed 12, St. Louis, 2012, Elsevier.)

position, the symphysis pubis can serve as a guide for shield placement over the testes. For safeguarding the ovaries of a female patient, the shield should be located approximately 2.5 cm (1 inch) medial to each palpable anterior superior iliac spine. If gonadal shields are placed incorrectly, the reproductive organs will not be fully properly protected, and necessary anatomic information in the image could be obscured.

Types of Gonadal Shielding Devices. The following four basic types of gonadal shielding devices are available:
- Flat contact shields
- Shadow shields
- Shaped contact shields
- Clear lead shields

Flat contact shields. Flat contact shields are made of lead strips or lead-impregnated materials 1 mm thick. These shields can be sited directly over the patient's reproductive organs (Fig. 12.6). They are most effective when used as protective devices for patients having anteroposterior (AP) or posteroanterior (PA) radiographs while in a recumbent position. Flat contact shields are not suited for nonrecumbent positions or projections other than AP or PA. If the flat contact shield is utilized during a typical fluoroscopic examination, it must be put under the patient to be effective because the x-ray tube is located beneath the radiographic table. However, some fluoroscopic tubes are located above the patient and are referred to as *remote rooms* because personnel set up the patient for the examination and then leave the room before activating the x-ray tube. In these rooms, the shield should be placed over the patient.

Shadow shields. Shadow shields are made of a radiopaque material (Fig. 12.7A). Suspended from above the radiographic beam-defining system, these shields hang above the area of clinical interest to cast a shadow in the primary beam over the patient's reproductive organs (see Fig. 12.7B and C). The clear lead filter illustrated in Fig. 12.8 functions as a shadow shield that is intended to shelter the breast and gonads. The beam-defining light casts the shadow of the shield over the anatomy. The light field must be accurately positioned to ensure correct positioning of the shield. When this is so, the device provides protection from the radiographic beam as efficiently as does the contact shield. The shadow shield is not suitable for use during fluoroscopy, though, because no localizing light field exists, and the field of view is usually moved about during a study. However, the shadow

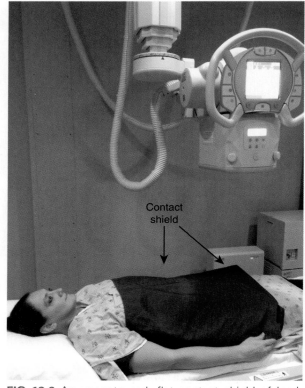

FIG 12.6 An uncontoured, flat contact shield of lead-impregnated material may be placed over the patient's gonads to provide protection from x-radiation during a radiographic procedure.

shield can be used effectively to provide gonadal protection in a sterile field or when incapacitated patients are examined. Shadow shields have the advantage of reducing patient embarrassment by generally eliminating the need for the radiographer to palpate the patient's anatomy in the area of the reproductive organs in order to place the shield in the appropriate position.

Shaped contact shields. Shaped contact shields, containing 1 mm of lead, are contoured to enclose the male reproductive organs. Disposable or washable athletic supporters or jockey-style briefs function as carriers for these shields. The carriers each contain a pouch into which the shield is placed (Fig. 12.9). The cup-like shape of the shield permits it to be placed comfortably over the scrotum and penis whether the patient is in a recumbent or a nonrecumbent position.

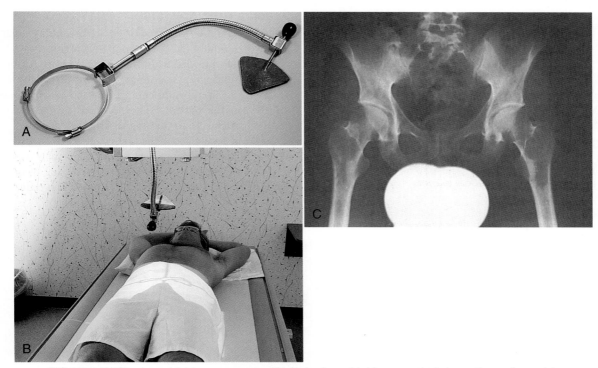

FIG 12.7 (A) Shadow shield components. (B) A shadow shield suspended above the radiographic beam-defining system casts a shadow over the protected body area, the gonads. (C) The radiographic image demonstrates effective gonadal shielding resulting from the use of a shadow shield. (Courtesy Fluke Biomedical.)

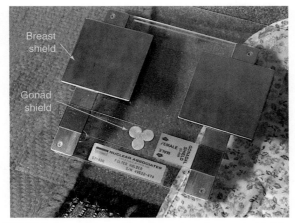

FIG 12.8 Lead filter with a breast and gonad shielding device. This shield functions as a shadow shield. (Courtesy Fluke Biomedical.)

Because the carrier securely holds the shaped contact shield in place, AP, oblique, and lateral projections may be obtained with maximal gonadal protection. This shield is also suitable for use during nonposterior fluoroscopic examinations. Shaped contact shields are not recommended for PA projections because the shield covers only the anterior and lateral surfaces of the reproductive organs.

Clear Lead shields. Accessories such as the previously described shaped contact shield and first-generation, or earliest type of, shadow shield are being replaced by transparent lead acrylic devices (see Fig. 12.8). These are impregnated with approximately 30% lead by weight. An example of their utilization is provided in Fig. 12.10, which demonstrates a full spinal scoliosis examination. For the latter procedure, along with the clear lead gonad and breast shields, a lightweight, fully transparent, clear lead filter is also incorporated so as to provide uniform density throughout the spinal canal (see Fig. 12.10).

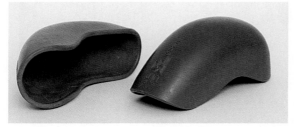

FIG 12.9 Shaped contact shields (cuplike in shape) may be held in place with a suitable carrier.

Specific Area Shielding

Need for Specific Area Shielding. Radiosensitive organs and tissues, other than the reproductive organs, may also be selectively guarded from the primary beam during a diagnostic radiographic examination. Shields for the lens of the eye are always of the contact type and are positioned directly on the patient.[2] They can reduce or entirely eliminate exposure to that highly sensitive area.

Areas of breast tissue may be safeguarded by using a clear lead shadow shield (see Fig. 12.8). This is of vital importance in providing protection during juvenile scoliosis examinations. It should be noted that radiation

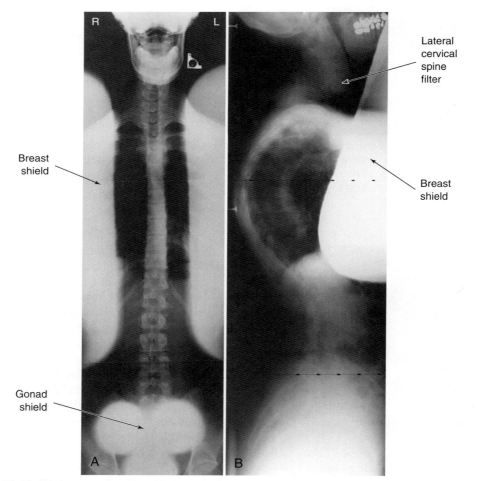

FIG 12.10 (A) Anteroposterior radiograph of a patient with full-spine scoliosis demonstrates a lead filter with breast and gonad shields. (B) Lateral radiograph of patient with full-spine scoliosis, with a lateral cervical filter and breast shield. (Courtesy Fluke Biomedical.)

dose to the breast of a young patient may be further reduced by performing the scoliosis examination with the radiographic beam entering the posterior surface of the patient's body instead of the anterior surface. The use of a PA projection results in a much lower radiation dose to the anterior body surface, thereby significantly reducing the dose to the patient's breasts.

Benefit of Specific Area Shielding. In summary, effective shielding programs can be established in any health care facility by providing and diligently using the appropriate shields. Patients with the potential to reproduce should be gonadally protected during x-ray procedures whenever the diagnostic value of the examination is not compromised. This action minimizes potentially deleterious x-ray–induced mutations expressed in future generations. Specific area shielding for selected radiosensitive body areas other than the gonads should also be employed whenever possible.

TECHNICAL EXPOSURE FACTORS

Selection of Appropriate Technical Exposure Factors

The selection of *scientifically correct* technical exposure factors for each x-ray examination is essential to ensure a useful diagnostic image with minimal patient dose. For both digital and non-digital imaging, a high-quality image has sufficient brightness or density to display anatomic structures, an appropriate level of subject contrast to differentiate among such structures, the maximum amount of spatial resolution,* and a minimal amount of distortion. In addition, with respect to digital imaging, limiting the amount of quantum noise, or mottle,† caused when too few x-rays reach the image receptor, is a concern.[3]

The appropriate technical factors are determined by considerations such as those listed in Box 12.1.

Use of Standardized Technique Charts

When a properly calibrated automatic exposure control (AEC) is not employed to obtain a uniform selection of

---

*Spatial resolution is the recorded detail in the radiographic image.

†Quantum noise, or mottle, is a blotchy radiographic image that results when an insufficient quantity of x-ray photons reaches the image receptor.

> **BOX 12.1** **Technical Exposure Factor Considerations**
>
> 1. Mass per unit volume of tissue of the area of clinical interest
> 2. Effective atomic numbers and electron densities of the tissues involved
> 3. Type of image receptor
> 4. Source-to–image receptor distance (SID)
> 5. Type and quantity of filtration employed
> 6. Type of x-ray generator used
> 7. Balance of radiographic density or brightness and contrast required

x-ray exposure factors, well-managed imaging departments make use of standardized technique charts that have been established for each x-ray unit. A digital image receptor is capable of responding to a large variance in x-ray intensities exiting the patient. As a result, the digital image receptor is said to have a wide dynamic range. Furthermore, computer processing produces acceptable images even when significant overexposure has occurred. Because of this, the standardization of technique charts has become even more important. Radiology departments cannot rely on vendors and other agencies to set technical standards. Establishing their own protocols helps radiology departments ensure consistency in the diagnostic quality of digital examinations and minimizes the potential for exposure technique selection errors.[3]

The radiographer is responsible for consulting the technique chart before making each radiographic exposure to ensure a diagnostic image with minimal patient dose. Neglecting to use standardized technique charts necessitates estimating the technical exposure factors, which may result in:
- Poor-quality images
- Repeat examinations
- Additional and unnecessary exposure of the patient
Standardizing exposure techniques, however, does not mean that radiographers use the same protocol for all patients in all situations. Exposure techniques must be adjusted for a patient's specific condition and history. Appropriate and consistent use of exposure technique charts, adequate peak kilovoltage (kVp), and a well-calibrated AEC are all essential to producing quality diagnostic images consistently while minimizing patient radiation exposure.[3]

Use of High-kVp and Low-mAs Exposure Factors to Reduce Dose to the Patient

Technique factors that minimize the radiation dose to the patient should be selected whenever possible. The use of higher kVp permits lower mAs settings, which reduces patient dose (Fig. 12.11A and B). For digital radiography (DR), kVp and mAs should be selected in the same manner as it was for screen-film imaging. For screen-film imaging, as kVp increases and mAs decreases, radiographic contrast is reduced. Consequently, the amount of diagnostically useful information in the recorded image is less. However, this is not the case in digital imaging, in which the amount of exposure (related to the mAs setting) to the digital image receptor does not directly affect the amount of brightness produced, because of computer processing. Adequate penetration of the anatomic part, which is kVp dependent, is needed

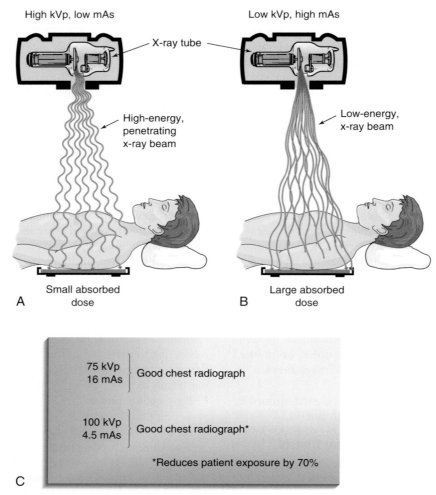

FIG 12.11 The use of higher kilovoltage (kVp) and lower milliamperage and exposure time in seconds (mAs) reduces patient dose. (A) The use of high kVp and low mAs results in a high-energy, penetrating x-ray beam and a small patient-absorbed dose. (B) The use of low kVp and high mAs results in a low-energy x-ray beam of greater intensity, the majority of which the patient will easily absorb. (C) Example of a higher kVp, lower mAs technique resulting in a 70% reduction in patient exposure without significantly compromising radiographic quality.

to create the differences in x-ray intensities exiting the part relative to that from adjacent structures to produce the desired level of contrast. As long as the part is adequately penetrated, changing kVp will have less of an effect on the contrast of the digital image. Consequently, the use of higher kVp than with screen film, along with an appropriate decrease in mAs, is an advocated practice. Increasing kVp by 15% with a corresponding decrease in mAs reduces patient radiation exposure significantly while yielding satisfactory image quality. Whether using digital imaging or screen film, the radiographer must always seek to achieve a balance in technical radiographic exposure factors to:

- Ensure the presence of adequate information in the recorded image
- Minimize patient dose (see Fig. 12.11C).

POSTPROCESSING OF THE RADIOGRAPHIC IMAGE

When digital images are acquired, correct image postprocessing is essential to produce a high-quality diagnostic image. For this, any artifacts produced by the image receptor, software, or patient-related problems must be controlled. Artifacts are unwanted densities in the image that are not part of the patient's anatomy and may negatively affect the ability of a radiologist to interpret the image correctly. Failure to eliminate these defects, or at least to reduce them significantly, can result in an unacceptable digital image and can therefore necessitate a repeat examination, thus increasing patient dose.

Quality Control Program

To ensure standardization in the processing of digital images, it is indispensable that every imaging department establish a *quality control program* that includes regular monitoring and maintenance of all processing and imaging display equipment in the facility. Such a program maximizes the likelihood of producing optimal-quality images. Radiographers are the operators of complex imaging equipment and therefore are the individuals who may first recognize any equipment malfunction. Problems that occur in digital imaging (either CR or DR) tend to be systematic, which can affect the quality of every image and the degree of radiation exposure of every patient until the problems are identified and corrected. Acceptance testing, regular calibration, and proactive and consistent quality control can prevent these systematic errors.[3]

Excellent reviews have been written on this subject. These reviews include step-by-step procedures for performance, monitoring, and continuing quality control.[2-7]

AIR GAP TECHNIQUE

Reduction of Scattered Radiation

The air gap technique is an alternative procedure to the use of a radiographic grid for reducing scattered radiation during certain examinations (e.g., cross-table lateral projection of the cervical spine, areas of chest radiography, and selected special procedures such as cerebral angiography in which some degree of magnification is acceptable). This technique works by using an increased object–to–image receptor distance (OID). Less scatter radiation at the detector decreases image blurring and thereby improves radiographic image contrast. If magnification is not desired, a complementary increase in source-to–image receptor distance (SID) may be made.

To perform an air gap technique, the image receptor is placed 10 to 15 cm (4 to 6 inches) from the patient, and the x-ray tube is placed approximately 300 to 366 cm (10 to 12 feet) away from the image receptor. The scattered x-rays from the patient are disseminated in many directions at acute angles to the primary beam when the radiographic exposure is made. Because of the increased distance between the anatomic structures being imaged and the image receptor, a higher percentage of the scattered x-rays produced is then less likely to strike the image receptor (Fig. 12.12). This air gap method effectively produces an adequate grid-type scatter cleanup effect. In general, the use of an air gap technique requires the selection of technical exposure factors that are comparable to those used with an 8:1 ratio grid. Therefore when patient dose is compared with a nongrid technique, it is higher, but when compared with the patient dose resulting from the use of a midratio grid (8:1), the dose from an air gap technique is about the same.

High Peak Kilovoltage Radiography

In high-kVp radiography that employs kVp settings of 90 or above, air gap techniques are, for the most part, not as effective. Still, some facilities that perform chest radiography by using kVp settings of 120 to 140 do successfully use air gap techniques. In general, when x-rays are scattered through greater angles, such as occurs for radiographs produced at less than 90 kVp, air gap techniques are more useful.

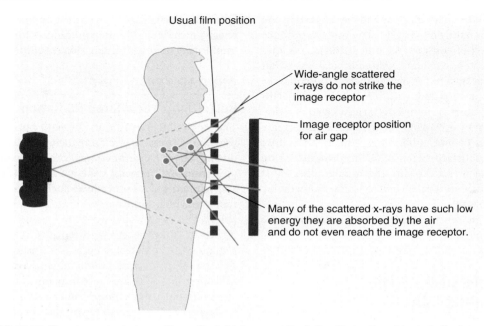

FIG 12.12 The air gap technique. (From *Radiobiology and Radiation Protection: Mosby's Radiographic Instructional Series,* St. Louis, 1999, Elsevier.)

REPEAT IMAGES

Consequence of Repeat Images

A repeat image is any image that must be performed more than once because of human or mechanical error during the production of the initial image. This additional imaging unfortunately increases patient dose. If the patient's gonads were included in the imaged area, then the gonads would have received a double dose. This is, of course, true for any other sensitive included areas. Occasionally, an additional image is permissible, when it is recommended by the radiologist for the purpose of obtaining additional diagnostic information. However, repeat exposures resulting from carelessness or poor judgment on the part of the radiographer must be eliminated. The radiographer should, from the beginning of the examination:

- Correctly position the patient
- Select the appropriate technical radiographic exposure factors that will ensure the production of optimal-quality images

Benefit of a Repeat Analysis Program

Health care facilities can gain significantly by implementing and maintaining a *repeat analysis program.*

Repeat analysis is particularly important in CR and DR. In these modalities repeating exposures because of improper technique is not usually necessary. Because the images are digital, overexposed or underexposed images can be adjusted by the computer to *appear technically normal.* Consequently, it is important for the delivery of nonexcessive patient exposures that a qualified medical physicist make exposure measurements for the techniques employed at the site to ensure that they are within acceptable ranges. With CR or DR, it is necessary to develop a policy whereby the digital files that correspond to retaken images can be recovered for analysis since this would not happen automatically. Analysis of the department's repeats rate:

- Provides valuable information for process improvement
- Helps minimize patient exposure
- Improves the overall performance of the department[3]
  Improving the overall performance of the department includes:
- Increasing awareness among staff and student radiographers of the need to produce optimal-quality images from the start
- Radiographers becoming more careful in producing radiographic images because they are aware that images are being reviewed

- When the repeat analysis program identifies problems or concerns, in-service education covering these specific topics may be designed for imaging personnel

Some categories for unacceptable images are listed in Box 12.2.

Benefit Versus Risk

Because the responsibility for ordering a radiologic examination lies with the referring physician, in making this decision, the physician must determine whether the benefit to the patient, in terms of medical information gained, sufficiently justifies subjecting the patient to whatever degree of risk is produced by the absorbed radiation resulting from the procedure.

Nonessential Radiologic Examinations

Some traditional radiographic examinations are very often just casually performed in the *absence of definite medical indications*. This practice unnecessarily exposes the patient to radiation because there is virtually no benefit to the patient in terms of useful information gained from the procedure. Examples of nonessential radiologic examinations are described in Box 12.3.

Concern About Risk of Exposure From Diagnostic Imaging Procedures

As a result of increased numbers of people in the United States undergoing diagnostic imaging procedures each year, concern about the *collective risk* of radiation exposure from these procedures continues to grow. Imaging personnel must therefore always strive to employ techniques that produce high-quality images with lower radiation exposure.

BOX 12.2 Reasons for Unacceptable Images

1. Patient mispositioning
2. Incorrect centering of the radiographic beam
3. Patient motion during the radiographic exposure
4. Incorrect collimation of the radiographic beam
5. Presence of external foreign bodies
6. Postprocessing artifacts

BOX 12.3 Unnecessary Radiologic Procedures

1. A chest x-ray examination automatically scheduled on admission to the hospital. This examination should not be performed without clinical indications of chest disease or another important concern that justifies exposing the patient to ionizing radiation. This includes presurgical patients. A panel of physicians appointed by the Food and Drug Administration (FDA)[8] concluded that a chest x-ray examination is not necessary for every presurgical patient. Patients admitted for treatment of pulmonary problems or diseases, however, may benefit from a preadmission chest x-ray examination.
2. A chest x-ray examination as part of a preemployment physical. Very little information about previous illness or injury can be gained through this examination, and it is unlikely to be useful to the employer.
3. Lumbar spine examinations as part of a preemployment physical. As with the preemployment chest x-ray examination, this examination provides minimum data about previous illness or injury that would be useful to an employer.
4. Chest x-ray examination or other unjustified x-ray examinations as part of a routine health checkup. Radiologic procedures should not be performed unless a patient exhibits symptoms that merit radiologic investigation.
5. Chest x-ray examination for mass screening for tuberculosis (TB). Such examinations are of negligible value for most people. Testing for TB may be done with more efficient procedures. However, some x-ray screening may still be acceptable for high-risk groups such as members of the medical and paramedical community, people working in fields such as education and food preparation, and selected groups of workers such as miners and workers dealing with material such as asbestos, beryllium, glass, and silica.[2]
6. Whole-body computed tomography (CT) screening. Patients may elect to undergo this type of CT procedure without an order from a referring physician. They can simply locate a facility that offers this service to the general public. Currently, the disease detection rate simply does not justify the relatively high radiation dose received by the patient from this procedure. Until there is evidence of a significant disease detection rate, whole-body CT screening should not be done.[2]

Specifying the Amount of Radiation Received by a Patient From a Diagnostic Imaging Procedure

In general, the amount of radiation received by a patient from diagnostic imaging procedures may be presented in three ways:

1. Entrance skin exposure (ESE) (includes skin and glandular)
2. Bone marrow dose
3. Gonadal dose

Although each type of specification has significance in estimating the risk to the patient, ESE is the most frequently reported because it is the simplest to determine.

Skin Dose. Skin dose is used in radiation safety terminology to refer to the dose to the *epidermis*, the most superficial layers of the skin. The thickness of the epidermis varies from one anatomic area to another. It is greater in areas such as the palms of the hands and soles of the feet. The primary function of the epidermis is to protect underlying tissues and structures.

Entrance Skin Exposure

Conversion of entrance skin exposure to patient skin dose. Entrance skin exposure (ESE) may be converted to patient skin dose by using well-documented multiplicative factors. These will be explicitly discussed and illustrated in several examples. When actual patient measurements are not available, reasonably accurate estimates can still be made, which is why ESE is so widely used in assessing the amount of radiation received by a patient.

Measuring skin dose directly. Thermoluminescent dosimeters (TLDs) are the sensing devices most often used to determine skin dose directly. A small, relatively thin pack of TLDs is secured to the patient's skin in the middle of the clinical area of interest and exposed during a radiographic procedure. Because lithium fluoride (LiF), the sensing material in the TLD, responds in a manner similar to human tissue when exposed to ionizing radiation, an accurate determination of surface dose can be made (see Table 2.5 for a list of permissible skin entrance exposures for various radiographic examinations). In fluoroscopy, the amount of radiation that a patient receives at the entrance surface of the skin (at the tabletop) is usually estimated by measuring the radiation exposure rate at the tabletop (based upon ionization chamber measurements as part of routine equipment surveys) and

multiplying by the fluoroscopy time. The placement of thermoluminescent dosimeters at that location can be used to verify that estimate.

Gonadal Dose

Difference in gonadal dose received by human male and female patients. Because genetic effects may result from exposure to ionizing radiation, protection of the reproductive organs is of particular concern in diagnostic radiology (see Table 2.5 for a list of typical gonadal doses from various radiographic examinations). For several examinations identified in Table 2.5, differences in dose received exist between male and female patients. Protection of the ovaries by overlying tissue accounts for these differences. In diagnostic radiology, the relatively low gonadal dose for a single human is considered unimportant. However, when the low gonadal dose is applied to the entire population, the dose becomes far more significant.

Genetically significant dose. The concept of genetically significant dose (GSD) is used to assess the impact of gonadal dose. GSD is the equivalent dose (EqD) to the reproductive organs that, if received by every human, would be expected to bring about an identical gross genetic injury to the total population, as does the sum of the actual doses received by exposed individual members of the population. In other words, if a maximum of 500 people inhabited the earth and each person were to receive an EqD of 0.005 Sv of gonadal radiation, the gross genetic effect would be identical to the effect that would occur if 50 individual inhabitants each were to receive 0.05 Sv of gonadal radiation and the other 450 inhabitants were not to receive an EqD. In simple terms, the GSD concept suggests that the genetic consequences of substantial absorbed doses of gonadal radiation become significantly less when averaged over an entire population rather than applied to just a few of its members.

Genetically significant dose considerations. The GSD takes into consideration that some people receive radiation to their reproductive organs during a given year, whereas others do not. In addition, it accounts for the fact that radiation exposure in members of the population who cannot bear children (e.g., those who are beyond reproductive years) has no genetic impact. Hence the GSD is the average annual gonadal EqD to members of the population who are of childbearing age. It includes the number of children who may be expected to be conceived by members of the exposed population in a given year.

According to the US Public Health Service, the estimated GSD for the population of the United States is approximately 0.20 millisievert (mSv).

Bone Marrow Dose. In humans, bone marrow is of great importance because it contains large numbers of stem, or precursor, blood cells that could be either depleted or, worse, even eliminated by substantial exposure to ionizing radiation. Because irradiation of bone marrow may be responsible for inducing leukemia, the dose to this organ becomes very significant.[2] **Bone marrow dose** may also be described in terms of a quantity called the *mean marrow dose,* which is defined as "the average radiation dose to the entire active bone marrow."[2] For example, if in the course of performing a specific radiographic procedure, 25% of the active bone marrow were in the useful beam and received an average absorbed dose of 0.8 mGy_t, the mean marrow dose would be 0.2 mGy_t. Because multiple bony areas span the entire body, the radiation dose absorbed by the organ that we call "bone marrow" cannot be measured accurately by a direct method; it can only be estimated. In diagnostic radiology, the bone marrow dose is one of the values that has been used to provide an approximation of patient-absorbed dose even though hematologic effects are generally negligible for doses associated with this modality.

Table 2.5 provides typical bone marrow doses for various radiographic examinations performed on human adults. The levels indicated in Table 2.5 are usually less for children because the active bone marrow is more evenly spread out, and significantly lower technical radiographic exposure factors are used. Although each dose listed in Table 2.5 results from fragmentary exposure of the human body, it is averaged over the whole body.

Fluoroscopically Guided Positioning

Fluoroscopically guided positioning (FGP) is the practice of using fluoroscopy to determine the exact location of the central ray before taking a radiographic exposure.[9] Some radiologic technologists (RTs) believe that the use of FGP results in less dose to the patient than does a repeat radiograph. However, the American Society of Radiologic Technologists (ASRT) adopted the following positioning statement:

The ASRT recognizes that the routine use of fluoroscopy to ensure proper positioning for radiography prior to making an exposure is an unethical practice that increases patient dose unnecessarily and should never be used in place of appropriate skills required of the competent radiologic technologist.[10]

Even though the ASRT does not condone FGP, some imaging facilities continue to allow RTs to use fluoroscopy as a positioning aid because they believe that it:
- Is faster than having a repeat exposure
- Reduces the number of repeat exposures
- Provides less radiation exposure to the patient

The Standard of Ethics as published by the American Registry of Radiologic Technologists (ARRT) serves as a guide for practicing technologists in maintaining a high level of ethical conduct and in providing for the protection, safety, and comfort of patients.[11]

Blind positioning, or positioning using the radiographer's skill and anatomic landmarks, without a repeat exposure, provides the patient with the lowest dose. However, some technologists argue that the chance of repeating the image is reduced when using FGP. This argument *does not hold true* according to the current repeat rates of 7% to 8%.[12] For example, if a technologist has a repeat rate of 10%, it would not be ethical to overexpose 90% of the patients in an attempt to lower the repeat rate. Thus the usage of FGP by technologists is a practice that should be avoided. It is, in fact, prohibited by many state regulatory agencies. Where FGP is permitted, the repeat rate depends on the:
- Technologist's skills in the operation of the fluoroscopic equipment
- Communication between the technologist and the patient
- Patient's cooperation
- Patient's condition

Therefore the chance of a repeat during an FGP examination is still present, and ultimately, it is the technologist's professional responsibility to reduce the amount of radiation exposure to all patients, not just those who may need to have a repeat examination.

Studies indicate that patient ESE increases with the use of FGP when a repeat exposure is needed.[13] Blind positioning provides the lowest patient ESE.

The current scientific consensus is that all dose levels of ionizing radiation have some detrimental effect. At the same time, however, procedures in radiology, such as fluoroscopy and other imaging modalities, are providing vital information to physicians for diagnosis or treatment of disease. Thus risk vs. benefit must always be weighed.

Exposure of patients to medical x-rays is commanding increasing attention in our society for two reasons:

1. The frequency of x-ray examinations, including many repetitive studies in short periods, among all age groups, is expanding annually. This increase indicates that physicians are relying more and more on radiographic examinations to assist them in patient care and diagnosis.
2. Concern among public health officials is growing regarding the risk of late effects associated with these multiple medical x-ray exposures.[2]

A review of the literature emphasized the following guidelines:

- No diagnostic procedure using ionizing radiation should be conducted unless its benefits outweigh its risks.
- Exposures should be kept ALARA, with the procedure optimized to reduce radiation hazards.
- The ESE dose levels set in regulations must not be exceeded.
- To maintain ALARA and follow the ASRT position statement and the ARRT code of ethics, *technologists must not use FGP positioning of patients.*

PROTECTING THE PREGNANT OR POTENTIALLY PREGNANT PATIENT

Position of the American College of Radiology on Abdominal Radiologic Examinations of Female Patients

Because much evidence suggests that the developing embryo-fetus is very radiation sensitive, special care is taken in radiography to prevent unnecessary exposure of the abdominal area of pregnant women. Unfortunately, many women are not aware that they are pregnant during the earliest stage of pregnancy, and this means that exposure of the abdominal area of potentially pregnant (i.e., fertile) women is a concern.[14,15] When the referring physician does not consider radiologic procedures urgent, they may be regarded as elective examinations and can be booked at an appropriate time to meet patients' needs and safety requirements. However, the official position of the ACR, the major professional organization of radiologists in the United States, is as follows: "Abdominal radiological exams that have been requested after full consideration of the clinical status of a patient, including the possibility of pregnancy, need *not* be postponed or selectively scheduled."[14] Although elective scheduling is not always attempted in departments with high workloads, it is some departments' policy that women of childbearing years should be made aware of the NCRP recommendations and given the choice as to when they want to have a nonurgent abdominal examination. The NCRP recommendation states that abdominal examinations should be performed during the first few days after the onset of menses to minimize the possibility of irradiating an embryo.[15,16]

Determining the Possibility of Pregnancy

Whenever a female patient of childbearing age is to undergo an x-ray examination, it is essential that the radiographer carefully question the patient regarding any possibility of pregnancy. Part of this questioning involves asking the patient for the date of her last menstrual period (LMP). If the patient is to receive substantial pelvic irradiation and there is some doubt about her pregnancy status, then, provided there are no overriding medical concerns, it is strongly recommended that the result of a pregnancy test be obtained before the pelvis is irradiated. For all female patients of childbearing age, using a gonadal shield when the uterus and ovaries are within the field of view is advisable, as long as the presence of the shield would not disrupt the interpretation of the image. A shield is also recommended if the ovaries and uterus are less than 5 cm from any edge of the field.

Irradiation During an Unknown Pregnancy

Even with precautionary steps, it is likely that a radiographer will encounter many occasions when a patient who was absolutely certain that she could not be pregnant later discovered that she was so at the time of her x-ray examination. This revelation usually is communicated to the imaging department by the patient's obstetrician and is accompanied by a request for the amount of radiation dose that the patient's embryo-fetus received from the x-ray study. The following discussion attempts to illustrate in a simplified manner how the radiography team can appropriately respond to such queries by presenting several case examples.

The first step in the process is to list the particulars of the x-ray examination in as much detail as possible. A useful form can be developed to assist in this process (Fig. 12.13). The information that is needed to fill out this form is listed in Box 12.4.

The following question sometimes arises in the event that a pregnant patient is inadvertently irradiated. Should

Facility: _____

Imaging Department

**REQUEST FOR PATIENT RADIATION DOSE
PATIENT X-RAY EXAM RECORD**

Patient's name: _____ X-ray study #: _____
Date of birth: _____ Exam date: _____
Date of last menstrual period: _____
Referring physician: _____
Physician requesting radiation dose: _____
Radiologist: _____ Radiographer: _____
Examination: _____ X-ray room unit: _____

RADIOGRAPHIC

Projection	Patient thickness	Film	kVp	mAs	SID	Number of images	Gonadal shield

FLUOROSCOPIC

Anatomic location	kVp (mean)	mA (mean)	Fluoro time	Exam description

SPOT FILMS

Anatomic location	kVp	mA	Time (msec)	Number of spots	Special details

FIG 12.13 Request for patient radiation dose form.

a therapeutic abortion be performed to prevent the birth of an infant because of radiation exposure during pregnancy? Studies of groups such as the atomic bomb survivors of Hiroshima have shown that damage to the newborn is unlikely for doses below 0.2 Gy. Because essentially all diagnostic medical procedures result in fetal exposures of less than 0.01 Gy (1 cGy), the risk of abnormality is very small. The position of the NCRP is stated in Box 12.5.[15]

Procedure to Follow and Responsibility for Absorbed Equivalent Dose Determination to the Patient's Embryo-Fetus

When the details of the x-ray examination have been collected and listed on an appropriate summary form, they must be conveyed to the radiation safety officer or to the medical physicist providing x-ray quality assurance services. It is then that person's task to determine the

BOX 12.4 Information Needed to Develop the Request for Patient Radiation Dose Form

1. The x-ray unit or units used for the study
2. The projections taken
3. The number of images associated with each examination
4. Each projection's technical exposure factors (kVp, mAs, image receptor size)
5. The source-to–image receptor distance (SID) for each projection
6. The patient's anteroposterior (AP) or lateral dimensions at the site of each projection
7. For fluoroscopic irradiation, the approximate kVp, mA, and especially the duration
8. For spot films, the number taken, the kVp and mA selected, and the approximate exposure time

BOX 12.5 Position of the National Council of Radiation Protection and Measurements Concerning Risk and Fetal Exposure With Regard to Termination of Pregnancy

This risk is considered to be negligible at a fetal absorbed dose of 5 cGy or less when compared with other risks during pregnancy. The chance of malformations is significantly increased above control levels only at doses beyond 15 cGy. Therefore the exposure of the fetus to radiation arising from diagnostic procedures would rarely be cause, by itself, for terminating a pregnancy. If there are reasons other than possible radiation effects to consider a therapeutic abortion, the attending physician should discuss those reasons with the patient so that it is clear that the radiation exposure is not being used as an excuse for terminating the pregnancy.

Adapted from National Council on Radiation Protection and Measurements (NCRP): *Radiation protection in pediatric radiology, Report No. 68,* Washington, DC, 1977, NCRP.

absorbed EqD to the patient's embryo-fetus. The calculation process makes use of actual measurements of radiation output on the involved x-ray unit or units and incorporating that with the examination data list supplied by the radiographer. It also uses published absorbed dose data tables. What eventually is obtained and presented by the medical physicist, radiologist, or radiation safety officer to the patient's physician is a calculated estimate of the approximate EqD to the embryo-fetus as a result of the x-ray examination.

Sample Cases to Estimate Approximate Equivalent Dose to the Embryo-Fetus

Several typical cases (somewhat simplified) are presented to illustrate one of the methods that may be used to obtain this calculated estimate. It is not the purpose here to provide an advanced presentation but rather to offer a basic method that makes use of fundamental principles and demonstrates the importance of the radiographer's input in the process. The most significant factor is the correction to the measured radiation output at a given kVp as a result of the patient's thickness and the distance from the image receptor to the tabletop. The product of radiation output at the patient's radiation entrance surface (mGy_a/mAs) at the kVp selected and the milliampere-seconds used for the x-ray projection considered yields the ESE_d for that view—the quantity that we seek to obtain for each x-ray exposure given to the patient. The most common measurements of milligray in air per milliampere-second are at a distance of 100 cm from the x-ray tube target. These values as a function of kVp and mAs are normally tabulated during each annual survey of the x-ray unit by a qualified medical physicist. For a patient with thickness T in centimeters and a *typical distance of 8 cm from the image receptor to the tabletop,* the radiation output at the patient's entrance surface for selected milliampere-seconds is determined as shown in Fig. 12.14, which illustrates all the geometric quantities of interest.

Because the skin surface is closer to the x-ray tube target, the milligray per milliampere-seconds value will be greater than it is at 100 cm. How much greater is determined from the inverse square law and given in Equation 12.1 below:

$$(mGy_a/mAs) \text{ at skin surface} = (mGy_a/mAs) \text{ at } 100 \text{ cm} \times (100/[92 - T])^2$$

As an example, assume the following values:

$$(mGy_a/mAs) \text{ at } 100 \text{ cm} = 0.06$$
$$T = 25 \text{ cm}$$

Then:

$$(mGy_a/mAs) \text{ at skin surface} = 0.06 \times (100/[92 - 25])^2$$
$$= 0.06 \times (100/67)^2$$
$$= 0.06 \times 2.23$$
$$= 0.13 \text{ mGy/mAs}$$

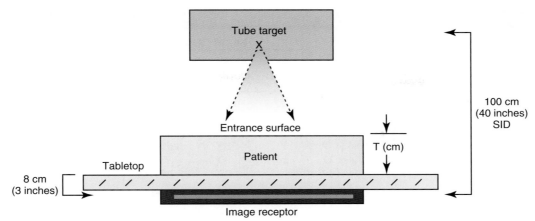

FIG 12.14 As the diagram shows, the distance from the tube target to the tabletop is 100 cm (40 inches) minus 8 cm (3 inches). The distance from the tube target to the top of the patient in centimeters is therefore equal to 100 − 8 − T where the patient's thickness, T, is specified in centimeters. To convert this value to inches just divide by 2.54.

The patient's ESE_d for an x-ray exposure is then given in Equation 12.2 below:

$$ESE_d = (mGy_a/mAs) \text{ at skin surface} \times mAs \text{ used}$$

Example:

$$mAs \text{ used} = 30$$

$$(mGy_a/mAs)_s = 0.13$$

$$ESE_d = 0.13 \times 30$$

$$= 3.9 \, mGy$$

After the ESE_d has been found for each x-ray exposure, it is necessary to obtain conversion factors that will yield a value for the uterine absorbed dose attributable to each exposure. In 1977 the NCRP published Report No. 54, *Medical Radiation Exposure of Pregnant and Potentially Pregnant Women*. Table 4 in this report has been a very useful resource for helping establish the uterine absorbed dose. Although other useful and more recent data tables exist, this table has been reproduced here as Table 12.1 to illustrate a simple method for fetal dose estimation. To use the table, it is necessary to know for each x-ray view the ESE_d, the anatomic location, the beam quality (half-value layer [HVL]), and the image receptor size.

Sample Cases to Obtain an Approximate Estimate of the Fetal Equivalent Dose

Two typical x-ray examinations will be considered and an approximate estimate of the fetal EqD resulting from each study obtained. These are presented in detail in Case 12.1 and Case 12.2.

Irradiating a Known Pregnant Patient

If the physician believes it is in the best interest of a pregnant or potentially pregnant patient to undergo a radiologic examination, the examination should be performed without delay and special efforts made to minimize the dose of radiation the patient receives to her lower abdomen and pelvic regions. This can be accomplished by consciously selecting the smallest technical exposure factors that will still yield a diagnostically useful image for the examination and by precisely collimating the radiographic beam to include only the anatomic area of interest. When the patient's lower abdomen and pelvic regions do not have to be included in the area to be irradiated, they should be protected with a lead apron or other suitable protective contact shield so that a developing embryo-fetus does not receive unnecessary radiation exposure (Fig. 12.15).

PEDIATRIC CONSIDERATIONS DURING RADIOGRAPHIC IMAGING

Vulnerability of Children to Radiation Exposure

Children are much more vulnerable to late effects of radiation than are adults. Hence children require special consideration when they undergo diagnostic x-ray

TABLE 12.1   Embryo (Uterine) Doses for Selected X-Ray Projections (mcGy/R)*[†]

Anatomy or Study	Projection	SID (Inches)	Image Receptor Size (Inches)[‡]	BEAM QUALITY (HVL MM ALUMINUM)					
				1.5	2.0	2.5	3.0	3.5	4.0
Pelvis, lumbopelvic	AP	40	17 × 14	142	212	283	353	421	486
	LAT	40	14 × 17	13	25	39	56	75	97
Abdominal[§]	AP	40	14 × 17	133	199	265	330	392	451
	PA	40	14 × 17	56	90	130	174	222	273
	LAT	40	14 × 17	13	23	37	53	71	91
Lumbar spine	AP	40	14 × 17	128	189	250	309	366	419
	LAT	40	14 × 17	9	17	27	39	53	69
Hip	AP (1)	40	10 × 12	105	153	200	244	285	324
	AP (2)	40	17 × 14	136	203	269	333	395	454
Full spine (chiropractic)	AP	40	14 × 36	154	231	308	384	457	527
Urethrogram	AP	40	10 × 12	135	200	265	327	386	441
Upper GI	AP	40	14 × 17	9.5	16	25	34	45	56
Femur (one side)	AP	40	7 × 17	1.6	3.0	4.8	6.9	9.4	12
Cholecystography	PA	40	10 × 12	0.7	1.5	2.6	4.1	6.0	8.3
Chest	AP	72	14 × 17	0.3	0.7	1.3	2.0	3.1	4.3
	PA	72	14 × 17	0.3	0.6	1.2	2.0	3.0	4.5
	LAT	72	14 × 17	0.1	0.3	0.5	0.8	1.2	1.8
Ribs, barium swallow	AP	40	14 × 17	0.1	0.3	0.5	0.9	1.4	2.0
	PA	40	14 × 17	0.1	0.3	0.5	0.9	1.5	2.2
	LAT	40	14 × 17	0.03	0.08	0.2	0.3	0.4	0.6
Thoracic spine	AP	40	14 × 17	0.2	0.4	0.8	1.4	4.1	3.0
	LAT	40	14 × 17	0.04	0.1	0.2	0.4	0.5	0.8
Skull, cervical spine, scapula, shoulder, humerus	—	40	—	<0.01	<0.01	<0.01	<0.01	<0.01	<0.01

AP, Anteroposterior; *GI*, gastrointestinal; *HVL*, half-value layer; *LAT*, lateral; *PA*, posteroanterior; *SID*, source-to–image receptor distance.

*Average dose to the uterus in millicentigray per roentgen entrance skin exposure (free-in-air) (ESE$_d$). The latter value in roentgens is essentially equal, in these energy ranges, to 10 mGy ESE$_d$ or 1 cGy ESE$_d$.

[†]Adapted from NCRP report No. 54 Rosenstein (1976).

[‡]Field size is collimated to the image receptor.

[§]Includes retrograde pyelogram; kidney, ureter, and bladder (KUB); barium enema, lumbosacral spine, intravenous pyelogram (IVP); renal arteriogram.

Data modified from National Council on Radiation Protection and Measurements (NCRP): *Medical radiation exposure of pregnant and potentially pregnant women, Report No. 54*, Washington, DC, 1977, NCRP.

studies. Some of these considerations are described in the following sections. Because children have a greater life expectancy, they may easily survive long enough to develop leukemia induced by radiation or develop a radiogenic malignancy such as lung or thyroid cancer. In fact, according to studies published in 1978, the risk of a radiation-induced leukemia in children after a substantial dose of ionizing radiation is approximately two times that of adults.[17] For low doses such as those generally encountered in ordinary diagnostic radiology,

CASE 12.1 Obstruction Series

X-ray projection details:

Although a 180-cm (72-inch) source-to–image receptor distance (SID) would normally be used for a posteroanterior (PA) upright chest projection, for purposes of simplifying the calculation, we will keep the SID = 100 cm (40 inches) the same for all x-ray projections in this series.

PA chest radiograph

(1) 80 kVp, 10 mAs, 100 cm SID, 35 × 43-cm cassette, 25-cm patient thickness

Erect anteroposterior (AP) abdomen

(1) 75 kVp, 32 mAs, 100 cm SID, 35 × 43-cm cassette, 20-cm patient thickness

Supine abdomen

(1) 70 kVp, 50 mAs, 100 cm SID, 35 × 43-cm cassette, 20-cm patient thickness

The first step is to obtain the value of mGy_a/mAs for each projection. To determine this value, a reference value $(mGy_a/mAs)_{100-cm}$ is needed for the x-ray unit involved and the kVp used. To comply with state rules and regulations, a medical physicist measures these values yearly for each x-ray tube. If the measured reference mGy_a/mAs values for the three projections are 0.01, 0.04, and 0.04, respectively, then substituting these numbers into Equation 12.1 along with the corresponding SIDs and patient thicknesses yields: $(mGy_a/mAs)_s$ PA chest = 0.02 $(mGy_a/mAs)_s$, erect AP abdomen = 0.08, and supine abdomen = 0.08, respectively. From Equation 12.2 the entrance skin exposure dose (ESE_d) value is then given by:

$$ESE_d \text{ PA chest: } 0.02 \times 10 = 0.2 \text{ mGy} = (0.02 \text{ cGy})$$

$$ESE_d \text{ erect AP abdomen: } 0.08 \times 32 = 2.6 \text{ mGy} \ (0.26 \text{ cGy})$$

$$ESE_d \text{ supine abdomen: } 0.08 \times 50 = 4 \text{ mGy} \ (0.4 \text{ cGy})$$

For the chest field, the half-value layer (HVL) is approximately 3 mm aluminum (Al), whereas for the abdominal fields, 2.5 and 2.0 mm Al, respectively, are used. Then from Table 12.1 the embryo/uterine dose conversion factors are 2 mcGy/cGy of ESE_d, 265 mcGy/cGy of ESE_d, and 199 mcGy/cGy of ESE_d. Multiplying these values by the ESE_d for each view gives a fetal dose estimate (FDE) for each, namely:

$$PA \text{ chest FDE} = 0.02 \times 2 = 0.04 \text{ mcGy (.04 millirads)}$$

$$\begin{aligned} \text{Erect AP abdomen FDE} &= 0.26 \times 265 \\ &= 69 \text{ mcGy (69 millirads)} \end{aligned}$$

$$\begin{aligned} \text{Supine abdomen FDE} &= 0.4 \times 199 \\ &= 79.6 \text{ mcGy (79.6 millirads)} \end{aligned}$$

(Note: 1 cGy = 1 rad and therefore 1 millicGy equals 1 millirad)

The total FDE is therefore 0.04 + 69 + 79.6 = 149 mcGy = 1.49 mGy. For diagnostic x-rays, 1 mGy is the same as an equivalent dose (EqD) of 1 mSv, and consequently the calculated approximate EqD to the patient's embryo-fetus from her obstruction series is 1.49 mSv (149 millirem).

For reference purposes, this value of EqD to the embryo-fetus is substantially less than the 5 mSv (500 mrem) recommended by the National Council on Radiation Protection and Measurements as a maximum EqD to the embryo-fetus during the 9-month gestation period.

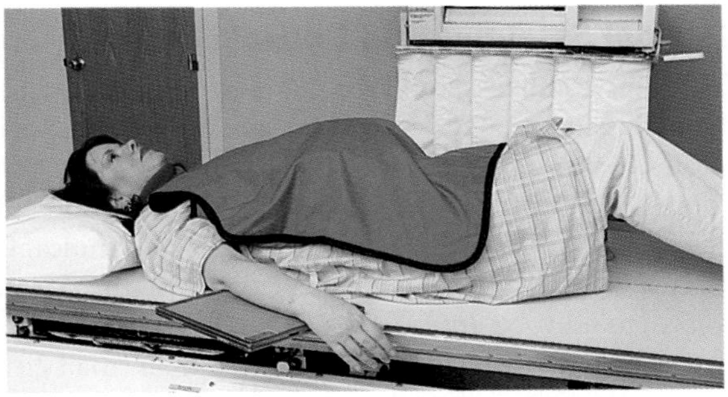

FIG 12.15 To protect a developing embryo-fetus from unnecessary radiation exposure, place a lead apron over the female patient's lower abdomen and pelvic regions when these sites do not have to be included in the area to be irradiated.

data are still inconclusive. With this consideration in mind, radiographers have to take every precaution to minimize exposure in all pediatric patients.

Children Require Smaller Radiation Doses Than Do Adults

In general, smaller doses of ionizing radiation are sufficient to obtain useful images in pediatric imaging procedures than are necessary for adult imaging procedures. For example, an entrance exposure below 5 mcGy results from an AP projection of an infant's chest,[18] whereas the same projection or a PA projection of an adult's chest yields an entrance exposure ranging from 10 to 25 mcGy.

CASE 12.2 Modified Upper Gastrointestinal Examination

X-ray projection details:
  Fluoroscopy: 115 kVp, 4.5 mA (mean values), 3.5 minutes
  Spot films (4): 110 kVp, 200 mA, 20 msec (mean values)
Calculation details:
  Suppose that from measured data on the involved fluoroscopic unit, the entrance exposure rate dose to the patient is about 12.5 mGy per milliampere minute. Therefore the entrance skin exposure dose (ESE$_d$) for the delivered fluoroscopic radiation is obtained from the product:

$$12.5\,mGy/mA\text{-}min \times 4.5\,mA \times 3.5\,min = 197\,mGy\ (19.7\,cGy)$$

  From measured spot film radiation output, for the technique factors used in this study, let the x-ray output at the patient's entrance surface be 0.5 mGy/mAs.* Therefore the total ESE$_d$ for the four spot films is given by:

$$4 \times 0.5\,mGy/mAs \times 200\,mA \times 0.020\,sec = 8\,mGy = (0.8\,cGy)$$

  Using half-value layer (HVL) values of 4.0 and 3.5 mm aluminum (Al), respectively, the uterine dose rates obtained from Table 12.1 are as follows:

Averaged fluoroscopic irradiation: 56 mcGy/cGy entrance = 56 mrem/cGy
Spot films: 45 mcGy/cGy entrance = 45 mrem/cGy
  The estimated approximate equivalent dose (EqD) to the embryo-fetus from this modified upper gastrointestinal (UGI) study is then:

$$56 \times 19.7 + 45 \times 0.8 = 1139\,mrem = 1.14\,rem = 11.4\,mSv$$

  For this modified UGI study on a heavy patient, we have obtained a fetal EqD estimate that is more than twice the National Council on Radiation Protection and Measurements recommended maximum fetal EqD of 5 mSv (0.5 rem). This result, however, is far below the range between 100 and 200 mSv (10 and 20 rem) at which therapeutic abortion has historically been considered. If the embryo-fetus were in its most sensitive stage (i.e., early first trimester), then possibly some genetic studies could be undertaken. Otherwise, in most situations, increased follow-up would be the course of action.

*For the spot films the entrance surface of the patient is only about 46 cm (18 inches) from the x-ray tube target, and that is why the value of mGy/mAs can be so high.

Patient Motion and Motion Reduction Methods

Patient motion is frequently a problem in diagnostic pediatric radiography. Because of the limited ability of children to understand the radiologic procedure and, in most cases, their imperfect ability to cooperate, children are less likely to remain still during a radiographic or fluoroscopic exposure. To solve or at least minimize this problem, the radiographer must employ very short exposure times by selecting a high-mA station and also make use of effective immobilization techniques. For some examinations, such as chest radiography, special pediatric motion restriction devices are available to hold the pediatric patient securely and safely in the required position (see Fig. 12.3). The use of such procedures and correct image postprocessing techniques greatly reduces or eliminates the need for repeat examinations that will increase patient dose.

Gaining Cooperation During the Procedure

The combination of technologists who have experience working with children and examination rooms specifically designed for pediatric studies is very beneficial. Such rooms contain not only the appropriate restraint devices but also suitable entertainment and distraction devices such as cartoon posters and puppets. The examination progresses most efficiently with the best chance of patient cooperation when the child feels less intimidated.

Gonadal Shielding and Gonadal Dose

The radiographer should be familiar with particular characteristics related to gonadal shielding in pediatric studies. First, if the gonadal tissue is more than 2 cm from the edge of the field of view (assuming good collimation), the use of a gonadal shield does not significantly affect the gonadal dose because in that case the dose is caused mainly by internal scatter. The shield can be dispensed with in such situations. Second, in small girls, the variation in anatomic location of the ovaries requires protection of the iliac wings as well as the sacral area when shielding is needed.[18] Effective shielding may not be possible, however, for some studies because it obscures the anatomic area of interest.

Collimation

Collimation is especially significant in pediatric studies. The automatic collimation system reduces the radiation field size to the dimensions of the image receptor, but because many pediatric patients are significantly smaller than the image receptor, further manual adjustment of collimation is often necessary. As in any other radiographic study, reducing the field size to the anatomic features of interest not only reduces patient exposure but also increases recorded image quality by decreasing scatter. Projection orientation also is important. Female patients who may be imaged in either PA or AP projection will receive significantly lower doses to the breast tissues in a PA projection.[19]

Patient Protection in Computed Tomography for Adults and Children: Similarities and Necessary Changes

Unfortunately, many facilities have in the past routinely used the same factors for both adults and small children and continue to do so today. There has been an apparent unwillingness to develop new scanning protocols because of the conflicting demands of multiple pediatric protocols. Mindful of the overall enhanced vulnerability of children to ionizing radiation, it is imperative that all facilities and imaging personnel make every conscious effort to develop and use low-dose pediatric protocols that are in the best interest of the children entrusted to their care.

IMAGE GENTLY CAMPAIGN

An initiative of the Alliance for Radiation Safety in Pediatric Imaging (as discussed in Chapter 1) is the Image Gently Campaign. The goal of this campaign is to change long-established practice by raising awareness about methods for lowering radiation dose during pediatric medical imaging examinations (Alliance for Radiation Safety in Pediatric Imaging, 2016).[20] The Image Gently website, www.imagegently.org, provides information about pediatric imaging examinations for RTs, medical physicists, radiologists, pediatricians, and parents. For RTs, the site includes protocols for reducing pediatric radiation dose during digital radiography, fluoroscopy, computed tomography exams, interventional radiology exams, and nuclear medicine procedures. Radiographers and imaging facilities can "pledge" to Image Gently (see

Appendix J for the pledge). As of 2015, over 35,000 RTs have taken the pledge.

IMAGE WISELY CAMPAIGN

A second initiative of the Alliance for Radiation Safety in Pediatric Imaging (as discussed in Chapter 1) is the Image Wisely Campaign. This campaign promotes lowering the amount of radiation used in medically necessary imaging procedures and eliminating unnecessary procedures in adult medical imaging. The Image Wisely Campaign includes on its website, www.imagewisely.org, information on radiography, fluoroscopy, computed tomography, and nuclear medicine examinations for radiologic technologists, medical physicists, radiologists, pediatricians, and parents. Radiographers can pledge to Image Wisely (see Appendix K for the pledge). As of 2015 over 47,000 RTs have taken the pledge.

▮ SUMMARY

- Effective communication with the patient is the first step in holistic patient care.
  - Imaging procedures should be explained in simple terms.
  - Patients must have an opportunity to ask questions and receive truthful and clear answers within ethical limits.
- Adequate immobilization of the patient is necessary to eliminate voluntary motion.
  - Restraining devices are available to immobilize either the whole body or the individual body part to be radiographed.
  - Involuntary motion can be compensated for by shortening exposure time with an appropriate increase in mA and by using very-high-speed image receptors.
- Protective shielding may be used to reduce or eliminate radiation exposure of radiosensitive body organs and tissues.
  - The reproductive organs should be protected from exposure to the useful beam when they are inside or within approximately 5 cm of a properly collimated beam, unless this would compromise the diagnostic value of the study.
  - Correctly placed, appropriate gonadal shielding can greatly reduce the exposure received by patients of both sexes (50% reduction for female patients, 90% to 95% reduction for male patients).

- The clear lead shadow shield and a PA projection can significantly reduce the dose to the breast of a young patient undergoing a scoliosis examination.
- Appropriate technical exposure factors for each examination that ensure a diagnostic image of optimal quality with minimal patient dose must be selected.
  - Standardized technique charts must be available for each x-ray unit to help provide a uniform selection of technical exposure factors. High kVp and lower mAs should be chosen whenever possible to reduce the amount of radiation received by the patient.
- When digital images are acquired, correct postprocessing is essential to produce a high-quality diagnostic image.
  - Imaging departments should establish a quality control program that ensures standardization in the postprocessing of digital images.
- An air gap technique can be used as an alternative to the use of a grid.
- Repeat radiographic exposures must be minimized to prevent the patient's skin and gonads from receiving a double dose of radiation.
- Radiographic examinations are to be performed only when patients will benefit from useful information gained from the procedure. Nonessential radiologic examinations should not be performed.
- The amount of radiation received by a patient from diagnostic imaging procedures may be specified as entrance skin exposure (ESE) (including skin and glandular), gonadal dose, or bone marrow dose.
  - ESE is the easiest quantity to obtain and the most widely used.
  - The estimated genetically significant dose (GSD) for the population of the United States is approximately 0.20 mSv.
- Fluoroscopically guided positioning is an unethical and unacceptable practice that leads to increased patient radiation dose.
- Abdominal radiologic examinations that have been requested after full consideration of the clinical status of a patient, including the possibility of pregnancy, need not be postponed or selectively scheduled.[14]
  - The NCRP recommendation for elective abdominal examinations of women of childbearing years states that such examinations should be performed during the first few days after the onset of menses to minimize the possibility of irradiating an embryo.[15,16]

- A radiographer must carefully question female patients of childbearing age regarding any possibility of pregnancy before they undergo an x-ray examination.
- If irradiation of an unknown pregnancy occurs, a calculated estimate of the approximate equivalent dose to the embryo-fetus as a result of the examination should be obtained. A radiologic physicist determines the fetal dose.
- Children are much more vulnerable to late effects of radiation than are adults.
  - Use a PA projection to protect the breasts of female patients.
  - In small girls, shielding of the ovaries requires protection of the iliac wings as well as the sacral area when shielding is needed.
  - Adequate collimation of the radiographic beam to include only the area of clinical interest is essential, and effective immobilization techniques should be used when necessary. The use of a high mA station and a short exposure time also helps minimize patient motion effects.
- A developing embryo-fetus is especially sensitive to exposure from ionizing radiation.
  - Use the smallest technical exposure factors that will generate a diagnostically useful radiographic image, carefully collimate the beam to include only the anatomic area of interest, and cover the lower abdomen and pelvic regions with a suitable contact shield if they do not need to be included in the examination.
  - The goal of the Image Gently Campaign is to change practice by increasing awareness about methods to lower radiation dose during pediatric medical imaging examinations.[20]
  - Radiographers and imaging facilities can pledge to Image Gently.
  - Radiographers can pledge to Image Wisely.

REFERENCES

1. Torres LS: *Basic medical techniques and patient care for radiologic technologists*, ed 5, Philadelphia, 1997, Lippincott Williams & Wilkins.
2. Bushong SC: *Radiologic science for technologists: physics, biology and protection*, ed 10, St. Louis, 2013, Mosby.
3. Herrman TL, et al: *White paper: best practices in digital radiography*, 2012. American Society of Radiologic

Technologists. Available at: http://www.asrt.org/docs/whitepapers/asrt12_bstpracdigradwhp_final.pdf.

4. Gray J, et al: *Quality control in diagnostic imaging*, Baltimore, 1983, University Park Press.

5. Hendee WR, et al: *Radiologic physics equipment and quality control*, Chicago, 1977, Year Book.

6. McKinney W: *Radiographic processing and quality control*, Philadelphia, 1988, Lippincott.

7. Carter CE, Veale BL: *Digital radiography and PACS*, St. Louis, 2008, Mosby.

8. US Food and Drug Administration (FDA): *Presurgical chest x-ray screening examinations*, Washington, DC, 1986, U.S. Government Printing Office. *FDA Publication No. 86-8265.*

9. Haynes K, Curtis T: Fluoroscopic vs. blind positioning: comparing entrance skin exposure. *Radiol Technol* 81:1, 2009.

10. American Society of Radiologic Technologists: *ASRT organizational issues: fluoroscoping for positioning.* Available at: http://www.asrt.org/docs/governance/hodpositionstatements66FE1F374C63.pdf.

11. American Registry of Radiologic Technologists: *ARRT Standards of Ethics.* Available at: http://arrt.org/pdfs/Governing-Documents/Standards-of-Ethics.pdf.

12. Adler A, et al: An analysis of radiographic repeat and reject rates. *Radiol Technol* 63:308, 1992.

13. Leeming BW, et al: A comparison of fluoroscopically controlled patient positioning and conventional positioning, including comparative dosimetry. *Radiology* 124:231, 1977.

14. Reynold FB: *Prepared remarks for the October 20, 1976.* American College of Radiology press conference.

15. National Council on Radiation Protection and Measurements (NCRP): *Medical x-ray, electron beam and gamma-ray protection up to 50 MeV (equipment design, performance and use), 1989. Report No. 102,* Bethesda, Md, NCRP.

16. National Council on Radiation Protection and Measurements (NCRP): *Medical exposure of pregnant and potentially pregnant women, 1977. Report No. 54,* Washington, DC, NCRP.

17. Ozasa K, et al: Studies of the mortality of atomic bomb survivors, Report 14, 1950-2003: an overview of cancer and noncancer diseases. *Radiat Res* 177(3):229–243, 2012. Paper published by, (doi:10,1667/RR2629.1) Iss14_e.pdf.

18. National Council on Radiation Protection and Measurements (NCRP): *Radiation protection in pediatric radiology, Report No. 68,* Washington, DC, 1981, NCRP.

19. Bontrager KL: *Textbook of positioning and related anatomy,* ed 4, St. Louis, 1997, Mosby.

20. *Alliance for Radiation Safety in Pediatric Imaging,* 2016. www.imagegently.org, Accessed 21 April 2017.

GENERAL DISCUSSION QUESTIONS

1. How does the patient benefit from effective communication with the radiographer during an imaging procedure?

2. What can the radiographer do to eliminate the problem of voluntary patient motion, and how can involuntary motion be compensated for during radiography?

3. When should gonadal shielding not be used during a diagnostic imaging procedure?

4. Why should a radiographer use a standardized technique chart to select technical exposure factors before performing an imaging procedure?

5. Why are correct radiographic image postprocessing and the establishment of a quality control program important for imaging departments that use digital imaging display equipment?

6. How does an air gap technique reduce scattered radiation?

7. How can the dose to the breast of a young female patient be reduced when a radiographic examination for scoliosis is performed?

8. When is a radiographic examination considered nonessential? Give some examples.

9. Describe three ways in which the amount of radiation received by a patient from diagnostic imaging procedures may be specified.

10. What does the genetically significant dose take into consideration?

11. Why is it unacceptable to use fluoroscopically guided positioning?

12. How should irradiation of an unknown pregnancy be handled?

13. What are the goals of the Image Gently Campaign and the Image Wisely Campaign?

14. When does the NCRP recommend the scheduling of elective examinations?

15. How do children compare with adults with regard to the potential for biologic damage from exposure to ionizing radiation?

16. What precautions should be taken by a radiographer who must perform a radiographic examination on a pregnant patient?

17. What is the position of the American College of Radiology (ACR) regarding abdominal radiologic examinations of pregnant or potentially pregnant patients?

18. What are the benefits of using a pediatric-designed x-ray room for young children?
19. How is a thermoluminescent dosimeter (TLD) used to measure skin dose?
20. What is meant by *standardized exposure techniques?*

REVIEW QUESTIONS

1. As a consequence of their anatomic location, the female reproductive organs receive about _____ exposure during a given radiographic procedure involving the pelvic region than do the male reproductive organs.
   A. Three times less
   B. Three times more
   C. Ten times less
   D. Ten times more
2. In fluoroscopy, how is the amount of radiation that a patient receives usually estimated?
   A. By having the patient wear an optically stimulated luminescence (OSL) dosimeter during the procedure
   B. By measuring the radiation exposure rate at tabletop and multiplying this by the milliamperage (mA) and kilovoltage (kVp) settings
   C. By measuring the radiation exposure rate at tabletop and multiplying this by the fluoroscopy time
   D. By placing an ionization-type survey meter next to the patient during the procedure to record the dose received
3. As part of the Image Gently Campaign, radiographers and imaging facilities can pledge to:
   A. Image Gently
   B. Image Wisely
   C. Image a patient only once in any given year
   D. Image a patient only when he or she is in danger of expiring
4. In which of the following projections will a young female patient receive a significantly lower dose to her breast tissue during a chest x-ray study?
   A. AP
   B. AP lordotic
   C. PA
   D. Lateral
5. A woman who is 3 months pregnant has been in a motor vehicle accident. The emergency room physician suspects there is injury to her cervical spine and thus feels justified in ordering an x-ray examination to aid in determining the extent of the patient's injury. Because the patient is pregnant, the radiographer should:
   1. Select the smallest technical exposure factors that will produce a diagnostically useful image
   2. Adequately and precisely collimate the radiographic beam to include only the anatomic area of interest
   3. Shield the patient's lower abdomen and pelvic region with a suitable protective contact shield
   A. 1 only
   B. 2 only
   C. 3 only
   D. 1, 2, and 3
6. Pediatric patients require special consideration and appropriate radiation protection procedures because they are much more vulnerable to which of the following?
   A. The late effects of radiation
   B. Only the late somatic effects of radiation
   C. Only the genetic effects of radiation
   D. Only the early somatic effects of radiation
7. The use of the PA projection during a juvenile scoliosis radiographic examination results in which of the following?
   A. Higher entrance exposure dose to the anterior body surface, thereby significantly increasing the dose to the breast
   B. Lower entrance exposure dose to the anterior body surface, thereby significantly reducing the dose to the breast
   C. Poorer-quality images that necessitate a repeat examination
   D. Images that do not adequately demonstrate spinal curvature
8. For protection of the ovaries of a female patient, the shield should be placed approximately:
   A. 5.0 cm (2 inches) medial to each palpable anterior superior iliac spine
   B. 2.5 cm (1 inch) medial to each palpable anterior superior iliac spine
   C. 5.0 cm (2 inches) lateral to each palpable anterior superior iliac spine
   D. 2.5 cm (1 inch) lateral to each palpable anterior superior iliac spine

9. Which of the following examinations are considered unnecessary radiologic procedures?
   1. Chest x-ray study as part of a preemployment physical
   2. Screening mammography
   3. Whole-body multislice spiral CT screening
   A. 1 and 2 only
   B. 1 and 3 only
   C. 2 and 3 only
   D. 1, 2, and 3

10. If a maximum of 500 people inhabited an island and each person were to receive an equivalent dose (EqD) of 0.005 Sv gonadal radiation, the gross genetic effect would be _____ the effect occurring if 50 individual inhabitants were each to receive 0.05 Sv of gonadal radiation and no equivalent dose were received by other inhabitants.
   A. Greatly different from
   B. Slightly different from
   C. Almost the same as
   D. Identical to

13

Special Considerations on Safety in Computed Tomography and Mammography

OBJECTIVES

- Define all key terms.
- Explain why computed tomography examinations are of greater concern in terms of radiation safety in comparison with routine radiographic examinations.
- List two concerns that relate to patient dose in CT scanning and explain each.
- Compare the entrance exposure from a CT examination with the entrance exposure from a routine fluoroscopic procedure.
- Describe how interslice scatter affects the radiation dose to a patient.
- State the reason why direct patient shielding is not necessary during a CT examination.
- For spiral, or helical, CT, state how patient dose is affected when pitch ratio is increased above 1 or decreased below 1.
- Identify various methods for reducing patient dose during a CT examination.
- Discuss the concept of computed tomography dose parameters.
- Explain how to calculate the effective CT dose.
- State the goal of CT imaging from a radiation protection point of view.
- Explain the value of mammography for the detection of breast cancer.
- State the maximum dose to the glandular tissue of a 4.5-cm compressed breast using a screen-film or digital system.
- Explain the reason why the age recommendation for a screening mammography is controversial.
- Cite examples of how radiation dose in mammography can be reduced.
- Recognize the value of digital mammography for imaging of patients with dense breasts.
- Identify the benefit of using the two most common metallic elements employed as filters in mammographic units.

CHAPTER OUTLINE

computed tomography (CT)
dose distribution
dose parameters
interslice scatter

iterative reconstruction
mammography
molybdenum filter
pitch ratio

rhodium filter
skin dose
spiral (helical) CT
tube current modulation

Some types of radiographic examinations require special consideration for radiation safety. This chapter addresses these concerns for computed tomography and for mammography.

PATIENT DOSE IN COMPUTED TOMOGRAPHY

Radiation Exposure

Computed tomography (CT) is defined as "the process of creating a cross-sectional tomographic plane of any part of the body."[1] This computer-reconstructed digital image of a patient is formed by an x-ray tube coupled with a precise arrangement of multiple detectors rotating around a selective area of anatomy. CT was previously referred to as *computed axial tomography (CAT)* because the first generation of scanners produced only axial images.* The term *computed tomography* is now more appropriate because "images can now be recreated in multiple planes."[1] Although a detailed discussion of CT equipment, function, and procedure is not within the scope of this text, patient dose resulting from exposure to ionizing radiation is relevant because CT is a frequently employed diagnostic x-ray imaging modality that is considered to be a relatively high radiation exposure examination. Currently, this is of even more concern because of the increasing use of multislice spiral (helical)* CT scanners utilizing *thin*** slice thickness, which relies

on markedly increasing the selected tube milliamperage per slice to keep under control the effect of ever-present random noise and thereby produce a high-quality image. With higher radiation exposure to the patient, there is an increased associated cancer risk. For this reason, physicians ordering such procedures must weigh the benefits of the procedure for the patient in terms of medical information gained and determine whether these benefits outweigh the risk.

Concerns Related to Patient Dose: Skin Dose and Dose Distribution

Two concerns relate to patient dose in CT scanning. One concern is the skin dose, and the other is the dose distribution during the scanning procedure. The dose at the edge of a beam does not decrease to zero immediately (i.e., there is no sharp cutoff of radiation at the beam boundary); some extra radiation is delivered at the edge of the slice. Because of this, the skin dose for a succession of adjacent scans is greater than the skin dose from a single scan. The neighboring slices contribute some dose from both sides as they overlap.

The skin dose from a CT scan is generally smaller than that for a radiographic or fluoroscopic image of the same region of the body. This is because the use of multiple views from many angles reduces the need for any one view to acquire enough x-ray exposure to achieve an acceptable image. Also, the use of smaller "field size" or collimation of any one view in CT as compared with radiography or fluoroscopy reduces scatter dose.

The dose distribution within the slice or tissue irradiated in a CT scan is not the same as the dose distribution occurring in routine radiologic procedures (Fig. 13.1). In radiography or fluoroscopy, skin dose at the entrance surface of the patient is much higher than at the exit surface. In abdominal imaging, for example, the entrance skin dose is approximately 100 times the exit dose. For CT, because the tube rotates around the patient, the dose is much more uniform throughout the patient. Because

---

*Axial images are images of the plane of the body perpendicular to the long (craniocaudal) axis of the patient. In spiral or helical image acquisition, the patient table moves during the acquisition so that a three-dimensional data set is obtained. The speed of table advance and the speed of rotation of the x-ray source are usually different and determine how much data are acquired (i.e., how densely the patient is sampled). Slower table speed allows thinner slices of the patient to be reconstructed.

**Some typical thin slice thickness values are 1.25 mm and 0.625 mm.

CT scanners use an x-ray beam that is tightly collimated, the amount of scatter radiation generated is lower than the scatter produced by the less tightly collimated radiographic beam. Also because of this, the mass of human tissue exposed to radiation falls off rapidly outside the plane of interest during the production of any given scan. Although in a single-slice scanner only one cross-sectional tomographic plane (slice) is exposed and imaged at a time,** a small overlap of the margins of the x-ray beam occurs when each single tomographic section is made. When a series of adjacent slices is obtained, some radiation will also scatter from the slice being made into the adjacent slices (**interslice scatter**). Both of these factors contribute to dose increase and are the reasons why a succession of adjacent tomographic sections (slices) imparts a higher absorbed dose than would a single tomographic section.

Direct Patient Shielding

Direct patient shielding is not typically used in CT. Because of the rotational nature of the exposure, a shield is no more effective than the collimators that already exist on the device. Because the beam is so tightly collimated to the slice thickness, any consequential exposure to the anatomy outside the field of view is usually caused only by internal scatter. Therefore generally in CT, anatomy does not appear in the primary x-ray beam unless it is part of the intended field of view.

Spiral, or Helical, Computed Tomography

Spiral CT presents a greater challenge for assessing patient dose than conventional CT. It may be defined as a data acquisition method that combines a continuous gantry rotation with a selectable speed of continuous table advance forming a spiral path of data acquisition[1] (Fig. 13.2). It is also called *helical CT.*

Spiral, or helical, scans may often be characterized by a quantity called the **pitch ratio** or just *pitch* for short. Pitch is the relationship between the movement or advance of the patient couch, also known as *table increment (I),* and the x-ray beam collimator dimension (Z). Mathematically, it is expressed as I/Z. When the spiral scan pitch ratio is approximately 1, the spiral CT patient dose is comparable to that produced by conventional or axial CT. However, when the pitch ratio is higher (e.g., 2:1), patient dose is reduced in comparison with conventional CT because the same number of x-rays produced during each rotation of the tube is spread out over more of the patient. The reverse also is true; patient dose increases at a lower pitch (Fig. 13.3).

**Note: In current scanners, multiple slices (e.g., 4, 8, 16, 32, 64, 128, 256, and even as many as 320)[1] can be acquired simultaneously.

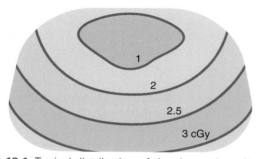

FIG 13.1 Typical distribution of the doses deposited in a single-slice computed tomography examination. For multiple contiguous slices, the doses may be twice these values.

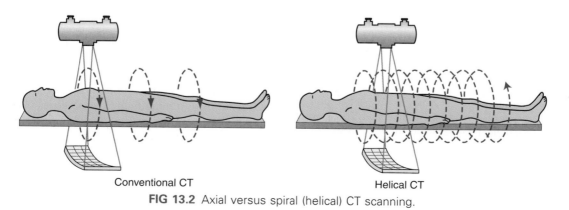

Conventional CT   Helical CT

FIG 13.2 Axial versus spiral (helical) CT scanning.

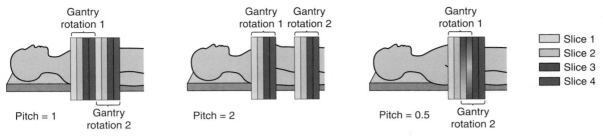

FIG 13.3 Illustration of different pitch value scan sequences.

BOX 13.1	**Optimization of Patient Dose in CT**

- Tube current modulation
  - Longitudinal
  - Angular
- Iterative reconstruction
- Optimization of tube voltage and other scan parameters
- Correct patient centering

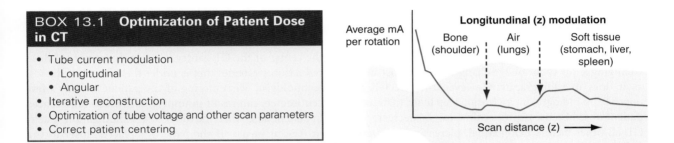

FIG 13.4 X-ray tube current as a function of position superimposed on a CT projection radiograph illustrating the principle of longitudinal dose modulation. (From McCollough CH, Bruesewitz MR, Kofler JM: CT dose reduction and dose management tools: overview of available options, *RadioGraphics* 26(2):503–512, 2006.)

METHODS FOR REDUCTION OF PATIENT DOSE IN CT

Box 13.1 provides a list of several dose reduction methods that lead to optimization of patient dose in CT. These methods are discussed in the sections that follow.

Tube Current Modulation

Recognizing that the x-ray tube current determines the rate of x-ray output from the tube, CT manufacturers utilize information from the initial "scout view" or "radiographic mode" image to modulate or change the current as the tube moves along the longitudinal axis of the patient, usually referred to as the *Z-axis*. Lower tube current is used in regions where there is decreased attenuation because the anatomy is thinner or less dense (e.g., the thorax), and higher tube current is used in regions where there is more attenuation due to the anatomy being thicker (e.g., the abdomen) (Fig. 13.4). Using this technique, patient dose will be lowered in regions where fewer photons are needed to acquire an image of acceptable quality. Tube current modulation is sometimes referred to as *automatic exposure control (AEC) for CT* in analogy with the AEC systems that are used in radiographic and fluoroscopic imaging systems.

Tube current may also be varied as the x-ray tube rotates about the patient to reduce dose to radiation-sensitive organs such as the breast that reside on the anterior surface of the patient rather than the midline. Angular-based tube current modulation reduces tube current while the x-ray tube is on the anterior side of the patient and maintains or increases dose as it rotates on the posterior side. This method has been shown to underdose the superficial anterior organs without adversely affecting image quality.[2]

In the past, external shields impregnated with radiopaque material such as bismuth have been used to reduce the dose to organs near the patient's surface. However, tube current modulation techniques have been found to be more effective and have less effect upon image quality.[3,4]

Iterative Reconstruction

Originally, CT scan data were reconstructed from data acquired during the scanning process through a technique known as *filtered back projection** that was applied only a single time. Recent advances in computer technology allow data to be acquired with lower dose. CT scan data can be reconstructed, modified, reconstructed again, modified, etc., until an image having the lowest noise possible is obtained. Such a repeated process is referred to as *iteration* and is used in iterative reconstruction techniques. With filtered back projection, decreasing tube current may decrease dose, but at a price of increased quantum noise in the final image. Iterative reconstruction techniques, however, can be used to reduce dose to levels below those of filtered back projection while maintaining acceptable noise levels.[5,6]

Optimization of Tube Voltage

Changing x-ray tube voltage changes patient dose in CT as it does in radiography. However, the effect is the opposite. In radiography, increasing kVp tends to decrease patient dose because exposure time can be decreased. In CT, all other factors being equal, increasing kVp tends to increase patient dose.[7] In radiography, increasing kVp tends to reduce the number of photoelectric interactions in the patient because the probability of photoelectric interactions decreases as photon energy is increased. So

---

**Filtered back projection:* The standard method of reconstructing CT slices is called *back projection.* This involves reflecting back the projection across the image at the angle it was acquired. By reflecting back all of the projections associated with a complete revolution of the x-ray tube and detector system, a composite image (i.e., a summary of more and less intense detector signals) can be built up, producing a reconstructed image. This image looks similar to the real picture but is blurry. In order to fix the blurring problem created by standard back projection, a filter is superimposed on all of the back projections, thereby producing what is known as a *filtered back projection image.* Filtering refers to changing the projection data before doing the back projections to remove the blurriness. The simplest filter employed is a high-pass filter, or a sharpening filter. This type of filter picks up sharp edges within the projection (and thus, in the underlying slice) and tends to ignore flat areas. Because the high-pass filter actually creates negative pixels at the edges, it subtracts out the extra smearing caused by plain back projection. Thus the end result is a correct reconstruction. The high-pass filter, however, accentuates the noise already present in a CT image. In order to obtain a "cleaner" image, other "softer" filters have been developed to replace the high-pass filter for images that do not have very high contrast (with appreciation from xrayphysics.com/ctsim.html).

more photons go through the patient to strike the image receptor, and the exposure time may be decreased. However, in CT, because of the higher effective energy of the x-ray beam, both photoelectric and Compton interactions contribute substantially to the image. Also, x-ray tubes are more efficient when operated at higher kVp. So, if kVp is increased, the output of the x-ray tube increases during a set scan time, and the patient exposure actually increases. Controlling the variables of kVp, scan time, and tube current is a major part of most CT protocols for optimum use of patient dose.[8]

Patient Centering

Verifying that the center of the patient coincides with the center of the CT gantry is a significant part of dose reduction strategies that is under the control of the CT technologist. Miscentering of the patient by only a few centimeters can result in unnecessarily large differences in patient dose when the tube current modulation system or AEC is in use. If the patient is placed closer to the x-ray tube when the scout view (radiographic) image is obtained, then the image of the patient is magnified, causing the tube current modulation system to increase the tube current, thereby overdosing the patient. A miscentering of 2 centimeters can produce as much as a 25% unnecessary increase in patient dose.[9] Automatic patient miscentering correction software is becoming available to alleviate this problem,[10] but there is no substitute for proper positioning.

COMPUTED TOMOGRAPHY DOSE PARAMETERS

In order to approximate the effective radiation dose to a patient who has undergone a CT study, the values of two CT-specific dose markers or quantities need to be determined for each scan series. The following discussion introduces and briefly defines all the relevant parameters, describes how their values can be obtained, and shows their relationships to one another. The relevant dose parameters are as follows:

- CT dose index (CTDI)
- $CTDI_W$
- $CTDI_{vol}$
- Dose length product (DLP)

The last two items are the required dose markers. Their values directly depend on the details of the performed CT scan and are displayed by the scanner's software for

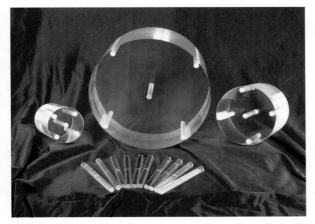

FIG 13.5 "Pencil" ionization chamber and acrylic body and head CTDI dosimetry phantoms.

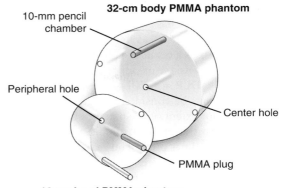

FIG 13.6 Demonstrates the measurement process for obtaining $CTDI_W$ for both the body and head phantoms. The pencil chamber will be successfully inserted into each of the four peripheral cavities and then into the central cavity and ionization measurements obtained. PMMA (poly methyl methacrylate) is an organic compound made up of carbon, hydrogen, and oxygen. It is the chemical name for what is commonly referred to as *acrylic* or *Lucite* or *Plexiglas*.

each completed patient scan. There is a direct progressive relationship among all four of the listed parameters, as demonstrated in the following paragraphs.

The CTDI is determined by an ionization measurement using a 1-cm diameter and 10-cm (100-mm) long, pencil-like, cylindric ionization chamber that has been inserted into a cylindrical acrylic phantom (Fig. 13.5). The phantom is similar in diameter to either a human head (16 cm diameter) or a human abdomen (32 cm diameter) and is scanned utilizing a single acquisition *axial* scan with technical factors (kVp, mAs, and slice thickness) that are equivalent to those used for a patient study. The irradiated pencil chamber is attached to an electrometer whose ionization charge reading, when multiplied by several correction factors, will then be given in milligray (mGy) units. Dividing this number by the scan direction collimation* will make this ionization measurement *representative* of the localized dose from a multiple slice examination. $CTDI_W$ is simply a weighted average of two measured CTDI values: one that is obtained with the pencil chamber placed in the central cavity of the acrylic phantom and the other derived from the average of

four peripheral (only 1-cm-deep) cavity measurements that are located at the 3, 6, 9, and 12 o'clock positions (Fig. 13.6).

$$CTDI_W = \frac{1}{3}(CTDI_{center}) + \frac{2}{3}(CTDI_{periph})$$

$CTDI_{VOL}$ is the average absorbed dose within the scanned volume. Its value is directly related to $CTDI_W$ by the following expression:

$$CTDI_{VOL} = CTDI_W / PITCH$$

For nonhelical or axial scans, such as those normally used in adult head scan sequences, the pitch (P) equals 1, and therefore $CTDI_{VOL} = CTDI_W$; but for typical helical scans, P is usually greater than 1 (e.g., 1.375 is quite common), so the magnitude of $CTDI_{VOL}$ will be less than that of $CTDI_W$.

The previous discussion demonstrates how a medical physicist can obtain a value for $CTDI_{VOL}$ by measurement. However, at the conclusion of each patient CT scan sequence, the built-in computer software accesses a database that supplies a numeric value of the $CTDI_{VOL}$ for that scan sequence. Also supplied is the value of a quantity called the *dose length product* (DLP).

DLP represents the product of the $CTDI_{VOL}$ and the irradiated scan length. It is expressed in milligray-centimeters

---

*Scan direction collimation is equal to the product of the number of data channels used during one axial acquisition (N) and the nominal slice width of one axial image (T). For example, in a single-slice scanner for a 10-mm slice thickness, N = 1 and T = 10, so NT = 10. In a multislice CT scanner with selected scan thickness parameters 5 mm, 4i (4i means four 5-mm slices acquired simultaneously), then N = 4, T = 5, and NT = 20.

(mGy-cm). DLP characterizes the volumetric extent along the patient's body that has been irradiated with an average absorbed dose. As such it has significance for estimating future cancer risk as a result of radiation doses unavoidably delivered to sensitive organs from CT examinations. Mathematically, **DLP = CTDI$_{VOL}$ × scan length.** Scan length, which may be considered as approximately the superior-inferior extent of the patient's irradiation, can be derived from the product of slice width times the number of slices times pitch. Thus a helical scan that is composed of 60 5-mm slices with a pitch of 1.5 has an approximate scan length of 60 × 0.5 × 1.5 = 45 cm. If instead, this were an axial scan, the scan length would be just 60 × 0.5 = 30 cm.

EFFECTIVE COMPUTED TOMOGRAPHY DOSE

What follows uses a table of scan region–specific conversion factors (Table 13.1) generated by the European Union[11] that when combined with the dose information supplied by the CT software for each delivered scan sequence will yield an effective dose (EfD) value for that CT scan. The simple expression to be used for calculation of EfD is given by the following equation:

$$EfD = DLP \times EfDLP$$

where EfDLP is the normalized EfD associated with a specific scan region of the body. EfDLP is expressed in millisieverts per milligray-centimeter (mSv/mGy-cm) and represents a conversion factor from a patient's CT scan dose length product to the effective dose received by the patient as a result of that scan. Experimentally determined numeric values for these factors are given in Table 13.1.

Using the values in Table 13.1 and the information displayed on the dose page printout for a patient's CT

scan, the EfD to the patient from that scan can be calculated. Several examples of using such data from actual patient CT scans are demonstrated in Cases 13.1 to 13.3. For greater ease of reading, some references to traditional units are included throughout the remainder of this chapter. Some typical effective dose values for computed tomography examinations can be found in Table 13.2.

In the early 2000s various publications calculated individual and population risks of cancer from CT based upon risk estimates from studies of the atomic bomb survivors. These studies were used to predict the number of cancers in large populations due to medical procedures such as CT by multiplying the small risk estimates for individual procedures by the large population of patients undergoing such studies every year. However, later analysis has shown no increase in risk of cancer or any other

TABLE 13.1   Scan Region Specific Conversion Factors

Body Region Scanned	Normalized Effective Dose (EfDLP) Factor
Head	0.0023
Neck	0.0054
Chest	0.017
Abdomen	0.015
Pelvis	0.019

CASE 13.1   Head Scan (Axial)

Scan data*: CTDI$_{VOL}$ = 60.8 mGy, DLP = 373 mGy-cm (portion of scan series at 140 kVp)
CTDI$_{VOL}$ = 49.1 mGy, DLP = 351 mGy-cm (portion of scan series at 120 kVp)
From Table 13.1, EfDLP = 0.0023.
Therefore the EfD to this patient is given by the following equation:

(373 + 351) × 0.0023 = 1.67 mSv (0.167 rem)

*See text for abbreviations.

CASE 13.2   Chest Scan (Helical)

Scan data*: CTDI$_{VOL}$ = 8.5 mGy, DLP = 323 mGy-cm
From Table 13.1, EfDLP = 0.017.
Therefore the EfD to this patient is given by the following equation:

323 × 0.017 = 5.49 mSv (0.549 rem)

*See text for abbreviations.

CASE 13.3   Abdominal Scan (Helical)

Scan data*: CTDI$_{VOL}$ = 10 mGy, DLP = 460 mGy-cm
From Table 13.1, EfDLP = 0.015.
Therefore the EfD to this patient is given by the following equation:

460 × 0.015 = 6.9 mSv (0.69 rem)

*See text for abbreviations.

measures of early death from effective doses below 100 mSv.[12,13] Routine head and body scans fall in the 1 to 10 mSv effective dose range, and CT angiography rarely exceeds 15 mSv. Because there is a very great uncertainty in the estimation of risk below 100 mSv, many of the major scientific and advisory bodies concerned with radiation bioeffects (UNSCEAR, ICRP, NCRP) have discredited this practice.[14-16] In 2011 the American Association of Physicists in Medicine issued a position statement[17] that includes the following:

> *"Discussion of risks related to radiation dose from medical imaging procedures should be accompanied by acknowledgement of the benefits of the procedures. Risks of medical imaging at effective doses below 50 mSv for single procedures or 100 mSv for multiple procedures over short time periods are too low to be detectable and may be nonexistent. Predictions of hypothetical cancer incidence and deaths in patient populations exposed to such low doses are highly speculative and should be discouraged."*

GOAL OF COMPUTED TOMOGRAPHY IMAGING FROM A RADIATION PROTECTION POINT OF VIEW

In summary, the goal of CT imaging should be to obtain the best possible image while delivering an acceptable level of ionizing radiation to the patient (i.e., optimize the dose to the patient). In the absence of specially designed scan protocols, the fulfillment of this responsibility lies with the technologist performing the examination.

PATIENT DOSE IN MAMMOGRAPHY

Mammography is used to detect breast cancer that is not palpable by physical examination (Fig. 13.7). Experts agree that yearly mammographic screening of women 50 years of age and older leads to earlier detection of breast cancer. Earlier treatment saves lives and reduces suffering. The value of mammography in younger women is somewhat controversial. The controversy has little to do with radiation risk (induction of breast cancer by radiation). Although it is still mentioned occasionally in the popular press, cancer researchers generally agree that radiation risk resulting from the small doses associated

TABLE 13.2   Typical Effective Dose Values for CT Examinations

Examination	Effective Dose (mSv)
Head	1–2
Chest	2–6
Abdomen	5–8
Pelvis	3–6
Coronary artery calcification	0.1–3
Coronary angiography	1–18

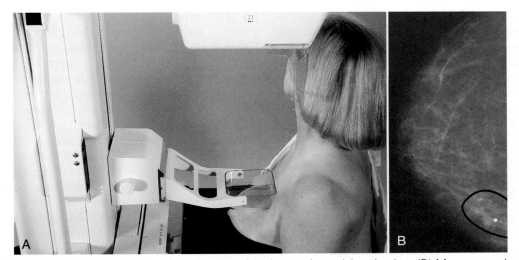

FIG 13.7 (A) Mammography of the breast using the craniocaudal projection. (B) Mammography can be used to detect breast cancer.

with mammography is negligible in all women.[18–20] Federal regulations for US Food and Drug Administration certification of screening mammography facilities state that the mean dose to the glandular tissue of a 4.5-cm compressed breast using a screen-film or digital mammography system should not exceed 3 mGy_t per view.[21] Studies have shown that well-calibrated mammographic systems are capable of providing excellent imaging performance with an average glandular dose of not more than 2 mGy_t.[22] The age recommendation for screening is controversial because mammography is less accurate in the detection of breast cancer in younger women and is likely to result in many false-positive readings, leading to unnecessary biopsies in that population. The increased density of the breast of younger women tends to reduce radiographic contrast, and therefore conventional screen-film mammography is frequently less sensitive in the average younger woman than in the average older woman. Digital mammography units, however, which can enhance contrast with image gray-level manipulation, offer substantial improvement for patients with dense breasts. Such units and the advent of a very new technique known as *Digital Tomosynthesis** will lower the percentage of false-positive readings caused by increased density and consequently permit a more effective screening of younger women. Earlier detection will save lives in general.

Mammography Screening

The authors of this textbook support the recommendations of the American College of Radiology, the American Cancer Society, and the American Medical Association. These groups advocate annual mammography screening or mammography screening at least every other year for women age 40 to 49 years. Before the onset of menopause, a baseline mammogram is also highly recommended for comparison with mammograms taken at a later age. The interested reader should contact these organizations for their latest policy statements on this subject.

---

*Digital Tomosynthesis is a method of breast imaging in which multiple (up to as many as 50) planar digital images, each at a slightly different angle, are acquired of a stationary compressed breast. Thus a series of different isocentric "slices" through the breast are obtained, which can be viewed either individually or in a sequence as a movie. The latter option allows a clinician to get an approximate three-dimensional view of the breast that permits a much more refined examination of suspicious architecture.

Dose Reduction in Mammography

Dose reduction in mammography can be achieved by limiting the number of projections taken or by lowering the dose associated with each projection. In standard mammography, axillary projections should be done only on request of the radiologist. If standard mammography is performed as a routine screening procedure, it is prudent to perform only craniocaudal and mediolateral projections of each breast with adequate compression to demonstrate breast tissue uniformly from the nipple to the most posterior portion.

Filtration for Mammographic Equipment

Appropriate attenuation is necessary for mammographic equipment, which produces photons with an energy range of 17 to 20 keV. Metallic elements such as molybdenum (Z = 42) and rhodium (Z = 45) are commonly employed as filters. When the x-ray tube target is made of molybdenum, either a 0.03-mm **molybdenum filter** or a 0.025-mm **rhodium filter** may be selected.[3] For rhodium x-ray tube targets, rhodium filters are used. These filtration and target materials facilitate a satisfactory level of contrast in the radiographic image over the clinical extent of compressed breast thickness. This is accomplished by preferentially selecting a particular range or window of energies from the x-ray spectrum emerging from the x-ray tube target that is very favorable for the photoelectric interaction. Molybdenum filters allow a lower energy window (17 to 20 keV) than rhodium filters (20 to 23 keV) (Fig. 13.8). Molybdenum filters are therefore suitable for small and average breast thickness, whereas rhodium filters used with a molybdenum or rhodium anode are better for larger or dense breasts[7] (i.e., compression thickness of 6 cm and greater) because they will produce an x-ray beam with higher or more penetrating energy. Systemic use of such materials has the effect of reducing the mean glandular dose in firm breast tissue. Maintaining and enhancing subject contrast are of paramount importance in mammography. Beryllium (Z = 4) takes the place of the glass in the window of the low-kVp x-ray producing mammographic x-ray tube to accommodate this need.[23] This light, strong metal permits the relatively soft characteristic radiation important for enhancing contrast to exit the tube without undergoing any significant attenuation.

Recently, it has been shown that newer, full-field digital mammography systems and digital tomosynthesis systems actually provide better images with tungsten targets with

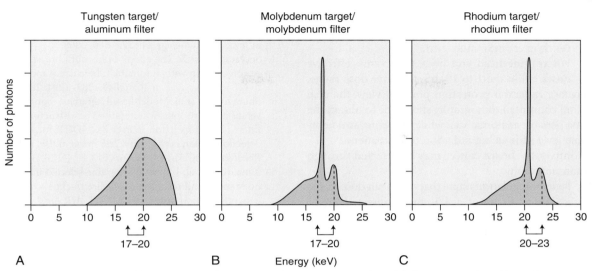

FIG 13.8 (A and B) X-ray emission spectra for tungsten and molybdenum anodes. Note that tungsten produces a high volume of x-ray photons above the 17 to 20 keV range considered ideal for mammography. These photons merely degrade the quality of the recorded image. The molybdenum anode, however, produces few x-ray photons above the ideal energy range, thereby initiating a higher contrast on the finished image. (C) A rhodium anode produces a higher average energy x-ray beam than does the molybdenum anode. The energy range for rhodium-produced photons is 20 to 23 keV. Photons from this energy range can provide better penetration of larger, denser breasts. (From Ballinger PW, Frank ED: *Merrill's Atlas of Radiographic Positions and Radiologic Procedures,* ed 9, St. Louis, 1999, Mosby.)

rhodium filtration (W/Rh) for most breast thicknesses and tungsten targets with silver filtration (W/Ag) for thicker breasts. Digital detectors are better able to separate out image features in mammography when presented with the broader spectra provided by the tungsten targets.

Molybdenum x-ray tube targets with molybdenum or rhodium filtration are being replaced in newer digital systems by tungsten targets with rhodium or silver filtration.[24,25]

■ SUMMARY

- Computed tomography is a frequently employed diagnostic x-ray imaging modality that is considered to be a relatively high radiation exposure examination.
  - With higher radiation exposure to the patient, there is potentially an increased associated cancer risk.
  - Skin dose and dose distribution are two concerns related to patient dose in CT scanning.
  - CT examinations generally expose a smaller mass of tissue than that exposed during an ordinary x-ray series.

- The entrance exposure from a CT examination may be compared with the entrance exposure received during a routine fluoroscopic examination.
  - When a series of adjacent slices is obtained, some radiation scatters from the slice being made into the adjacent slices. This is called *interslice scatter.*
  - Direct patient shielding is not typically used in CT.
  - When the spiral scan pitch ratio is approximately 1, the spiral CT patient dose is comparable to that produced by conventional or axial CT.
  - Tube current modulation in CT scanning can help to reduce patient dose.
- Recent advances in computer technology allow scan data to be reconstructed, modified, reconstructed again, modified, etc., until an image having the lowest noise possible is obtained. Such a repeat process is referred to as *iteration* and used in iterative reconstruction in CT.
  - In CT, all other factors being equal, increasing kVp tends to increase patient dose.
  - A miscentering of 2 centimeters can produce as much as a 25% increase in patient dose.[9]

- CTDI$_{VOL}$ and DLP are required dose markers.
- EfDLP is expressed in millisieverts per milligray-centimeter (mSv/mGy-cm).
- For routine head and body CT exams, effective doses fall in the 1 to 10 mSv effective dose range.
- From a radiation protection point of view, the goal of all computed tomography should be to obtain the best possible anatomic scan while delivering an acceptable level of ionizing radiation to the patient.
- Nonpalpable breast cancer may be detected through mammography.
  - Federal regulations state that the mean dose to the glandular tissue of a 4.5-cm compressed breast using a screen-film or digital mammography system should not exceed 3 mGy$_t$ per view.
  - Studies have shown that well-calibrated mammographic systems are capable of providing excellent imaging performance with an average glandular dose of not more than 2 Gy$_t$.[22]
  - Digital mammography units with the ability to enhance contrast with image gray-level manipulation offer substantial visualization improvement for patients with dense breasts.
  - Dose reduction in standard mammography can be achieved by limiting the number of projections taken.
  - Axillary projections in mammography should only be done on request of the radiologist.
  - Metallic elements such as molybdenum (Z = 42) and rhodium (Z = 45) are commonly employed as filters in mammography. However, molybdenum x-ray tube targets with molybdenum or rhodium filtration are being replaced in newer digital systems by tungsten targets with rhodium or silver filtration.
  - Beryllium (Z = 4) takes the place of glass in the window of the low kVp mammographic x-ray tube.

REFERENCES

1. Long BW, et al: *Merrill's atlas of radiographic positioning and procedures* (vol 3). ed 13, St. Louis, 2016, Elsevier/Mosby.
2. Schimmöller L, et al: Evaluation of automated attenuation-based tube potential selection in combination with organ-specific dose reduction for contrast-enhanced chest CT examinations. *Clin Radiol* 69:721–726, 2014.
3. Leswick DA, et al: Thyroid shields versus z-axis automatic tube current modulation for dose reduction at neck CT. *Radiology* 249:572–580, 2008.
4. Servaes S, Zhu X: The effects of bismuth breast shields in conjunction with automatic tube current modulation in CT imaging. *Pediatr Radiol* 43:1287–1294, 2013.
5. Shuman WP, et al: Model-based iterative reconstruction versus adaptive statistical iterative reconstruction and filtered back projection in liver 64-MDCT: focal lesion detection, lesion conspicuity, and image noise. *AJR Am J Roentgenol* 200(5):1071–1076, 2013.
6. Kanal KM, et al: Impact of operator-selected image noise index and reconstruction slice thickness on patient radiation dose in 64-MDCT. *AJR Am J Roentgenol* 189(1):219–225, 2007.
7. Pooley RA: Is it possible for a patient with a pacemaker to undergo MRI? *AJR Am J Roentgenol* W230, February, 2016. doi:10.2214/AJR.15.15696.
8. Lutz M, et al: Automated tube voltage selection in thoracoabdominal computed tomography at high pitch using a third-generation dual-source scanner: image quality and radition dose performance. *Invest Radiol* 50:352–360, 2015.
9. Mayo-Smith, et al: How I do it: managing radiation dose in CT. *Radiology* (vol 273). Number 3-December 2014, pp 657–672.
10. Auto Couch Height Positioning Compensation, Toshiba America Medical Systems, Inc: 2441 Michelle Dr., Tustin, CA 927890, 800-421-1968. Available for download from: http://medical.toshoba.com/downloads/ct-aq-one-fam-wp-sureexposure. (Last accessed 21 October 2016).
11. European Union, EUR 16262 EN: European guidelines on quality criteria for computed tomography, May, 1999. http://w3.tue.nl/fileadmin/sbd/Documenten/Leergang/BSM/European_Guidelines_Quality_Criteria_Computed_Tomography_Eur_16252.pdf.
12. Preston DL, et al: Solid cancer incidence in atomic bomb survivors: 1958-1998, *Radiat Res* 168:1–64, 2007.
13. Ozasa K, et al: Studies of the mortality of atomic bomb survivors: report 14, 1950-2003 – an overview of cancer and noncancer diseases. *Radiat Res* 177:229–243, 2012.
14. United Nations Scientific Committee on the Effects of Atomic Radiation (UNSCEAR): Report of the United Nations Scientific Committee Nations Scientific Committee on the Effects of Atomic Radiation (UNSCEAR). New York, NY; 2012.
15. (no author listed). The 2007 recommendations of the International Commission on Radiological Protection: ICRP publication 103. *Ann ICRP* 37:1–332, 2007.
16. Health Physics Society Website: Radiation risk in perspective. Position statement of the Health Physics

Society (PS010-1). http://hps.org/documents/riskps010-2.pdf. Revised 2010.

17. American Association of Physicists in Medicine website: AAPM position statement on radiation risks from medical imaging procedures: policy no. pp 25-A. www.aapm.org/org/policies/details.asp?id=318&type=pp. Published 2011.

18. Huda W, et al: Radiation doses due to breast imaging in Manitoba: 1978-1988. *Radiology* 177:813, 1990.

19. Ritenour ER, Hendee WR: Screening mammography: a risk vs. risk decision. *Invest Radiol* 24:17, 1989.

20. Taubes G: The breast-screening brawl. *Science* 275:1056, 1997.

21. Office of the Federal Register: Federal Register 67FR (5446) subpart B, section 900.12, e5 (vi), Feb 6, 2002, Washington, DC, U.S. Government Printing Office.

22. Yaffe M, Mawdsley GE: Equipment requirements and quality control for mammography, in specification, acceptance testing and quality control of diagnostic x-ray imaging equipment. In Siebert JA, Barnes GT, Gould RG, editors: *American Association of Physicists in Medicine medical physics monograph*, No. 20, College Park, Md, 1994, American Association of Physicists in Medicine.

23. Carlton RR, Adler AM: *Principles of radiographic imaging: an art and a science*, ed 5, Albany, NY, 2013, Delmar Cengage Learning, pp 578–579.

24. Baldelli P, Phelan N, Egan G: Investigation of the effect of anode/filter materials on the dose and image quality of a digital mammography system based on an amorphous selenium flat panel detector. *Br J Radiol* 83(988):290–295, 2010. doi:10.1259/bjr/60404532.

25. Williams MB, et al: Optimization of exposure parameters in full field digital mammography. *Med Phys* 36:2414–2423, 2008.

GENERAL DISCUSSION QUESTIONS

1. Why do CT examinations generally expose a smaller mass of tissue than what occurs during an ordinary x-ray series?

2. What is interslice scatter?

3. Recent advances in computed tomography allow scan data to be reconstructed, modified, reconstructed again, modified again, etc., until an image having the lowest noise possible is obtained. What is this repeat process referred to as?

4. What filters are recommended for use with a molybdenum anode when a mammographic examination is performed on a patient with larger or dense breasts? Why are they recommended?

5. Why is the age recommendation for screening mammography so controversial?

6. What are two concerns related to patient dose in CT scanning?

7. Why should ordering physicians weigh the benefits and risks of a CT scan procedure for a patient?

8. What is tube current modulation?

9. What are two required dose markers used in CT?

10. In what unit is EfDLP expressed, and how is EfDLP determined?

11. In the early 2000s various publications calculated individual and population risk of cancer due to CT based upon risk estimates from studies of what group of people?

12. What is the goal of CT imaging from a radiation protection point of view?

REVIEW QUESTIONS

1. Direct patient shielding is not typically used in:
   A. Computed tomography
   B. Digital fluoroscopy
   C. Computed radiography
   D. Digital radiography

2. As much as what percent of unnecessary increase in patient dose can a miscentering of 2 centimeters cause during a CT examination?
   A. 15%
   B. 25%
   C. 50%
   D. 75%

3. In CT examinations, which of the following interactions of x-radiation with matter contribute to the image?
   A. Coherent scattering and photodisintegration
   B. Compton scattering and pair production
   C. Photoelectric and Compton interactions
   D. Photoelectric and coherent interactions

4. In what mSv effective dose range do routine head and body CT examinations fall?
   A. 1 to 10
   B. 15 to 25
   C. 30 to 40
   D. 45 to 60

5. The entrance exposure from a CT examination may be compared with which of the following procedures?
   A. An interventional x-ray procedure
   B. A mammography examination

C. A single chest x-ray performed with a mobile x-ray unit

D. A routine fluoroscopic examination

6. When the spiral CT scan pitch ratio is approximately 1, to what is the spiral CT patient dose comparable?
   A. To that produced by conventional or axial CT unit
   B. To that produced by a magnetic resonance imaging machine
   C. To that produced by a dedicated mammographic unit
   D. To that produced by a routine diagnostic x-ray unit

7. Studies have shown that well-calibrated mammographic systems are capable of providing excellent imaging performance with an average glandular dose of not more than:
   A. 10 mGy$_t$
   B. 7 mGy$_t$
   C. 5 mGy$_t$
   D. 2 mGy$_t$

8. Digital mammography units, which can enhance contrast with image gray-level manipulation, offer substantial improvement for patients with:
   A. Thin breast tissue
   B. Sparse breast tissue
   C. Porous breast tissue
   D. Dense breast tissue

9. Axillary projections of the breast should be done only at the request of the:
   A. Administrator of the imaging facility
   B. Patient
   C. Radiologist
   D. Radiographer

10. What material takes the place of glass in the window of the low-kVp-producing mammographic x-ray tube?
    A. Aluminum
    B. Beryllium
    C. Copper
    D. Lead

14

Management of Imaging Personnel Radiation Dose During Diagnostic X-Ray Procedures

OBJECTIVES

After completing this chapter, the reader will be able to perform the following:

- Define all key terms.
- State the annual occupational effective dose limit for whole-body exposure of diagnostic imaging personnel during routine operations.
- Explain why occupational exposure of diagnostic imaging personnel must be limited, and state the most important reason for allowing a larger equivalent dose for radiation workers than for the population as a whole.
- Identify the type of x-radiation that poses the greatest occupational hazard in diagnostic radiology, and explain the various ways this hazard can be significantly reduced.
- Explain how the various methods and techniques that reduce patient exposure during a diagnostic examination can also reduce exposure for the radiographer and any other personnel.
- Discuss the responsibilities of the employer for protecting declared pregnant diagnostic imaging personnel from radiation exposure.
- Describe the three basic principles of radiation protection that can be used for personnel exposure reduction.
- State and explain the inverse square law, and solve mathematical problems applying this concept.
- Differentiate between a primary and a secondary protective barrier, and list examples of such barriers.

- Describe the construction of protective structural shielding, and list the factors that govern the selection of appropriate construction materials.
- Discuss the protective garments that may be worn to reduce whole-body or partial-body exposure and also the circumstances in which such garments are worn.
- List and explain the various methods and devices that may be used to reduce exposure for personnel during routine fluoroscopic examinations and during interventional procedures that use high level control fluoroscopy.
- Specify the techniques that are useful for reducing the radiographer's exposure when performing a mobile radiographic examination.
- Explain the variation in dose rate caused by scatter radiation near the entrance and exit surfaces of the patient during C-arm fluoroscopy, and speak about methods of dose reduction for C-arm operators.
- List the three categories of radiation sources that may be generated in an x-ray room, list the considerations on which the design of radiation-absorbent barriers should be based, and explain the importance of each.
- Differentiate between a controlled area and an uncontrolled area.
- Discuss current approaches to shielding design.
- Describe radiation warning signage.

KEY TERMS

Bucky slot shielding device
control-booth barrier
controlled area
cumulative effective dose
   (CumEfD) limit
distance

inverse square law (ISL)
leakage radiation
occupancy factor (T)
primary protective barrier
primary radiation
scatter radiation

secondary protective barrier
shielding
time
uncontrolled area
use factor (U)
workload (W)

Some x-ray procedures increase the radiographer's risk of exposure (Box 14.1) due to scatter radiation. This chapter presents an overview of methods that can be used to reduce exposure for imaging professionals during diagnostic x-ray procedures. In addition, a brief explanation of diagnostic x-ray suite radiation protection design is presented.

ANNUAL LIMIT FOR OCCUPATIONALLY EXPOSED PERSONNEL

Effective Dose Limits

Federal government standards, following a recommendation of the National Council on Radiation Protection and Measurements (NCRP), permit diagnostic imaging personnel to receive an "annual occupational effective dose (EfD) of 50 millisievert (mSv)"[1] for whole-body exposure during routine operations. However, in keeping with the ALARA policy and diligent supervision of personnel cumulative radiation exposure records, no radiographer should ever approach this effective dose level. To be clear, the dose level referred to here includes only occupational dose and not personal medical exposure that an employee may receive or the background exposure that all people receive.

To ensure that the lifetime risk of occupationally exposed personnel remains acceptable, an additional recommendation is that the *lifetime effective dose* in millisieverts should not exceed 10 times the person's age in years. Hence a **cumulative effective dose (CumEfD) limit** has been established for the whole body.

Annual Occupational and Nonoccupational Effective Dose Limits

The annual occupational effective dose limit of 50 mSv is an upper boundary limit. It is much greater than the annual effective dose limit allowed for individual members of the general population not occupationally exposed. That limit is:

BOX 14.1 Imaging Procedures That Increase the Radiographer's Risk of Exposure

- General fluoroscopy
- Interventional procedures that employ high level control fluoroscopy (HLCF)
- Mobile examinations
- C-arm fluoroscopy

- 1 mSv for *continuous or frequent* exposures from artificial sources other than medical irradiation and natural background radiation[1]
- 5 mSv for *infrequent* annual exposure[1]

The 1 mSv annual effective dose limit set for members of the general public is designed to limit that exposure "to reasonable levels of risk comparable with risks from other common sources—i.e., about 10^{-4} to 10^{-6} annually"[1] (10^{-4} to 10^{-6} means an excess cancer risk of 1 chance in 10,000 to 1 chance in 1 million per year). The 5 mSv maximal annual effective dose limit recommendation "is made because annual exposures in excess of the 1 mSv recommendation, usually to a small group of people, need not be regarded as especially hazardous, provided it does not occur often to the same groups and that the average exposure to individuals in these groups does not exceed an average annual effective dose of about 1 mSv."[1] Both these limits "will keep the annual equivalent dose to those organs and tissues that are considered in the effective dose system below levels of concern for tissue reactions."[1]

Allowance for a Larger Equivalent Dose for Radiation Workers

Valid reasons exist for permitting radiation workers to accumulate a larger equivalent dose (EqD). Among the most important of these reasons is that the workforce in radiation-related jobs is small when compared with the population as a whole. Therefore the expectation of any measurable increase in disease in the population, in individuals, or in impact upon the gene pool is negligible. Thus the amount of radiation received by this workforce can be larger than the amount received by the general public without alteration in the genetically significant dose, the average annual gonadal EqD to members of the population who are of childbearing age. Although the radiographer and other diagnostic imaging personnel are allowed to absorb more radiation, the EqD received must be minimized whenever possible. This reduces the potential for:
- Somatic damage
- Genetic damage

ALARA CONCEPT

The as low as reasonably achievable (ALARA) principle has been discussed elsewhere in the text (see Chapters 1 and 10). The best method for radiologists and radiographers to apply ALARA is to conscientiously employ all

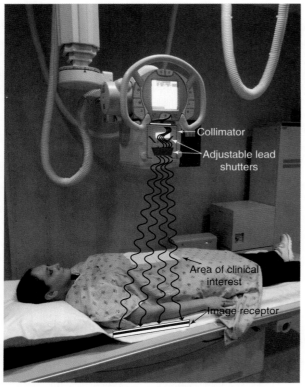

FIG 14.1 Radiographic beam collimation (restricting the x-ray beam to the area of clinical interest) limits the production of scattered radiation. This radiation-control procedure helps keep the radiographer's occupational exposure as low as reasonably achievable (ALARA).

appropriate radiation-control procedures to keep their exposure levels ALARA. Personnel should employ radiation control procedures such as:

- Applying the principles of time, distance, and shielding
- Adequately collimating the radiographic beam (Fig. 14.1)

DOSE-REDUCTION METHODS AND TECHNIQUES

Avoiding Repeat Imaging

Methods and techniques that reduce patient exposure can also reduce exposure for the radiographer, thereby limiting occupational exposure. Whenever a repeat image is performed because of human or mechanical error, the patient receives a double dose of primary radiation, while increasing the radiographer's potential for exposure to scattered radiation.

The Patient as a Source of Scattered Radiation

During any diagnostic x-ray examination, the patient becomes a source of scattered radiation as a consequence of the Compton interaction process. At a 90-degree angle to the primary x-ray beam, at a distance of 1 m, the scattered x-ray intensity is generally approximately 1/1000th of the intensity of the primary x-ray beam. This characteristic should always be kept in mind as an additional method of radiation protection.

Scattered Radiation—Occupational Hazard

Because scattered radiation poses the greatest occupational hazard in diagnostic radiology, the use of any device or imaging technique that lessens the amount of scattered radiation will significantly reduce occupational exposure of diagnostic imaging personnel. Beam constraint devices, such as automatic collimation or positive beam limitation, restrict the dimensions of the radiographic beam so that its margins do not extend beyond the image receptor. This reduction in beam size decreases the number of x-ray photons available to undergo Compton scatter. Because scatter is reduced, the radiographer's potential for occupational exposure is diminished.

Filtration of the Diagnostic X-Ray Beam

When a radiographic beam is properly filtered, nonuseful low energy photons are removed from the primary beam. Without proper filtration, a relatively high percentage of the normally excluded low energy photons will interact with the tissues of the patient's body. Some of these photons undergo Compton scatter. The radiographer's EqD could therefore increase as a result of exposure to this excess scattered radiation. Most of these low energy photons, however, are absorbed in the patient, thereby increasing the patient's absorbed dose and contributing nothing to the radiographic image. Thus filtration primarily benefits the patient.

Protective Apparel

Protective lead aprons (Fig. 14.2A) and, in their absence, shielded barriers (Fig. 14.2B) function as gonadal shields for diagnostic imaging personnel. These devices protect personnel from both scatter and leakage radiation, which are types of secondary radiation.

Like protective gloves that are used to cover the hands of radiologists or radiographers when they must be in or near the primary x-ray beam, lead aprons are available

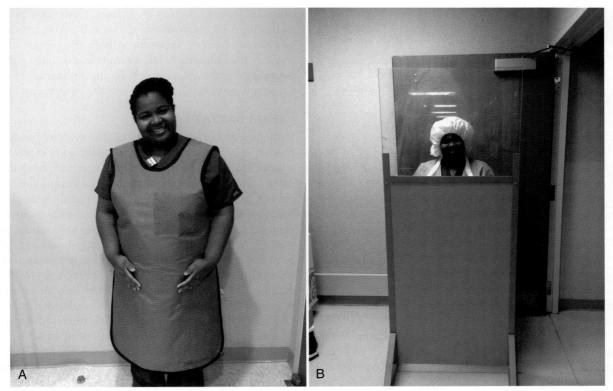

FIG 14.2 (A) A lead apron protects occupationally exposed personnel from scattered radiation. (B) A lead mobile x-ray barrier of 0.5- or 1.0-mm lead equivalent provides protection from scattered radiation. It may be used during special procedures, in the operating room, and in cardiac units.

in various thicknesses such as 0.25, 0.5, and 1 mm of lead equivalent.[2] Higher lead equivalents in protective apparel provide greater protection from radiation exposure. However, for practical use in the clinical setting, the weight of the garment must also be considered, along with the approximate length of time that it will be worn. An apron containing 1-mm lead equivalent may weigh as much as 12 kg.[2] Wearing this protective device for a lengthy procedure can therefore result in considerable back strain.* Depending on the energy range of the radiation for a specific procedure, an apron containing the lead equivalent of 0.5 mm or an apron containing

the minimum required lead equivalent of 0.25 mm may be sufficient for use. The standard 0.5-mm lead equivalent apron, which has traditionally been worn during routine fluoroscopic procedures, weighs 3 to 7 kg, whereas the 0.25 mm minimum lead equivalent apron can weigh 1 to 5 kg.[2] Some physical attributes of protective lead aprons, including the percentage of x-ray attenuation at selective peak kilovoltages (kVps), are listed in Table 14.1.

In the event that any personnel could have the posterior surface of their body turned toward the x-ray source during a radiologic procedure, a *wraparound style apron* would afford the best protection. When taking into consideration both the amount of protection provided by an apron and its weight, the 0.5-mm lead equivalent apron provides a good compromise for general use.

To preserve integrity, all protective apparel must be stored correctly when not in use. Lead aprons should be hung on racks or draped over a bar designed for storage to prevent unnecessary damage. They are never to be folded or crunched up in any fashion because this

---

*To reduce the possibility of back or neck problems, other materials may be used in the protective apron to lessen its weight. Some garments, for example, are impregnated with tin[2] or similar metals because the electron shell structures of these substances offer advantages in terms of a more probable photoelectric interaction attenuation than does lead in the lower diagnostic x-ray energy range.

TABLE 14.1   **Physical Attributes of Protective Lead Aprons**

Lead Equivalent Thickness (mm)	Weight (kg)	PERCENTAGE X-RAY ATTENUATION		
		KILOVOLTS AT PEAK		
		50	75	100
0.25	1–5	97	66	51
0.50	3–7	99.9	88	75
1.00	5–12	99.9	99	94

At 100 kVp, x-ray attenuation for a 0.50-mm lead equivalent apron and a 1-mm lead equivalent apron is 75% and 94%, respectively.

Modified from Bushong SC: *Radiologic Science for Technologists: Physics, Biology and Protection*, ed 10, St. Louis, 2013, Mosby.

will lead to cracks or breaks in the lead-impregnated material, thus compromising the device's effectiveness for protection from radiation. To be sure of the continued reliability of protective apparel, regulatory requirements state that all aprons be inspected on a yearly basis for cracks or other defects either by fluoroscopy or by radiographing each area of the apparel with a high kVp technique.

Technical Exposure Factors

Technical exposure factors can influence the quantity of scattered radiation produced and thereby reaching imaging personnel. For lower kVps, more mA is needed to secure a high quality image, and therefore greater numbers of low-energy photons are present. These characteristics of the x-ray beam lend themselves to the production of increased large-angle scatter radiation. Conversely, higher kVp techniques:

- Increase the mean energy of the photons comprising the radiographic beam, leading to a decrease in large angle scatter
- Require lower photon beam intensity (i.e., lower mAs)

Therefore less side-scattered radiation is available to strike imaging personnel, and the potential EqD is reduced.

Repeats in Digital Imaging

Because image contrast and overall brightness in digital imaging can be manipulated after image acquisition, the need for almost all repeats as a result of improper technical

exposure factors has been eliminated. However, repeats necessitated by mispositioning can still occur, causing additional radiation exposure to both the patient and possibly the radiographer. Care must be taken from the beginning of the examination by the radiographer to accurately position the patient and the equipment.

Patient Restraint

Radiographers must never stand in the primary (useful) beam to restrain a patient during a radiographic exposure (Fig. 14.3A). When patient restraint is necessary, mechanical restraining devices should be used to immobilize the patient whenever possible. If mechanical means of restraint are not feasible, nonoccupationally exposed persons, wearing appropriate protective apparel, are to perform this function. These individuals should be positioned so that their lead-protected torsos are not struck by the primary, or direct, beam (Fig. 14.3B). Holding patients may be necessary when they are unable to support themselves. For example, a weak elderly male patient may be unable to stand without assistance and raise his arms above his head for a lateral chest x-ray examination. In this situation, a nonoccupationally exposed person (relative or friend) equipped with a lead apron can hold the patient in position during the exposure. A mechanical restraining device is often used to hold an infant in the upright position for chest radiographs. If such a device is not available, the child has to be physically held (usually by a parent) during the exposure. Pregnant women are never to be permitted to assist in holding a patient during an exposure.

PROTECTION FOR PREGNANT PERSONNEL

Imaging Department Protocol

Pregnant staff members should be able to continue performing their duties without interruption of employment if they follow established radiation safety practices. Most health care facilities have policies for protecting pregnant personnel from radiation. Under these policies, an imaging professional who becomes pregnant first informs her supervisor. After this voluntary declaration has been made, the health care facility officially recognizes the pregnancy. The facility, through its radiation safety officer:

- Provides essential counseling
- Furnishes an appropriate additional radiation dosimeter

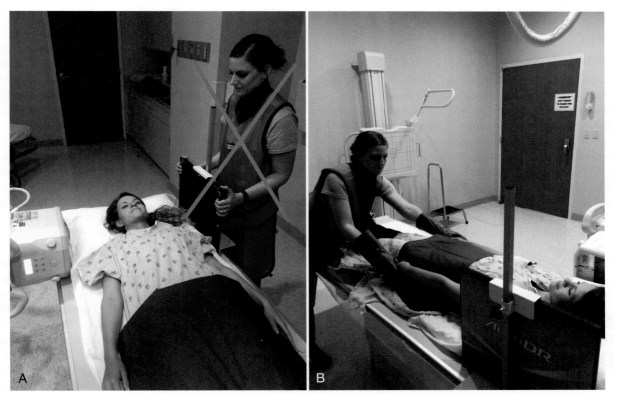

FIG 14.3 (A) The radiographer should never stand in the primary (useful) beam to restrain the patient. (B) A nonoccupationally exposed person restraining a patient during a radiographic exposure should wear a lead apron, gloves, and thyroid shield and stand outside the primary beam.

This additional dosimeter is to be worn at the waist level during all radiation procedures. When a protective lead apron is used, the dosimeter should be worn at waist level beneath the garment. The purpose of this additional monitor is to ensure that the monthly EqD to the embryo-fetus does not exceed 0.5 mSv. This EqD limit excludes:

- Medical radiation
- Natural background radiation

It is designed to significantly restrict the total lifetime risk of leukemia and other malignancies in persons exposed in utero.

Acknowledgment of Counseling and Understanding of Radiation Safety Measures

After receiving radiation safety counseling, the pregnant radiologic technologist must read and sign a form acknowledging that she has received counseling and understands the practices to be followed to ensure the safety of the embryo-fetus. For monitoring of pregnant personnel, a separate monthly report is provided to track the exposure of the worker and the embryo-fetus. A copy of this report is sent to the health care facility's radiation safety officer.

Protective Maternity Apparel

Protective maternity apparel, when needed, should be available for pregnant radiologists and radiographers. Specially designed maternity protective aprons consist of 0.5-mm lead equivalent over their entire length and width and have an extra 1-mm lead equivalent protective panel that runs transversely across the width of the apron to provide added safety for the embryo-fetus.

Wraparound protective aprons of 0.5-mm lead equivalent can also be used during pregnancy. The overall physical size of the apron must be appropriate for the pregnant worker to ensure safety and provide reasonable comfort.

Work Schedule Alteration

In accordance with ALARA guidelines, work schedules are designed to distribute radiation exposure risk evenly to all employees. If a declared pregnant radiographer is reassigned to a lower radiation exposure risk area (e.g., removed from interventional fluoroscopy and assigned to general radiography), then the remaining radiographers in the higher risk area who must fill in can be subject to increased risk. Therefore the declared pregnant radiographer does not necessarily need to be reassigned to a lower radiation exposure position as a direct consequence of a declared pregnancy. However, it is imperative that, while remaining in her current position, the EqD to the embryo-fetus from occupational exposure of the mother not exceed the NCRP recommended monthly EqD limit of 0.5 mSv or a limit of 5.0 mSv during the entire pregnancy.

BASIC PRINCIPLES OF RADIATION PROTECTION FOR PERSONNEL EXPOSURE REDUCTION

As previously stated, the three basic principles of radiation protection are:
- Time
- Distance
- Shielding

Occupational radiation exposure of imaging personnel can be minimized by the use of these cardinal principles.

Time

The amount of radiation a worker receives at a particular location is directly proportional to the length of time the individual is in the path of ionizing radiation. During fluoroscopy, reduced exposure time will decrease both:
- Patient exposure
- Personnel exposure

For this reason, most fluoroscopic x-ray units are equipped with 5-minute timers to alert the radiologist or other authorized equipment operator that a specific amount of time has elapsed. To minimize radiation exposure, a radiographer therefore should be present in a fluoroscopy room only when needed to perform relevant patient care and to fulfill the respective duties associated with the procedure. Otherwise, the radiographer should remain behind a protective barrier.

Distance

Distance is the most effective means of protection from ionizing radiation. Because there is a significant decrease in the radiation level as a consequence of the dispersion or spread of the radiation beam with distance, imaging personnel will receive significantly less radiation exposure by standing farther away from a source of radiation.

Application of the Inverse Square Law. The inverse square law (ISL) expresses the relationship between distance and intensity (quantity) of radiation and is significant as a tool to be used in governing the dose received by personnel. The law is stated as follows: "The intensity of radiation is inversely proportional to the square of the distance from the source."

To be more explicit, as the separation between the radiation source and a measurement point increases, the quantity of radiation measured at the more distant position decreases by the square of the ratio of the original distance from the source to the new distance from the source (Fig. 14.4). This lowering of radiation concentration physically occurs because the area, which the same flux of x-rays at the original location now covers at the new location, has increased by the square of the relative distance change. For example, when the distance from the x-ray target, a point source* of radiation, is doubled, the radiation at the new location spans an area four times larger than the original area. However, because the same amount of radiation exists to cover this larger area, the intensity at the new distance consequently decreases by a factor of four (Fig. 14.5).

The ISL may be stated as a formula, shown in the equation in Box 14.2. A mathematical example is also provided. The ISL should be used whenever possible to reduce the radiographer's exposure from sources of x-radiation. (This law also may be applied to sources of gamma and neutron radiation.)

---

*Point source: To be able to correctly treat finite-sized radioactive sources as "point sources" so as to facilitate the calculation of exposure rates at points of interest, it is necessary that the distance of such points from the radioactive source be at least equal to 10 times the largest dimension of the source. As an example of this concept, consider a spherical radioactive source whose diameter is 2.5 cm. Then the smallest distance away from this source at which it may be accurate enough to regard it mathematically as a "point source" will be 25 cm.

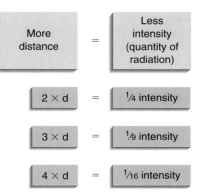

FIG 14.4 As the distance between the source of radiation and any given measurement point increases, radiation intensity (quantity) measured at that point decreases by the square of the relative change in distance between the new location and the old.

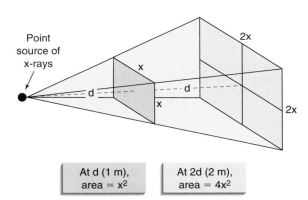

| At d (1 m), area = x^2 | At 2d (2 m), area = $4x^2$ |

FIG 14.5 When the distance from a point source of radiation is doubled, the radiation at the new location spans an area four times larger than the original area. However, the intensity at the new distance is only one-fourth of the original intensity.

The ISL also implies that if a radiographer moves closer to a source of radiation, his or her radiation exposure can dramatically increase. For example, if the radiographer stands 2 meters away from an x-ray source instead of 6 meters away, the radiographer's radiation exposure increases by a factor of $(6/2)^2 = 9$.

Shielding

When it is not possible to use the principles of time and/or distance to minimize occupational radiation exposure, **shielding** of appropriate thickness may be used to provide

---

BOX 14.2   Inverse Square Law Formula and Example

$$\frac{I_1}{I_2} = \frac{(d_2)^2}{(d_1)^2}$$

where I_1 expresses the exposure (intensity) at the original distance, I_2 expresses the exposure (intensity) at the new distance, d_1 expresses the original distance from the source of radiation, and d_2 expresses the new distance from the source of radiation.

Example: If a radiographer stands 1 m away from an x-ray tube and is subject to an exposure rate dose* of 2 mGy$_a$ per hour, what will it be if the same radiographer moves to a position located 2 m from the x-ray tube? Answer:

$$\frac{I_1}{I_2} = \frac{(d_2)^2}{(d_1)^2}$$

$$\frac{2}{I_2} = \frac{(2)^2}{(1)^2}$$

$$\frac{2}{I_2} = \frac{4}{1} \text{ (cross-multiply)}$$

$$4I_2 = 2$$

$$I_2 = 0.5 \, mGy_a/hr$$

*Exposure rate dose given in units of mGy$_a$ per hour is the same quantity as air kerma rate.

adequate protection from radiation. The most common materials used for structural protective barriers are:
- Lead
- Concrete

Accessory protective devices are made of lead-impregnated vinyl. These accessory devices include:
- Aprons
- Gloves
- Thyroid shields
- Protective eyeglasses

This apparel is to be used when it is not possible to remain wholly behind either a stationary or movable protective barrier. The ability of materials to attenuate radiation depends on their atomic number, density, and thickness.

Protective Structural Shielding. Structural barriers such as walls and doors in an x-ray room have been designed to provide radiation shielding for both:
- Imaging department personnel
- The general public

These barriers are necessary to ensure that occupational and nonoccupational annual effective dose limits are not exceeded. Lead sheets of appropriate thickness that are placed in the walls of the radiography or fluoroscopy room are generally used to provide proper shielding. A qualified medical physicist determines the exact protection requirements for a particular imaging facility. Although radiographers should understand the concept of shielding, they are not responsible for determining barrier thickness.

Primary protective barrier. The purpose of a **primary protective barrier** is to prevent direct, or unscattered, radiation from reaching personnel or members of the general public on the other side of the barrier. The primary beam is made up of the x-ray photons that follow straight-line paths through all sets of collimator shutters. Primary protective barriers are located perpendicular to the undeflected line of travel of the x-ray beam (Fig. 14.6).

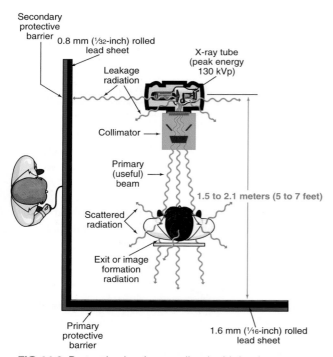

Secondary protective barrier
0.8 mm (1/32-inch) rolled lead sheet
X-ray tube (peak energy 130 kVp)
Leakage radiation
Collimator
Primary (useful) beam
1.5 to 2.1 meters (5 to 7 feet)
Scattered radiation
Exit or image formation radiation
Primary protective barrier
1.6 mm (1/16-inch) rolled lead sheet

FIG 14.6 Protective barriers are lined with lead to protect personnel and the general public from radiation. The primary protective barrier is located perpendicular to the undeflected line of travel of the x-ray beam. The walls that are not in the direct line of travel of the primary beam are called *secondary protective barriers* because they are designed to shield only against secondary (leakage and scattered) radiation.

If the peak energy of the beam is 120 kVp, the primary protective barrier in a typical installation:
- Consists of 1.6 mm (1/16 inch) lead
- Extends 2.1 m upward from the floor of the x-ray room, when the x-ray tube is 1.5 to 2.1 m from the wall in question

Secondary protective barrier. Secondary radiation consists of radiation that has been deflected from the primary beam. Leakage from the tube housing (photons that pass through the housing because the lead shielding around the tube for practical reasons cannot be made perfect) and scatter (primarily from the patient) make up the secondary radiation. A **secondary protective barrier** protects against leakage and scatter radiation. Any wall or barrier that is never struck by the primary x-ray beam is classified as a secondary barrier (see Fig. 14.6). This does not mean that secondary radiation cannot hit primary barriers as well. A secondary barrier should overlap the primary protective barrier by approximately 1.27 cm (1/2 inch). In a typical installation, the secondary barrier consists of 0.8 mm (1/32 inch) of lead.

Radiographic and fluoroscopic exposures should be made only when the doors to x-ray rooms are closed. This practice affords a substantial degree of protection for persons in areas adjacent to the room door because in most facilities room doors have attenuation for diagnostic energy x-rays equivalent to that provided by 0.8 mm (1/32 inch) of lead.

Control-booth barrier. X-ray rooms housing permanent radiographic equipment contain a **control-booth barrier** for the protection of the radiographer. This barrier must:
- Extend at least 2.1 m upward from the floor
- Be permanently secured to the floor

Diagnostic x-rays should scatter a minimum of two times before reaching any area behind this barrier. Because this booth is situated so that it intercepts leakage and scattered radiation only, it may be regarded as a secondary protective barrier. To ensure maximum protection during radiographic exposures, personnel must remain *completely* behind the barrier. The radiographer may observe the patient through the lead glass window* in the booth (Fig. 14.7). This window typically consists of 1.5-mm (~ 1/6-inch) lead equivalent. With the appropriate degree

---

*The wall barrier of the control booth should be at least 46 cm (18 inches) beyond the edge of the view window.

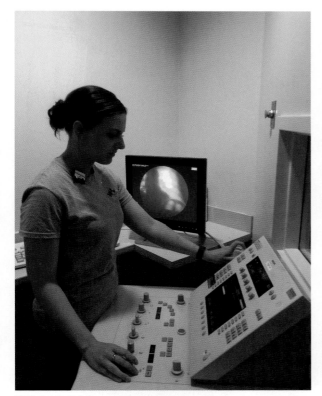

FIG 14.7 While making a radiographic exposure with a stationary radiographic unit, the radiographer must remain completely within the control-booth barrier (behind the fixed protective barrier) for safety. The radiographer may observe the patient through the lead glass observation window in the control booth.

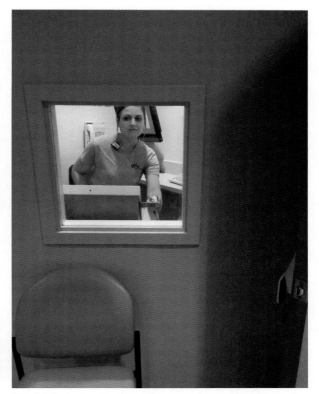

FIG 14.8 A clear lead acrylic secondary protective barrier impregnated with approximately 30% lead lends a modern appearance to the facility.

of shielding in the barrier, exposure of the radiographer will not exceed a maximum allowance of 1 mSv per week; in actual practice in a well-designed facility, exposure should not exceed 0.02 mSv per week. For further protection, the exposure cord, if one is present, must be short enough that the exposure switch can be operated only when the radiographer is completely behind the control-booth barrier.

Clear lead–acrylic secondary protective barrier. Clear lead–acrylic material impregnated with approximately 30% lead by weight may be fashioned into an effective secondary protective barrier, such as for the control booth (Fig. 14.8). This creates a modern appearance for the facility and permits a panoramic view, allowing diagnostic imaging personnel to observe the patient more completely. Modular x-ray barriers:

- Are shatter resistant
- Can extend 2.1 m upward from the floor
- Are available in lead equivalency from 0.3 to 2 mm

Clear lead–acrylic overhead protective barrier. Clear lead–acrylic protective barriers also can be used as overhead x-ray barriers to provide an open view during special procedures and cardiac catheterization (Fig. 14.9). This shielding typically offers 0.5-mm lead equivalency protection.

Accessory Protective Devices. Accessory protective shielding includes aprons, gloves, and thyroid shields made of lead-impregnated vinyl. These protective garments are available in a variety of:

- Shapes
- Sizes
- Thicknesses

As lead equivalent thickness increases, attenuation of the x-ray beam also increases when kVp remains the same.

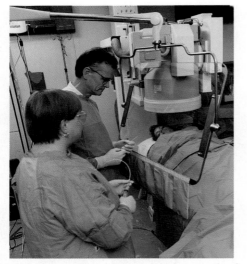

FIG 14.9 A clear lead acrylic overhead protective barrier used during special procedures and cardiac catheterization. (From Fluke Biomedical.)

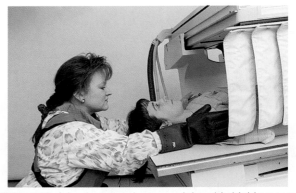

FIG 14.10 A lead apron, gloves, and thyroid shield protect the radiographer from scattered radiation.

Requirements for lead aprons and gloves. If the radiographer's hands will be near the x-ray beam, leaded gloves should be used. A suitable lead apron is to be worn whenever the radiographer cannot remain behind a protective barrier during an exposure (Fig. 14.10). Historically, from regulatory doctrine, if the peak energy of the x-ray beam was 100 kVp, then a protective apron's attenuation must be equivalent to at least a 0.25 mm thickness of lead. An apron of 0.5-mm lead equivalent, however, affords much greater security and is the most widely used and recommended thickness in diagnostic imaging and, in fact, is the minimum lead equivalent required for a protective garment worn by occupationally exposed individuals during fluoroscopic or interventional procedures. Thus regardless of the regulatory mention of 0.25 mm thicknesses of lead for some purposes, the need for 0.5-mm lead equivalent for fluoroscopy and interventional cases and the recommendations from various authorities that 0.5-mm lead aprons are desirable for all purposes have induced most facilities to stock personal shielding devices of this nature only. This eliminates the possibility of personnel inadvertently selecting the wrong apron. Therefore 0.5-mm has become the all-purpose apron of choice and in many cases, should also be in a wraparound style. A lead apron with 0.25 mm of lead is, however, very appropriate for use in mammography.

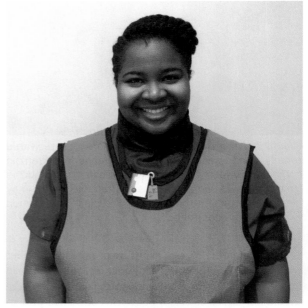

FIG 14.11 The neck and thyroid gland can be protected from radiation exposure through the use of a 0.5-mm lead equivalent protective shield.

Neck and thyroid shield. A neck and thyroid shield (Fig. 14.11) is employed to guard the thyroid area of occupationally exposed personnel during:
• General fluoroscopy
• X-ray special procedures
The neck and thyroid shield should be a minimum of 0.5-mm lead equivalent.

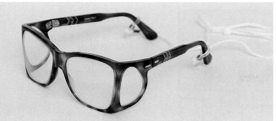

FIG 14.12 Eyeglasses protect the lens of the eyes during general fluoroscopy and special procedures. (Shown are glasses with wraparound frames; other styles are also available.)

Protective eyeglasses. Scatter radiation to the lens of the eyes of diagnostic imaging personnel can be substantially reduced by the use of protective eyeglasses (Fig. 14.12), fitted with optically clear lenses that contain a minimal lead equivalent protection level of 0.35 mm. Side shields on the glasses are also available for procedures that require turning of the head. A wraparound frame containing optically clear lenses with 0.5-mm lead equivalent may also be acquired.

X-RAY TUBE HOUSING CABLES

Although the x-ray tube housing is also designed to protect the operator from the hazard of electric shock, the radiographer must be careful when handling this piece of equipment and its adjoining part, the collimator. While manipulating the tube housing for a radiographic examination, the radiographer should avoid handling or severely bending the high-tension cables that connect to the positive and negative terminals of the x-ray tube. No one should touch the tube housing or high-tension cables while a radiographic exposure is in progress.

PROTECTION DURING FLUOROSCOPIC PROCEDURES

Personnel Protection

To ensure protection from scattered radiation emanating from the patient during a fluoroscopic examination, the radiographer should:
- Stand as far away from the patient as is practical
- Move closer to the patient only when assistance is required

A protective apron of at least 0.5-mm lead equivalent must be worn during all fluoroscopic procedures.

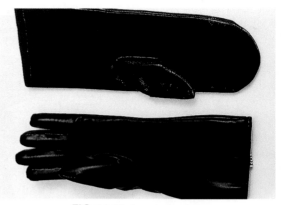

FIG 14.13 Lead gloves.

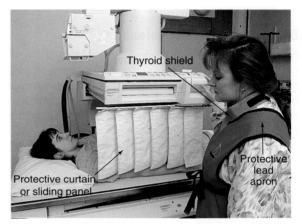

FIG 14.14 Scattered radiation produced during a fluoroscopic examination can be absorbed by a protective curtain or sliding panel, with a minimum of 0.25-mm lead equivalent placed between the fluoroscopist and the patient.

Protective lead gloves of at least 0.25-mm lead equivalent should be worn whenever the hands must be placed near the fluoroscopic field (Fig. 14.13). Imaging personnel assisting during a fluoroscopic examination also should wear thyroid shields of 0.5-mm lead equivalent, especially if they are standing in close proximity to the patient being examined (Fig. 14.14). If immediate presence assisting a radiologist during a fluoroscopic examination is not required near the x-ray table, the radiographer should either stand behind the radiologist, who is also wearing protective apparel, or stand behind the control-booth barrier until his or her services are required. To protect

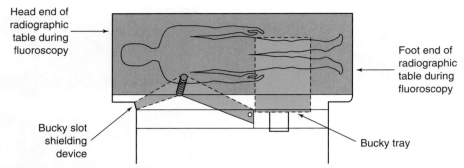

FIG 14.15 To provide protection at the gonadal level for the fluoroscopist, the Bucky slot shielding device should be at least 0.25-mm lead equivalent.

personnel who must move around the x-ray room during a fluoroscopic examination, a wraparound protective apron is recommended.

Dose-Reduction Techniques

Many of the methods and devices that reduce the radiographer's exposure when operating stationary (fixed) radiographic equipment also reduce the dose received by the radiographer and the radiologist during a fluoroscopic procedure. These methods and devices include:

- Adequate beam collimation
- Adequate filtration
- Control of technical exposure factors
- Appropriate source-to-skin distance
- Use of a cumulative timing device
- Diagnostic-type protective x-ray tube housing

Some additional requirements are included in the federal government specifications for the use of fluoroscopic equipment to ensure adequate protection for both the radiographer and the radiologist.

Remote Control Fluoroscopic Systems

The remote control unit provides imaging personnel the best radiation protection opportunity. It permits the radiologist and assisting radiographer to remain outside of the fluoroscopic room at a control console located behind a protective barrier until their presence within the room is needed. This system consequently further improves imaging personnel safety because the added distance from the x-ray tube makes use of the inverse square law.

Protective Curtain

A protective curtain, or sliding panel, with a minimum of 0.25-mm lead equivalent should normally be positioned between the fluoroscopist and the patient to intercept scattered radiation above the tabletop (see Fig. 14.14).

Bucky Slot Shielding Device

A Bucky slot shielding device of at least 0.25-mm lead equivalent must automatically cover the Bucky slot opening in the side of the x-ray table during a standard fluoroscopic examination when the Bucky tray is positioned at the foot end of the table (Fig. 14.15). This shielding device protects the radiologist and radiographer at the gonadal level. Without this device and the protective curtain in place, the exposure rate for the fluoroscopist would exceed 1 mGy$_a$/hr at a distance of 0.6 m from the side of the x-ray table.

Rotational Scheduling of Personnel

Diagnostic imaging personnel are potentially subjected to the highest occupational exposure during:

- Fluoroscopy
- Mobile radiography
- Special procedures
- Interventional surgery

Scheduling radiographers to spend less time in these higher radiation tasks by arranging assignments to clinical areas in a rotational pattern can decrease this exposure. This practice therefore uses the cardinal safety principle of *time* as a means of additional radiation protection.

PROTECTION DURING MOBILE RADIOGRAPHIC EXAMINATIONS

Use of Protective Garments

Mobile radiographic systems create special radiation protection considerations for the radiographer. Some states require radiographers to wear lead aprons whenever they are performing mobile radiographic or fluoroscopic examinations. A protective apron should be assigned to each mobile unit so that it is immediately available for the radiographer.

Distance as a Means of Protection

Some mobile units are equipped with a remote control exposure device. This permits the radiographer to leave the immediate vicinity and uses the cardinal principle of *distance* as an effective means of protection from radiation. Most mobile units are not remote controlled. For them the cord leading to the exposure switch must be long enough to permit the radiographer to stand at least 2 m from the:
- Patient
- X-ray tube
- Useful beam

Where the Radiographer Should Stand During a Mobile Radiographic Procedure

If possible, the radiographer should also attempt to stand at a right angle (90 degrees) to the x-ray beam–scattering object (the patient) line. This is the location at which the least amount of scattered radiation is received (Fig. 14.16). However, because distance and shielding have much more influence on the reduction of exposure to the technologist, these factors should be addressed first.

PROTECTION DURING C-ARM FLUOROSCOPY

Personnel Exposure From Scattered Radiation

Safety procedures are particularly important when mobile fluoroscopy (C-arm) systems are used. Because patterns of exposure direction are less predictable and the equipment is frequently operated by physicians whose training and experience in radiation safety may not match those of an experienced radiologist, the radiographer should exercise special vigilance. For C-arm devices with similar fields of view, the dose rate for personnel located within a meter of the patient is comparable to that in routine fluoroscopy—approximately several milligray in air (mGy_a) per hour. Exposure of personnel is caused by scattered radiation from the patient. During operating room procedures in which cross-table exposures are used

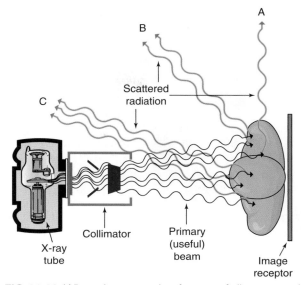

FIG 14.16 When the protective factors of distance and shielding have been accounted for, the radiographer will receive the least amount of scattered radiation by standing at a right angle (90 degrees) to the scattering object (the patient) (in position A). The most scattered radiation would be received at point C because of backscatter coming from the patient. (Intensity, or quantity, of x-ray exposure at any given point is indicated in this picture by the number of scattered x-rays reaching that point.)

(Fig. 14.17), an understanding of the patterns of x-ray scatter is particularly useful. The exposure rate caused by scatter near the entrance surface of the patient (the x-ray tube side) exceeds the exposure rate caused by scatter near the exit surface of the patient (the image intensifier side). The difference in the amount of scatter, typically a factor of 2 or 3, is caused by the higher radiation intensity at the entrance surface of the patient. Thus the location of the lower potential scatter dose is on the side of the patient away from the x-ray tube (i.e., the image intensifier side). Obviously, the radiographer should never encounter the actual useful beam.

Need for Protective Apparel for All Personnel and Monitoring of Imaging Personnel

The C-arm fluoroscope can be manipulated into almost any position and remain in an energized state for lengthy periods to accommodate, for example, an orthopedic surgeon performing an open reduction of a fractured

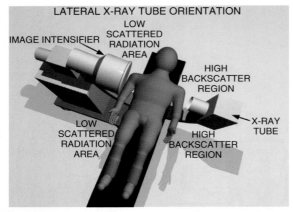

FIG 14.17 Cross-table exposure during use of a C-arm fluoroscope. The exposure rate caused by scatter near the entrance surface of the patient (the x-ray tube side) exceeds the exposure rate caused by scatter near the exit surface of the patient (the image intensifier side). The location of lower potential scatter dose is on the side of the patient away from the x-ray tube (i.e., the image intensifier side). (From Mark Rzeszotarski.)

hip in the operating room or a vascular surgeon performing an interventional procedure. When radiographers and other medical personnel participate in procedures that require this unit to be energized for significant durations, they are subject to increased radiation exposure. In addition, the physical configuration of a C-arm fluoroscopic unit limits the methods that can be used to achieve protection from scattered radiation. For this reason, personnel who routinely operate a C-arm fluoroscope or those who are in the immediate area of the unit when it is energized must wear a lead apron instead of crowding behind a portable lead–acrylic shield. This garment should be 0.5-mm lead equivalent to ensure adequate protection. A neck and thyroid shield of 0.5-mm lead equivalent should also be worn. Appropriate monitoring of imaging personnel who are normally involved in C-arm fluoroscopic procedures is mandatory.

Positioning of the C-Arm Fluoroscope

The positioning of a C-arm fluoroscope with the x-ray tube over the table and the image intensifier underneath the table results in higher exposure of the patient and increased scatter radiation. From the perspective of increased radiation safety, it is best to reverse the C-arm to place the x-ray tube under the table and the image intensifier over the table (see Fig. 11.24).

Exposure Reduction for Personnel

At the start of each procedure, the equipment operator should set the unit's cumulative timer to zero so that it will be possible to be aware of the amount of beam-on time actually used.[3] When some type of image storage device (e.g., last image hold) is used in conjunction with the unit, beam-on time decreases and therefore exposure reduction increases. If the image intensifier is positioned as close to the patient as possible, the required fluoroscopic x-ray beam intensity is minimized. This equipment–patient arrangement also permits the image intensifier to function more effectively as a scatter barrier between the patient and the person operating the C-arm fluoroscope. All these methods can lead to significant exposure reduction to both personnel and patient.

During a procedure involving the use of a C-arm fluoroscope, it is imperative that the patient's anatomic region of interest be oriented correctly with a minimal use of "positioning" fluoroscopy.[3] Furthermore, collimating the x-ray beam to the smallest area possible that includes the anatomic area of interest will decrease the amount of scattered radiation produced from the interaction of the x-ray beam with the patient, the actual scattering object.

Because distance from the source of radiation is the simplest method of protection for occupationally exposed personnel, C-arm operators should use it to their advantage whenever possible. Usually, this can be accomplished by using the foot pedal or the handheld exposure switch with the cables extended away from the machine as far as possible when making x-ray exposures.

For better visualization of small body parts, C-arm fluoroscopes have the capability to magnify the image. However, the use of magnification usually requires greater mA, which produces additional radiation exposure. *Mag mode* should be used only on the request of the physician performing the procedure.[3]

PROTECTION DURING HIGH LEVEL CONTROL INTERVENTIONAL PROCEDURES

Increased Importance of Radiation Safety Techniques

All the standard precautions and procedures for the reduction of dose to personnel are applicable during interventional procedures. Here, these techniques take on an increased importance because of the extended length of some of these procedures, the large number of digital images that may be taken, and, in certain studies, the frequent use of the high level control (boost) mode of operation. In boost mode, the exposure rate may significantly exceed the rate used in routine fluoroscopy (e.g., maximum allowed entrance exposure rate dose to a patient in regular fluoroscopy is 10 cGy/minute, whereas in high level or boost mode this value can range upward to 20 to 40 cGy/minute).

Knowledge of Dose-Reduction Techniques Required by the Radiographer

Although the duration of the procedure and the number of the exposures taken are under the control of the radiologist or other interventional physician, the radiographer should verify that all dose-reducing features are available and in good working order. These include the presence of:

- High-quality, low-dose fluoroscopy mode
- Pulsed beam operation (e.g., using 7.5, 15, or 30 radiation pulses/second in place of continuous fluoroscopy radiation)
- Manual collimation
- Correct beam filtration
- Removable grids
- Road mapping*
- Time interval differences†
- Last image hold mode

Road mapping is a method of digital image subtraction in which the frame that contains the greatest amount of contrast material in vessels is identified and is then subtracted from all subsequent images. Live fluoroscopic images of the catheter moving through the vasculature can then be seen even after the vessels contain less contrast. By using this equipment feature, overlaying of two images can be accomplished (e.g., a stored image and a current image). Thus there is a decrease of procedure time because fewer mask images are needed. This leads to some reduction in radiation dose. Choosing the road-mapping feature in place of cineradiography can also result in a lower radiation dose.

†*Time-interval difference* is a method of digital image subtraction in which each image is subtracted from an image a few frames in advance. This technique reveals vessels containing material and suppresses soft tissue in the images. It is less sensitive to patient motion than when the first image is subtracted from all successive images. Employing this feature results in a reduction of fluoroscopy "on time" because there is a time interval between the images. Less beam-on time decreases radiation dose.

As we discussed previously, using the last image hold mode feature, the operator does not need to be exposed again simply to review the position of a catheter in relation to landmarks when no new information is needed. Also, if possible, the beam entry side could be changed during the procedure to reduce the total dose to any one area of skin.

High level control is to be used sparingly and only when increased visualization is necessary during a critical maneuver such as embolization or deployment of devices such as stents.[4] Many standard and C-arm interventional fluoroscopic systems now possess the technical capability for standardized dose structure reporting.[5] This is accomplished through printouts from these units that yield an actual exposure record for every examination. For older equipment that does not have printout capability, records should be kept so that the cumulative fluoroscopic exposure time may be determined.

How the Radiologist or Other Interventional Physician Can Reduce Radiation Exposure

The radiologist or other interventional physician can reduce radiation exposure by the following means:

- Decreasing the duration of the procedure, thereby shortening fluoroscopic beam-on time
- Taking fewer digital images
- Reducing the use of continuous fluoroscopic mode relative to the pulsed mode of operation
- Retaining the protective curtain, if available, on the image intensifier or keeping the scatter shield in place during a procedure
- Regularly using the last image hold feature to view the most recent fluoroscopic image

These practices will substantially decrease exposure not only to all participating personnel but to the patient as well.

Extremity Monitoring

Because the hands and forearms of physicians performing interventional procedures can be subjected to large radiation exposures if the safety protocol is not carefully followed—and sometimes this may not be possible—it is important that extremities be monitored. Physicians need to be aware of the recommended dose limits that have been established for extremities. The NCRP currently recommends an annual EqD limit to localized areas of the skin and hands of 500 mSv. To avoid even remotely approaching this quite large limit and consequently increasing the possibility of future adverse effects, protective gloves should be worn whenever feasible by any physician whose hands will, of necessity, often be close to the fluoroscopic beam.

DIAGNOSTIC X-RAY SUITE PROTECTION DESIGN

Requirement for Radiation-Absorbent Barriers

To reduce the EfD to radiographers, nonoccupationally exposed personnel, and the general public to levels deemed statistically safe by both federal and international bodies, every room in which a diagnostic x-ray unit is housed must be equipped with radiation-absorbent barriers. The design of these barriers is based on considerations listed in Box 14.3.

Reason for Overshielding

The shielding designer must take all the factors identified in Box 14.3 into account to meet necessary radiation protection standards. In addition, the designer should plan conservatively to satisfy future regulatory limits that may be more stringent. This and the ALARA principle are two reasons why many diagnostic x-ray facilities are overshielded. Spending extra money up front for additional shielding is far easier and much less expensive than adding it after the suite has been completed.

BOX 14.3   Radiation-Absorbent Barrier Design Considerations

- The mean energy of the x-rays that will strike the barrier
- Whether the barrier is of a primary or a secondary nature
- The distance from the x-ray source to a position of occupancy 0.3 m from the barrier
- The workload of the unit
- The use factor of the unit
- The occupancy factor behind the barrier
- The intrinsic shielding (e.g., tube housing attenuation) of the x-ray unit
- Whether the area beyond the barrier is "controlled" or "uncontrolled"

Radiation Shielding Categories

As mentioned in previous discussions, three categories of radiation sources are generated in an x-ray room. They are classified as follows:
1. Primary radiation
2. Scatter radiation
3. Leakage radiation

The last two categories are collectively known as *secondary radiation.*

Primary Radiation. Primary radiation emerges directly from the x-ray tube collimator (Fig. 14.18) and moves without deflection toward a wall, door, viewing window, and so on. Because of this property, primary radiation also is known as *direct radiation*. Energy from direct radiation has not been degraded by scatter, and substantial portions of the initial beam may not have been attenuated. Therefore a wall in the path of direct radiation requires the most protective shielding to ensure the safety of personnel and the public. In a typical x-ray suite, the most important primary radiation barrier is that behind the wall Bucky unit.

Scatter Radiation. Scatter radiation results whenever a diagnostic x-ray beam passes through matter. Compton interactions between the x-ray photons and the electrons of the atoms within the attenuating object deflect x-ray photons from their initial trajectories. As a result, photons emerge from the object in all directions (Fig. 14.19). Scattered radiation is greatly reduced in intensity relative to the incident beam. It also is quite weakened in energy and consequently in penetrating power. The amount of

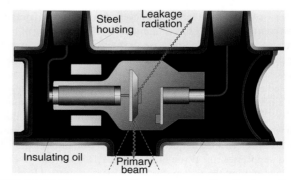

FIG 14.18 Primary radiation emerges directly from the collimator and spreads throughout the room.

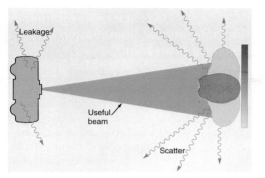

FIG 14.19 Scatter radiation emerges from the patient and spreads in all directions.

shielding required to protect against scatter radiation is therefore almost always much less than that for primary radiation. In general, the patient is the major source of scatter radiation.

Leakage Radiation. Leakage radiation is radiation generated in the x-ray tube that does not exit from the collimator opening but rather penetrates the protective tube housing and, to some degree, the sides of the collimator (see Figs. 14.18 and 14.19). Leakage radiation is therefore always present in some amount. When shielding is planned for a secondary barrier, the potential contributions from leakage radiation must be added to those from the scatter radiation reaching that barrier.

Calculation Considerations

Workload. Because a diagnostic x-ray unit does not produce radiation 24 hours a day, 7 days a week, a parameter that reflects the unit's radiation-on time has been used in the determination of barrier shielding requirements. The quantity is called its **workload (W)**. The workload is essentially the radiation output-weighted time that the unit is actually delivering radiation during the week. Workloads are specified either in units of milliampere-seconds (mAs) per week or milliampere-minutes (mA-min) per week. The following example illustrates this concept.

Example: A radiographic x-ray suite is in operation 5 days per week. The average number of patients per day is 20, and the average number of images per patient is 3. The average technical exposure factors are 90 kVp, 300 mA, and 0.1 sec. Find the weekly workload.

$$W = (300\,\text{mA} \times 0.1\,\text{sec}) \times (5\,\text{days/wk})$$
$$\times (20\,\text{patients/day}) \times (3\,\text{images/patient})$$
$$= 9000\,\text{mAs/wk}$$
$$= 150\,\text{mA-min/wk}$$

Note that the kVp is not used in the workload calculation. It is, however, an important parameter in the calculation of barrier-shielding thickness. (This is explicitly seen in an example illustrating the calculation of shielding for a wall in an x-ray suite.)

Inverse Square Law. Just as the perceived brightness of a light source decreases with separation from its origin, the intensity of an x-ray beam is lessened as the distance from its source increases. The ISL, introduced earlier in this chapter, is the mathematical relation describing this property and is a fundamental component of radiation protection. As such, the ISL plays a major role in the design of radiation safety barriers. An example of its use for this purpose is shown here.

Example: At a distance of 1 m from an x-ray tube target, the dose rate measured by a radiation survey meter was 4.5 mGy per hour. What would that instrument read if it were moved back an extra 2 m? As already seen, the ISL is mathematically given by the following proportion:

$$\frac{I_1}{I_2} = \frac{(d_2)^2}{(d_1)^2}$$

If the given data are substituted into the relation and cross-multiplied, the following result is obtained:

$$3^2 \times I_2 = 4.5 \times 1^2$$
$$9\,I_2 = 4.5$$
$$I_2 = 0.5\,\text{mGy/hr}$$

This result demonstrates a substantial reduction in radiation intensity. Its direct consequence is a greatly reduced barrier shielding thickness requirement.

The inverse square law is actually built into the combined mathematical and empiric (i.e., experimentally derived) formulas that determine primary barrier thickness values and secondary barrier thickness values. Because these relations are constructed to give answers for broad-beam attenuation* rather than just for a localized area, the ISL effect is slightly less than it would be for an idealized situation. A short discussion with an example illustrating the usage of this for a primary barrier is presented in the following pages. However, before this discussion, several other concepts of fundamental importance in the design of appropriate shielding have to be introduced.

Use Factor. If radiation, whether primary or secondary, is never directed at a particular wall or structure, then ordinary or existing construction is sufficient. Most structures in a diagnostic x-ray suite, however, are struck by radiation to some degree for some fraction of the weekly beam-on time. The use factor (U) is a quantity that was introduced to select this fractional contact time.

For primary radiation, the use factor represents the portion of beam-on time that the x-ray beam is directed at a primary barrier during the week. Consider a typical radiographic suite with a wall Bucky unit. If 50% of the x-ray examinations involve this device, the wall behind the Bucky unit has a U (*primary*) = ½.

Because scatter and leakage radiation emerge in all directions in the x-ray room, every wall, door, viewing window, and other surface will always be struck by some quantity of radiation. Therefore U (*secondary*) = 1 for all radiation-accessible structures. Furthermore, if a particular wall is considered a primary barrier and its required shielding is designed on that basis, then in virtually all situations no supplementary shielding need be added for the secondary radiation that may also be striking this barrier.

Table 14.2 presents the most current recommended use factor values. The use factor also can be referred to as the *beam direction factor*.

Occupancy Factor. Radiation barriers are installed to protect personnel and the general public from radiation that otherwise would reach them uninhibited. If no one will ever be present beyond an existing wall in a particular area while the x-ray unit is being operated, the addition of supplementary shielding to that wall is unnecessary.

---

*As defined in NCRP Report 147 (see later), broad-beam attenuation refers to that effect occurring when the field area is large at the barrier and the point of measurement is near the barrier's exit surface.

TABLE 14.2   Use Factors Recommended by the International Commission on Radiological Protection

Use Factor	Primary Barrier
Full use (U = 1)	Floors of radiation rooms except dental installations, doors, walls, and ceilings of radiation rooms exposed routinely to the primary beam
Partial use (U = ¼)	Doors and walls of radiation rooms not exposed routinely to the primary beam; also floors of dental installations
Occasional use (U = ¹⁄₁₆)	Ceilings of radiation rooms not exposed routinely to the primary beam; because of the low use factor, shielding requirements for a ceiling usually determined by secondary rather than primary beam considerations

From International Commission on Radiological Protection (ICRP): *Report of Committee III on protection against x-rays up to energies of 3 MeV and beta and gamma rays from sealed sources,* ICRP Publication No. 3, New York, 1960, Pergamon Press.

This shielding design statement would be that *existing construction is sufficient.* An example of this is an outside wall facing a courtyard that "always" has zero occupancy. The opposite extreme is an area in which someone is always present. When planning radiation protection shielding for a diagnostic x-ray suite, the designer must consider not only zero and full occupancy cases but also the more common partial occupancy situation. The occupancy factor (T) is used to modify the shielding requirement for a particular barrier by taking into account the fraction of the work week during which the space beyond the barrier is occupied. Table 14.3 lists the latest recommended values for T.

Controlled and Uncontrolled Areas. If a region adjacent to a wall of an x-ray room is used only by occupationally exposed personnel (e.g., radiographers), that location is designated a controlled area. Conversely, a nearby hall or corridor that is frequented by the general public is classified as an uncontrolled area. For the latter, the weekly maximum permitted equivalent dose (MPED) is

TABLE 14.3 Suggested Occupancy Factors*†

Location	Occupancy Factor (T)
Administrative or clerical offices; laboratories, pharmacies, and other work areas fully occupied by an individual; receptionist areas, attended waiting rooms, children's indoor play areas, adjacent x-ray rooms, film reading areas, nurses' stations, x-ray control rooms	1
Rooms used for patient examinations and treatments	$\frac{1}{2}$
Corridors, patient rooms, employee lounges, and staff rest rooms	$\frac{1}{5}$
Corridor doors‡	$\frac{1}{8}$
Public toilets, unattended vending areas, storage rooms, outdoor areas with seating, unattended waiting rooms, patient holding areas	$\frac{1}{20}$
Outdoor areas with only transient pedestrians or vehicular traffic, unattended parking lots, vehicular drop-off areas (unattended), attics, stairways, unattended elevators, janitors' closets	$\frac{1}{40}$

*For use as a guide in planning shielding where other occupancy data are not available.
†When using a low occupancy factor for a room immediately adjacent to an x-ray room, care should be taken to also consider the areas farther removed from the x-ray room. These areas may have significantly higher occupancy factors than the adjacent room and may therefore be more important in shielding design despite the larger distances involved.
‡The occupancy factor for the area just outside a corridor door can often be reasonably assumed to be lower than the occupancy factor for the corridor.
Adapted from National Council on Radiation Protection and Measurements (NCRP): *Structural shielding design for medical x-ray imaging facilities, Report No. 147,* Bethesda, MD, 2004, NCRP.

equal to 20 microsieverts (20 μSv); for controlled areas, it is a much larger amount—1000 μSv or 1 millisievert (1 mSv). The main reason for this disparity lies in the fact that the occupationally exposed population is only a tiny fraction of the overall population. Therefore the potential for detrimental radiobiologic effects in the general public as a whole as a result of the higher MPED to occupationally exposed personnel is statistically

negligible. Whether the area beyond a structure is designated as controlled or uncontrolled is very significant in determining the amount of radiation shielding to be added to that structure. The following sections discuss the use of these concepts in the determination of radiation shielding requirements.

Calculating Barrier Shielding Requirements

For each wall, door, and other barrier in an x-ray room that is to provide protection against radiation, the product of mA-minutes $\times$ U $\times$ T must be determined. The number of mA-minutes or workload is generally fixed by the overall use of the x-ray unit, whereas the use and occupancy factors are typically different among various barriers. The protection planner also must know whether the barrier is primary or secondary and whether the area beyond the barrier is controlled or uncontrolled.

With the publication of NCRP Report No. 147,[6] entitled *Structural Shielding Design for Medical Imaging Facilities*, the objective of a shielding calculation is now described as determining the thickness of a barrier sufficient to reduce the *air kerma** in a full or partially occupied area to a value that is less than or at most equal to the ratio **P/T**. The quantity **P** refers to the permissible weekly radiation dose (note: for diagnostic x-rays, dose and dose equivalent are numerically equal) to that location, and **T** is the area's occupancy factor.

Primary Barrier Calculation. Using material from NCRP Report No. 147, the combined mathematic and empiric relation that was briefly mentioned in the section on the ISL is introduced. For primary or direct radiation only, the relation is given by $B = P\,(d_p)^2/(K_r\,NUT)$, where B is by definition the broad-beam x-ray transmission factor and is in fact the ratio of air kerma (K_a) behind a barrier of material thickness "x" to the value of K_a at the same location with no intervening barrier; d_p is the distance from the x-ray source to a representative location and distance behind the direct radiation barrier (e.g., one-third of a meter beyond the barrier is typical); K_r is the average unshielded air kerma per patient at a reference distance of 1 m from the source; N is the expected number of patients examined in the room per week; U and T are,

---

*Recall that air kerma (K_a) is essentially absorbed dose in air resulting from the passage of an x-ray beam through it. Its numeric value is specified in units of gray.

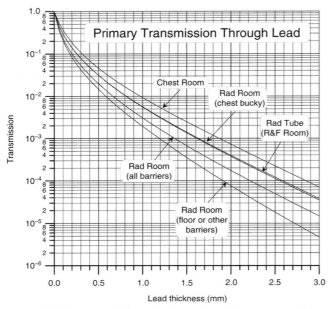

FIG 14.20 Assorted plots of primary broad-beam transmission through lead. (From National Council on Radiation Protection and Measurements [NCRP]: *Structural shielding design for medical x-ray imaging facilities, Report No. 147*, Bethesda, MD, 2004.)

as we have seen, respectively, the use and occupancy factors; and P depends on whether the barrier is for a controlled or uncontrolled area. Once the value of B has been calculated for a particular situation, then plots of transmission factors versus attenuating material thickness supplied in Appendix B of NCRP Report No. 147 may be used to obtain the required shielding thickness for the barrier. Such a graph is shown in Fig. 14.20.

The primary radiation intensity for a selected kVp at the barrier location for an x-ray suite may be determined by making air kerma measurements on the suite's x-ray unit at a reference distance (e.g., 100 cm) from the x-ray tube target with the aid of a calibrated ionization chamber. This information can then be used to determine the amount of shielding necessary to attenuate the radiation to permissible levels for that x-ray energy. The following example demonstrates determination of the primary barrier-shielding requirement associated with a wall Bucky from an average-usage radiographic room.

Example: Let the average kVp for the x-rays striking the barrier = 100.

Let the area behind the wall be an uncontrolled area. Therefore $P = 0.02$ mGy/wk.

Let the total distance from x-ray source to occupied area d_p (including one-third of a meter beyond the shielding barrier) be 3 m.

Let there be 100 patients per week in this x-ray room. Let $U = 1/2$ and $T = 1/4$.

From measurements on the x-ray unit, we find that at 1 m for 100 kVp, the value of K_r is 6 mGy per mA-min.

Solution: Substituting the foregoing information into the expression for the transmission factor gives:

$$B = (0.02)(3)^2/(6)(0.5)(0.25)(100)$$
$$= 0.0024$$

From the graph in Fig. 14.20, using the curve for radiographic room chest Bucky, we obtain a shielding requirement of approximately 1.3 mm lead. Currently, in the United States shielding is specified in fractions of an inch of lead, most commonly, 1/32 and 1/16. The standard 1/32 inch is approximately 0.8 mm, and the standard 1/16 inch is equal to 1.58 mm. Because our calculation of shielding for our primary barrier required 1.3 mm lead, then in the United States the choice would be to conservatively install 1/16-inch lead shielding for this barrier.

Secondary Barrier Calculation. Secondary barriers intercept both scatter and leakage radiation. No additional shielding against secondary radiation is needed for areas already protected against primary radiation. Because scatter and leakage radiation emerge in all directions, the use factor for these is always 1.

Scatter radiation. The intensity and energy of the scatter radiation at the location of a barrier are generally unknown. Therefore the following have been assumed for the determination of barrier shielding requirements:
1. The energy of the scatter radiation is equal to the primary radiation.
2. The intensity of radiation scattered at 90 degrees at a distance of 1 m from its source is reduced by a factor of 1000 relative to the primary radiation for a field size of 400 cm^2 (20 cm × 20 cm).

The greater the x-ray field dimension at the source of the scatter radiation (usually the patient), the larger the amount of generated scatter radiation will be. Also significant are the primary beam photon energy and the location of the x-ray beam on the patient. The ISL again plays an important role in shielding determination, but in the case of scatter radiation the distance is measured from the center of the irradiated portion of the patient rather than from the x-ray tube target.

Leakage radiation. Leakage radiation does not emerge directly from the collimator opening but rather penetrates through the x-ray tube housing walls or through the sides of the collimator when the x-ray beam is on. Leakage radiation is therefore an additional radiation output component that shielding designers must consider. Regulatory standards mandate that the maximum permissible leakage exposure rate at 1 m from the target of a diagnostic x-ray tube in all directions cannot exceed 100 mR/hour when the tube is being operated continuously at its maximal permitted kVp and mA combination.

Leakage radiation is always present when the x-ray tube is on, even if the collimator shutters are tightly closed. Because of the attenuation that occurs when leakage radiation penetrates the tube housing walls, it is essentially a monoenergetic beam; thus the concept of half-value layer (HVL) may be used at barriers to reduce leakage radiation levels to permissible values. Data tables incorporating this concept have been devised to specify the amount of shielding needed to attenuate leakage radiation sufficiently at various distances from the x-ray tube. This shielding should be compared with that necessary to attenuate scatter radiation satisfactorily. Traditionally, if both requirements do not differ substantially (i.e., are less than 3 HVLs apart) then the conservative decision would be to install a composite shielding that is the sum of the shielding for each radiation source. However, if the barrier shielding for the two differs substantially (i.e., more than 3 HVLs), then conservatively one can just use the larger value. The following example illustrates the method used in most existing diagnostic x-ray rooms for determining leakage radiation shielding requirements.

Example: Suppose that shielding must be added to a wall that is subject only to secondary radiation to protect a controlled area. Given the following information, find the total thickness of lead needed.

HVL for scatter and leakage radiation: 0.2 mm lead each

Shielding requirement for scatter radiation alone for a particular barrier: 0.75 mm lead

Shielding requirement for leakage radiation alone for that barrier: 0.3 mm lead

Solution: The difference in barrier shielding requirements for scatter and leakage = 0.45 mm lead, which is less than 3 HVL, which = 3 × 0.2 mm lead, or 0.6 mm lead. Therefore the conservative total shielding thickness for the barrier would be 0.75 + 0.3 = 1.05 mm lead.

TABLE 14.4 Brief Summary of National Council on Radiation Protection and Measurements Report No. 147 New Shielding Guidelines

Item	New Approach
Workload	More realistic use of contemporary survey data
Leakage and scatter	Explicit barrier calculations
Use factor	Adjusted for beam direction data reflecting actual usage patterns
Occupancy factor	Realistic assumptions of occupancy of low-occupancy areas (e.g., stairwells)

Adapted from National Council on Radiation Protection and Measurements (NCRP): *Structural shielding design for medical imaging facilities, Report No. 147,* Bethesda, MD, 2004, NCRP.

New Approaches to Shielding

Among the new approaches to shielding design detailed in NCRP Report No. 147, a more rigorous workload analysis incorporates the range of kVps actually used. In addition, the true role of leakage radiation in state-of-the-art equipment is now modeled explicitly, along with scatter. The traditional rule of adding an HVL if leakage and scatter barrier requirements are similar has been abandoned in favor of exact calculations. Use factors now reflect a true percentage of the time that the beam is directed at various barriers. Some existing shielding that was generally ignored in older design calculations, such as the patient table, Bucky, and cassette holder, is included in the new designs. Finally, the suggested occupancy factors have been reevaluated to approximate more closely the percentage of the time that workers are expected to be present (see Table 14.3). In NCRP Report No. 49,[7] a minimal occupancy factor of at least 1/16 was assumed. Under the revised guidelines, occupancy factors for areas such as closets and stairways may be placed as low as 1/40. Some of the changes in the revision of NCRP Report No. 49 are listed in Table 14.4.

RADIATION WARNING SIGNAGE

Signage is an important component of safety in a radiology department. However, after becoming familiar with the "feel" of being in a department, staff sometimes forget to notice the presence of warning indicators. In the

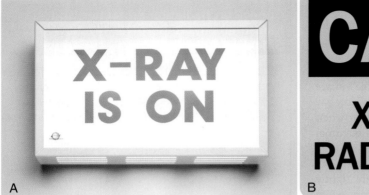

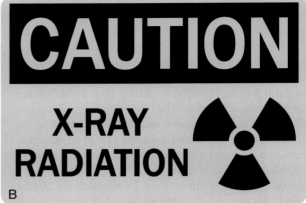

A   B

FIG 14.21 Radiation warning signs typically found in a diagnostic radiologic facility. (A) A self-illuminated sign used outside the door to a CT scanner. (B) A general radiation warning sign used to indicate the potential for exposure that may exceed 0.05 mSv at 30 cm from a source of radiation. (A, From Brian Struble/DigitalMomentStudios.com, © 2017.)

material that follows, some general guidelines for warning signs and other indicators of the potential for radiation exposure are given. Specific rules and regulations vary somewhat according to the jurisdiction of the facility (i.e., state, federal, military, etc.). However, the main points concerning the type of signs and the circumstances under which posting is required are essentially the same. Each radiographer should check with his or her own institution's radiation safety officer concerning specific regulations that govern the facility where they work.

Beam-On Indicator Sign

Some states require specific imaging equipment installations, primarily computed tomography (CT) scanners, to include warning lights that are conspicuous near the door to the examination room from any corridor. The sign should read "x-ray beam on" or the equivalent. It should be self-illuminating whenever the x-ray equipment is energized. Some states require an interlock such that exposure is terminated if the door is opened.

General Posting

Radiation warning signs are posted within controlled areas of the hospital or facility and are typically found on the door to CT and interventional x-ray rooms, linear accelerator treatment rooms, and storage areas for radioactive materials. An example of the familiar radiation warning sign is shown in Fig. 14.21. Such signs are

required to be magenta or purple or black on a yellow background. Further specifications may be found in Recommended State Regulations of the Conference of Radiation Control Program Directors.[8] A sign reading "Caution Radiation Area" is usually adequate for rooms containing fixed diagnostic equipment. A radiation area is generally taken to mean an area in which radiation exposures may exceed 0.05 mSv in 1 hour at 30 cm from a source. Other categories of caution signage exist for areas in which radiation exposures may exceed those encountered in diagnostic radiology. These signs are required in radiation oncology or nuclear medicine departments and include the labels High Radiation, Very High Radiation, Airborne Radioactivity, and Radioactive Materials.

■ SUMMARY

- An annual occupational effective dose of 50 mSv for whole-body exposure during routine operations and an annual effective dose of 1 mSv for individuals in the general population have been established.
- A cumulative effective dose (CumEfD) limits a radiation worker's whole-body lifetime effective dose to his or her age in years times 10 mSv.
- Radiation workers can receive a larger equivalent dose than the general public without altering the GSD.
- Occupational exposure must be kept ALARA.

- The following methods of reducing scatter radiation also reduce the occupational hazard for the radiographer:
  - Use of beam-limitation devices, higher kVp and lower mA techniques, appropriate beam filtration, and adequate protective shielding
  - Proper utilization of protective apparel (lead aprons, gloves, thyroid shields)
  - Reduction of repeat images
- The basic principles of time, distance, and shielding are to be employed to minimize occupational radiation exposure.
- Pregnant radiographers can wear an additional monitoring device at waist level to ensure that their monthly equivalent dose does not exceed 0.5 mSv.
- Primary and secondary protective barriers must be designed so that annual effective dose limits are not exceeded.
- A lead-lined, metal, diagnostic-type protective tube housing protects the radiographer and the patient from leakage radiation.
- The following practices are important in protecting the radiographer during routine fluoroscopy:
  - The radiographer, in addition to wearing appropriate protective apparel, should stand as far away from the patient as is practical and move closer to the patient only when assistance is required.
  - A protective curtain and Bucky slot shielding device must be used.
  - The x-ray beam must be adequately collimated, and a cumulative timing device should be used.
- The following are required to protect the radiographer during mobile radiographic examinations:
  - The radiographer must wear protective garments.
  - The radiographer should stand at least 2 m from the patient, x-ray tube, and useful beam.
  - If possible, the radiographer should also stand at a right angle to the x-ray beam–scattering object (the patient) line.
- Limited exposure time and dose reduction features are required to protect the radiographer during high level control fluoroscopy.
- Distance is the most effective means of protection from ionizing radiation.
- If the peak energy of the x-ray beam is 100 kVp, a lead apron of at least 0.25 mm lead equivalent thickness should be worn if the radiographer cannot remain behind a protective barrier. A lead apron of 0.5- or 1-mm lead equivalent thickness affords much greater protection.
- Lead gloves, a thyroid shield, and protective glasses are sometimes required.
- Radiographers should never stand in the primary beam to hold a patient during a radiographic exposure.
- When designing diagnostic x-ray suites, equivalent dose to radiation workers, nonoccupationally exposed personnel, and the general public must be taken into consideration.
  - Facilities must be equipped with radiation-absorbent barriers.
  - Occupancy factor, workload, and use factor must be considered when thickness requirements for a protective barrier are being determined. Whether an area beyond a structure is designated as a controlled or uncontrolled area is significant in determining the amount of radiation shielding to be added to that structure.
- Radiation warning signs are an important component of safety in a radiology department.

REFERENCES

1. National Council on Radiation Protection and Measurements (NCRP): *Limitation of exposure to ionizing radiation, Report No. 116,* Bethesda, MD, 1993, NCRP.
2. Bushong SC: *Radiologic science for technologists: physics, biology and protection,* ed 10, St. Louis, 2013, Mosby.
3. Femia J: It pays off in safety to know your C-arm. *Adv Imaging Radiat Ther Prof* 20:19, 2007.
4. Marx MV: *Interventional procedures: risks to patients and personnel, in radiation risk,* Reston, VA, 1996, American College of Radiology Commission on Physics and Radiation Safety.
5. Center for Devices and Radiological Health, U.S. Food and Drug Administration: White paper: Association for Medical Imaging Management, 2011.
6. National Council on Radiation Protection and Measurements (NCRP): *Structural shielding design for medical x-ray imaging facilities, Report No. 147,* Bethesda, MD, 2004, NCRP.
7. National Council on Radiation Protection and Measurements (NCRP): *Structural shielding design and evaluation for medical use of x-rays and gamma rays with energies up to 10 meV, Report No. 49,* Washington DC, 1976, NCRP.
8. Website of the Conference of Radiation Control Program Directors, http://www.crcpd.org/page/SSRCRs. (Last accessed 1 November 2016).

GENERAL DISCUSSION QUESTIONS

1. Why has a cumulative effective dose limit for the whole body been established for radiation workers?
2. Why can radiation workers receive a larger equivalent dose than members of the general population?
3. What can a radiographer do during a radiographic procedure to reduce scattered radiation from a patient?
4. When an additional radiation dosimeter is worn by a pregnant radiographer to monitor the equivalent dose to the embryo-fetus, where should the dosimeter be placed if a protective lead apron is worn?
5. Why is it *not* necessary to reassign a declared pregnant radiographer to a lower radiation exposure risk area?
6. Why is the control-booth barrier considered a secondary protective barrier?
7. During a fluoroscopic procedure, when a radiographer's presence is *not* immediately required, where should this person stand until his or her services are needed?
8. How can the use of a remote control exposure device on a mobile radiographic unit reduce exposure for the radiographer?
9. Why is it best to position the image intensifier of a C-arm fluoroscope close to the patient during any x-radiation procedure?
10. How can the radiologist reduce radiation exposure for himself or herself and for assisting personnel during a high level control interventional procedure?
11. During a high level control interventional procedure, how can a record of radiation exposure be obtained?
12. When should the radiographer stand in the primary beam to restrain a patient during a radiographic exposure?
13. What factors must the shielding designer take into account to meet necessary radiation protection standards?
14. What quantity *best* describes the weekly radiation usage of a diagnostic x-ray unit?
15. What mathematical relationship plays a major role in the design of radiation safety barriers?

REVIEW QUESTIONS

1. When performing a mobile radiographic examination, if the protection factors of distance and shielding are equal, the radiographer should stand at a _____ to the scattering object (the patient) line.
   A. 30-degree angle
   B. 45-degree angle
   C. 75-degree angle
   D. 90-degree angle
2. Diagnostic imaging personnel may receive an annual occupational effective dose of _____ for whole-body exposure during routine operations.
   A. 1 mSv
   B. 5 mSv
   C. 25 mSv
   D. 50 mSv
3. At a 90-degree angle to the primary x-ray beam, at a distance of 1 m, the scattered radiation is what fraction of the intensity of the primary beam?
   A. $\frac{1}{10}$
   B. $\frac{1}{100}$
   C. $\frac{1}{1000}$
   D. $\frac{1}{10,000}$
4. If a radiographer stands 6 m away from an x-ray tube and receives an exposure rate dose of 4.0 mGy$_a$/hr, what will the exposure rate dose be if the same radiographer moves to stand at a position located 12 m from the x-ray tube?
   A. 1 mGy$_a$/hr
   B. 2 mGy$_a$/hr
   C. 3 mGy$_a$/hr
   D. 4 mGy$_a$/hr
5. Which of the following are methods that can be used by a C-arm operator to reduce occupational exposure for himself or herself and other personnel?
   1. Collimate the x-ray beam to include only the anatomy of interest.
   2. Use the foot pedal or the handheld exposure switch with their cables extended away from the machine as far as possible whenever making an exposure.
   3. Use magnification whenever possible to visualize body parts better.
   A. 1 and 2 only
   B. 1 and 3 only
   C. 2 and 3 only
   D. 1, 2, and 3
6. If the Bucky slot shield and protective curtain or sliding panel were *not* in the correct position during a routine fluoroscopic examination, what exposure dose rate would the fluoroscopist experience?

A. Exceed 1 mGy$_a$/hr at a distance of 0.6 m from the side of the x-ray table

B. Not exceed 1 mGy$_a$/hr at a distance of 0.6 m from the side of the x-ray table

C. Exceed 2.5 mGy$_a$/hr at a distance of 0.6 m from the side of the x-ray table

D. Exceed 5 mGy$_a$/hr at a distance of 0.6 m from the side of the x-ray table

7. Units of either mAs/wk or mA-min/wk are used to determine the _____ for a specific x-ray room.

A. Distance factor

B. Occupancy factor

C. Use factor

D. Workload

8. A Bucky slot shielding device of at least _____ must automatically cover the Bucky slot opening in the side of the x-ray table during a fluoroscopic examination when the Bucky tray is positioned at the foot end of the table.

A. 0.25-mm aluminum equivalent

B. 0.25-mm lead equivalent

C. 0.5-mm aluminum equivalent

D. 0.5-mm lead equivalent

9. For mobile radiographic units, which are not equipped with remote control exposure devices, the cord leading to the exposure switch must be long enough to permit the radiographer to stand *at least* _____ from the patient, the x-ray tube, and the useful beam to reduce occupational exposure.

A. 1 m

B. 2 m

C. 3 m

D. 5 m

10. Of the following factors, which are specifically considered when determining thickness requirements for protective barriers?

1. Occupancy factor (T)

2. Workload (W)

3. Use factor (U)

4. kVp

A. 1 and 2 only

B. 2 only

C. 1, 2, and 3 only

D. 1, 2, 3, and 4

15

Radioisotopes and Radiation Protection

OBJECTIVES

After completing this chapter, the reader will be able to perform the following:

- Define all key terms.
- Explain how cancerous growths or tumors can either be eliminated or at least controlled by irradiation.
- Name some therapeutic isotopes, understand their properties, and describe how they are used.
- Explain the process of electron capture.
- Identify the two best radiation safety practices to follow for patients having therapeutic prostate seed implants.
- Explain the process of beta decay.
- Discuss the radiation hazards that may be encountered by personnel caring for a patient who is receiving iodine-131 therapy treatment for thyroid cancer.
- Explain how isotopes that are used as radioactive tracers in nuclear medicine work.
- Discuss how residual isotopes and radioactive materials may be properly disposed of.
- Identify the most common radioisotope used in nuclear medicine diagnostic studies.
- Identify and describe the types of radiation events that are used in positron emission tomography (PET).
- Identify the most common isotope used for PET scanning.
- Explain the benefit of the combined imaging device called a PET/CT scanner.
- Describe radiation safety concerns associated with the design of a PET/CT imaging suite, and explain how radiation protection has been provided.
- Discuss the reasons for concern over the use of radiation as a terrorist weapon, and identify what action most hospitals have taken for handling emergency situations involving radioactive contamination.
- Explain what a radioactive dispersal device, or "dirty bomb," is, and mention the possible consequences of the detonation of such a device.
- Describe the procedure for external decontamination from radioactive materials.
- State the dose limit per event for individuals engaged in both nonlifesaving and lifesaving activities during a radiation emergency.
- State the reason why the Environmental Protection Agency (EPA) sets limits for radioactive contamination.
- Discuss the medical management of persons experiencing radiation bioeffects.
- Describe various strategies used to treat internal radiation contamination.

CHAPTER OUTLINE

KEY TERMS

annihilation radiation	half-value layer (HVL)	positron emission tomography
beta decay	internal contamination	(PET)
computed tomography (CT)	iodine-123 (^{123}I)	radiation emergency plans
decontamination	iodine-125 (^{125}I)	radiation therapy
electron capture	iodine-131 (^{131}I)	radioactive contamination
Environmental Protection Agency	isotopes	radioactive dispersal device, or
(EPA)	neutrino	"dirty bomb"
fluorine-18 (^{18}F)	nuclear medicine	radioisotopes
fluorodeoxyglucose (FDG)	PET/CT scanner	surface contamination
Geiger–Müller (GM) detectors	positron	technetium-99m (^{99m}Tc)

Atoms that have the same number of protons within the nucleus but have different numbers of neutrons are called isotopes. Most elements in the periodic table (see Appendix C) have some associated isotopes, and quite a few of them have many. However, not all the nuclei of these isotopes represent stable groupings of protons and neutrons (i.e., the most secure bonding or the lowest energy configuration). A few have too many protons for stability, whereas others have too many neutrons, and some are just formed in higher energy states. Because of this, such isotopes spontaneously undergo processes or transformations to rectify their unbalanced arrangement or to achieve a lower state of energy. All atoms whose nuclei behave in this manner are referred to as radioisotopes.

This chapter provides a brief description of the use of radioisotopes in both diagnostic and therapeutic medical procedures and discusses some relevant radiation safety issues. The use of radiation as a terrorist weapon is also considered, and the chapter includes some fundamental principles for dealing with radioactive contamination in a health care setting.

To assist the learner, both English and metric units are used in this chapter.

MEDICAL USAGE

Radiation Therapy

As discussed in previous chapters, well-oxygenated, rapidly dividing cells are very sensitive to damage by radiation. This sensitivity is the foundation on which the branch of medicine commonly known as radiation therapy is

based. Cancerous growths or tumors can be either eliminated, or at least controlled, by sufficient irradiation of the area containing the growth. Radiation treatments are normally delivered externally using high energy accelerators. However, for certain types of cancer or cancerous locations, radiation can be advantageously delivered internally by infusion or implantation of certain radioisotopes. These therapeutic isotope procedures comprise a branch of radiation therapy known as *brachytherapy*. The utilized isotopes are characterized by relatively long half-lives that are measured in terms of multiple days or multiple years and, with the exception of a few of them, by relatively high energy radiation emissions. The radiation may be in the form of gamma rays* or fast electrons (beta radiation). Several of the most important therapeutic radioisotopes are briefly described here.

Iodine-125. Iodine-125 (^{125}I) is an unstable and therefore radioactive isotope of the element iodine. It has been used quite extensively since 2000 in the form of titanium-encapsulated cylindrical seeds (4.5 mm long and in cross-section about the diameter of a paper clip [Fig. 15.1]) to give a tumoricidal radiation equivalent dose to cancers that are confined within the prostate gland. With the aid of computerized treatment planning and real-time

---

*Gamma rays are high energy photons (particles of electromagnetic radiation) that are emitted by the nucleus as a result of an unstable situation. They differ from x-ray photons, which are also particles of electromagnetic radiation, only in the method of how they are produced.

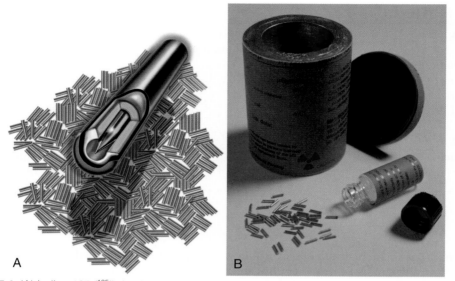

FIG 15.1 (A) Iodine-125 (^{125}I) titanium–encapsulated cylindrical seed. (B) ^{125}I seeds before encapsulation. (From Implant Sciences Corporation.)

ultrasound imaging, the seeds are permanently inserted into the gland in a calculated prescribed arrangement. The goal is to deliver 145 gray (Gy) to at least 90% of the prostate's volume while limiting radiation dose as much as possible to adjacent structures such as the urethra, bladder, and anterior rectal wall. The insertion process is done in the operating room and typically takes about 2 hours. This is a same-day procedure, and the patient is usually discharged within 4 to 5 hours afterward.

^{125}I has 53 protons and 72 neutrons in its nucleus and has a half-life of 59.4 days. It decays by a process called **electron capture,** wherein an inner-shell electron is captured by one of the nuclear protons, followed directly by the two combining to produce a neutron. There is also the emission of characteristic energy in the form of a 27 keV x-ray generated because of the filling of the inner-electron shell vacancy by an outer low-energy electron. The nucleus now has one less proton, and thus the decay process has led to the formation of a different element called *tellurium-125* (^{125}Te). ^{125}Te, which has 52 protons and 73 neutrons, is produced in an unstable excited energy state; this instability is immediately relieved as its nucleus emits energy in the form of a 35 keV gamma ray. Both the 27 keV characteristic x-rays and the 35 keV gamma rays deliver the radiation equivalent dose to the prostate gland. The decay process leading to the useful therapeutic radiation can be written as:

$$^{125}I_{53} + e^- \rightarrow {}^{125}Te_{52}^\bullet + xray_{(27\,KeV)} \rightarrow {}^{125}Te_{52} + \gamma_{(35\,KeV)} + xray_{(27\,KeV)}$$

where the • refers to an excited state and the symbol γ signifies a gamma ray.

Because these radiation emissions have little penetrating power, a very high percentage of the radiation energy remains concentrated in the prostate gland. Essentially all of the remaining radiation is absorbed by the patient except for some small but detectable amount on the patient's physique, which emerges. At a distance of 1 meter, the radiation exposure rate for virtually all prostate seed implants is less than 0.5 milliroentgens per hour (mR/hr), increasing, however, to 15 to 20 mR/hr at the patient's lower abdominal surface. In terms of international units these values correspond to equivalent dose rates of approximately 5 microsieverts/hr at 1 meter and 150 to 200 microsieverts/hr at the abdominal surface.

The concepts of distance and time are the best radiation safety practices to be followed for these types of therapeutic implants. A typical safety recommendation is that patients with ^{125}I implants should significantly limit durations of close contact (less than 30 cm or less than 1 foot) with small children and pregnant women for a period of 6 months (three half-lives) after the implant procedure. They may then resume completely normal behavior.

Iodine-131. Iodine-131 (^{131}I) is another unstable isotope of the element iodine, with 53 protons and 78 neutrons in its nucleus. It has a half-life of 8 days. As a consequence of its radioactive decay process (**beta decay***), it generates both electrons with an approximate mean energy of 192 keV and relatively high-energy assorted gamma rays (mean energy of 365 keV).

^{131}I can be joined chemically with sodium to form the chemical compound sodium iodide ^{131}I (NaI^{131}), which is radioactive and can be orally administered in the form of tablets. For a patient who has thyroid cancer, it is desirable to strongly irradiate any residual thyroid tissue not removed by surgery in order to destroy any remaining cancerous areas while significantly sparing surrounding tissue and other organs. Because the thyroid gland tends to highly absorb any iodine in the blood, administration of ^{131}I-labeled sodium iodide tablets is an efficient way of delivering a destructive radiation dose to the remainder of the thyroid. The relatively low energy electrons mainly cause the destruction.

Although the much more penetrating gamma rays deliver some radiation dose to more distant body sites, these rays primarily exit the body and present a radiation protection hazard to both:

- Nursing personnel
- Nuclear medicine technologists

As discussed in earlier chapters, the concepts of time, distance, and shielding should be applied. If the patient is hospitalized (usually no more than 2 days), a large, up to 25 mm or 1 inch-thick, rolling lead shield can be positioned between the patient and any attending personnel for protection. Such patients are also encouraged to drink lots of fluids so that as much ^{131}I, and therefore high-energy gamma radiation, can be removed from the body by urination in as short a time as possible.

The radioiodide tablets dissolve in the bloodstream, thus permitting an escape of some radioactivity through the pores of the skin, through urination, and in some special cases from vomiting. Therefore this poses another radiation safety hazard and a possible lengthy cleanup task. As a result, hospital rooms for ^{131}I therapy patients are usually isolated with restricted entry for general safety considerations and carefully prepared with well-placed absorbent cloths on top of nonporous flooring to facilitate a relatively easy cleanup of any radioactively contaminated surfaces. Only trained oncology nurses and nuclear medicine personnel should be allowed in the patient's room. Both groups should be wearing personnel dosimeters when they do so.

Handling and Disposal of Radioactive Materials

Radioisotopes and items that they have contaminated require that an institution follows appropriate procedures for their handling and disposal. Such procedures should be detailed within the radiation safety program of the institution. They must be in complete accord with the guidelines provided by state and federal regulations (e.g., Part 20 of Title 10 of the Code of Federal Regulations). All personnel involved in the handling and dispensing of radionuclides, as well as the removal of any remaining isotopes and any radioactively contaminated items, must wear gloves if the isotopes are in liquid form, be equipped with personnel dosimeters (whole body and extremity, the latter in the case of close handling), and follow the cardinal rules of radiation protection (time, distance, and shielding) where applicable. No solid encapsulated radioactive source is ever to be touched directly by hand. Instead, long tongs, which add distance as a safety measure, should be used.

At the conclusion of a brachytherapy or diagnostic radionuclide procedure, any residual isotope is to be returned to its shielded container. That container should then be labeled with how much activity remains and the current date. Also, any contaminated items as detected by a survey meter (e.g., gloves, clothing articles, absorbent pads, etc.) are to be placed in a sealed plastic bag that is labeled with the name of the radioisotope and the current date. After this is done, all involved personnel are to be checked with the survey meter to ensure that they have not been contaminated. Then the remaining isotope (if it is not to be returned to its supplier) and the packaged contaminated items are to be placed into a secure, shielded, and posted*

---

*Beta decay is the process wherein a nucleus relieves an instability by one of its neutrons, transforming itself into a combination of a proton and an energetic electron (called a *beta particle*). There is also emission of another particle called a *neutrino* (discussed later on).

*Posting should include a prominent display at the entrance of the storage area of the standard Caution Radioactive Materials sign, as well as emergency contact numbers for key personnel and regulatory agencies such as the state department of environmental protection and/or the Nuclear Regulatory Commission local office.

storage area where they must be held for a period of 10 half-lives** before being suitable for disposal in ordinary trash. An exit survey, which should indicate background radiation levels, is to be conducted at that time. Otherwise, the disposal must be delayed. A record of the storage and disposal of the residual radionuclide and contaminated items should be kept for review by regulatory inspectors.

Nuclear Medicine

Nuclear medicine is the branch of medicine that employs radioisotopes to study organ function in a patient, to detect the spread of cancer into bone, and to treat certain types of diseases. Diagnostic techniques in nuclear medicine typically make use of short-lived radioisotopes as radioactive tracers. These radionuclides have been attached to biologically active substances or chemicals and form radioactive compounds that predominantly diffuse into certain regions or organs where it is medically desired to scrutinize particular physiologic processes.

Iodine-123. One of the most common examples of process monitoring makes use of iodine-123 (^{123}I), yet another unstable isotope of the element iodine. ^{123}I undergoes radioactive decay by the process of *electron capture* (described in the section on iodine-125) and has an average half-life of 13.3 hours. When chemically coupled with sodium, it forms the radiotracer compound sodium iodide ^{123}I. This compound preferentially passes into the thyroid gland and achieves levels of concentration there that can be directly correlated with the thyroid gland's performance status. Thus measurement of radioactivity in the region of the thyroid gland, which results from the relative degree of uptake by the thyroid of ^{123}I-labeled sodium iodide, makes it possible to determine the percentage of remaining functioning thyroid tissue.

Technetium-99m. By far the most common radioisotope used in nuclear medicine diagnostic studies (as much

---

** For example, for an iodine-125 brachytherapy case, any unused seeds would have to be held for a period of 10 × ($T^{1/2}$ = 60 days) or 1.64 years before permissible disposal in ordinary trash, whereas for nuclear medicine procedures, which use radionuclides containing technetium 99m (see the following discussions), $T^{1/2}$ = 6 hours, and therefore the required storage time is 60 hours or 2.5 days.

as 80% of all procedures) is technetium-99m (^{99m}Tc). This radionuclide is generated from the radioactive decay of another unstable isotope (molybdenum-99 [^{99}Mo]), which relieves its instability by beta decay, during which (as discussed previously) an excess neutron transforms itself into a proton, with the emission of a fast electron from the nucleus. An additional proton within the nucleus means a change in atomic number and consequently a different element. The new element in this case is ^{99m}Tc, with 43 protons and 56 neutrons. Because the beta decay of ^{99}Mo produces technetium in a higher energy state than normal, it, too, is unstable. Most isotopes generated in this manner immediately shed their excess energy. However, some do not do so for a short period, and these relatively more enduring isotopes are given the designation *m*, which stands for *metastable* (meaning "more lasting"). ^{99m}Tc has a half-life of 6 hours and decays primarily by emission from its nucleus of a gamma ray photon with energy of 140 keV. The decay process can be depicted as:

$$_{42}Mo^{99} \rightarrow {}_{43}Tc^{99m} + e^- \rightarrow {}_{43}Tc^{99} + \gamma + e^- \ (T^{1/2} = 6 \ hr)$$

^{99m}Tc is an extremely versatile radioisotope because it can be incorporated into a wide variety of different compounds or biologically active substances, each with a specificity for different tissues or organs of the body. For example, in combination with a tin compound, it binds to red blood cells and is useful for mapping circulatory system disorders; in combination with a sulfur compound, it is absorbed by the spleen, thus making it possible to image the structure of the spleen; in another chemical combination, it concentrates in bone and permits evaluation of potential cancer spread to bony areas; it can also be used to evaluate heart function. All these studies are possible because either a deficiency of radioisotope uptake (i.e., a cold spot in radioactivity) or an excessive uptake of radioisotope-labeled compound (i.e., hot spots of radioactivity) signals abnormal organ behavior. Because of such capabilities, nuclear medicine offers diagnostic input relating to *function* that goes substantially beyond the information provided by ordinary x-ray techniques.

Positron Emission Tomography and Computed Tomography

In Chapter 3, in which the pair production interaction is discussed, a diagnostic modality called positron emission tomography (PET) is also mentioned. Although this modality does not require the occurrence of pair production interactions, it does make use of the annihilation radiation events that are a by-product of this interaction. However, in the case of PET, the annihilation radiation is initiated by the radioactive decay of the nucleus of an unstable isotope. The instability in this case is associated with too many protons residing within the nucleus. Nuclei such as these usually spontaneously undergo a reaction in which the excess proton is transmuted into a neutron and a positively charged electron (positron). This conserves electric charge because the neutron has none. To conserve energy as well, the process includes the emission of an additional particle called the neutrino. A neutrino has no electric charge and almost negligible mass, but its energy of motion (kinetic energy) balances the energy of the reaction. This requirement for energy balancing, in accordance with satisfying the law of conservation of energy, was the main reason for postulating the existence of the neutrino. Neutrinos almost never interact and are therefore nearly impossible to detect.

A positron, classified as antimatter, when passing close to an electron—normal matter—will interact destructively with the electron. In the process, both particles will disappear, having *annihilated* one another. Their respective masses are converted into energy that will be carried off by two photons emerging from the annihilation site in opposite directions, each with a kinetic energy of 511 keV. These energies correspond to the mass energies of the former positron and electron.

Imaging. If there is a volume (e.g., a human torso) in which many of these annihilation events are taking place, and if this volume is surrounded by a ring of densely packed detectors that are specifically tuned to 511 keV photon energies, then it is possible, in a manner analogous to that used in computed tomography (CT), to reconstruct useful images of the regions within the encompassed volume from which the annihilation photons are coming. Such images can reveal the performance status of a physical process. This is the concept of PET scanning.

Fluorine-18. By far the most important isotope in PET scanning is the positron emitter fluorine-18 (^{18}F), which symbolically can be depicted as $_9$F^{18}. Thus nine protons and nine neutrons are present in its nucleus. Nine neutrons are not enough to maintain a stable arrangement of protons and neutrons within this nucleus. More

neutrons are needed, and so the unstable nucleus will undergo a change in which, as described previously, one less proton is present. This can be represented as:

$$p \rightarrow n + e^+ + \nu$$

where the Greek character "ν" is the symbol for a neutrino. The positron will subsequently come into contact with an ordinary electron, resulting in an annihilation reaction leading to the production of two high energy photons.

The process as a whole can be summarized as:

$$_9F^{18} \rightarrow {}_8O^{18} + \nu + 2 \text{ annihilation energy photons}$$

where $_8$O^{18} is a stable isotope of oxygen with 8 protons and 10 neutrons.

PET is a very important imaging modality because it can be used to examine metabolic processes within the body. This is particularly relevant to the proliferation of cancer cells. Such cells seek to reproduce without end and to do so require a great deal of sugar, or glucose, to supply the energy for this unlimited growth. Therefore if it were possible to introduce within the body a radioactive molecule that was very similar to a glucose molecule, then the presence of excessive glucose metabolism sites associated with cancer cell proliferation could be discerned by detecting areas of abnormally high radioactivity.

The great significance of the isotope ^{18}F is that it can be attached to a glucose molecule, yielding a compound called fluorodeoxyglucose (FDG). FDG is a *radioactive tracer* that is very similar in chemical behavior to ordinary glucose, and so it is readily taken up or metabolized by cancerous cells. As such it reveals the locations of these cells through its positron emission decay and subsequent generation of oppositely traveling annihilation photons. These annihilation event sites are physically localizable through the PET scanner's patient-surrounding ring of coincidence detectors.

If a PET scanner is mechanically joined in a tandem configuration (e.g., like a two-person bicycle) with a CT scanner to produce a single joint imaging device, then in essence a facility gains not only the ability to detect the presence of abnormally high regions of glucose metabolism, yielding evidence of cancer spread (metastasis) into other body areas, but also the means to obtain detailed information about the anatomic location and extent of these lesions or growths. Such a combined imaging device is called a PET/CT scanner (Fig. 15.2).

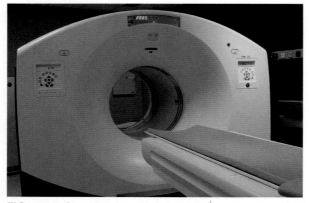

FIG 15.2 Combined positron emission tomography/computed tomography (PET/CT) system. (From Long BW, Rollins JH, Smith BJ: *Merrill's Atlas of Radiographic Positioning and Procedures,* ed 13, St. Louis, 2016, Elsevier.)

Radiation Protection

Positron emitters result in the production of high energy radiation. Each ^{18}F nuclear transformation by positron decay yields two highly penetrating 511 keV photons. These cannot be shielded by an ordinary lead apron. In fact, because the thickness of lead needed to attenuate such high energy radiation by 50% (i.e., its **half-value layer [HVL]**) is approximately 0.5 cm (0.2 in.), adequate shielding at close distances could require up to 2.5 cm or an inch of lead. Therefore the design of a PET/CT imaging suite is complex, involving significant radiation safety concerns. A discussion of the radiation safety design difficulties with respect to the PET/CT technologist for a minimal, but not zero, radiation exposure facility follows.

Unlike the usual diagnostic imaging suites in which the designer concentrates on protection from the radiation produced by an x-ray machine, the design of a PET/CT imaging suite presents unique additional radiation safety problems. In this situation, the scatter radiation generated by the CT scanner portion is the least of the designer's difficulties. Of much more importance is the high energy annihilation photons emanating in all directions from the patient having the PET/CT scan. Furthermore, the presence of yet a third source of radiation, also of high energy, must be considered. Every patient who is to have a PET/CT scan requires what is called a "prep" time. During this time ^{18}F, in the form of FDG with an initial activity usually of approximately 15 millicuries (555 megabecquerels [MBq]) is injected into the patient. The patient typically remains in the injection or prep room in a semireclining position for 45 to 60 minutes so that the FDG gets distributed throughout the body. This implies that to have a smooth-flowing, coordinated patient throughput, it will be necessary that while one "hot" patient is being scanned, a second "hot" patient is reclining in a nearby room *waiting* to be scanned. Therefore during this procedure the technologist and other personnel, as well as the general public, must be protected from at least two sources of high energy photon radiation in addition to the scatter x-radiation from the CT scanner.

All of this makes the calculations for a practical space-limited shielding design anything but trivial. These problems are greatly simplified, however, when a facility can be designed from scratch instead of being retrofitted into limited existing space. Unfortunately, most often the latter is the case. Earlier it was stated that it takes a considerable amount of lead to attenuate photons with 511 keV energy. Thus unless other potentially mitigating factors can be applied, the amount of lead shielding needed to ensure acceptable radiation safety could become unreasonable. However, such mitigating factors do exist. They involve the concepts of weekly workload (W) and occupancy factor (T), the decay in activity of the ^{18}F during the prep and scan times, self-attenuation by the patient, and, significantly, the distance to each area of occupancy, which brings into play the *inverse square law*. Requirements for the protection of a radiographer in a new PET/CT suite will now be briefly considered.

A potential workload for an average facility could be 7 PET/CT patients per daily shift, which amounts to 35 patients per work week, with each patient receiving at the start of prep time an activity of 15 mCi of ^{18}F doped FDG. The larger the weekly workload becomes, the greater the shielding that will be needed to maintain permissible maximum equivalent dose levels to personnel and the public and vice-versa, of course, for lesser workloads. ^{18}F has a physical half-life of 110 minutes; therefore the patient's degree of radioactivity will diminish naturally throughout the prep time, losing approximately 25% to 30% by the time of scanning. This process will continue during the 45- to 50-minute scan time, with the amount of ^{18}F having decreased through physical decay alone to approximately 50% of its initial activity at the conclusion of the scan. The patient's radioactivity is further lessened by any voiding that may take place just before the scanning procedure. The two processes taken together constitute what is known as an *effective half-life* (T_{eff}), which can be much less than the physical half-life of 110 minutes. Consequently, the patient's remaining radioactivity will typically be about one-fourth of its initial value after the scan is completed. This is important for radiation safety of the general public and any family members at the patient's home.

Such patients at discharge produce a measured midline *surface* radiation exposure rate of 40 to 50 mR/hr, which corresponds to about 0.4 to 0.5 millisieverts per hour equivalent dose rate, and *at a distance of 30 cm (1 foot)* to approximately 15 mR/hr exposure rate or 0.15 mSv/hr equivalent dose rate. Usually, it is recommended that such patients maintain a 1-meter separation from others as much as possible for the remainder of the day. After returning home, the patient is encouraged to drink plenty of fluids so that with frequent urination and little permanent tissue retention, the patient's residual ^{18}F activity will be so small that emitted radiation will be almost negligible 1 day later. After this time, the patient may resume full contact with all.

A well-designed facility should be arranged so that no areas of full occupancy are immediately adjacent to a high energy radiation source; the prep room and scanning location of the patient are the most important of these sites from which to have adequate separation. A secondary but less significant site is the patient's toilet, which could easily acquire some contamination.

To determine the equivalent dose rate (specified in μSv/hr at a particular distance from a person injected with a specific amount of ^{18}F), the shielding planner must make use of a measured quantity called the *dose rate constant*. Its value is 6.96 μSv/hr at a distance of 1 meter per millicurie (mCi) of ^{18}F. Thus if the patient did not self-attenuate any of the ^{18}F radiation, then just after a 15 mCi injection, the equivalent dose rate at 1 meter would be approximately $7 \times 15 = 105$ μSv/hr. At greater distances, the inverse square law can be applied to obtain a value. For example, at a distance of 4 meters (approximately 13 feet), the equivalent dose rate without any shielding present diminishes to:

$$105/4^2 = 6.6 \, \mu Sv/hr$$

Distance is thus seen to be a very powerful tool of radiation protection. A well-designed facility takes good advantage of this. Returning to the injected patient, there are other facilitators of radiation protection at hand. Both the patient and nature are generators of these facilitators.

It has been found that the body can absorb a substantial amount of ^{18}F annihilation radiation.

The mean maximum equivalent dose rate at 1 m from the patient per mCi (37 MBq) injected just after the injection is *not* 6.96 μSv/hr, as it would be for an unshielded point source of radiation; rather, it has been determined to be approximately 3 μSv/hr per mCi due to patient self-attenuation.* At a distance of 4 m from the patient just after a 15 mCi injection, the equivalent dose rate is now given by:

$$(15 \times 3)/4^2 = 2.8 \, \mu Sv/hr$$

Nature's contribution to the radiation protection effort is that ^{18}F has a short half-life. Therefore the 15 mCi dose injected at 2 p.m. will be approximately 70% (decay factor is obtained from $e^{-(0.693 \times 60/110)} = 0.69$) as strong at 3 p.m. (the approximate time that a scan will start) because of natural radioactive decay. Thus in actuality, the equivalent dose delivered by the "hot" patient while waiting during the prep time at a distance of 4 m is less than 2.8 microsieverts. If not this amount, then what dose equivalent would a person at this 4-meter distance effectively receive in 60 minutes? It must be a percentage of the whole, between 100% and 70%. Doing the mathematics of radioactive decay** yields a value of approximately 83%, or a correction factor of 0.83. Consequently, the equivalent dose at a distance of 4 m that could be received by a technologist who is continuously present at this location (i.e., occupancy level T = 1) from a 1-hour prep patient in the absence of any added shielding is:

$$0.83 \times 2.8 = 2.3 \, \mu Sv$$

Over the course of a week, assuming a total of 35 patients, then, with all other conditions remaining the same, this technologist will accumulate from prep patients an equivalent dose of:

$$35 \times 2.3 = 81 \, \mu Sv \, (8.1 \, millirem)$$

Over 50 weeks, this would add up to about 4000 μSv (400 mrem) from prep patients alone. However, prep

---

*The information discussed in this paragraph is based on material presented at the 2004 American College of Medical Physics Annual Meeting in Scottsdale, Arizona, by Melissa C. Martin, MS, FACR, in a workshop entitled *PET/CT-Site Planning and Shielding Design*.
**Decay correction factor = $1.443 \times (110/60) \, (1 - e^{-[0.693 \times 60/110]})$ = 0.83.

patients are not the only sources of high energy radiation dose to PET/CT personnel. There is also the scan patient and, to a much lesser extent, the patient's toilet. The contributions of these sources of radiation dose also need to be factored into the facility's design and shielding plan.

Consider the scan patient in some detail. As always, it is desirable to have a good distance, if at all possible, between personnel and the radiation source. That may not be feasible if the facility is being fit into a preexisting area. So let it be assumed that there is a separation of only 3.3 m from the scan patient's midline to the location of the PET/CT technologist. In the absence of additional shielding, what could be the equivalent dose rate from the scan patient? The first factor to be aware of is the lesser activity remaining in the scan patient due to physical decay, namely, 70% of the original 15 mCi. However, this is not the whole story. The prep patient is encouraged to void just before being scanned. What this means is that the residual ^{18}F in the patient's body at the start of the scan is less than 70% of the original activity. If it is assumed that approximately 20% more was removed by voiding, then at the start of the scan, the activity within the patient is just 50% of the original activity, namely, 0.5 × 15 = 7.5 mCi. If there were no other considerations,* then *at the start of the scan* the equivalent dose rate at the location of the technologist with no shielding would be:

$$(7.5 \text{ mCi} \times 3 \text{ μSv/hr per mCi})/(3.3)^2 = 2 \text{ μSv/hr}$$

However, as seen previously, the radioactivity within the patient continues to decay all throughout the approximate 1 hour between voiding and his or her departure. Therefore the equivalent dose to the technologist from the scan patient will actually be 0.83 × 2 μSv/hr, or 1.7 μSv. Over the course of a week, this amounts to 35 × 1.7 = 60 μSv. At 50 weeks, this equals 3000 μSv (300 mrem). Assuming that all other sources (e.g., patient's toilet and possibly the "hot" laboratory) of radiation dose to the technologist could contribute an additional 500 μSv annually, then the unshielded technologist could receive an annual equivalent dose of 7500 μSv (4000 + 3000 + 500) or 750 mrem in this facility.

Shielding can be installed to decrease this amount significantly. Let us seek to reduce this value to a total of 2500 μSv (250 mrem), or 50 μSv/wk (5 mrem/wk).

Fig. 15.3 depicts a facility layout schematic that will be referred to for shielding calculations. For simplicity, these calculations will be restricted to protection of the PET/CT radiographer. In addition, the task will be further confined to just the contributions from the patient occupying the prep room and the patient being scanned. Beginning with the scan patient, let it be required as an exercise that both the viewing window and its surrounding wall be shielded so that the 3000 μSv (300 mrem) annual equivalent dose contribution decreases to one-third of its value, namely to 1000 μSv (100 mrem). As mentioned earlier, the amount of lead needed to decrease the intensity of this high-energy radiation by 50% is called its *half-value layer* (HVL). The HVL is equal to 0.5 cm (0.2 inch) of lead. One HVL will bring the equivalent dose down to 1500 μSv (150 mrem), and 2 HVLs will cut it to 750 μSv (75 mrem). Therefore less than 2 HVLs would be needed. Doing the mathematics:

The number "*n*" of required HVLs is determined from the equation:

$$2^{-n} = \frac{1}{3}$$
$$\log 2^{-n} = \log(1/3)$$
$$-n \log 2 = \log 1 - \log 3 = -\log 3$$
$$n = \log 3 / \log 2$$
$$n = 1.56$$

Thus 1.56 HVLs, which amounts to 1.56 × (0.5 cm of lead per HVL) = 0.78 cm (approximately 5/16 inch) of lead, must be placed in the wall surrounding the view window, and the view window itself must be composed of this amount of lead acrylic to achieve the goal. This amount of lead is far more than would be required to shield the operator from the much less penetrating CT scatter radiation. Therefore this scatter radiation does not have to be additionally accounted for. For the patient in the prep room, the goal is to interpose shielding so that the 4000 μSv (400 mrem) annual equivalent dose contribution to the technologist decreases to 1000 μSv (100 mrem); this decrease by a factor of 4 clearly requires 2 HVLs, or 1 cm (0.4 inches) of lead. Examining the diagram, it is evident that this amount of shielding can be distributed between the prep room corridor wall and door (labeled *A* and *D,* respectively) and the scan suite corridor wall (labeled *B*). Excluding personnel other than the operator and any other circumstances, a practical

---

*In this discussion, any shielding provided by the scanner itself is being neglected.

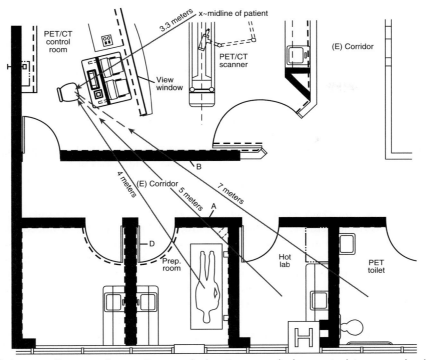

FIG 15.3 Layout diagram of a positron emission tomography/computed tomography (PET/CT) imaging facility.

solution is to place 6 mm ~¼ in. of lead in *A* and *D* and 5 mm ~³⁄₁₆ in. of lead in *B*.

In conclusion, it is obvious that there is much to be considered when radiation shielding is designed for a PET/CT facility. Other personnel and the general public must also be protected from the high-energy radiation. Their protection involves lower permissible equivalent dose limits than for the occupationally exposed radiographer. If there is the opportunity to construct the facility from the beginning, then with intelligent design the required shielding can be greatly reduced; if not, then the calculations and the amount of needed shielding can be sizable.

RADIATION EMERGENCIES: USE OF RADIATION AS A TERRORIST WEAPON

After the attack on the World Trade Center by hijacked airplanes on September 11, 2001, the possibility of the use of other terrorist weapons, such as radiation, became a public health concern. Today, most hospitals have radiation emergency plans for handling emergency

situations involving radioactive contamination. Radiologic technologists should become aware of the radiation emergency plans that exist in the facilities in which they work. In this section, some fundamental principles of dealing with radioactive contamination in a health care environment are discussed.

Contamination

A radioactive dispersal device, or "dirty bomb," is a radioactive source mixed with conventional explosives. It is intended to contaminate an area with radioactive material and thereby cause panic. The actual long-term health effects of a dirty bomb are likely to be minimal. If the radioactive material remains in a small area, few people may be affected. However, if enough explosives are used to spread the radioactive material over a broad area, then the radioactivity will be diluted and may not be much higher than background levels.

For example, it would be difficult for terrorists to accumulate as much radioactive material as existed in the Chernobyl nuclear reactor. Even if they were able to do this and were to explode the device with the same force as the explosion at Chernobyl, the actual number of radiation injuries would probably be quite small. At Chernobyl, no cases of acute radiation syndrome (ARS) were caused by exposure outside the immediate vicinity of the reactor. The only cases occurred in emergency workers, primarily firemen, who worked very near the reactor. They had little training and essentially no protective gear to prepare them for a radioactive emergency. In the United States at the present time, emergency responders are equipped to monitor and assess personnel exposure on-site.

After an explosion of a dirty bomb, some individuals would be contaminated with dust and debris, some of which could contain radioactive materials. The procedure for **decontamination** is surprisingly simple. Removal of contaminated clothing and immersion in a shower comprise the best method. If a wound contains radioactive material, a simple rinse of the area is usually sufficient to allow medical personnel to provide medical attention. Most hospitals are stocked with **Geiger–Müller (GM) detectors** (described in Chapter 5), and emergency personnel are trained to provide guidance concerning contamination levels. The facility's radiation safety officer would also be available to assess contamination levels.

It is unlikely that a dirty bomb would cause contamination with so much radioactive material that a victim could not receive medical attention. The key here is that the same personnel need not be near patients for any length of time. Most emergency room treatments do not require the staff to be near patients for as long as an hour. Even if a GM detector shows readings of two to five times natural background radiation, this means an effective dose rate of only 0.03 to 0.15 mSv/hr would be experienced by a physician who is in direct contact with the patient. Therefore a physician could treat this patient under these circumstances without exceeding normal dose limits. In fact, normal dose limits do not apply in radiation emergency situations.

The **Environmental Protection Agency (EPA)** suggests that during an emergency situation, individuals engaged in nonlifesaving activities work under a dose limit of 50 mSv per event. For individuals engaged in lifesaving activities, the dose limit rises to 250 mSv per event.[1] Because it may be difficult to monitor all workers involved in a radiation emergency, a dose rate criterion is often used. In this case, if the dose rate in the area is less than 0.1 mSv/hr, emergency personnel may enter an area to perform critical tasks. If the dose rate exceeds 0.1 mSv/hr, emergency personnel should await specific instructions from radiation experts on how to proceed.[2]

Cleanup of a Contaminated Urban Area

The EPA sets limits for radioactive contamination that assume that a *1 in 10,000* risk of causing a fatal cancer is unacceptable. This type of regulation requires hospitals, educational facilities, and industries to control accidental exposures so that the health of the population cannot be measurably affected. It also assumes that many other carcinogens are present and that all are regulated to a similar low level.

However, if radioactive contamination were to result from a dirty bomb, it is hoped that a more realistic evaluation of actual risk would be used. Unnecessary use of resources to clean a large inhabitable area (e.g., at the heart of a major city) to unreasonably stringent standards would be an unfortunate outcome requiring the expenditure of vast resources that could be used to benefit the public elsewhere. For example, *a 1 in 10,000 probability of causing a fatal cancer corresponds approximately to a 2 mSv effective dose.* Recall from Chapter 2 that the annual effective dose resulting from average natural background radiation is approximately 3 mSv. Therefore cleanup of a contaminated site to levels associated with normal radiation protection standards would require heroic measures, such as:

- Removal of topsoil
- Digging up of roadways

A practical compromise should be made to allow land use after a reasonable cleanup.

Medical Management of Persons Experiencing Radiation Bioeffects

If **surface contamination** is suspected, personnel should wear gowns, masks, and gloves when working with the patient. The same procedures that control the spread of infection are useful to prevent the spread of radioactive contamination. The clothing of individuals who have been contaminated should be placed in plastic containers and set aside for later evaluation. Removal of surface contamination involves removal of the patient's clothing and the use of a shower to cleanse the skin.

The various stages of ARS are discussed in Chapter 8. (A complete discussion of procedures for handling acute radiation syndrome is beyond the scope of this text. The interested reader is referred to recent publications

TABLE 15.1   Dose Effect Relation After Acute Whole-Body Radiation From Gamma Rays or X-Rays*

Whole-Body (Gy$_t$)	Absorbed Dose Effect
0.05	No symptoms
0.15	No symptoms but possible chromosomal aberrations in cultured peripheral blood lymphocytes
0.5	No symptoms (minor decreases in white blood cell and platelet counts in a few persons)
1	Nausea and vomiting in approximately 10% of patients within 48 hr after exposure
2	Nausea and vomiting in approximately 50% of persons within 24 hr, with marked decreases in white blood cell and platelet counts
4	Nausea and vomiting in 90% of persons within 12 hr and diarrhea in 10% within 8 hr; 50% mortality in the absence of treatment
6	100% mortality within 30 days because of bone marrow failure in the absence of treatment
10	Approximate dose that is survivable with the best medical therapy available
>10–30	Nausea and vomiting in all persons in less than 5 minutes; severe gastrointestinal damage; death likely in 2 to 3 weeks in the absence of treatment
>30	Cardiovascular collapse and central nervous system damage, with death in 24 to72 hours

*Data from Gusev I, Guskova AK, Mettler FA Jr, editors: *Medical Management of Radiation Accidents*, ed 2, Boca Raton, FL, 2001, CRC Press.

on this subject.[3,4]) In dealing with patients with ARS, some estimate of the amount of exposure they have received helps predict the clinical course of the syndrome (Table 15.1). For exposures localized to specific regions of the body, medical management involves the prevention of infection and control of pain and potential skin grafts. If beta-emitting radioactive material settles on a patient's skin, the dose is superficial, and skin grafts may be successful. Gamma-emitting materials can produce a deeper dose that could interfere with healing.

During the first 48 hours of ARS, symptoms such as nausea and vomiting occur. Medical management at this time is simply to treat the symptoms and try to prevent dehydration. The bone marrow becomes depleted (leukopenia and thrombocytopenia) after a few weeks. Bone marrow transplantation has been attempted in individuals such as severely exposed Chernobyl emergency workers. However, this strategy has not been successful. The current plan is to administer drugs that stimulate activity in any remaining bone marrow.

In the event of **internal contamination**, various strategies are used, depending on the clinical and radiologic form of contamination. Some of these methods include:
- Dilution (forcing fluids)
- Blocking absorption in the gastrointestinal tract (administration of emetics, charcoal, laxatives)

If the radionuclide is iodine, administration of potassium iodide to block further uptake in the thyroid is possible if no more than a few hours have elapsed since the contamination.

The National Library of Medicine and the National Institutes of Health maintain a website that contains a wealth of information on dealing with radiation emergencies. It contains:
- Both basic and advanced methods for decontamination
- Methods to reduce exposure
- Specific medical emergency procedures for various situations

The website may be found at www.nlm.nih.gov/medlineplus/radiationemergencies.html.

■ SUMMARY

- Isotopes are atoms that have the same number of protons within the nucleus but have different numbers of neutrons.
- Some nuclei of isotopes have too many neutrons or too many protons for stability.
- Radioactive isotopes spontaneously undergo changes or transformations to rectify their unstable arrangement.
- Rapidly dividing cells that are well oxygenated are very radiosensitive.
- When cells are radiosensitive, cancerous growths or tumors can be either eliminated, or at least controlled, by irradiation of the area containing the growth.

- Therapeutic isotopes generally have relatively long half-lives compared with diagnostically employed isotopes.
- Fast electrons are beta radiation.
- Gamma rays and x-ray photons differ only in their point of origin.
- Iodine-125 decays with a half-life of 59.4 days by a process called *electron capture.*
- The most practical radiation protection to follow for patients having therapeutic prostate seed implants is use of the concepts of distance and time.
- When iodine-131 is being administered to treat a hospitalized patient for thyroid cancer, a large, up to 2.5 cm or 1-inch thick, rolling lead shield can be positioned between the patient and any attending personnel for protection.
- Residual unused nonreturned radioisotopes, as well as radioactively contaminated items, must be held in a secure, shielded, and posted storage area for a period of 10 half-lives of the isotope before being able to be discarded in ordinary trash. Proper record keeping is to be kept of storage and disposal.
- Diagnostic techniques in nuclear medicine typically make use of short-lived radioisotopes as radioactive tracers.
- Technetium-99m is the most common radioisotope used in nuclear medicine.
- Positron emission tomography (PET) makes use of annihilation radiation events.
- When matter–antimatter annihilation occurs, a positron and an electron interact destructively and disappear. Their respective masses are converted into energy that will be carried off by two photons emerging from the annihilation site in opposite directions, each with a kinetic energy of 511 keV.
- A neutrino is a particle that has almost negligible mass and no electric charge but carries away any excess energy from the nucleus of the atom in processes such as beta and positron decay.
- Fluorine-18 is the most important isotope used for PET scanning.
- PET is an important imaging modality because it can examine metabolic processes within the body.
- Fluorodeoxyglucose (FDG) is a radioactive tracer that is taken up or metabolized by cancerous cells and that reveals their location through positron emission decay and subsequent generation of oppositely traveling annihilation photons.

- A PET/CT scanner can detect the presence of regions of abnormally high glucose metabolism, thus providing evidence of cancer metastasis to other body areas, and at the same time can obtain detailed information about the location and size of these lesions or growths.
- Positron emitters result in the production of high energy radiation, and for this reason, the design of a PET/CT imaging suite involves significant radiation safety concerns.
- Most hospitals have radiation emergency plans for handling emergency situations involving radioactive contamination.
- A radioactive dispersal device, or "dirty bomb," is a radioactive source mixed with conventional explosives, the actual long-term health effects of which will most likely be minimal.
- If radioactive material from a dirty bomb remains in a small area, only a few people may be seriously affected.
- Conversely, if enough explosives are used to spread the radioactive material over a broad area, radioactivity will be diluted and may not be much higher than background levels.
- If a dirty bomb were to explode with the same force as the explosion at Chernobyl, the actual number of radiation injuries could be quite small.
- The United States currently has emergency responders who are prepared and equipped to monitor and assess personnel exposure on-site in an emergency situation.
- After an explosion of a dirty bomb, externally contaminated individuals can be decontaminated by removal of contaminated clothing and immersion in a shower.
- Geiger–Müller (GM) detectors may be used by trained emergency personnel to monitor contamination levels.
- During an emergency situation, individuals engaged in nonlifesaving activities are to work under a dose limit of 50 mSv per event, whereas those persons performing lifesaving activities have a dose limit of 250 mSv.
- If surface contamination is suspected, emergency personnel should protect themselves by wearing gowns, masks, and gloves while working with the patient.
- Handling of patients with internal contamination varies depending on the clinical and radiologic form of contamination. Strategies may include dilution and blocking absorption in the gastrointestinal tract. Potassium iodide can be administered to block further uptake of radioactive iodine in the thyroid gland.

REFERENCES

1. Mettler FA, Voelz GL: Major radiation exposure: what to expect and how to respond. *N Engl J Med* 346:1554, 2002.
2. National Council on Radiation Protection and Measurements (NCRP): *Management of terrorist events involving radioactive material, Report No. 138*, Bethesda, MD, 2001, NCRP.
3. Gusev I, et al, editors: *Medical management of radiation accidents*, ed 2, Boca Raton, FL, 2001, CRC Press.
4. Jarrett D, editor: *Medical management of radiation casualties: handbook, AFRRI Special Publication 99-92*, Bethesda, MD, 1999, Armed Forces Radiobiology Research Institute. Also available at: www.afrri.usuhs.mil.

GENERAL DISCUSSION QUESTIONS

1. Why do isotopes that have too many neutrons or too many protons spontaneously undergo changes or transformations?
2. What causes cancerous growths or tumors to be eliminated or controlled by irradiation?
3. What difference exists between gamma rays and x-ray photons?
4. What are the best radiation safety practices to follow for patients having therapeutic prostate seed implants?
5. While caring for a hospitalized patient receiving iodine-131 therapy for cancer, what can hospital personnel do to minimize occupational exposure?
6. What radiation safety concerns are associated with the design of a PET/CT imaging suite, and how is radiation protection provided to meet these concerns?
7. What is a radioactive dispersal device, or "dirty bomb," and what are the possible consequences if such a device is detonated?
8. If a wound contains radioactive material, what should be done to decontaminate the wound?
9. What dose level may an individual engaged in lifesaving activities during a radiation emergency receive?
10. If surface contamination is suspected, what should medical personnel wear when working with a contaminated patient?

REVIEW QUESTIONS

1. Well-oxygenated rapidly dividing cells are:
   A. Very insensitive and are not damaged by radiation
   B. Very sensitive to damage by radiation
   C. Moderately sensitive to damage by radiation
   D. Somewhat sensitive to damage by radiation
2. Iodine-125 decays with a half-life of 59.4 days by a process called:
   A. Attenuation
   B. Electron capture
   C. Pair production
   D. Photodisintegration
3. Which of the following steps should be taken for external decontamination from radioactive materials?
   1. Removal of contaminated clothing
   2. Immersion of contaminated person in a shower
   3. Monitoring of the contaminated individual with a Geiger–Müller detector
   A. 1 and 2 only
   B. 1 and 3 only
   C. 2 and 3 only
   D. 1, 2, and 3
4. What dose level may an individual who is engaged in nonlifesaving activities during a radiation emergency safely receive?
   A. 10 mSv per event
   B. 30 mSv per event
   C. 50 mSv per event
   D. 250 mSv per event
5. The clothing of individuals that has been contaminated should be:
   A. Aired out on a clothesline to decontaminate
   B. Burned immediately
   C. Placed in plastic containers and set aside for later evaluation
   D. Shaken out and put back on
6. All of the following statements are true *except*:
   A. In dealing with patients with acute radiation syndrome (ARS), some estimate of the amount of exposure they have received helps predict the clinical course of the syndrome.
   B. If beta-emitting radioactive material settles on a patient's skin, the dose is very deep and skin grafts will not be very successful.

C. Gamma-emitting radioactive materials can produce a deep dose that may interfere with healing.

D. Current strategy for an ARS patient is to administer drugs that stimulate any remaining bone marrow.

7. Some of the strategies used to treat internal radiation contamination include:
    1. Dilution (forcing fluids)
    2. Blocking absorption in the gastrointestinal tract (administration of emetics, charcoal, laxatives)
    3. Administration of potassium iodide to block further uptake in the thyroid if the radionuclide is iodine and no more than a few hours have elapsed since the contamination
    A. 1 only
    B. 2 only
    C. 3 only
    D. 1, 2, and 3

8. A well-designed PET/CT facility should be arranged so that there are no areas of full occupancy immediately adjacent to a:

A. High energy radiation source

B. Low energy radiation source

C. Patient waiting area

D. Public corridor

9. Which of the following are almost impossible to detect?
    A. X-rays
    B. Gamma rays
    C. Positrons
    D. Neutrinos

10. Patients receiving iodine-125 should *significantly* limit durations of close contact (<30 cm or 1 foot) with small children and pregnant women for a period of:
    A. Six days after the implant procedure
    B. Six weeks after the implant procedure
    C. Six months after the implant procedure
    D. Six years after the implant procedure

Relationships Between Systems of Units

As has been shown throughout this textbook, various quantities are necessary for describing physical processes. Well-known examples of such quantities are length, mass, force, energy, and time. If one also includes electric charge, then virtually all of the fundamental constants of nature can be found to be included within combinations of these physical quantities or, more precisely, *the units associated with them.* The purpose of this appendix is to tabulate quantities and units, including those that pertain to ionizing radiation that may be encountered by the student. It should be emphasized that a concerted effort has long been under way to just have one system of units in place throughout the world, namely the Systeme International, or SI. There are strong pockets of resistance to this, especially in the United States, which is firmly wedded to the English system. However, in official communities such as radiation protection regulations, educational materials, and registry and licensing examinations, SI units have become the norm and will be used in this text as much as possible.

Three basic systems of physical units have been in existence for a long time and are familiar to varying degrees, depending on what part of the world one lives in and perhaps one's field of work. They are the English system, the CGS system, and the MKS (SI) system. The following tables specify for each important physical quantity the corresponding associated fundamental unit in each of the three systems and the relationship among these units when possible. Boxes demonstrating calculations for conversions among units and for equivalent and effective dose are also provided.

English System

Quantity	Unit
Length	Foot, inch
Force (weight)	Pound (lb.)
Mass	Slug (an object of mass; 1 slug weighs 32 lb.)
Energy	Foot-pound
Power	Horsepower (hp)
Pressure	Lb/in^2
Time	Second
Electric charge	Coulomb
Temperature	Degrees Fahrenheit (°F)
Absorbed dose	No specific unit
Exposure	Roentgen*

*The roentgen is defined as the photon (either x-ray or gamma ray) exposure that, under standard conditions of pressure and temperature, produces a total positive or negative charge of 2.58×10^{-4} C/kg of dry air.

CGS System

Quantity	Unit
Length	Centimeter (cm)
Force (weight)	Dyne (1 gm-cm/sec^2)
Mass	Gram (g)
Energy	Erg (1 gm-cm^2/sec^2)
Power	Ergs per second
Pressure	Barye (Ba) (1 Ba = 1 dyne/cm^2)
Time	Second
Electric charge	Statcoulomb or ESU (ESU means electrostatic unit of charge)
Temperature	Degrees Centigrade (Celsius) (°C)
Absorbed dose	Rad (1 rad = 100 ergs/gram)
Equivalent dose	Rem**

**Rem stands for "radiation equivalent man." It is defined as the dose that is equivalent to any type of ionizing radiation that produces the same biologic effect as 1 rad (radiation absorbed dose) of x-radiation.

MKS (SI) System

Quantity	Unit
Length	Meter (m)
Force (weight)	Newton (1 N = 1 kg-m/sec²)
Mass	Kilogram (kg)
Energy	Joule (1 J = 1 kg-m²/sec²)
Power	Watt (1 W = 1 joule/sec)
Pressure	N/m²
Time	Second
Electric charge	Coulomb (C)
Temperature	Degrees Centigrade (Celsius), degrees Kelvin
Absorbed dose	Gray (Gy) (1 Gy = 1 J/kg)
Equivalent dose	Sievert (Sv)

Relationships Among Units

Quantity	Unit Conversions
Length	1 m = 100 cm = 39.37 inches; 2.54 cm = 1 inch
Force (weight)	1 N = 0.225 lb = 10^5 dynes
Mass	1 kg = 1000 g; 1 slug = 14.6 kg
Energy	1 J = 10^7 ergs = 0.738 ft-lb
Power	1 W = 0.738 ft-lb/sec; 1 hp = 550 ft-lb/sec = 746 W = 0.746 kW
Pressure	1 N/m² = $1.45(10)^{-4}$ lb/in² =10 Ba; 1 atmosphere = 14.7 lb/in² = $1.013(10)^5$ N/m²
Time	1 second = 1/3600 hour = approximately 1/100,000 day
Electric charge	1 ESU = 1 statcoulomb = $3.34(10)^{-10}$ C
Temperature	$T_F = \frac{9}{5} T_C + 32$, $T_K = T_C + 273$
Exposure	1 coulomb/kg = 1 R / $2.58(10)^{-4}$ C/kg per R = 3876 R (a very large exposure)
Absorbed dose	1 Gy = 100 rad, 1 cGy = 1 rad
Equivalent dose	1 Sv = 100 rem, 10 mSv = 1 rem 1 mSv = 0.1 rem = 100 mrem

Conversion of Roentgens (R) to Coulombs per Kilogram (C/kg)

Example: To convert 100 R to C/kg:

$$100\,R = 100/3876 = 0.0258\ C/kg = 2.58(10)^{-2}\ C/kg$$

Conversion of Coulombs per Kilogram (C/kg) to Roentgens (R)

Example: To convert 0.01 C/kg to R:

$$C/kg = 0.01 \times 3876 = 38.8\,R$$

Conversion of Rad to Gray (Gy)

Example: 5000 rad = 5000 / 100 = 50 Gy

Conversion of Gray (Gy) to Rad or cGy

Example: 10 Gy = 10 × 100 = 1000 rad = 1000 cGy

Conversion of Millisievert (mSv) to Millirem (mrem)

Conversion of millisievert (mSv) to millirem (mrem)
Example: 3 mSv = 3 × 100 = 300 mrem

Determining and Expressing Equivalent Dose (EqD) Using Rad and Rem

Example: An individual received the following absorbed doses: 10 rad of x-radiation, 5 rad of fast neutrons, and 20 rad of alpha particles. What is the *total* equivalent dose in rem? In SI units?

Solution: We make use of the expression:

$$EqD = (D \times W_R)_1 + (D \times W_R)_2 + (D \times W_R)_3$$

in which W_R stands for radiation weighting factor. The radiation weighting factor for each radiation type in question may be obtained from Table 4.2.

Answer:

Radiation Type	D	X	W_R	=	EqD
X-radiation	10 rad	×	1	=	10 rem
Fast neutrons	5 rad	×	20	=	100 rem
Alpha particles	20 rad	×	20	=	400 rem
	Total EqD			=	510 rem

The number of Sieverts = 510 rem / 100 = 5.1 Sv

Determining and Expressing Effective Dose (EfD) in Rem

Example: The W_R for x-radiation is 1 (see Table 4.2), and the W_T for the gonads is 0.20 (see Table 4.3). If the gonads receive an absorbed dose (D) of 10 rad from exposure to x-radiation, what is the EfD in rem?

Answer:

$$EfD = D \times W_R \times W_T$$
$$= 10 \times 1 \times 0.20$$
$$= 0.2 \, rem$$
$$= 0.2/100 = 0.002 \, Sv$$

Traditional and SI Equivalents

1 roentgen (R) equals	2.58×10^{-4} C/kg of air
1 milliroentgen (mR) equals	$\frac{1}{1000}$ R or 10^{-3} R
1 rad equals	100 erg/g
	$\frac{1}{100}$ J/kg
	$\frac{1}{100}$ Gy
	1 cGy
1 millirad equals	10^{-3} rad
1 rem equals	$\frac{1}{100}$ J/kg (for x-radiation, Q = 1)
	$\frac{1}{100}$ Sv
	1 cSv
	10 mSv
1 millirem equals	$\frac{1}{1000}$ rem

B APPENDIX

Standard Designations for Metric System Lengths, Electron Volt Energy Levels, and Frequency Spectrum Ranges

Metric System Equivalents for Length

Length	Symbol	Power of 10 Fractional Form	Power of 10 Decimal Form	Scientific Notation
Yottameter	Ym	1,000,000,000,000,000,000,000,000	1,000,000,000,000,000,000,000,000	10^{24} (m)
Zettameter	Zm	1,000,000,000,000,000,000,000	1,000,000,000,000,000,000,000	10^{21} (m)
Exameter	Em	1,000,000,000,000,000,000	1,000,000,000,000,000,000	10^{18} (m)
Petameter	Pm	1,000,000,000,000,000	1,000,000,000,000,000	10^{15} (m)
Terameter	Tm	1,000,000,000,000	1,000,000,000,000	10^{12} (m)
Gigameter	Gm	1,000,000,000	1,000,000,000	10^{9} (m)
Megameter	Mm	1,000,000	1,000,000	10^{6} (m)
Kilometer	km	1000	1000	10^{3} (m)
Hectometer	hm	100	100	10^{2} (m)
Dekameter	dam	10	10	10^{1} (m)
Meter	m	1	1	10^{0} (m)
Decimeter	dm	1/10	0.1	10^{-1} (m)
Centimeter	cm	1/100	0.01	10^{-2} (m)
Millimeter	mm	1/1000	0.001	10^{-3} (m)
Micrometer	μm	1/1,000,000	0.00001	10^{-6} (m)
Nanometer	nm	1/1,000,000,000	0.000000001	10^{-9} (m)
Picometer	pm	1/1,000,000,000,000	0.000000000001	10^{-12} (m)
Femtometer	fm	1/1,000,000,000,000,000	0.000000000000001	10^{-15} (m)
Attometer	am	1/1,000,000,000,000,000,000	0.000000000000000001	10^{-18} (m)
Zeptometer	zm	1/1,000,000,000,000,000,000,000	0.000000000000000000001	10^{-21} (m)
Yoctometer	ym	1/1,000,000,000,000,000,000,000,000	0.000000000000000000000001	10^{-24} (m)

Electron Volt Common Energy Designations

The abbreviation *eV* stands for *electron volt*; 1 eV is defined as the energy acquired by an electron when it is moved through a 1-V potential difference by a battery or some other mechanism.

The following terms designate various powers of 10 multiples of 1 eV:

1 KeV = 1000 eV = 10^3 eV
1 MeV = 1,000,000 eV = 10^6 eV
1 GeV = 1,000,000,000 eV = 10^9 eV

The following terms designate various powers of 10 fractions of 1 eV:

1 meV = 0.001 eV = 10^{-3} eV
1 μeV = 0.000001 eV = 10^{-6} eV
1 neV = 0.000000001 eV = 10^{-9} eV

Common Frequency Spectrum Designations

The abbreviation *Hz* stands for *hertz,* which is the standard unit for frequency; 1 Hz is, by definition, equal to one repeatable cycle of a phenomenon or event (e.g., a water wave rising from flat to crest, descending to trough, and returning to flat) occurring in 1 second. Ten hertz corresponds to 10 such cycles occurring every second, whereas 0.1 Hz corresponds to only 1/10th of a cycle occurring each second.

The following terms designate frequency ranges that constitute various powers of 10 multiples of 1 Hz:

1 KHz = 10^3 Hz
1 MHz = 10^6 Hz
1 GHz = 10^9 Hz
1 THz = 10^{12} Hz
1 PHz = 10^{15} Hz
1 EHz = 10^{18} Hz

Periodic Table of Elements

Periodic Table of the Elements

Key:

Atomic number	11
Element symbol	Na
Element name	Sodium
Atomic weight	22.990

Legend:
- Alkali metals
- Alkaline earth metals
- Lanthanides
- Actinides
- Transition metals
- Post-transition metals
- Metalloids
- Other nonmetals
- Halogens
- Noble gases
- Unknown properties

Period	Group 1 / 1A	2 / 2A	3 / 3B	4 / 4B	5 / 5B	6 / 6B	7 / 7B	8 / 8B	9 / 8B	10	11 / 1B	12 / 2B	13 / 3A	14 / 4A	15 / 5A	16 / 6A	17 / 7A	18 / 8A
1	1 H Hydrogen 1.0078																	2 He Helium 4.0026
2	3 Li Lithium 6.938	4 Be Beryllium 9.0122											5 B Boron 10.806	6 C Carbon 12.009	7 N Nitrogen 14.006	8 O Oxygen 15.999	9 F Fluorine 18.998	10 Ne Neon 20.180
3	11 Na Sodium 22.990	12 Mg Magnesium 24.305											13 Al Aluminum 26.982	14 Si Silicon 28.084	15 P Phosphorus 30.974	16 S Sulfur 32.059	17 Cl Chlorine 35.446	18 Ar Argon 39.948
4	19 K Potassium 39.098	20 Ca Calcium 40.078	21 Sc Scandium 44.956	22 Ti Titanium 47.867	23 V Vanadium 50.942	24 Cr Chromium 51.996	25 Mn Manganese 54.938	26 Fe Iron 55.845	27 Co Cobalt 58.933	28 Ni Nickel 58.693	29 Cu Copper 63.546	30 Zn Zinc 65.38	31 Ga Gallium 69.723	32 Ge Germanium 72.63	33 As Arsenic 74.922	34 Se Selenium 78.96	35 Br Bromine 79.904	36 Kr Krypton 83.798
5	37 Rb Rubidium 85.468	38 Sr Strontium 87.62	39 Y Yttrium 88.906	40 Zr Zirconium 91.224	41 Nb Niobium 92.906	42 Mo Molybdenum 95.96	43 Tc Technetium 98.9062	44 Ru Ruthenium 101.07	45 Rh Rhodium 102.91	46 Pd Palladium 106.42	47 Ag Silver 107.87	48 Cd Cadmium 112.41	49 In Indium 114.82	50 Sn Tin 118.71	51 Sb Antimony 121.76	52 Te Tellurium 127.60	53 I Iodine 126.90	54 Xe Xenon 131.29
6	55 Cs Cesium 132.91	56 Ba Barium 137.33	57 La Lanthanum 138.91	72 Hf Hafnium 178.49	73 Ta Tantalum 180.95	74 W Tungsten 183.84	75 Re Rhenium 186.21	76 Os Osmium 190.23	77 Ir Iridium 192.22	78 Pt Platinum 195.08	79 Au Gold 196.97	80 Hg Mercury 200.59	81 Tl Thallium 204.38	82 Pb Lead 207.2	83 Bi Bismuth 208.98	84 Po Polonium (209)	85 At Astatine (210)	86 Rn Radon (222)
7	87 Fr Francium (223)	88 Ra Radium (226)	89 Ac Actinium (227)	104 Rf Rutherfordium (261)	105 Db Dubnium (262)	106 Sg Seaborgium (266)	107 Bh Bohrium (264)	108 Hs Hassium (269)	109 Mt Meitnerium (268)	110 Ds Darmstadtium (268)	111 Rg Roentgenium (268)	112 Cn Copernicium (268)	113 Uut Ununtrium (268)	114 Fl Flerovium (268)	115 Uup Ununpentium (268)	116 Lv Livermorium (268)	117 Uus Ununseptium (268)	118 Uuo Ununoctium (268)

Lanthanides:

58 Ce Cerium 140.12	59 Pr Praseodymium 140.91	60 Nd Neodymium 144.24	61 Pm Promethium (145)	62 Sm Samarium 150.36	63 Eu Europium 151.96	64 Gd Gadolinium 157.25	65 Tb Terbium 158.93	66 Dy Dysprosium 162.50	67 Ho Holmium 164.93	68 Er Erbium 167.26	69 Tm Thulium 168.93	70 Yb Ytterbium 173.04	71 Lu Lutetium 174.97

Actinides:

90 Th Thorium 232.04	91 Pa Protactinium 231.04	92 U Uranium 238.03	93 Np Neptunium (237)	94 Pu Plutonium (244)	95 Am Americium (243)	96 Cm Curium (247)	97 Bk Berkelium (247)	98 Cf Californium (251)	99 Es Einsteinium (252)	100 Fm Fermium (257)	101 Md Mendelevium (258)	102 No Nobelium (259)	103 Lr Lawrencium (262)

(Source: Tate K: Periodic table of the elements. www.LiveScience.com.)

Chance of a 50-KeV Photon Interacting With Atoms of Tissue as It Travels Through 5 cm of Soft Tissue

Let N_0 be the number of x-ray photons incident on a uniform slab of tissue of thickness "y." The probability that there will be an interaction of any sort between a photon and an atom within the slab is, in the simplest case, proportional to the slab thickness and the number of incident photons and the mean target size presented by a slab atom to an x-ray photon.

Mathematically, one may proceed as follows:

1. Let dN be the change in the number of photons in the x-ray beam after the beam has passed through an infinitesimal distance, dy. Because the number of photons decreases with every interaction, dN is a negative quantity.

2. At any depth within the phantom, the number of interactions that will occur in the next incremental thickness, dy, is proportional to the remaining number of photons, N, at that depth and the distance of penetration, dy. In mathematical terms:

$$dN = -\mu N dy$$

where the symbol μ is the constant of proportionality and is known as the *linear attenuation coefficient*. It is defined by the previous equation and has the following unit: 1/cm.

3. Rearranging the previous equation, one performs the following integration:

$$\int_{N_0}^{N} dN/N = -\mu \int_{0}^{y} dy$$

which leads to the following relation:

$$\ln(N/N_0) = -\mu y$$

4. If one uses the properties of logarithms and raises both sides of the last equation to the power e, the x-ray attenuation equation is as follows:

$$N = N_0 e^{-\mu y}$$

5. For 50-KeV photons passing through 5 cm of soft tissue:

$$\mu_{soft\ tissue} = 0.214 \text{ and } y = 5$$

Substituting these values into the last equation and rearranging the equation a bit, the following is obtained:

$$N/N_0 = e^{-(0.214 \times 5)} = 0.34$$

which shows that only 0.34, or 34%, of the initial number of photons in the 50-KeV beam remain (i.e., have not undergone an interaction) after traversing a 5-cm slab of tissue. In other words, 66% of the incident x-ray beam has interacted with a tissue atom.

Relationship Among Photons, Electromagnetic Waves, Wavelength, and Energy

Before 1900, all attempts to use current theories and concepts in physics to explain the measured energy distribution of radiation from a heated body failed grievously. In that year, a German physicist, Max Planck, introduced the concept of a "quantum," or discrete unit of energy, to resolve these discrepancies. According to Planck's theory, whenever radiation is emitted or absorbed by a hot object, the energy of that radiation is not emitted or absorbed continuously but rather in discrete amounts, which he called *quanta*.

Mathematically, a single such amount or energy quantum is given by the following equation:

$$E = hf$$

where **f** is the frequency of the radiation and **h** is a proportionality constant called, appropriately, *Planck's constant*. This quantum of energy has since received the name *photon*. Thus the energy of a photon varies directly as the frequency of the associated radiation. Because the frequency **f** and the wavelength **w** of any type of radiation are related by the simple expression

$$c = fw$$

where **c** is the speed of light (300,000,000 m/sec in a vacuum), then

$$E = hf = hc/w$$

This result shows that the energy of a photon decreases as the wavelength of the radiation increases (e.g., photons of infrared light are less energetic than those of ultraviolet light because infrared wavelengths are longer than ultraviolet wavelengths). Einstein used these ideas to successfully explain the emission of electrons from a metallic surface when visible light radiation was directed at it. This process is called the *photoelectric effect*. The light-produced electrons, or photoelectrons, were found to have *energies that depended on the wavelength of the focused light* but were completely independent of the intensity or brightness of that light. This phenomenon could not be explained by traditional physics. However, it was fully explicable in terms of the new concept of radiation energy (quanta or photons) and the energy relation given in the last equation. That relation contains *no reference to the brightness of the light* and, instead, shows that the incident light's energy, and consequently its ability to eject electrons from the metallic surface, is dependent upon the light's wavelength. For his work in this area, Einstein received the Nobel Prize in Physics in 1921.

To summarize, photons are the particles associated with the electromagnetic (EM) radiation spectrum (within which visible light and x-rays are included). When energy is transferred from an EM wave through interaction with matter, the energy is transferred by photons in discrete, or integral, amounts. Each such discrete amount is directly proportional to the frequency of the EM radiation or inversely proportional to its wavelength.

Electron Shell Structure of the Atom

Other than the hydrogen atom, all atoms contain more than one electron. The purpose of this appendix is to describe, without delving too extensively into the details of modern physics, specifically quantum mechanics: how electrons are arranged—that is, ordered—in multielectron atoms. To do so we must introduce two discovered principles that serve as the foundations for our discussion. These are, simply, that electrons in undisturbed or stable atoms are always distributed in the lowest overall energy configuration or energy states and that no two electrons can ever occupy the exact same energy level (in more precise terminology, no two electrons in an atom can exist in the exact same quantum state). The latter restriction was postulated from careful analysis of observed atomic spectral lines by the German physicist Wolfgang Pauli in 1925 and has since been known as the *Pauli Exclusion Principle.*

Early in the 20th century it was discovered that the distribution of electrons within an atom relative to the nucleus is not continuous or equally spaced but rather is specifically "discrete." This means that atomic electrons do not locate in a uniform way about the nucleus as marbles in a bowl or stack up one right after the other according to distance from the nucleus. Rather it was determined that their "most probable" allowable locations are in certain concentric "shells" of limited capacity that radially fan out from the nucleus. The existence of these electron shells was first determined experimentally from x-ray absorption studies—that is, missing spectral lines (absent wavelengths or frequencies) that are observed as black segments in an atom's energy spectrum after a beam of x-rays is passed through samples of that atom or element. And this has been found to be true for all elements. These missing wavelengths (w) or frequencies (f) are directly related to the energies of x-ray photons ($E = hf = hc/w$) that have been absorbed by the atoms within

the target samples. Through examination of such spectra in detail, it became possible to map out the actual pattern of electron energy levels within various atoms. This led to a direct correlation between the Bohr solar system model of the atom, in which groups of electrons were believed to orbit the nucleus at certain distances, and the concept of electron shells that were formed by these orbiting electron groups. Each electron shell was associated with a particular orbital radius at which some electrons were *most likely* to be found. The smaller the radius, the more tightly were these electrons held in their orbits about the nucleus, or in terms of energy, the greater was their binding energy and, consequently, the effort needed to free them from the attraction of the nucleus. For electron groups or electron shells farther away from the nucleus, the binding energies progressively decreased with distance until one reached the outermost shell, in which electrons needed only a few electron volts of additional energy to escape the atom. These electrons are therefore the predominant category of atomic electrons removed by ionizing radiation and also, quite importantly, the electrons most often involved in chemical reactions. For this reason they are given the special name "valence" electrons.

The electron shells were labeled in order of increasing distance from the nucleus with capital letters, beginning with the letter *K*, designating the innermost electron shell, and progressing through *L, M, N, O, P,* and *Q.* Again, from exhaustive spectral analysis, it was found that each electron shell except for the K shell was composed of multiple subshells labeled with lowercase letters *s, p, d, f, g, h,* and *i,* and these subshells were limited in the maximum number of electrons they could contain (s, 2; p, 6; d, 10; f, 14; g, 18; h, 22; i, 26). The theoretical rules that govern this are beyond the scope of this appendix. The following table demonstrates the electron shell occupancies for a number of atoms.

Atom	Atomic Number	Electron Shells	Electron Subshells and Electron Occupancy	
Hydrogen	1	K	s	1
Helium	2	K	s	2
Lithium	3	K	s	2
		L	s	1
Carbon	6	K	s	2
		L	s	2
			p	2
Oxygen	8	K	s	2
		L	s	2
			p	4
Sodium	11	K	s	2
		L	s	2
			p	6
		M	s	1
Argon	18	K	s	2
		L	s	2
			p	6
		M	s	2
			p	6
Calcium*	20	K	s	2
		L	s	2
			p	6
		M	s	2
			p	6
		N	s	2
Krypton	36	K	s	2
		L	s	2
			p	6
		M	s	2
			p	6
			d	10
		N	s	2
			p	6

*Because the electrons in an unexcited atom will always be arranged in the lowest overall energy configuration, there will be situations in which small subshells of higher shells will begin filling up before large subshells of lower shells are completely filled.

G | APPENDIX

Compton Interaction

The principle of conservation of mass–energy is that for an isolated system (i.e., a system on which no external energy source or energy drain is active), the total mass plus energy of all the particles comprising the system remains constant. This restraint, however, does not prevent mass–energy transfers between individual particles within the system.

The *linear momentum* of a particle is defined as the product of its mass and its velocity. A photon, which is the particle associated with electromagnetic radiation, moves at the speed of light; consequently, according to Einstein's theory of relativity, a photon must be a massless entity. Because of the equivalence between mass, m, and energy, E, given by the famous relation

$$E = mc^2$$

where c is the speed of light in a vacuum, one can associate with the photon a mass equivalent given by

$$E/c^2$$

Then the photon can be considered to have a linear momentum given by the product of the "mass equivalent" and the velocity of the photon.* The principle of conservation of linear momentum states that, for an isolated system, the sum of the linear momenta of all its particles

is constant. Exchanges of linear momentum between particles within the system can, of course, occur.

The Compton interaction is, most simply, a collision between an incident x-ray photon and the weakly bound outer electron of a target atom. Application of the principles of conservation of mass–energy and the conservation of linear momentum to the x-ray photon and outer electron system leads to equations that can be used to predict the energies and angles of scattering of both particles after their collision. If the energy of the incident photon is E, the following energy balance relation can be written:

$$E = E' + K$$

where E' is the photon's energy after the collision and K is the recoil energy of the "struck" electron.

Several important types of Compton interactions will now be described. These effects depend on the magnitude of the photon's incident energy, E, and the angle at which the photon interacts with the electron.

Case 1: The photon makes a head-on collision with the electron.

Result: The electron travels or scatters directly forward, and the photon travels or scatters backward (180-degree scatter angle).

Energy Situations:

a. $E \ll 511$ keV (low energy range):
   E' is approximately equal to E
   K is almost zero

b. $E = 511$ keV:
   $E' = E/3$
   $K = (2/3)$ E

c. $E \gg 511$ keV (high energy range):
   E' is approximately zero
   $K = E$ to good approximation

---

*Linear momentum = mass times velocity

Photon mass equivalent = E/c^2
Magnitude of photon velocity = speed of light, c
Photon linear momentum, p, therefore is given by:
$$\mathbf{p} = (E/c^2)\,c = \mathbf{E/c}$$
Since E = hc/w (see Appendix E), then we can also write that:
$$\mathbf{p} = E/c = (hc/w)/c = \mathbf{h/w}$$

Case 2: The photon grazes the electron.

Result: The photon emerges from the collision nearly undeflected from its initial direction, and the electron scatters at right angles.

Energy Situation:

E′ is approximately equal to E

K is approximately zero

Collisions of this nature, in which the incident photon loses little or no energy, are especially important in the planning of radiation shielding for therapeutic x-ray suites.

Revision of 10 CFR Part 35*

§ 35.50 Training for Radiation Safety Officer

Except as provided in § 35.57, the licensee shall require an individual fulfilling the responsibilities of the Radiation Safety Officer (RSO) as provided in § 35.24 to be an individual who:

(a) Is certified by a specialty board whose certification process includes all of the requirements in paragraph (b) of this section and whose certification has been approved by the Commission or;

(b) (1) Has completed a structured educational program consisting of both:

    (i) 200 hours of didactic training in the following areas:

        (A) Radiation physics and instrumentation;

        (B) Radiation protection;

        (C) Mathematics pertaining to the use and measurement of radioactivity;

        (D) Radiation biology; and

        (E) Radiation dosimetry; and

    (ii) One year of full-time radiation safety experience under the supervision of the individual identified as the RSO on a Commission or Agreement State license that authorized similar types(s) of use(s) of byproduct material involving the following:

        (A) Shipping, receiving, and performing related radiation surveys;

        (B) Using and performing checks for proper operation of dose calibrators, survey meters, and instruments used to measure radionuclides;

        (C) Securing and controlling byproduct material;

        (D) Using administrative controls to avoid mistakes in the administration of byproduct material;

        (E) Using procedures to prevent or minimize radioactive contamination and using proper decontamination procedures; and

        (F) Disposing of byproduct material; and

    (2) Has obtained written certification, signed by a preceptor RSO, that the requirements in paragraph (b)(1) of this section have been satisfactorily completed and that the individual has achieved a level of competency sufficient to independently function as an RSO for medical uses of byproduct material; and

    (3) Following completion of the requirements in paragraph (b) of this section, has demonstrated sufficient knowledge in radiation safety commensurate with the use requested by passing an examination given by an organization or entity approved by the Commission in accordance with Appendix A of this part; or

(c) Is an authorized user, authorized medical physicist, or authorized nuclear pharmacist identified on the licensee's license and has experience with the radiation safety aspects of similar types of use of byproduct material for which the individual has RSO responsibilities.

---

*Training is the same as described in current 10 CFR Part 35.

Consumer-Patient Radiation Health and Safety Act of 1981*

SUBTITLE I—CONSUMER-PATIENT RADIATION HEALTH AND SAFETY ACT OF 1981

Short Title

[42 USC 10001.] note
SEC. 975. This subtitle may be cited as the "consumer-patient radiation health and safety act of 1981."

Statement of Findings

[42 USC 10001.]
SEC. 976. The congress finds that . . .
(1) it is in the interest of public health and safety to minimize unnecessary exposure to potentially hazardous radiation due to medical and dental radiologic procedures;
(2) it is in the interest of public health and safety to have a continuing supply of adequately educated persons and appropriate accreditation and certification programs administered by state governments;
(3) the protection of the public health and safety from unnecessary exposure to potentially hazardous radiation due to medical and dental radiologic procedures and the assurance of efficacious procedures are the responsibility of state and federal governments;
(4) persons who administer radiologic procedures, including procedures at federal facilities, should be required to demonstrate competence by reason of education, training, and experience; and
(5) the administration of radiologic procedures and the effect on individuals of such procedures have a substantial and direct effect upon United States interstate commerce.

Statement of Purpose

[42 USC 10002.]
SEC. 977. It is the purpose of this subtitle to—
(1) provide for the establishment of minimum standards by the federal government for the accreditation of education programs for persons who administer radiologic procedures and for the certification of such persons; and
(2) ensure that medical and dental radiologic procedures are consistent with rigorous safety precautions and standards.

Definitions

[42 USC 10003.]
SEC. 978. Unless otherwise expressly provided, for purposes of this subtitle, the term—
(1) "radiation" means ionizing and nonionizing radiation in amounts beyond normal background levels from sources such as medical and dental radiologic procedures;
(2) "radiologic procedure" means any procedure or article intended for use in—
   (A) the diagnosis of disease or other medical or dental conditions in humans (including diagnostic x-rays or nuclear medicine procedures); or
   (B) the cure, mitigation, treatment, or prevention of disease in humans that achieves its intended purpose through the emission of radiation;
(3) "radiologic equipment" means any radiation electronic product that emits or detects radiation and is used or intended for use to—
   (A) diagnose disease or other medical or dental conditions (including diagnostic x-ray equipment); or
   (B) cure, mitigate, treat, or prevent disease in humans that achieves its intended purpose through the emission or detection of radiation;

---

*Modified from Consumer-Patient Radiation Health and Safety Act of 1981, Chapter 107, Secs. 10001-8 (Aug. 13, 1981).

(4) "practitioner" means any licensed doctor of medicine, osteopathy, dentistry, podiatry, or chiropractic who prescribes radiologic procedures for other persons;

(5) "persons who administer radiologic procedures" means any person, other than a practitioner, who intentionally administers radiation to other persons for medical purposes and includes medical radiologic technologists (including dental hygienists and assistants), radiation therapy technologists, and nuclear medicine technologists;

(6) "Secretary" means the Secretary of Health and Human Services; and

(7) "State" means the several states, the District of Columbia, the Commonwealth of Puerto Rico, the Commonwealth of the Northern Mariana Islands, the Virgin Islands, Guam, American Samoa, and the Trust Territory of the Pacific Islands.

Promulgation of Standards

[Regulation. 42 USC 10004.]
SEC. 979.

(a) Within 12 months after the date of enactment of this act, the Secretary, in consultation with the Radiation Policy Council, the Administrator of Veterans' Affairs, the Administrator of the Environmental Protection Agency, appropriate agencies of the States, and appropriate professional organizations, shall by regulation promulgate minimum standards for the accreditation of educational programs to train individuals to perform radiologic procedures. Such standards shall distinguish between programs for the education of (1) medical radiologic technologists (including radiographers), (2) dental auxiliaries (including dental hygienists and assistants), (3) radiation therapy technologists, (4) nuclear medicine technologists, and (5) such other kinds of health auxiliaries who administer radiologic procedures as the Secretary determines appropriate. Such standards shall not be applicable to educational programs for practitioners.
[Regulation.]

(b) Within 12 months after the date of enactment of this act, the Secretary, in consultation with the Radiation Policy Council, the Administrator of Veterans' Affairs, the Administrator of the Environmental Protection Agency, interested agencies of the States, and appropriate professional organizations, shall by regulation promulgate minimum standards for the certification of persons who administer radiologic procedures. Such standards shall distinguish between certification

of (1) medical radiologic technologists (including radiographers), (2) dental auxiliaries (including dental hygienists and assistants), (3) radiation therapy technologists, (4) nuclear medicine technologists, and (5) such other kinds of health auxiliaries who administer radiologic procedures as the Secretary determines appropriate. Such standards shall include minimum certification criteria for individuals with regard to accredited education, practical experience, successful passage of required examinations, and such other criteria as the Secretary shall deem necessary for the adequate qualification of individuals to administer radiologic procedures. Such standards shall not apply to practitioners.

Model Statute

[42 USC 10005.]
SEC. 980. In order to encourage the administration of accreditation and certification programs by the states, the Secretary shall prepare and transmit to the states a model statute for radiologic procedure safety. Such model statute shall provide that—

(1) it shall be unlawful in a state for individuals to perform radiologic procedures unless such individuals are certified by the state to perform such procedures; and

(2) any educational requirements for certification of individuals to perform radiologic procedures shall be limited to educational programs accredited by the state.

Compliance

[42 USC 10006.]
SEC. 981.

(a) The Secretary shall take all actions consistent with law to effectuate the purposes of this subtitle.

(b) A state may utilize an accreditation or certification program administered by a private entity if—

    (1) such state delegates the administration of the state accreditation or certification program to such private entity;

    (2) such program is approved by the state; and

    (3) such program is consistent with the minimum federal standards promulgated under this subtitle for such program.

(c) Absent compliance by the states with the provisions of this subtitle within 3 years after the date of enactment of this act, the Secretary shall report to the Congress recommendations for legislative changes considered necessary to ensure the states' compliance with this subtitle.

[Report to Congress.]

(d) The Secretary shall be responsible for continued monitoring of compliance by the states with the applicable provisions of this subtitle and shall report to the Senate and the House of Representatives by January 1, 1982, and January 1 of each succeeding year the status of the states' compliance with the purposes of this subtitle.

(e) Notwithstanding any other provision of this section, in the case of a state that has, prior to the effective date of standards and guidelines promulgated pursuant to this subtitle, established standards for the accreditation of educational programs and certification of radiologic technologists, such state shall be deemed to be in compliance with the conditions of this section unless the Secretary determines, after notice and hearing, that such state standards do not meet the minimum standards prescribed by the Secretary or are inconsistent with the purposes of this subtitle.

Federal Radiation Guidelines

[42 USC 10007.]

SEC. 982. The Secretary shall, in conjunction with the Radiation Policy Council, the Administrator of Veterans' Affairs, the Administrator of the Environmental Protection Agency, appropriate agencies of the states, and appropriate professional organizations, promulgate Federal radiation guidelines with respect to radiologic procedures. Such guidelines shall—

(1) determine the level of radiation exposure due to radiologic procedures that is unnecessary and specify the techniques, procedures, and methods to minimize such unnecessary exposure;

(2) provide for the elimination of the need for retakes of diagnostic radiologic procedures;

(3) provide for the elimination of unproductive screening programs;

(4) provide for the optimum diagnostic information with minimum radiologic exposure; and

(5) include the therapeutic application of radiation to individuals in the treatment of disease, including nuclear medicine applications.

Applicability to Federal Agencies

[42 USC 10008.]

SEC. 983.

(a) Except as provided in subsection (b), each department, agency, and instrumentality of the executive branch of the federal government shall comply with standards promulgated pursuant to this subtitle.

[Regulations.]

[38 USC 101 *et seq.*]

(b) (1) The Administrator of Veterans' Affairs, through the Chief Medical Director of the Veterans' Administration, shall, to the maximum extent feasible consistent with the responsibilities of such Administrator and Chief Medical Director under subtitle 38, United States Code, prescribe regulations making the standards promulgated pursuant to this subtitle applicable to the provision of radiologic procedures in facilities over which the Administrator has jurisdiction. In prescribing and implementing regulations pursuant to this subsection, the Administrator shall consult with the Secretary in order to achieve the maximum possible coordination of the regulations, standards, and guidelines, and the implementation thereof, which the Secretary and the Administrator prescribe under this subtitle.

[Report to congressional committees.]

(2) Not later than 180 days after standards are promulgated by the Secretary pursuant to this subtitle, the Administrator of Veterans' Affairs shall submit to the appropriate committees of Congress a full report with respect to the regulations (including guidelines, policies, and procedures thereunder) prescribed pursuant to paragraph (1) of this subsection. Such report shall include—

(A) an explanation of any inconsistency between standards made applicable by such regulations and the standards promulgated by the Secretary pursuant to this subtitle;

(B) an account of the extent, substance, and results of consultations with the Secretary respecting the prescription and implementation of regulations by the Administrator; and

(C) such recommendations for legislation and administrative action as the Administrator determines are necessary and desirable.

[Publication in Federal Register.]

(3) The Administrator of Veterans' Affairs shall publish the report required by paragraph (2) in the Federal Register.

Image Gently Pledge

Yes, I want to *image gently*.

Recognizing that every member of the health care team plays a vital role in caring for the patient and wants to provide the best care, I pledge:

- To make the image gently message a priority in staff communications this year
- To review the protocol recommendations and, where necessary, implement adjustments to our processes
- To respect and listen to suggestions from every member of the imaging team on ways to ensure changes are made
- To communicate openly with parents

Thank you for committing to the goal to image gently when you image or treat children.

Spread the word in your department, practice, hospital, or clinic.

Take the pledge at https://radsociety.wufoo.com/forms/image-gently-pledge/

Image Wisely Pledge

PLEDGE FOR IMAGING PROFESSIONALS

Yes, I want to **image wisely.**
I wish to optimize the use of radiation in imaging patients and thereby pledge:

1. To *put my patients' safety, health, and welfare first* by optimizing imaging examinations to use only the radiation necessary to produce diagnostic-quality images
2. To *convey the principles of the Image Wisely program* to the imaging team in order to ensure that my facility optimizes its use of radiation when imaging patients
3. To *communicate optimal patient imaging strategies to referring physicians* and to be available for consultation
4. To *routinely review imaging protocols* to ensure that the least radiation necessary to acquire a diagnostic-quality image is used for each examination
5. To *monitor examination radiation dose indices* to enable comparison to established diagnostic reference levels

Take the pledge at http://www.imagewisely.org/Pledge/Imaging-Professionals-Pledge

GLOSSARY

A

Aberration Deviation from normal development or growth; a lesion or anomaly.

Absolute risk Model predicting that a specific number of excess cancers will occur as a result of exposure to ionizing radiation.

Absorbed dose (D) The amount of energy per unit mass absorbed by an irradiated object (e.g., the patient's body tissue). This absorbed energy is responsible for any biologic damage resulting from the tissues being exposed to radiation. The gray (Gy) is the SI unit of this radiation quantity.

Absorption Transference of electromagnetic energy from an x-ray beam to the atoms or molecules of the matter through which it passes (e.g., the patient's biologic material).

Acid–base balance State of equilibrium or stability between acids and bases.

Acids Hydrogen-containing compounds that can attack and dissolve metal (e.g., HNO_3, nitric acid).

Action limits Limits for occupational exposure that are set by the medical facility well below the regulatory values as they appear in state or federal regulations. These limits are set at levels, typically a tenth of the action limit, that are not routinely exceeded by personnel. They are meant to trigger an investigation that should uncover the reason for any unusually high exposure.

Acute Something that begins suddenly and runs a short but severe course (e.g., an acute disease).

Acute radiation syndrome (ARS) Radiation sickness, or early somatic tissue reactions, occurring in humans soon after whole-body reception of large doses of ionizing radiation delivered over a short period.

Added filtration Sheets of aluminum (or its equivalent) of appropriate thickness interposed outside the glass window of the x-ray tube housing above the collimator shutters.

Adenine (A) One of two purine bases found in both DNA and RNA.

Agreement states Individual states of the United States that have entered into an agreement with the Nuclear Regulatory Commission (NRC) to assume responsibility for enforcing radiation protection regulations through their respective health departments.

Air gap technique An alternative procedure to the use of a radiographic grid for reducing scattered radiation during certain examinations.

Air kerma SI quantity that can be used to express radiation energy transferred to a point, such as the surface of a patient's or radiographer's body. Air kerma is kinetic energy released in a unit mass (kilogram) of air and is expressed in metric units of joule per kilogram (J/kg).

ALARA concept/principle Precept holding that occupational exposure of the patient, occupationally exposed persons, and the general public should be kept "as low as reasonably achievable." Radiation exposure should always be kept ALARA for all medical imaging procedures.

Alkali A member of a group of elements that includes lithium, sodium, and potassium.

Alkaline earth A member of a group of elements including calcium, magnesium, and strontium.

Alliance for Radiation Safety in Pediatric Imaging A partnership of medical societies, founded in 2007, whose overall common purpose is to reduce dose for pediatric patients.

Alopecia See *Epilation.*

Alpha particle A positively charged particle of radiation that is emitted from nuclei of very heavy elements such as uranium and plutonium during the process of radioactive decay. An alpha particle contains two protons and two neutrons and therefore carries an electric charge of plus two.

Aluminum (Al) The metal most frequently used as a filter material to efficiently remove low-energy (soft) x-rays from a polyenergetic beam.

Aluminum oxide (Al_2O_3) Sensing material found in optically stimulated luminescence dosimeters.

American Association of Physicists in Medicine (AAPM) Professional organization that is the primary scientific and educational body for medical physicists and is also responsible for accrediting laboratories that calibrate instruments used to measure radiation exposure in medical radiology.

American College of Radiology (ACR) Major professional organization of radiologists in the United States.

American Registry of Radiologic Technologists Nongovernmental credentialing organization that tests and certifies radiologic technologists on a national level. The intention is to "seek and ensure quality patient care in radiologic technology."

American Society of Radiologic Technologists The "premier professional association" of persons employed in medical imaging and radiation therapy. It provides education, advocacy, and research for the membership.

Amino acids The structural units of protein.

Amorphous selenium A noncrystalline grouping of silicon atoms in which, rather than a regular geometric pattern, the silicon atoms are distributed in a continuous random fashion.

Ampere The SI unit of electrical charge. One ampere represents the quantity of electrons amounting to a charge of 1 coulomb crossing unit area per second.

Analog image A visible image produced by x-radiation on a finished radiographic film.

Anaphase The phase of mitosis during which the duplicate centromeres migrate in opposite directions along the mitotic spindle and carry the chromatids to opposite sides of the cell.

Anemia A condition characterized by a lack of vitality and caused by a decrease in the number of red blood cells in the circulating blood.

Anion A negatively charged ion.

Annihilation radiation Radiation in the form of two oppositely moving 511-keV photons generated as the result of the mutual annihilation of matter and antimatter (i.e., an electron and a positron).

Annual occupational effective dose (EfD) limit An upper boundary limit for radiation workers for yearly whole-body exposure (excluding personal medical and natural background exposure) of 50 millisieverts (mSv). There is also an added recommendation that the lifetime EfD in mSv should not exceed 10 times the occupationally exposed person's age in years.

Anode The positively charged target in the x-ray tube.

Antibodies Materials developed by the body in response to the presence of foreign antigens such as bacteria or a virus. Once the skin is penetrated, they provide a primary defense mechanism against such antigens.

Antigens Any substance that causes an immune system to produce antibodies against it; usually a foreign substance, such as a toxin or a component of a virus, bacterium, or parasite.

Antimatter Matter composed of the counterparts of ordinary matter that does not exist freely in the universe and is unstable in the presence of ordinary matter.

Aplastic anemia Anemia resulting from bone marrow failure.

Apoptosis A nonmitotic or nondivision form of cell death that occurs when cells die without attempting division during the interphase portion of the cell life cycle. Also known as *programmed cell death* (formerly called *interphase death*).

Artifact A structure or an appearance that is not normally present on the radiograph and is produced by artificial means.

Artificial radiation See *Manmade radiation*.

Ataxia An inability to coordinate voluntary muscular movements.

Atom The smallest portion of an element that has all of its chemical properties.

Atomic number The number of protons contained within the nucleus of an atom.

ATP (adenosine triphosphate) A type of molecule found in every cell. It stores and supplies the cell with energy.

Atrophy A shrinkage of any body part that may follow substantial partial-body radiation exposure.

Audible sound system An audio amplifier and speaker, such as in a Geiger–Müller detector.

Auger effect When an inner-shell vacancy occurs in an atom, the energy liberated when this vacancy is filled can be transferred to another electron of the atom, thereby ejecting the electron. The process is known as the *Auger effect,* and the emitted electron is known as an *Auger electron.*

Automatic collimation See *Positive beam limitation (PBL).*

Axon A long, single tentacle from the cell body that carries impulses away from it.

B

Background equivalent radiation time (BERT) Method to compare the amount of radiation received from a radiologic procedure with natural background radiation received over a specified period such as days, weeks, months, or years.

Backscatter Photons that have interacted with the atoms of an object and as a result are deflected backward (toward the x-ray tube).

Bases Alkali or alkaline earth OH compounds that can neutralize acids.

Beam direction factor See *Use factor (U).*

Beam limiting device See *X-ray beam limitation device.*

Becquerel The SI unit of radioactivity. It is equal to 1 disintegration (decay) per second.

Beta decay The process wherein a nucleus relieves instability by a neutron transforming itself into a combination of a proton and an energetic electron (called a *beta particle*). There is also emission of another particle called a *neutrino,* which has negligible mass and no electric charge but carries away any excess energy.

Beta particles High-speed electrons ejected from a nucleus that undergoes beta decay. They are also known as *beta rays.*

Binding energy Force that holds the components of an atom or a nucleus together.

Biologic dosimetry A method of dose assessment in which biologic markers or effects of radiation exposure are measured and the dose to the organism is inferred from previously established dose–effect relationships. Examples include white blood cell counts and chromosomal aberrations.

Biology A science that explores living things and life processes.

Birth defects See *Embryologic effects.*

Blebs Tiny membrane-enclosed structures that are produced when cells shrink in apoptosis.

Bone marrow syndrome See *Hematopoietic syndrome.*

Bragg–Gray theory Relates the ionization produced in a small cavity within an irradiated medium or object to the energy absorbed in that medium as a result of its radiation exposure.

Bremsstrahlung Polyenergetic ionizing electromagnetic radiation that is produced when a beam of electrons in an x-ray tube

undergoes deceleration by interaction with the nuclei of the x-ray tube target atoms.

Bucky grid An assembly of moving lead strips resembling a venetian blind, placed between a patient being x-rayed and the image receptor to improve the collimation and reduce scatter radiation on the detector.

Bucky slot shielding device A protective device made of at least 0.25-mm lead equivalent that automatically covers the Bucky slot opening in the side of the x-ray table during a fluoroscopic examination when the Bucky tray is positioned at the foot end of the table. This protects the radiographer and the radiologist from gonadal radiation exposure.

Bureau of Radiological Health (BRH) See *Center for Devices and Radiological Health (CDRH).*

C

Calibrated instrument Any device that is compared with a generally accepted (nationally or internationally) standard device so that its accuracy has been determined. Radiation survey instruments are usually calibrated every 1 to 2 years.

Candela per square meter Unit used to describe luminance. One candela corresponds to 3.8 million billion photons per second being emitted from a light source through a cone-like field of view.

Carbohydrates Compounds composed of only carbon, hydrogen, and oxygen. Carbohydrates such as sugars and starches are involved in energy-releasing processes in animals and plants. Also known as *saccharides.*

Carbon Nonmetallic element that is the basic constituent of all organic matter.

Carbon fiber Material used in the tops of radiographic tables. It has a lower x-ray absorption potential when compared with materials such as aluminum but has the strength to support adult patients. The use of carbon fiber results in lower radiographic techniques for producing the recorded image, thereby lowering patient dose.

Carcinogenesis The production or origin of cancer.

C-arm fluoroscope A portable device for producing real-time (motion) images of a patient. The opposite ends of the C-shaped support arm hold the x-ray tube and the image receptor.

Catabolism The breaking down in living organisms of more complex molecules into simpler ones, with the release of energy.

Catalyst Agent that affects the speed of a chemical reaction without being altered itself.

Catalytic failure The inability to influence the speed of a required chemical reaction (e.g., during protein synthesis).

Cataract Opacity of the lens of the eye.

Cataractogenesis The production or origin of cataracts.

Cathode A negative electrode. The cathode is the source of the high-speed electrons in an x-ray tube.

Cation A positively charged ion.

Cell division The process whereby one cell divides to form two or more cells.

Cell membrane The frail, semipermeable, flexible structure encasing and surrounding the human cell. It functions as a barricade to protect cellular contents from their outside environment and controls the passage of water and other materials into and out of the cell.

Cell metabolism The series of chemical reactions that modifies foods for cellular use.

Cell survival curve A method of displaying the sensitivity of a particular type of cell to lethal effects of radiation.

Cells The basic units of all living matter.

Cellular life cycle The passage of a cell through the phases G1, S, G2, and M.

Center for Devices and Radiological Health (CDRH) Known before 1982 as the *Bureau of Radiological Health (BRH)*, this agency is responsible for conducting an ongoing electronic product radiation control program.

Centigray (cGy) One one-hundredth of a gray (1/100 Gy).

Centrioles A pair of small, hollow, cylindrical structures oriented at right angles to each other and embedded in a material mass of more than 100 proteins. They play a significant role in the formation of the mitotic spindle during cell division.

Centromere A clear region on a chromosome serving as a joining point; it is actually the center of the chromosome.

Centrosomes Structures located in the center of the cell near the nucleus that contain the centrioles.

Cerebrovascular syndrome Form of acute radiation syndrome that results when the central nervous system and cardiovascular system receive doses of 50 Gy, or more of ionizing radiation. A dose of this magnitude can cause death within a few hours to 2 or 3 days after exposure.

Characteristic photon A quantum or quantity of radiant energy given off by an atom when an electron from an outer-shell drops down to fill an inner-shell vacancy. The energy of a characteristic photon is equivalent to the difference in energy level between the two electron shells. Also known as *characteristic x-ray* or *fluorescent radiation*.

Characteristic radiation Radiation consisting of characteristic photons. In a general-purpose x-ray tube characteristic radiation comprises about 10% of the primary radiation beam for tube voltages between 80 and 100 kVp.

Charge-coupled device (CCD) A device that, when struck by visible light, produces electrical signals in proportion to the brightness of the light. CCDs are used in indirect types of digital x-ray detectors. Indirect digital detectors use a phosphor to convert the x-ray energy to visible light, after which the CCD converts the visible light into electrical signals.

Chernobyl nuclear power plant accident Massive explosion that blew apart the Unit 4 reactor at the nuclear power plant in Chernobyl, Russia, on April 26, 1986.

Chromatid A highly coiled strand; one of the two duplicate portions of DNA in a replicated chromosome that appear during cell division.

Chromatid aberrations Deviation from normal development or growth. Lesions that result when irradiation of individual chromatids occurs later in interphase, after DNA synthesis has taken place.

Chromatin The substance distributed in the nucleus of a cell that condenses to form chromosomes during cell division.

Chromosome aberrations Deviation from normal development or growth. Lesions that result when irradiation occurs early in interphase, before DNA synthesis takes place.

Chromosome breakage The breaking of one or both of the sugar–phosphate chains of a DNA ladder-like structure, which is a potential outcome when ionizing radiation interacts with a DNA macromolecule.

Chromosomes Tiny, rod-shaped bodies that contain genes.

Chronic Something that continues for a long time (i.e., a chronic disease).

Classical scattering See *Coherent scattering.*

Clear lead shields Transparent lead–acrylic material that has been impregnated with approximately 30% lead by weight. It is used for viewing windows and pull-down or roll-away x-ray room shielding.

Cleaved chromosome A broken chromosome.

Code of Standards for Diagnostic X-Ray Equipment Effective August 1, 1974, this code applies to complete systems and major components manufactured after that date.

Coherent scattering The process wherein a low-energy photon (typically less than 10 keV) interacts with an atom of human tissue and does not lose kinetic energy. The atom responds by releasing the energy it has received in the form of a scattered photon that has the same wavelength and energy as the original incident photon. The emitted photon changes direction by 20 degrees or less. No ionization of the biologic atom occurs. Also known as *classical scattering, elastic scattering, unmodified scattering, and Rayleigh scattering.* Thompson scattering is also another type of coherent scattering.

Collective effective dose (ColEfD) Designated for use in the description of a population or group exposed to different individual amounts of ionizing radiation. It is equal to the sum of all of the doses times the number of individuals exposed and would be expressed in units such as person-Sv.

Collimation Limiting all the margins of the useful x-ray field to a specific size and shape to confine the beam to the anatomic area of interest. This reduces the dose the patient receives and improves contrast of the radiographic image.

Committed effective dose equivalent (CEDE) A measure of the probabilistic health effect on an individual as a result of intake of radioactive material into the body. It takes into account the length of time that the radioactive material may stay within the body.

Compensating filter A material such as aluminum, lead–acrylic, or other suitable material inserted between the x-ray source and the patient to modify the quality (penetrating power, spectrum) of the beam across the field of view.

Compton scattered electron An energetic electron dislodged from the outer shell of an atom of the irradiated object as a result of a Compton interaction with an incoming x-ray photon. Also known as a *secondary,* or *recoil, electron.*

Compton scattered photon X-ray photon of weaker energy emerging from an atom, usually in a new direction, following a Compton interaction with that atom.

Compton scattering An interaction between an incoming x-ray photon and a loosely bound outer-shell electron of an atom in the irradiated object. The photon surrenders a portion of its kinetic energy to dislodge the electron from its outer-shell orbit, thereby ionizing the atom, and then continues in a new direction. This process accounts for most of the scattered radiation produced during diagnostic procedures. Also known as *incoherent scattering, inelastic scattering,* or *modified scattering.*

Computed axial tomography (CAT) See *Computed tomography (CT).*

Computed radiography (CR) Process in which an image is captured on a removable digital storage cassette, using storage phosphor technology. The cassette is then taken to a "reader" that interprets the stored signal and transfers it in a digital matrix to a picture archiving and communication system (PACS) system. CR has been largely replaced by digital radiography, or DR.

Computed tomography (CT) "The process of creating a cross-sectional tomographic plane of any part of the body." This computer-reconstructed image of a patient is created by "an x-ray tube and detector assembly rotating 360 degrees about a specified area of the body." CT has also been referred to as *computerized axial tomography (CAT).*

Cone A circular metal tube that attaches to the x-ray tube housing or variable rectangular collimator to limit the beam to a predetermined size and shape.

Congenital abnormalities Defects existing at birth that are not inherited but rather acquired during development in utero.

Console See *Control panel.*

Consumer-Patient Radiation Health and Safety Act of 1981 Provides federal legislation requiring the establishment of minimal standards for accreditation of educational programs for persons who perform radiologic procedures and the certification of such persons.

Contrast media (negative) The use of air or gas to enhance visualization of body structures during a radiologic procedure.

Contrast media (positive) A liquid solution containing an element with a higher atomic number than surrounding tissue (e.g., barium or iodine) that is either ingested or injected into biologic tissues or structures to be visualized.

Control monitor Dosimeter provided by the monitoring company with each batch of dosimeters to serve as a basis for comparison with the remainder of the dosimeters after they have been returned to the monitoring company for processing. The control monitor determines whether the batch of dosimeters has been exposed to radiation in transit to or from the health care facility.

Control panel Where technical exposure factors such as milliamperes (mA) and peak kilovoltage (kVp) are selected and visually displayed. Also called a *console.* Besides having buttons for initiating the exposure, it indicates the conditions of exposure and shows when the x-ray tube is energized.

Control-booth barrier A permanently secured protective barrier for imaging personnel that is located in an x-ray room that contains housing for permanent or nonportable radiographic equipment. It may be regarded as a secondary protective barrier.

Controlled area A region that is occupied only by occupationally exposed personnel and others under their direct supervision.

Conventional radiography The use of a screen-film system to produce an image on radiographic film.

Cosmic radiation (cosmic rays) Very-high-energy particles and photons. They result from nuclear interactions that have taken place throughout the universe, including the sun and other stars.

Coulomb (C) Basic SI unit of electrical charge. It represents the quantity of electrical charge flowing past a point in a circuit in 1 second when an electrical current of 1 ampere is used.

Coulomb per kilogram (C/kg) SI unit of radiation exposure: 1 coulomb per kilogram (C/kg) of air equals 1 SI unit of exposure, or $1/(2.58 \times 10^{-4})$ R = 3.88×10^3 R. C/kg (traditional unit: roentgen) is used for x-ray equipment calibration because x-ray output intensity is measured directly with an ionization chamber.

Covalent bond A chemical union created between atoms by the sharing or transfer of one or more electrons.

Covalent cross-link See *Covalent bond.*

Crookes tube Vacuum discharge tube used by Wilhelm Conrad Roentgen when he discovered x-rays.

Crossover Process occurring during meiosis in which the chromatids exchange some chromosomal material (genes).

CTDI CT dose index (CTDI) is a standardized measure of radiation dose output of a CT scanner that allows the user to compare radiation output of different CT scanners. It refers to the dose to a standard 16-cm (head) or 32-cm (body) plastic phantom.

Cumulative effective dose (CumEfD) limit A radiation worker's lifetime EfD must be limited to his or her age in years times 10 mSv. This limit pertains to the whole body.

Cumulative timing device A required resettable device on a fluoroscopic x-ray unit that times the x-ray beam-on time and sounds an audible alarm after the fluoroscope has been activated for 5 minutes.

Curie The standard unit of radioactivity in use before the SI system of units was established. One curie is equal to 3.7×10^{10} nuclear disintegrations per second.

Cutie pie Nickname for an ionization chamber–type survey meter.

Cyclotrons Units that, with the aid of a strong static magnetic field and rapidly varying electric fields, produce in a circular evacuated cavity beams of high-energy charged particles such as 150-MeV proton beams.

Cytogenetics The study of cell genetics with emphasis on analysis of chromosomes.

Cytoplasm The protoplasm that exists outside of the cell's nucleus.

Cytoplasmic organelles Miniature cellular components present in the cytoplasm that enable the cell to function.

Cytosine (C) One of two pyrimidine bases found in both DNA and RNA.

D

Daughter cell A cell resulting from division of an individual parent cell.

Dead-man–type fluoroscopic exposure switch A fluoroscopic exposure switch (operated by foot pressure) that requires continuous pressure from the operator. If the operator becomes incapacitated, the exposure automatically terminates.

Deep equivalent dose External whole-body exposure at a tissue depth of 1 cm (1000 mg/cm^2).

Deletion A part of the chromosome or chromatid is lost at the next cell division, thus creating an aberration known as an *acentric fragment.* This will result in a cell mutation.

Dendrites Tentacle-like extensions from a nerve cell body that carry impulses toward the cell.

Deoxyribonucleic acid (DNA) A type of nucleic acid that carries the genetic information necessary for cell replication and regulation of cellular activity needed to direct protein synthesis. It is often referred to as the *master chemical* in the cell because it contains all the information that the cell needs to function.

Deoxyribose A five-carbon sugar molecule.

Dermis Middle layer of skin composed of connective tissue.

Desquamation Shedding of the outer layer of skin; occurs after high radiation doses.

Diagnostic efficacy The degree to which a diagnostic study accurately reveals the presence or absence of disease in the patient.

Diagnostic-type protective tube housing The lead-lined metal housing enclosing the x-ray tube that protects both the radiographer and the patient from leakage radiation by restricting the emission of the x-rays to the area of the useful, or primary, beam.

Dicentric chromosomes Chromosomes that have two centromeres.

Diffusion The motion of liquid, gas, or solid particles from an area of relatively high concentration to an area of lower concentration.

Digital fluoroscopy A technique in which the fluoroscopic image exists in digital form at some point in the image acquisition process. In nondigital fluoroscopy, an image intensifier and an analog television camera are used. Typical approaches to digital fluoroscopy include replacement of the image intensifier with a digital detector, replacement of the analog television camera with a digital video camera, and digitization of the analog signal from an analog television camera.

Digital image Image produced by computer representation of anatomic information.

Digital radiography The use of a flat panel detector to record a radiographic image and render it in digital form without developing or scanning the image receptor.

Direct action Biologic damage that occurs as a result of ionization of atoms on essential molecules, which may cause these molecules to become either inactive or functionally altered.

Direct radiation See *Primary radiation.*

Direct transmission Primary x-ray photons that traverse a patient without interacting.

Dirty bomb See *Radioactive dispersal device.*

Distance A very important method of protection from ionizing radiation. Imaging personnel receive significantly less radiation exposure by standing farther away from a source of radiation because an inverse square law governs the decrease in the radiation level.

DNA synthesis The building up of DNA macromolecules.

Dominant mutation A genetic mutation that will probably be expressed in offspring.

Doppler shift Refers to the apparent change in the frequency of any wave as the observer and the source move toward or away from each other.

Dose The amount of radiant energy absorbed by an irradiated object per unit mass.

Dose area product (DAP) The sum total of air kerma over the exposed area of the patient's surface.

Dose commitment The dose that could ultimately be delivered from a given intake of radionuclide given that it may remain in the body for some time.

Dose length product A measure of the dose for an entire CT scan. It is mathematically equal to the product of the volume CTDI and the scan length. It has the units of mGy-cm.

Double-strand break The ionization of a DNA macromolecule that results in the rupture of both of the two sugar–phosphate chains of the DNA ladderlike molecular structure. This results in breakage of a chromosome.

Doubling dose The radiation dose that causes the number of spontaneous mutations occurring in a given generation to increase to two times their original number.

E

Early somatic tissue reactions Reactions in biologic tissues that are dependent on the duration of time after the exposure to ionizing radiation. Subject to their nature, they appear within minutes, hours, days, or weeks of the time of exposure. These reactions are precipitated by cell death.

Edema Swelling caused by excess fluid trapped in body tissue.

Effective atomic number (Zeff) A composite Z value for when multiple chemical elements comprise a material.

Effective dose (EfD) Quantity that is used for radiation protection purposes to provide a measure of the overall risk of exposure to humans from ionizing radiation. Effective dose takes into account the dose from all types of ionizing radiation (e.g., alpha, beta, gamma, x-ray) to various irradiated organs or tissues in the human body (skin, gonadal tissue, thyroid). By including a specific weighting factor for each of those parts of the body mentioned, EfD takes into account the chance or risk of each of those body parts to develop a radiation-induced cancer (or in the case of the reproductive organs, the risk of genetic damage).

Effective dose (EfD) limit Concerns the upper boundary dose of ionizing radiation that results in a negligible risk of bodily injury or hereditary damage. These limits may be expressed for whole-body exposure, partial-body exposure, and exposure of individual organs. Separate limits are set for occupationally exposed individuals and for the general public.

Effective dose (EfD) limiting system The current method for assessing radiation exposure and associated risk of biologic damage to radiation workers and the general public. It is a set of numeric dose limits that are based on calculations of the various risks of cancer and genetic effects to tissues or organs exposed to radiation.

Effective half-life (T$_{eff}$) The actual half-life of a radioactive material in a patient's body resulting from a combination of natural decay and physical removal by bodily functions.

Elastic scattering See *Coherent scattering.*

Elective examinations Nonurgent x-ray examinations that can be scheduled at an appropriate time to meet patient needs and safety requirements.

Electric charge The physical property of matter that causes it to experience a force when placed in an electromagnetic field. There are two types of electric charges: positive and negative. Like charges repel, and unlike charges attract.

Electrical potential difference (voltage difference) A potential difference or voltage is required to give energy to charged particles. The energy acquired by an electric charge when it is placed in a potential difference of one volt is equal to one electron-volt (eV) of energy. An electron in a potential difference of 100,000 volts acquires an energy of 100,000 eV or 100 keV.

Electrical potential energy The electrical energy acquired by a charged particle as a result of the voltage to which it is exposed. Electrical potential energy may be measured in units of joules or electron-volts. When an x-ray tube uses an applied voltage of 100,000 volts, it accelerates electrons toward its anode with an energy of 100 keV.

Electrolytes See *Salts*.

Electromagnetic radiation Radiation composed of interacting, varying electric and magnetic fields that propagate through space at the speed of light. Examples include radio waves, microwaves, visible light, ultraviolet rays, x-rays, and gamma rays.

Electromagnetic spectrum The full range of frequencies and wavelengths of electromagnetic waves.

Electromagnetic wave Electric and magnetic fields that fluctuate rapidly as they travel through space, including radio waves, microwaves, visible light, and x-rays.

Electrometer A device used to measure electrical charge.

Electron capture A process wherein an inner-shell electron is captured by one of the nuclear protons, followed directly by the two combining to produce a neutron.

Electron volt (eV) A unit of energy equal to the quantity of kinetic energy an electron acquires as it moves through a potential difference of 1 volt.

Electrons Negatively charged atomic particles.

Element A substance made up of atoms that all have the same atomic number and hence the same chemical properties.

Emaciation The state of being extremely thin.

Embryologic effects Damage to an organism that occurs as a result of exposure to some agent (such as ionizing radiation) during the embryonic stage of development. Also known as *birth defects*.

Endoplasmic reticulum A vast, irregular network of tubules and vesicles spreading and interconnecting in all directions throughout the cytoplasm, thus enabling the cell to communicate with the extracellular environment and transfer food from one part of the cell to another.

Energy The ability to do work.

Enhanced natural sources Natural sources of ionizing radiation that grow larger because of accidental or deliberate human actions.

Entrance exposure Quantity of radiation—given in SI units, coulombs per kilogram, or traditional units (roentgens)—incident on an object.

Entrance skin exposure (ESE) X-ray exposure to the skin of the patient.

Entrance skin exposure dose rates Limited by federal standards of general-purpose intensified fluoroscopic units to a maximum of 100 mGy$_a$ per minute. Measured at tabletop with the image intensifier entrance surface at a prescribed 30 cm above.

Environmental Protection Agency (EPA) US government agency that facilitates the development and enforcement of regulations pertaining to the control of radiation in the environment. It directs federal agencies, oversees the general area of environmental monitoring, and has authority over specific areas such as determining the action level for radon.

Enzymatic proteins Proteins that control the cell's various physiologic activities by functioning as catalysts. Also known as *enzymes*.

Epidemiology "Science that deals with the incidence, distribution, and control of disease in a population."

Epidermis Outer layer of skin.

Epilation Loss of hair. Also called *alopecia*.

Epithelial tissue A substance that lines and covers body tissue; the cells that comprise this tissue are highly radiosensitive because the body constantly regenerates this tissue.

Equivalent dose (EqD) A radiation quantity used for radiation protection purposes when a person receives exposure from various types of ionizing radiation. This quantity attempts to numerically specify the differences in transferred energy and therefore potential biologic harm that are produced by different types of radiation. EqD is the product of the average absorbed dose in a tissue or organ in the human body and its associated radiation weighting factor chosen for the type of radiation in question. Equivalent dose enables the calculation of the effective dose (EfD).

Erg A unit of energy and work that is equal to 10^{-7} joules.

Erythema Diffused redness over an area of skin after irradiation.

Erythroblasts Red blood stem cells.

Erythrocytes Red blood cells that, through their hemoglobin, carry oxygen from the lungs to all body tissues and cells as blood circulates.

Europium-activated barium fluorohalide The most commonly employed photostimulable phosphor used in computed radiography imaging plates as the image receptor.

Excess cancers Cancers that would not have occurred in a population without exposure to ionizing radiation.

Excitation The addition of energy to a system, thereby transforming it from a calm, or low energy, state to an excited, or higher-energy state.

Exit, or image formation, radiation All the x-ray photons that reach their destination (the image receptor) after passing through the patient being radiographed; previously known as *remnant radiation*.

Exposure The total electric charge of one sign, either all pluses or all minuses, per unit mass that x-ray and gamma ray photons with energies up to 3 million electron volts (MeV) generate in dry (i.e., nonhumid) air at standard temperature and pressure (760 mm Hg or 1 atmosphere at sea level and 22°C); the amount of ionizing radiation that may strike an object, such as the human body, when in the vicinity of a radiation source. In the SI system it can be measured in coulombs per kilogram (C/kg).

Exposure linearity Consistency in output radiation intensity at any selected kVp settings when generator settings are changed from one milliamperage and time combination to another. (See *Linearity* for additional information.)

Exposure rate dose Given in units of mGy$_a$ per hour; the same quantity as air kerma rate.

Exposure reproducibility Consistency in output in radiation intensity for identical generator settings from one individual exposure to subsequent exposures. This means that the x-ray unit must have the ability to duplicate certain radiographic exposures for any given combination of kilovolts at peak (kVp), milliamperes (mA), and time. A variance of 5% or less is acceptable.

Extremity dosimeter A device that monitors the equivalent dose of radiation to the hands.

Eye equivalent dose Radiation equivalent dose to the lens of the eye at a tissue depth of 0.3 cm (300 mg/cm^2).

F

Fallout Radiation produced as a consequence of nuclear weapons testing.

Fats Compounds composed of carbon, hydrogen, and oxygen, with the ratio of hydrogen atoms to oxygen atoms much greater than 2:1; a rich energy source. (See *Lipids*.)

Fatty acids   Compounds formed when fat combines with an acidic group of atoms (e.g., the carboxyl group); a constituent of amino acids from which proteins are built.

Fetus   A developing human in utero.

Fiber   A protracted, threadlike structure.

Fibrils   Minute fibers or strands that are frequently part of a compound fiber.

Fibrosis   Abnormal formation of fibrous tissue.

Filtration   Elements that are part of or added to the x-ray tube to reduce exposure to the patient's skin and superficial tissue by absorbing most of the lower-energy photons from the heterogeneous beam and thereby increasing the mean energy, or quality, of the x-ray beam.

Fission   The splitting of the nuclei of atoms whereby some mass is converted into energy.

Fixed radiographic equipment   Radiologic equipment that is installed in and cannot be moved from a specific place in an imaging facility. It may also be referred to as *stationary equipment*.

Flat contact shield   Uncontoured lead strip or lead-impregnated material 1 mm thick placed directly over the patient's reproductive organs to provide protection from exposure to ionizing radiation.

Fluorescent radiation   See *Characteristic photon* or *Characteristic radiation*.

Fluorescent yield   The number of x-rays emitted by an atom per inner-shell vacancy.

Fluorine-18   Radioactive isotope used for positron emission tomography (PET) scanning. It decays by positron emission and has a half-life of 110 minutes.

Fluorodeoxyglucose (FDG)   Radioactive tracer that is very similar in chemical behavior to ordinary glucose and so will be taken up or metabolized by cancerous cells. As such it will reveal their locations through its positron emission decay and subsequent generation of oppositely traveling annihilation photons.

Fluoroscopic-guided positioning (FGP)   The practice of using fluoroscopy to determine the exact location of the central ray before taking an exposure.

Fluoroscopy   Process in which an x-ray examination is performed that demonstrates dynamic, or active, motion of selected anatomic structures by producing a temporary image of these structures on a television monitor working in conjunction with an image intensifier system under low-light conditions.

Focal spot   The area on the anode of the x-ray tube from which the x-rays emanate.

Follicle   In the female reproductive system, an ovarian follicle is a fluid-filled sac that contains an immature egg, or oocyte.

Food and Drug Administration   See *US Food and Drug Administration (FDA)*.

Foot-candle   A unit of illuminance on a surface that is everywhere 1 foot from a uniform point source of light of one candle and equal to one lumen per square foot.

Forward scatter   Photons that have interacted with the atoms of an object and consequently are deflected forward (toward the radiographic image receptor). (See also *Small-angle scatter*.)

Free air ionization chamber   An instrument used in a calibration laboratory to obtain a precise measurement of exposure to x-radiation.

Free radicals   Solitary atoms, or most often a combination of atoms, that are very chemically reactive as a result of the presence of unpaired electrons.

Frequency   The number of vibrations or cycles per second (given in units of hertz [Hz]).

G

Gamma rays   Short wavelength, high energy electromagnetic waves emitted by the nuclei of radioactive substances. Although they are generally shorter in wavelength than x-rays and have a different point of origin, their other characteristics are identical to those of diagnostic x-rays.

Gastrointestinal (GI) syndrome   A form of acute radiation syndrome that appears in humans at a whole-body threshold dose of approximately 6 Gy_t and that peaks after a dose of 10 Gy_t.

Geiger–Müller (GM) detector   A device that detects individual radioactive particles or photons and that serves as the primary portable radiation survey instrument for area monitoring in nuclear medicine facilities.

Genes   Segments of DNA that serve as the basic units of heredity.

Genetic cells (germ cells)   Cells of the human body associated with reproduction.

Genetic code   The set of rules by which information encoded within genetic material (DNA or mRNA sequences) is translated into proteins by living cells.

Genetic damage   Radiation damage to generations yet unborn.

Genetic death   See *Mitotic death*.

Genetic effects   Biologic effects of ionizing radiation on future generations due to irradiation of germ cells in previous generations. Also known as *hereditary effects*.

Genetic mutations   See *Mutations*.

Genetically significant dose (GSD)   Concept used to assess the impact of gonadal dose. GSD is the equivalent dose to the reproductive organs that, if received by every human, would be expected to bring about an identical gross genetic injury to the total population, as does the sum of the actual doses received by exposed individual members of the population. For the US population, this dose is estimated to be about 0.20 mSv.

Germ cells   Male and female reproductive cells.

Glow curve   A graphic plot that demonstrates the relationship of light output to temperature variation for a thermoluminescent (TL) material, such as is used in a TL dosimeter (TLD).

Glucose   A form of sugar that is the primary energy source for the cell.

Glycerine   A sweet, colorless, odorless, syrupy liquid obtained from fats that are soluble in water; often used as a moistening agent.

Glycoproteins   Proteins with a sugar attached to them. They give structural support to cells, help to form connective tissues, and are key molecules involved in immune response within the immune system.

Golgi apparatus   Minute vesicles that extend from the nucleus to the cell membrane. They consist of tiny sacs located near the nucleus. The Golgi apparatus unites large carbohydrate molecules and then combines them with proteins to form glycoproteins. These minute vesicles transport enzymes and hormones through the cell membrane so that they can exit the cell, enter the bloodstream, and be carried to the areas of the body where they are required.

Gonadal dose   Radiation exposure received by the male and female reproductive organs.

Gonadal shielding devices   Devices used during diagnostic x-ray procedures to protect the reproductive organs from exposure to the useful beam, when they are in or within approximately 5 cm of a properly collimated beam. Gonadal shielding is used unless it would compromise the diagnostic value of the examination.

Gonads   Male and female reproductive organs.

Gram (g) A unit of mass of the metric system. An object near the earth's surface that has a mass of 454 grams will weigh 1 pound.

Granules Small, insoluble, nonmembranous particles found in cytoplasm.

Granulocyte A scavenger type of white blood cell that fights bacteria.

Gray (Gy) SI unit of absorbed dose and air kerma. One Gy equals an energy absorption of one joule (J) per kilogram (kg) of matter in the irradiated object. In the traditional system 100 rad equals one Gy.

Grenz rays X-rays in the energy range of 10 to 20 kVp.

Grid ratio The ratio of the height of the lead strips in the grid to the distance between them.

Guanine (G) One of two purine bases found in both DNA and RNA.

H

Half-life Statistical quantity equal to the amount of time associated with a 50% decrease in the radioactivity of a sample containing radioactive atoms.

Half-value layer (HVL) The thickness of a designated absorber (customarily a metal such as aluminum) required to decrease the intensity of the primary beam by 50% of its initial value.

Helical CT See *Spiral computed tomography.*

Hematopoietic syndrome A form of acute radiation syndrome that occurs when humans receive whole-body doses of ionizing radiation ranging from 1 to 10 Gy_t and in which the reduction of the number of blood cells in the circulating blood results in a loss of the body's ability to clot blood and fight infection; also called *bone marrow syndrome.*

Hematopoietic system Blood-forming system.

Hemoglobin A protein; the oxygen-carrying pigment of the red blood cells (erythrocytes).

Hemorrhage Abnormal escape of blood; heavy bleeding.

Hereditary effects See *Genetic effects.*

High contrast resolution The ability of a system to make two dissimilar adjacent objects visually distinguishable. On radiographic film the image will only have few shades of gray.

High-LET radiation Includes particles that possess substantial mass and charge such as alpha particles, ions of heavier nuclei, and charged particles released from interactions between neutrons and atoms. Low energy neutrons, which carry no electric charge, are also high linear energy transfer (LET) radiation.

High-level control fluoroscopy (HLCF) An operating mode for state-of-the-art fluoroscopic equipment in which exposure rates are substantially higher than normally allowed for routine procedures. The higher exposure rate allows visualization of smaller and lower contrast objects that do not usually appear during standard fluoroscopy. HLCF is also known as *"boost"* mode.

High-speed image receptor system A relative term that describes an image receptor that requires less exposure to obtain a response, such as generation of a digital image or production of a chemical change displayed as an increase in optical density (darkening) of film.

Highly differentiated cells Mature or more specialized cells.

Holistic approach to patient care Treating the whole person, rather than just the area of concern.

Homeostasis A state of equilibrium between the different elements of an organism or a tendency toward such a state; the ability of the body to return to and maintain normal functioning despite the changes it has undergone.

Hormones Chemical secretions manufactured by various endocrine glands and carried by the bloodstream to influence activities of other parts of the body, such as regulating growth and development.

Human genome The total amount of genetic material (DNA) contained within the chromosomes of a human being.

Hydrocephaly Abnormal fluid in the brain.

Hydrogen peroxide A cellular poison that can result from the radiolysis of water.

Hydroperoxyl radical A substance toxic to the cell that can result from the radiolysis of water.

Hyperbaric oxygen High-pressure oxygen sometimes used in radiation therapy treatment of certain types of cancerous tumors to increase their radiosensitivity.

Hypodermis A subcutaneous layer of fat and connective tissue.

Hypoxic cells Cells that lack an adequate amount of oxygen.

I

Image intensification fluoroscopy Use of an image intensifier to enormously increase the brightness of the real-time image produced on a fluorescent screen during fluoroscopy.

Image intensifier tube An "electronic device that receives the image forming x-ray beam and converts it into a visible light image of high intensity" (e.g., a gain of 5000 or more is possible).

Image matrix The array of pixels that comprises a digital image. Examples of matrix sizes are 512×512 and 1024×1024.

Image receptor Any device that captures a radiographic image. Examples include radiographic film or phosphorescent screens and digital detectors.

Image receptor (IR) exposure The radiation exposure of any image receptor that is stored and converted into an image.

Incident photon Incoming photon.

Incoherent scattering See *Compton scattering.*

Indirect action The effect produced by free radicals that are created by the interaction of radiation with water molecules; cell death can result.

Indirect transmission Primary photons that undergo Compton and/or coherent interactions and are scattered or deflected while passing through a patient and then still reach the image receptor.

Inelastic scatter The interaction of an incident photon with a loosely bound outer-shell electron of the target atom in which the photon surrenders some of its kinetic energy to free the electron from its orbit and then continues on its way in a new direction.

Inherent filtration The glass envelope (0.5-mm aluminum equivalent) encasing the x-ray tube, the insulating oil surrounding the tube, and the glass window in the tube housing.

Inorganic compounds Compounds that do not contain carbon. The inorganic compounds found in the human body occur in nature independent of living things.

Instant cell death Instant death of large numbers of cells occurs when a volume is irradiated with an x-ray or gamma ray dose of about 1000 Gy_t in a period of seconds or a few minutes.

Integral dose Product of dose and volume of tissue irradiated.

Intensity (of radiation) Quantity, or amount, of radiation crossing unit area per unit time.

Intermittent fluoroscopy Manual activation of the fluoroscopic tube by the fluoroscopist or automatic periodic activation (also known as *pulsed fluoroscopy*), rather than lengthy or continuous activation.

Internal contamination Ingestion or inhalation of radioactive material within the body.

Internal radiation Radiation from radioactive atoms (also known as *radionuclides*) that make up a small percentage of the tissues of the human body.

International Commission on Radiological Protection (ICRP) Radiation protection standards organization considered to be the international authority on the safe use of sources of ionizing radiation. The ICRP is responsible for providing clear and consistent radiation protection guidance through its recommendations on occupational and public dose limits.

International system of units (SI) System of units that makes possible an interchange of units among all branches of science throughout the world.

Interphase The period of cell growth that occurs before actual mitosis.

Interphase death See *Apoptosis.*

Interslice scatter Radiation that scatters from the CT slice being scanned into adjacent slices.

Interstrand cross-link A cross-link formed between complementary DNA strands or between entirely different DNA molecules.

Interventional procedures Medical procedures, such as inserting catheters into vessels or tissues for the purpose of drainage, biopsy, or alteration of vascular occlusions, performed by a physician during an imaging procedure such as digital fluoroscopy.

Intrastrand cross-link A cross-link formed between two places on the same DNA strand.

Inverse square law (ISL) Expresses the relationship between distance and intensity (quantity) of radiation. The law states: "The intensity of radiation is inversely proportional to the square of the distance from the source."

Investigational levels Defined as level I and level II in the ALARA concept. These are badge reading levels at which the Radiation Safety Officer investigates the reason for excess exposure even though the excess is still within legal limits. In the United States, these levels are traditionally one tenth to three tenths the applicable regulatory limits.

Involuntary motion Motion that cannot be willfully controlled. It is caused by muscle groups such as those of the digestive organs and the heart.

Iodine-123 (^{123}I) Unstable isotope of the element iodine used for monitoring thyroid gland function.

Iodine-125 (^{125}I) A radioactive isotope of the element iodine with a half-life of approximately 60 days. It decays by the method of electron capture, emitting a low energy gamma ray and a low energy characteristic photon in the process.

Iodine-131 (^{131}I) An unstable isotope of the element iodine with 53 protons and 78 neutrons in its nucleus. It undergoes beta decay with a half-life of 8 days.

Ionization The conversion of atoms to ions.

Ionization chamber A device that measures the amount of electric charge resulting from the ions produced by irradiation of a volume of air.

Ionization chamber–type survey meter ("cutie pie") This instrument is both a rate meter device (for exposure rate or dose rate in air) used for area surveys and an accurate integrating or cumulative exposure or dose measurement instrument for x-radiation and gamma radiation and, if equipped with a suitable window, for recording beta radiation as well.

Ionize To remove one or more electrons from an atomic orbit.

Ionizing radiation Radiation that produces positively and negatively charged particles (ions) when passing through matter.

Ion pair Two oppositely charged particles.

Ions Positively and negatively charged particles.

Isotopes Atoms that have the same number of protons within the nucleus but have different numbers of neutrons (e.g., helium-3 and helium-4, whose nuclei contain one and two neutrons, respectively). Radioactive isotopes of atoms that make up biologic materials may be used in medical imaging nuclear medicine studies.

J

Joule (J) A unit of energy. The work done or energy expended when a force of 1 newton acts on an object along a distance of 1 meter.

K

Karyotype A chromosome map that consists of a *photograph*, or *photomicrograph*, that is taken of the human cell

nucleus during metaphase, when each chromosome can be individually demonstrated. It is used to provide a cytogenetic analysis of chromosomes.

Kiloelectron volt (keV) A unit used to measure the kinetic energy of an individual electron in the high speed electron beam within the x-ray tube; equivalent to 1000 electron volts. Also used to measure the energies of x-rays.

Kilogram (kg) 1000 grams (g).

Kilovolt (kV) Electrical potential equal to 1000 volts.

Kinetic energy Energy of motion.

L

Last image hold feature An equipment feature in digital fluoroscopy units in which the most recent fluoroscopic image remains in view as a guide to the radiologist when the x-ray beam is not activated. The use of this feature permits dose reduction for the patient and is required by the FDA on all fluoroscopes manufactured for use in the United States.

Late stochastic (probabilistic) somatic effects Late effects that do not have a threshold, that occur in an arbitrary or probabilistic manner, whose severity does not depend on dose, and that occur months or years after high level and possibly after low level radiation exposure.

Late tissue reactions Nongenetic consequences of radiation exposure that appear months or years afterward. These effects may be either stochastic or tissue reactions.

Latent period The period of about 1 week after the prodromal stage of acute radiation syndrome, during which no visible symptoms of radiation exposure occur.

Law of Bergonié and Tribondeau The radiosensitivity of cells is directly proportional to their reproductive activity and inversely proportional to their degree of differentiation.

LD 50/30 A quantitative measurement signifying the whole-body dose of radiation that can be lethal to 50% of the exposed population within 30 days. It is fairly precise when applied to experimental animals.

LD 50/60 A quantitative measurement signifying the whole-body dose of radiation that can be lethal to 50% of the exposed population within 60 days. It may be more accurate when applied to humans.

LD 100/60 A quantitative measurement signifying the whole-body dose of radiation that can be lethal to 100% of the exposed population within 60 days.

Lead-equivalent Thickness of radiation-absorbing material that produces an attenuation equivalent to that which would be accomplished by a specified amount of lead.

Leakage radiation Radiation generated in the x-ray tube that does not exit from the collimator opening but rather penetrates the protective tube housing and, to some degree, the sides of the collimator.

LET See *Linear energy transfer [LET]*.

Leukemia Neoplastic overproduction of white blood cells.

Leukemogenesis The production or origin of leukemia.

Leukocytes White blood cells.

Leukopenia An abnormal decrease of white blood corpuscles, usually to less than 5000/mm³.

Lifetime effective dose limit Dose that does not exceed 10 times the occupationally exposed person's age in years.

Light-localizing, variable-aperture rectangular collimator A x-ray beam limitation device that permits the equipment operator to adjust the size and shape of the x-ray beam either automatically or manually.

Linear dose–response curve A model used to calculate the occurrence of cancer by extrapolating from information associated with high levels of radiation to determine the risk associated with low doses: the linear dose–response curve describes current high dose information satisfactorily but exaggerates the actual risk or danger at low doses and dose rates.

Linear energy transfer (LET) The average of energy deposited by ionizing radiation in an object per unit length of track as it passes through the object. It is expressed in units of keV/μm.

Linearity The ratio of the difference in mR/mAs values between two successive generator stations to the sum of those mR/mAs values. It must be less than 0.1. When changing from one mA station to a neighboring mA station, the most that linearity can vary is 10%. (Also see *Exposure linearity.*)

Linear nonthreshold curve of radiation dose–response This curve implies that the chance of a biologic response to ionizing radiation is directly proportional to the dose received. The use of this curve is recommended for most types of cancers.

Linear-quadratic dose–response curve A model used to calculate the occurrence of cancer by extrapolating from information associated with high levels of radiation to determine the risk associated with low doses. This model fits the current high dose information satisfactorily but may underestimate risk at low doses. Therefore it can estimate only the risk associated with low dose radiation.

Linear, threshold dose–response relationship The relationship between dose and response is such that a biologic response does not occur below a specified level of radiation dose.

Lipids Water insoluble, organic macromolecules that consist only of carbon, hydrogen, and oxygen; lipids store energy in the body for long periods. Also known as *fats*.

Lithium fluoride (LiF) The sensing material of the thermoluminescent dosimeter (TLD).

Local tissue damage A response in biologic tissue that can occur when any part of the human body receives a high radiation dose.

Log, or logarithmic, scale A method used to graph data that cover several orders of magnitude (the powers of 10; e.g., 1, 10, 100, 1000).

Long scale of radiographic contrast Radiographic contrast containing many shades of gray. A wide range of exposures will produce a wide range of shades of gray when a long scale image receptor or display is used.

Low-LET radiations External radiations such as x-rays and gamma rays that produce sparse ionization per unit length of path (LET = linear energy transfer).

Low-level radiation "An absorbed dose of 0.1 Sv or less delivered over a short period of time" and as "a larger dose delivered over a long period of time, for instance 0.5 Sv in 10 years."

Luminance A scientific term referring to the brightness of a surface. Luminance quantifies the intensity of a light source (i.e., the amount of light per unit area coming from its surface).

Lymphocytes A subgroup of white blood cells that play an active role in producing immunity for the body by producing antibodies to combat disease; the most radiosensitive blood cells in the human body.

Lymph A colorless fluid containing white blood cells that bathes the tissues and ultimately drains into the bloodstream.

Lymph nodes Small, bean-shaped organs important in the function of the immune response and that also store special cells that can trap cancer cells or bacteria that are traveling through the body through the lymph.

Lysosomes Small, pealike sacs or single-membrane spherical bodies that are of great importance for digestion within the cytoplasm. Their primary function appears to be the breaking down of large molecules.

M

M On a personnel monitoring report, this letter signifies that an equivalent dose below the minimum measurable quantity of radiation has been received during the interval of time covered by the report. Doses less than 0.1 mSv (10 mrem) are not usually detected and are reported as (M) on a personnel monitoring report.

Macromolecule Large molecule built up from smaller chemical structures.

Magnification mode Refers to a selectable smaller but enhanced field of view of an area displayed by the output phosphor of an image intensification system.

Mammography Radiographic study of the breast.

Manifest illness The stage of acute radiation syndrome when symptoms that affect the hematopoietic, gastrointestinal, and cerebrovascular systems become visible again after a latent period.

Manmade radiation Ionizing radiation created by humans for various uses, including nuclear fuel for generation of power, consumer products containing radioactive material, air travel security, and medical radiation. Also called *artificial radiation*.

mAs See *Milliampere-seconds (mAs)*.

Mass density Quantity of matter per unit volume. It is generally specified in units of kilograms per cubic meter (kg/m³) or grams per cubic centimeter (g/cc).

Master molecule A molecule vital to the survival of the cell that maintains normal cell function. It is also referred to as a *key molecule*.

Maximum permissible dose (MPD) A term used *in the past* to indicate the maximum dose equivalent of ionizing radiation that an occupationally exposed person could absorb in a specified time period without sustaining appreciable bodily injury.

Mean energy The average energy of an x-ray beam.

Mean glandular dose The average dose to the glandular tissue, considered the "tissue at risk," within a breast. For a 4.2-cm compressed breast consisting of 50% fat and 50% glandular tissue, the maximum permitted dose is 3 mGy.

Mean marrow dose "The average radiation dose to the entire active bone marrow." Also known as *bone marrow dose*.

Medical exposure Exposure to ionizing radiation incurred for the purpose of obtaining medical diagnosis or undergoing treatment.

Megaelectron volts (MeV) A unit of energy equal to 1 million electron volts.

Megakaryocytes Platelet stem cells.

Meiosis The process of germ (genetic) cell division that reduces the number of chromosomes in each daughter cell to half the number of chromosomes in the parent cell.

Meningitis An inflammation of the membranes (meninges), surrounding the brain and spinal cord.

Mesons Penetrating, unstable, subatomic particles that are components of cosmic radiation.

Messenger RNA (mRNA) The substance that directs the process for making proteins out of amino acids.

Metabolism Chemical reactions that modify foods for cellular use. Metabolism enables the cell to perform the vital functions of synthesizing proteins and producing energy.

Metaphase The phase of cell division during which the mitotic spindle is completed. It is also the phase of cell division in which chromosome damage caused by radiation exposure can be evaluated.

Microcephaly Abnormally small head circumference.

Microwaves An electromagnetic wave with a wavelength in the range 0.001 to 0.3 m, shorter than that of a normal radio wave but longer than those of infrared radiation.

Milliampere (mA) Unit of measurement. X-ray tube current.

Milliampere-seconds (mAs) The product of electron tube current and the amount of time in seconds that the x-ray tube is activated.

Milligray (mGy) A subunit of a gray equal to one one-thousandth of a gray (1/1000 Gy).

Millirad (mrad) A subunit of a rad equal to one one-thousandth of a rad (1/1000 rad).

Millirem (mrem) A subunit of a rem equal to one one-thousandth of a rem (1/1000 rem).

Millisievert (mSv) A subunit of a sievert equal to one one-thousandth of a sievert (1/1000Sv).

Mineral salts See *Salts*.

Mitochondria Large, double-membranous, oval or bean-shaped structures containing highly organized enzymes in their inner membranes that supply the energy for cells. Because of this they are referred to as "powerhouses" of the cell.

Mitosis The process of somatic cell division wherein a parent cell divides to form two daughter cells identical to the parent cell.

Mitotic death Cell death that occurs when a cell dies after one or more divisions. This can happen after irradiation. Mitotic death is also known as *genetic death*.

Mitotic delay The failure of a cell to start dividing on time; this can occur when a cell is exposed to as little as 0.01 Gy_t of ionizing radiation just before it begins dividing.

Mitotic spindle The delicate fibers attached to the centrioles and extending from one side of the cell to the other.

Mobile C-arm fluoroscopic unit A portable fluoroscopic x-ray unit that is C-shaped. It has an x-ray tube attached to one end of its arm and an image intensifier attached to the other end.

Mobile radiographic equipment Manually portable radiographic equipment.

Modified scattering See *Compton scattering*.

Molecular change An alteration in the basic structure of a molecule caused by some type of destructive process, such as exposure to ionizing radiation. Molecular damage results in the formation of structurally changed molecules that may impair cellular function.

Molecular damage Injury on the molecular level resulting from exposure to ionizing radiation.

Molecular lesions See *Point lesions*.

Molecule The smallest unit of a specific substance composed of one or more atoms.

Molten Melted or liquefied by heat.

Monitoring A means of overseeing occupational radiation exposure to ensure that such exposure is kept well below the annual effective dose limit.

Monomers A molecule that can combine with others of the same kind to form a polymer. Glucose molecules, for example, are monomers that can combine to form the polymer cellulose.

Muscle tissue Tissue that contains fibers that affect movement of an organ or part of the body; muscle tissue does not divide and is relatively insensitive to radiation.

Mutagenesis Birth defects that can be caused by irradiation of reproductive cells (sperm and ova) before conception.

Mutagens Agents that increase the frequency of occurrence of mutations, such as elevated temperatures, ionizing radiations, viruses, and chemicals.

Mutation frequency The number of spontaneous or mutagen-caused mutations that occur in a given generation.

Mutations Changes in genes caused by the loss or change of a nitrogenous base on the DNA chain. It is generally the result of the interaction of high-energy radiation with a DNA molecule.

Myeloblasts Precursors of granulocytes, a type of white blood cell.

N

NARM Stands for "naturally occurring and/or accelerator produced materials."

National Academy of Science/National Research Council Committee on the Biological Effects of Ionizing Radiation (NAS/NRC-BEIR) An advisory group that reviews studies of the biologic effects of ionizing radiation and risk assessment and provides the information to other organizations for evaluation.

National Council on Radiation Protection and Measurements (NCRP) In the United States the NCRP is a nongovernmental, nonprofit, private corporation that reviews the recommendations formulated by the International Commission on Radiological Protection (ICRP). The NCRP determines the way ICRP recommendations are incorporated into US radiation protection criteria; recommendations are published in the form of various NCRP Reports.

National Institute of Standards and Technology (NIST) Professional organization responsible for accrediting calibration laboratories that measure radiation exposure in medical radiography.

Nationwide Evaluation of X-Ray Trends (NEXT) Program Conducted by the US Food and Drug Administration and the Conference of Radiation Control Program Directors and most state health departments to provide data on systems as they exist in the United States on the latest survey. These groups have compiled reference values for patient dose. They are usually based upon large-scale surveys of actual measurements of x-ray machines in hospitals.

Natural background radiation Ionizing radiation from environmental sources, including radioactive materials in the earth, cosmic radiation from space, and radionuclides deposited in the human body via the food chain.

Necrosis Death of areas of tissue or bone surrounded by healthy parts.

Negative contrast media Agents such as air or gas that result in areas of increased density on a completed radiographic image.

Negatron A normal electron carrying a negative charge.

Negligible individual dose (NID) An annual effective dose that provides a low exposure cutoff level so that regulatory agencies may dismiss a level of individual risk as negligible.

Neonatal death Death at birth.

Nervous tissue Conductive tissue found in the brain and spinal cord.

Neuron A nerve cell consisting of a cell body and two kinds of very fine, string-like tissue segments, called processes, that extend outward, namely, dendrites and the axon.

Neuron organogenesis In the embryo-fetus, a period of development and change of the nerve cells that extends into the beginning of the fetal period.

Neutrino A particle that has no electric charge but carries away excess energy and has an almost negligible mass. The neutrino shows an exceedingly small tendency to interact with any type of matter and is therefore nearly impossible to detect.

Neutron An electrically neutral particle located within the nucleus of the atom; one of the fundamental constituents of the atom. It has approximately the same mass as a proton.

Neutrophils Leukocytes that fight infection.

Newton Unit of force in the meter-kilogram-second system of physical units.

One newton corresponds to approximately one-fourth of a pound.

Nit See *Candela per square meter.*

Nitrogen A tasteless, odorless, colorless, gaseous chemical element found free in the air; an integral part of protein and nucleic acids and thus found in every living cell.

Nitrogenous bases Organic bases that contain the element nitrogen.

Noble gas Any of a group of rare gases that include helium, neon, argon, krypton, xenon, and usually radon and that exhibit great stability and extremely low reaction rates—also called *inert gases.*

Nonagreement states Individual US states in which both the state departments of environmental protection and the Nuclear Regulatory Commission (NRC) enforce radiation protection regulations. These states have decided to maintain their own designed independent radiation protection programs for radioactive materials.

Nonessential radiologic examinations Radiologic examinations performed in the absence of definite medical indications.

Nonionizing radiation Radiation that does not have sufficient energy to eject electrons from atoms.

Nonoccupational exposure Radiation exposure received by members of the general population who are not employed as radiation workers.

Nonoccupational person Any person not employed as a radiation worker.

Non–self-reading pocket dosimeter A pocket ionization chamber that requires a special accessory electrometer to read the device and is used for personnel monitoring in areas of low radiation exposure when immediate readout is not necessary.

Nonspecific life span shortening A reduction in the life cycle of small laboratory animals resulting from nonlethal exposure to ionizing radiation. Early demise actually resulted from radiation-induced cancer.

Nonthreshold Any radiation dose has the capability of producing a biologic effect. No radiation dose can be considered absolutely safe.

Nonverbal messages Unconscious actions, or body language.

Nuclear medicine Branch of medicine that employs radioisotopes to study organ function in a patient, to detect the spread of cancer into bone, and to treat certain types of diseases.

Nuclear medicine procedure The administration, either orally or intravenously, of a radioactive isotope for the purpose of conducting a diagnostic study of a body area.

Nuclear reactor A mechanism for creating and continuing a controlled nuclear chain reaction in a fissionable fuel for the production of energy or supplementary fissionable material.

Nuclear Regulatory Commission (NRC) A federal agency (formerly known as the *Atomic Energy Commission*) that has the authority to control the possession, use, and production of atomic energy in the interest of national security. This agency also has the power to enforce radiation protection standards.

Nucleic acids Very large, complex macromolecules made up of nucleotides.

Nucleolus A small body in the nucleus of a cell that contains protein and RNA and is the site for the synthesis of ribosomal RNA and for the formation of ribosomal subunits.

Nucleoplasm A gelatinous liquid within the nucleus that surrounds the chromosomes and the nucleoli.

Nucleotides Units formed from the following: a nitrogenous base such as adenine, guanine, cytosine, or thymine; a five-carbon sugar molecule, deoxyribose; and a phosphate molecule. Several nucleotides make up a nucleic acid.

Nucleus The center of the cell; a spherical mass of protoplasm containing the genetic material (DNA), which is stored in its molecular structure.

O

Occupancy factor (T) A factor used to modify the shielding requirement for a particular barrier by taking into account the fraction of the work week during which the space beyond the barrier is occupied.

Occupational and nonoccupational dose limits Upper boundary doses of ionizing radiation for which there is a negligible risk of bodily injury or genetic damage.

Occupational exposure Radiation exposure received by radiation workers in the course of exercising their professional responsibilities.

Occupational risk (1) The probability of injury, ailment, or death resulting from an activity that takes place in the workplace; (2) the possibility of developing a radiogenic cancer or the induction of a genetic defect as a consequence of the radiation exposure received.

Occupational Safety and Health Administration (OSHA) A monitoring agency functioning in places of employment, predominantly in industry, OSHA regulates occupational exposure to radiation.

Occupationally exposed person Individual employed as a radiation worker.

Off-focus radiation X-rays emitted from parts of the tube other than the focal spot. Also called *stem radiation*.

Oncology Branch of medicine dealing with cancer.

Oocytes Immature female germ cells.

Oogonium Female germ cell.

Optically stimulated luminescence (OSL) dosimeter A device for monitoring occupational exposure that contains an aluminum oxide detector. The dosimeter is "read out" by using laser light at selected frequencies. When such laser light is incident on the sensing material, it becomes luminescent in proportion to the amount of radiation exposure that was received.

Optimal-quality image High-quality, diagnostic radiographic digital or film image of a part of the human body.

Optimization for radiation protection (ORP) See *ALARA concept/principle*.

Organic acids Organic compounds containing the carboxyl (COOH) group.

Organic compounds All compounds that contain carbon, hydrogen, and oxygen.

Organogenesis (1) Period of gestation that corresponds to approximately 10 days to 12 weeks after conception. During this time, the nerve cells in the brain and spinal cord of the fetus are most susceptible to radiation-induced congenital abnormalities; (2) the stage in which undifferentiated cells are implanted in the uterine wall.

Osmosis When water tends to move across cell surfaces or membranes into areas in which a high concentration of potassium ions is present.

Osmotic pressure The force created when a semipermeable membrane separates two solutions of different concentrations.

Osteogenic sarcoma Bone cancer.

Osteoporosis Decalcification of the bone.

Ovum The mature reproductive cell of female animals and human females produced in the ovaries. Also called the *egg*, the ovum contributes one chromosome of each pair to the fertilized cell.

Oxidation Most simply, the combining of a substance with oxygen. The definition of oxidation, however, has been broadened to include reactions in which electrons are lost by an atom.

Oxygen enhancement ratio (OER) The ratio of the radiation dose required to cause a particular biologic response of cells or organisms in any oxygen-deprived environment to the radiation dose required to cause an identical response under normally oxygenated conditions.

Oxygen fixation Refers to nonreparable DNA lesions produced by x-rays with the chemical participation of oxygen.

P

Pair production Interaction between an incoming photon of at least 1.022 MeV and an atom of irradiated biologic tissue in which the photon approaches, strongly interacts with the nucleus of the atom of the irradiated tissue, and disappears. In the process, the energy of the incoming photon is transformed into two new particles—a negatron and a positron—after which these particles exit from the atom and carry away some of the momentum of the absorbed photon when the photon's energy is greater than 1.022 MeV.

Parenchymal cells The distinguishing or specific cells of a gland or organ, contained in and supported by the connective tissue framework.

Particulate radiation As opposed to x-rays and gamma rays, which are electromagnetic radiations, particulate radiation is a form of radiation that includes alpha particles (nuclei of helium), beta particles (electrons), neutrons, and protons that are ejected from atoms at very high speeds.

Patient restraint Immobilization of the patient by a mechanical device or human restraint during an imaging procedure.

Peak kilovoltage (kVp) The highest energy level of photons in the x-ray beam.

Peak voltage Maximum voltage directed across an x-ray tube.

Peptic bond Chemical bond connecting two amino acids.

Peptide bond A chemical link that connects each amino acid in long, chain-like molecular complexes.

Permeable Penetrable.

Personnel dosimeter A device that provides an indication of the working habits and working conditions of diagnostic imaging personnel. It determines occupational exposure by detecting and measuring the quantity of ionizing radiation to which the dosimeter has been exposed over a period of time.

Personnel dosimetry Monitoring of any person occupationally exposed on a regular basis to ionizing radiation.

Personnel monitoring report A written report of occupational radiation exposure of personnel prepared by a monitoring company.

Person-sievert SI unit for the radiation quantity collective effective dose (ColEfD).

PET/CT scanner A unit in which a positron emission tomography (PET) scanner is mechanically joined in a tandem configuration with a computed tomography (CT) scanner to produce a single imaging device. This unit can detect the presence of abnormally high regions of glucose metabolism, yielding evidence of cancer spread (metastasis) in other body areas, but also, at the same time, obtain detailed information about the anatomic location and extent of these lesions or growths.

Photodisintegration An interaction that occurs above 10 MeV in high-energy radiation therapy treatment machines. In this interaction, a high energy photon collides with the nucleus of an atom, which directly absorbs all the photon's energy. This energy excess in the nucleus creates an instability that in most cases is alleviated by the emission of a neutron from the nucleus. Also, if sufficient energy is absorbed by the nucleus, another type of emission is possible, such as a proton or proton–neutron combination (deuteron) or even an alpha particle.

Photoelectric absorption Process whereby the kinetic energy of the incident photon is completely absorbed as it interacts with an atom and ejects an inner-shell electron in its orbit.

Photoelectron The electron ejected from its inner-shell orbit during the process of photoelectric absorption. It possesses kinetic energy and can ionize other atoms it encounters until its energy is spent.

Photomultiplier tube An electron tube that converts the computed radiography (CR) stored latent image, thus transforming visible light photons into an amplified electronic signal.

Photon A particle associated with electromagnetic radiation that has neither mass nor electric charge.

Photopic vision Cone vision (daytime vision).

Photostimulable phosphor The image receptor of a computed radiography (CR) system. When struck by x-rays, electrons within the phosphor become trapped at energy levels that are quasistable. When a laser strikes the surface of the phosphor, visible light is emitted in proportion to the x-ray exposure that had been received by the phosphor. A photomultiplier tube then records the visible light intensity, which corresponds to the brightness of a picture element, or pixel, in the CR image.

Picocurie A very small quantity of radioactivity equivalent to one-trillionth (10^{-12}) of a curie.

Pitch (pitch ratio) Table distance traveled in one 360-degree gantry rotation divided by beam collimation. For example, if the table traveled 5 mm in one rotation and the beam collimation was 5 mm, then pitch equals 5 mm/5 mm = 1.0.

Pixels Each miniature square box in the image matrix of the digital image is an individual picture element. When taken together, they represent the total information contained in a slice or a volume of tissue.

Platelets Circular or oval disks found in the blood of all vertebrates. Platelets initiate blood clotting and prevent hemorrhage.

Pluripotential stem cell A single precursor cell from which all of the cells of the hematopoietic system develop.

Pocket ionization chamber (pocket dosimeter) A personnel monitoring device that contains two electrodes, one positively charged (the central electrode) and one negatively charged (the outer electrode). When these electrodes are exposed to ionizing radiation, the air surrounding the central electrode (+) becomes ionized and discharges the mechanism in direct proportion to the amount of radiation to which it has been exposed.

Point lesions Altered areas in molecules caused by the breaking of a single chemical bond.

Point mutations Genetic mutations at the molecular level. The chromosome is not broken, but the DNA within it is damaged. (See *Single-strand break*.)

Polymer A large molecule, or macromolecule, composed of many repeated subunits called *monomers*.

Polysaccharides Polymeric carbohydrate molecules composed of long chains of monosaccharides.

Portable radiographic equipment See *Mobile radiographic equipment*.

Positive beam limitation (PBL) A feature of current radiographic collimators that automatically adjusts the collimators so that the radiation field size matches the size of the image receptor. Also known as *automatic collimation*.

Positive contrast media Solutions containing elements that have a higher atomic number than surrounding soft tissue (e.g., barium or iodine based) that are either ingested or injected into the body tissues or structures to be visualized.

Positron A positively charged electron, which is a form of antimatter.

Positron emission tomography (PET) A nuclear medicine imaging technique that produces a three-dimensional picture of functional processes within the body. It does this with a detection system or camera that records pairs of oppositely traveling photons (annihilation radiation) indirectly produced by a positron-emitting radionuclide. Images in three-dimensional space of heightened activity can be generated using mathematic reconstruction techniques similar to those employed by x-ray computed tomography.

Potential difference The difference in electrical potential or voltage between two points in a circuit.

Potential risk The possibility of inducing a radiogenic cancer or genetic defect after irradiation.

Precursor cells See *Stem cells*.

Preimplantation stage Approximately 0 to 9 days after conception. In this stage the fertilized ovum divides and forms a ball-like structure containing undifferentiated cells.

Primary beam See *Primary radiation*.

Primary protective barrier (1) A barrier designed to prevent primary, or direct, radiation from reaching personnel or members of the general public on the other side of the barrier; (2) a barrier located perpendicular to the undeflected line of travel of the primary x-ray beam.

Primary radiation Radiation that emerges directly from the x-ray tube collimator and moves without deflection toward a wall, door, viewing window, and so on. Also called *direct radiation* or the *useful beam*.

Probabilistic effects See *Stochastic effects*.

Prodromal syndrome The first stage of acute radiation syndrome, which occurs within hours after a whole body absorbed dose of 1 Gy_t or more; characterized by

nausea, vomiting, diarrhea, fatigue, and leukopenia. Also called the *initial stage of ARS*.

Programmed cell death See *Apoptosis*.

Prophase The first phase of cell division, during which the nucleus and the chromosomes enlarge and the DNA begins to take structural form.

Proportional counter A radiation survey instrument generally used in a laboratory setting to detect alpha and beta radiation and small amounts of other types of low level radioactive contamination.

Protective apparel Special garments such as aprons, gloves, and thyroid shields that are conventionally made of lead-impregnated vinyl and worn during fluoroscopic and certain selective radiographic procedures.

Protective barrier Any medium of adequate composition and thickness that absorbs primary and/or secondary radiation, thereby reducing the exposure of persons located on the other side of the barrier.

Protective curtain A sliding panel with a minimum of 0.25-mm lead equivalent that can be positioned between the fluoroscopist and the patient to intercept scattered radiation above the tabletop.

Protective eyeglasses Eyeglasses with optically clear lenses that contain a minimum lead-equivalent protection of 0.35 mm.

Protective shielding A structure or device made of certain materials such as concrete, lead, or lead-impregnated material that will adequately attenuate ionizing radiation.

Protein Amino acids linked in various patterns and combinations. Proteins contain carbon, hydrogen, nitrogen, oxygen, and occasionally other elements, such as sulfur. Proteins are the most elementary building blocks of cells.

Protein synthesis The making of new proteins.

Proton One of the three main constituents of an atom, the proton carries a positive electric charge equal in magnitude to that of an electron.

Protoplasm The chemical building material for all living things, protoplasm consists of inorganic substances, such as water and mineral salts, and organic substances, including proteins, carbohydrates, lipids, and nucleic acids.

Pulsed fluoroscopy See *Intermittent fluoroscopy*.

Purines A class of nitrogenous bases found in DNA and RNA. These bases include adenine (A) and guanine (G).

Pyrimidines A class of nitrogenous bases found in DNA and RNA. These bases include cytosine (C), thymine (T), and, in the case of RNA, uracil (U), which replaces thymine.

Q

Quality control program A method used in imaging departments to ensure standardization in film processing and processing of digital images. It includes monitoring and maintenance of all processing and image display equipment in the facility.

Quality factor An adjustment multiplier that was used in the calculation of dose equivalence to specify the ability of a dose of any kind of ionizing radiation to cause biologic damage. Also known as a *modifying factor*.

Quantum mottle Faint blotches (image noise) in the recorded radiographic image produced by an intrinsic fluctuation in the incident photon intensity. This effect can degrade the radiographic image.

R

Rad (radiation absorbed dose) The traditional unit that has been used to indicate the amount of radiant energy transferred to an irradiated object by any type if ionizing radiation. The rad is equivalent to an energy transfer of 100 ergs per gram to an irradiated object and numerically is equal to 1/100 gray.

Radiant energy Energy that moves in the form of a wave and is transmitted by radiations such as x-rays and gamma rays.

Radiation Kinetic energy that passes from one location to another; a transfer of energy that results from either a change occurring naturally within an atom (see *Radiation decay*) or a process caused by the interaction of a particle with an atom.

Radiation biology The science concerned with the effects of ionizing radiations on living systems.

Radiation Control for Health and Safety Act of 1968 Law passed by the US Congress to protect the public from the hazards of unnecessary radiation exposure resulting from electronic products such as microwave ovens, color televisions, and diagnostic x-ray equipment.

Radiation decay A naturally occurring process in which atoms with unstable nuclei relieve that instability by various types of nuclear spontaneous emissions, including charged particles, uncharged particles, and photons.

Radiation dose The amount of radiation received by an individual. The amount of energy transferred to electrons in biologic tissue by ionizing radiation is the basis of this concept.

Radiation dose–response curve A graph that maps out the effects of radiation observed in relation to the dose of radiation received.

Radiation dose–response relationship The relationship between radiation and dose–response. The information obtained can be used to attempt to predict the risk of occurrence of malignancies in human populations exposed to low levels of ionizing radiation.

Radiation emergency plan Plan that hospitals can implement for handling emergency situations involving radioactive contamination.

Radiation hormesis Effect that is a beneficial consequence of radiation for populations continuously exposed to moderately higher levels of radiation.

Radiation monitoring device A device worn by diagnostic imaging personnel to indicate occupational exposure by measuring the quantity of radiation to which it has been exposed over time.

Radiation permeability The ability of a structure to be penetrated by radiation.

Radiation protection Effective measures employed by radiation workers to safeguard patients, personnel, and the general public from unnecessary exposure to ionizing radiation.

Radiation safety committee (RSC) Group that assists in the development of the radiation safety program in a health care facility; provides guidance for the program and facilitates its ongoing operation.

Radiation safety officer (RSO) An individual such as a medical physicist, health physicist, radiologist, or other individual qualified through adequate training and experience. It is the responsibility of the RSO to ensure that state, federal, and internationally accepted guidelines for radiation protection are followed in the facility.

Radiation safety program An effective and detailed program conducted in facilities that provide imaging services to ensure adequate radiation safety of patients and radiation workers.

Radiation survey instruments Area monitoring devices that detect and/or measure radiation.

Radiation therapy Use of x-rays or gamma rays, usually with energies much greater than those employed for diagnostic purposes, to destroy the cells comprising a tumor while sparing the surrounding nontumor tissues.

Radiation weighting factor (W_R) A dimensionless factor (a multiplier) that was chosen for radiation protection purposes to account for differences in biologic impact among various types of ionizing radiations. This factor places risks associated with biologic effects on a common scale.

Radiation-induced malignancy Cancerous neoplasm caused by exposure to ionizing radiation.

Radicals Groups of atoms that remain together during a chemical change and behave almost like a single atom. Atoms in a radical are held together by covalent bonding.

Radioactive contamination Radioactive material that is attached to or associated with dust particles or is in liquid form on various surfaces. Removal of the liquid or dust accomplishes removal of the radioactive material. Radioactive contamination may consist of surface, internal (inhaled, ingested), internal wound, or external wound contamination.

Radioactive dispersal device A radioactive source mixed with conventional explosives. When detonated, this device explodes, spreading radioactive material through a specific area and causing contamination and panic; also called a *dirty bomb*.

Radiodermatitis Redening of the skin caused by exposure to ionizing radiation.

Radiogenic malignancies Cancerous neoplasms induced by exposure to ionizing radiation.

Radiographer A person qualified through formal education and certification to practice medical imaging procedures and provide related patient care.

Radiographic beam–light beam coincidence Both physical size (length and width) and alignment between the radiographic beam and the localizing light beam must correspond to within 2% of the source-to–image distance (SID).

Radiographic contrast Differences in gray levels between adjacent anatomic structures on a completed image. Image receptor contrast and subject contrast combined produce radiographic contrast.

Radiographic fog Undesirable additional darkness on a completed radiographic image caused by scattered radiation reaching the image receptor.

Radiographic grid A device made of parallel radiopaque lead strips alternately separated with low-attenuation strips of aluminum, plastic, or wood. It is placed between the patient and the radiographic image receptor to remove scattered x-ray photons that emerge from the patient before they reach the image receptor. Use of a grid improves radiographic contrast and visibility of detail, but it also increases patient dose.

Radiographic grid ratio The ratio of the height to the width of the gaps between lead strips.

Radiographic image receptor Phosphor plate, digital radiography receptor, or radiographic film.

Radioisotopes Isotopes of a particular element that are unstable because of their neutron–proton configuration.

Radiologist A qualified physician who specializes in diagnosis and treatment through the use of radiant energy.

Radiolucent Transparent to radiation; a material that allows radiation to pass through it.

Radiolysis of water Ionization interaction of radiation with water molecules resulting in a separation into other components.

Radionuclide An unstable nucleus that emits one or more forms of ionizing radiation to achieve greater stability. The emissions may include alpha particles, beta particles, and gamma rays.

Radiosensitivity Comparable sensitivity of human cells, tissues, and organs to the injurious action of ionizing radiation.

Radio waves A very low frequency electromagnetic wave (from roughly 30 kilohertz to 100 gigahertz).

Radium This element (Z = 88) has an unstable nucleus and decays with a half-life of 1622 years by alpha particle emission to the radioactive element radon (Z = 86).

Radon The first decay product of radium; a colorless, odorless, heavy radioactive gas that, along with its own decay products, polonium-218 and polonium-214 (solid form), is always present to some degree in the air. It comprises the largest component of natural background radiation.

Rayleigh scattering See *Coherent scattering.*

Recessive mutation A genetic mutation that probably will not be expressed for several generations because both parents must possess the same genetic defect.

Recoil electron See *Compton scattered electron.*

Recovery When the cell is able to recover after exposure to sublethal doses of ionizing radiation.

Relative biologic effectiveness (RBE) Describes the relative capabilities of radiation with differing linear energy transfers (LETs) to produce a particular biologic reaction. Simply defined, it is the ratio of the dose of a reference radiation (conventionally, 250kVp x-rays) to the dose of radiation of the type in question that is necessary to produce the same biologic reaction in a given experiment. The reaction is produced by a dose of the test radiation delivered under the same conditions.

Relative risk Model predicting that the number of excess cancers will increase as the natural incidence of cancer increases with advancing age in a population.

Rem (radiation equivalent man) Traditional unit for the radiation quantity equivalent dose (EqD); defined as the dose that is equivalent to any type of ionizing radiation that produces the same biologic effect as 1 rad (radiation absorbed dose) of x-radiation.

Remnant radiation See *Exit,* or *image formation, radiation.*

Repair enzymes Enzymes that can mend damaged molecules and are therefore capable of helping the cell to recover from a small amount of radiation-induced damage.

Repeat analysis program An attempt to record the various causes of inadequate quality on occasions when an image has to be retaken.

Repeat image Any radiographic image that must be performed more than once because of a human or mechanical error during the production of the initial image.

Reproductive cells Male and female germ cells (relatively radiosensitive).

Reproductive death The permanent loss of a cell's ability to divide because of exposure to doses of ionizing radiation in the range of 1 to 10 Gy. The cell itself does not die but continues to metabolize and synthesize nucleic acids and proteins.

Restitution A process in which chromosome breaks rejoin in their original configuration with no visible damage.

Retina The rod and cone containing area of the eye; the retina receives the image formed by the lens.

Ribonucleic acid (RNA) Type of nucleic acid that carries genetic information from the DNA in the cell nucleus to the ribosomes located in the cytoplasm.

Ribosomal RNA (rRNA) Type of RNA that assists in the linking of messenger RNA to the ribosome to facilitate protein synthesis.

Ribosomes Very small, spherical, cytoplasmic organelles that attach to the endoplasmic reticulum; they are the assembly sites where mRNA and tRNA combine amino acids into proteins. They are the cell's "protein factories."

Right-to-Know Act (Employee) A series of statutes passed by individual states requiring that employees be made aware of the hazards in the workplace. This act covers hazardous substances, infectious agents, ionizing radiation, and nonionizing radiation.

Risk In general terms, the probability of injury, ailment, or death resulting from an activity. In the medical industry with reference to the radiation sciences, risk is the possibility of inducing a radiogenic cancer or genetic defect after irradiation.

Road mapping A method of digital image subtraction in which the frame that contains the greatest amount of contrast material in vessels is identified and is then subtracted from all subsequent images. Live fluoroscopic images of the catheter moving through the vasculature can then be seen even after the vessels contain less contrast.

Roentgen (R) Internationally accepted traditional unit of measurement of exposure to x-radiation and gamma radiation. One roentgen is the photon exposure that under standard conditions of pressure and temperature produces a total positive or negative ion charge of $2.58 \times (10)^{-4}$ coulombs per kilogram of dry air.

Rung A step in the DNA ladder-like structure composed of a pair of nitrogenous bases.

S

Saccharides See *Carbohydrates.*

Salts Chemical compounds resulting from the action of an acid and a base on each other. They are sometimes referred to as *electrolytes.*

Sarcophagus   Large concrete shelter constructed by the Soviet Union atop the remains of the Reactor 4 building after the Chernobyl nuclear accident to provide protection from radiation exposure.

Scan direction collimation   The product of the number of data channels used during one axial acquisition (N) and the nominal slice width of one axial image (T).

Scattered radiation   All the radiation that arises from the interaction of an x-ray beam with the atoms of a patient or any other object in the path of the beam.

Scattering   The process wherein x-ray photons undergo a change in direction after interacting with the atoms of an object.

Scintillator   A substance that glows when hit by high-energy particles or photons.

Scotopic vision   Rod vision (night vision).

Scout view   A preliminary radiographic image of a portion of a patient's anatomy in either the coronal or sagittal direction obtained before performing a CT scan in that region.

Secondary electron   See *Compton scattered electron.*

Secondary protective barrier   A barrier that affords protection from secondary radiation (leakage and scattered radiation) only; as such, it is not designed to intercept the direct x-ray beam or to provide adequate attenuation of the beam.

Secondary radiation   The radiation that results from the interaction between primary radiation and the atoms of the irradiated object and the off-focus or leakage radiation that penetrates the x-ray tube protective housing.

Self-reading pocket dosimeter   A pocket ionization chamber that contains a built-in electrometer and provides an immediate exposure readout for radiation workers who work in high-exposure areas.

Semipermeable membrane   A film that permits the passage of a pure solvent such as water but does not allow material dissolved by the solvent to pass through it.

Shadow shield   A shield of radiopaque material suspended from above the radiographic beam-defining system; these shields hang over the area of clinical interest to cast a shadow in the primary beam over the patient's reproductive organs.

Shallow equivalent dose   The external exposure of the skin or extremity at a tissue depth of 0.007 cm (7 mg/cm^2) averaged over an area of 1 cm^2.

Shaped contact shield   A cup-shaped radiopaque shield, containing 1 mm of lead that is contoured to enclose the scrotum and penis to protect the male reproductive organs from exposure to ionizing radiation.

Shielding   Radiation-absorbent barrier of appropriate thickness used to provide protection from radiation. The most common materials used for structural barriers are lead and concrete. Accessory devices such as aprons, gloves, and thyroid shields are made of lead-impregnated vinyl to provide shielding from radiation exposure when individuals cannot remain behind a protective structural barrier during certain imaging procedures.

Side scatter   Photons that interact with the atoms of an object and consequently are deflected to the side.

Sievert (Sv)   The SI unit of measure for the radiation quantities, equivalent dose (EqD), and effective dose (EfD). It is the product of the absorbed dose and the radiation weighting factor. For x-radiation (Q = 1) one sievert equals one joule of energy absorbed per kilogram of tissue. This unit is used *only* for radiation protection purposes. It provides a common scale whereby varying degrees of biologic damage caused by equal absorbed doses of different types of ionizing radiation (Q equals one or greater) can be compared with the degree of biologic damage caused by the same amount of x-radiation or gamma radiation. In the traditional system, 100 rem equals 1 sievert.

Sigmoid or "S-shaped" (nonlinear), threshold curve of radiation dose–response   Generally employed in radiation therapy to demonstrate high-dose cellular response. This curve indicates the existence of a threshold. Different effects require different minimal doses.

Signal-to-noise ratio (SNR)   The comparison of the average computed tomography (CT) number in a region with the statistical variation of CT number in that region.

Single-strand break   The ionization of a DNA macromolecule resulting in a break of one of its chemical bonds, thereby severing one of the sugar–phosphate chain side rails or strands of the ladderlike DNA molecular structure.

Skin dose   In general represents the absorbed dose to the most superficial layers of the skin.

Skin erythema dose   The received quantity of radiation (corresponding roughly to a moderate dose of several gray) that causes diffused redness over an area of skin after irradiation.

Small angle scatter   Photons that pass through the patient being radiographed, interact with the atoms of the body, and are deflected at such a small angle that they can reach the image receptor, thereby degrading the completed radiographic image by producing small amounts of radiographic fog.

Somatic cells   All the cells in the human body other than female and male germ cells.

Somatic effects   Biologic damage experienced by living organisms (such as humans) as a result of exposure to ionizing radiation. (See either *Early somatic tissue reactions* or *Late somatic tissue reactions.*)

Somatic tissue reactions   Biologic reactions in tissues of the body that were irradiated that can be directly related to the dose of ionizing radiation received. These are cell-killing responses that exhibit a threshold dose below which the reactions are absent and above which the severity of the early tissue reactions increases as the radiation dose increases.

Source-to–image receptor distance (SID)   The distance from the anode focal spot to the radiographic image receptor.

Source-to-skin distance (SSD)   The distance from the anode focal spot to the skin of the patient.

Source-to-tabletop distance   The distance from the anode focal spot to the top of the radiographic table.

Spacer bar   A device that projects down from the housing of some collimators to prevent the collimators from being closer than 15 cm to the patient.

Specific area shielding   The use of lead or lead-impregnated material to protect selective body areas from exposure to ionizing radiation.

Spermatocytes   Sperm cells at their infancy. They divide by meiosis to produce cells with half the number of chromosomes.

Spermatogonium   The male germ cell.

Spiral computed tomography   In computed tomography (CT), a "data acquisition method that combines a continuous gantry rotation with a continuous table movement to form a spiral path of scan data." It is also known as *helical CT.*

Spontaneous mutations   A natural phenomenon involving alterations in genes and DNA. These mutations occur at random and without a known cause.

Standardized dose reporting A system of standardizing a patient's radiation dose by having the dose dictated into the patient's report and then tracking this dose.

Stem cells Immature or precursor cells.

Stem radiation See *Off-focus radiation.*

Stochastic effects Mutational or randomly occurring biologic changes, independent of dose, in which the chance of occurrence of the effect rather than the severity of the effect is proportional to the dose of ionizing radiation. These effects occur months or years after high level, and possibly also after low level, radiation exposure. Examples include cancer and genetic effects. Also called *probabilistic effects.*

Structural proteins Those proteins from which the body acquires its shape and form. They also are a source of heat and energy.

Sunspots Dark spots that occasionally appear on the surface of the sun. Sunspots indicate regions of increased electromagnetic field activity and are sometimes responsible for ejecting particulate radiation into space.

Surface contamination External contamination of the skin or clothing of an individual with radioactive material.

Surface integral dose (SID) The total amount of radiant energy transferred by ionizing radiation to the human body during a radiation exposure.

Syndrome A collection of symptoms.

T

Target theory Concept of radiation damage resulting from discrete and random events. If a critical location on the master molecule (believed to be DNA) is a target receiving multiple hits from ionizing radiation, it may well be inactivated. Normal cell function will then cease, and the cell will die. If, on the other hand, it receives only a single hit, then the master molecule most likely will still be operational. The target theory concept may be useful for explaining cell death and nonfatal cell abnormalities caused by exposure to radiation.

Technetium-99m (⁹⁹ᵐTc) A gamma-emitting radioisotope with a 6-hour half-life that is produced from the radioactive decay of another unstable isotope, molybdenum-99, which relieves its instability by beta decay. It is the most common radioisotope used in nuclear medicine studies.

Telangiectasia Dilation of capillaries and sometimes of terminal arteries of an organ.

Telophase The phase of mitosis during which cell division is completed with the formation of two new daughter cells, each of which contains exactly the same genetic material as the parent cell.

Teratogenesis Birth effects induced by irradiation in utero.

Terrestrial radiation Long-lived radioactive elements such as uranium-238, radium-226, and thorium-232 that emit densely ionizing radiations. These sources are present in variable quantities in the crust of the earth.

Therapeutic ratio The ratio obtained by dividing the effective therapeutic dose by the minimum lethal dose; a comparison of the amount of a therapeutic agent that causes the therapeutic effect to the amount that causes toxicity.

Thermal neutron Nominally classified as a neutron whose kinetic energy is approximately less than or equal to 1 eV. Typically, these are neutrons whose kinetic energy has been significantly degraded as a result of multiple energy loss collisions.

Thermoluminescent dosimeter (TLD) A personnel monitoring device that most often contains a crystalline form of lithium fluoride as its sensing material. When this device is placed in a TLD analyzer and heated, the crystals emit visible light in proportion to the amount of radiation to which the TLD dosimeter was exposed. A graphic plot of this light intensity (also known as *thermoluminescence intensity*) versus the heating temperature is known as a "glow curve." The glow curve represents a unique signature of the exposure received by the TLD dosimeter.

Thompson scattering The elastic scattering of an x-ray photon by a free electron.

Thoron A radioactive decay product of an isotope of radon, namely radon-220, with a half-life of 54.5 seconds. It is given the name *thoron* because radon-220 was itself derived from the radioactive decay of thorium-232, a naturally occurring material.

Threshold (1) The point at which a response or reaction to an increasing stimulation first occurs; (2) with reference to ionizing radiation, this means that below a certain radiation level or dose, no biologic effects are observed.

Thrombocytes See *Platelets.*

Thrombocytopenia A disorder in which there is a relative decrease of thrombocytes, commonly known as *platelets,* present in the blood. A normal human platelet count ranges from 150,000 to 450,000 platelets per microliter of blood.

Thymine (T) A pyrimidine base found only in DNA.

Thymus gland An organ of the lymphatic system, located in the mediastinal cavity anterior to and above the heart. It plays a critical role in the body's defense against infection.

Thyroid gland A gland located in the neck just below the larynx. The hormone produced by this gland helps regulate the body's metabolic rate and the process of growth.

Thyroid shield See *Protective apparel.*

Time The amount of radiation a worker receives is directly proportional to the length of time that the individual is exposed to ionizing radiation.

Time interval difference A method of digital image subtraction in which each image is subtracted from an image a few frames in advance. This technique reveals vessels containing contrast material and suppresses soft tissue in the images. It is less sensitive to patient motion than when the first image is subtracted from all successive images.

Tissue reactions Any radiation effects on organ or organ systems that increase with increasing dose and below which the effect rarely or never occurs. They may occur as early effects, immediately after irradiation, or late effects, after some latent period.

Tissue weighting factor (W$_T$) A value that denotes the percentage of the summed stochastic (cancer plus genetic) risk stemming from irradiation of tissue (T) to the all-inclusive risk when the entire body is irradiated in a uniform fashion.

Title 10 of the Code of Federal Regulations, Part 20 A document prepared and distributed by the US Office of the Federal Register. The rules and regulations of the Nuclear Regulatory Commission (NRC) and fundamental radiation protection standards governing occupational radiation exposure are included in this document.

TLD analyzer A device that measures the amount of ionizing radiation to which a TLD badge has been exposed.

TLD ring badge See *Extremity dosimeter.*

Tolerance dose A radiation dose to which occupationally exposed persons could be continuously subjected without any apparent harmful acute effects, such as erythema of the skin.

Total effective dose equivalent (TEDE) A system of units and quantities used to monitor occupationally exposed personnel such as nuclear medicine technologists and interventional radiologists. TEDE is the sum of effective dose equivalent from external radiation exposures and the committed effective dose equivalent (CEDE) from internal sources. It is designed to take into account all possible causes of radiation exposure.

Total filtration Inherent filtration plus added filtration.

Traditional units Special units associated with radiation protection and dosimetry, namely, the roentgen and the rem.

Transfer RNA (tRNA) Type of RNA that combines with individual amino acids from different areas of the cell and attaches them to the ribosomes.

Trimester A 3-month period of gestation (i.e., first, second, and third trimesters).

Tubules Small tubes.

Tungsten A metal with a high melting point (greater than 3400°C) and a high atomic number ($Z = 74$). The anode in the x-ray tube is usually made primarily of this metal. It is also the principal component of the filament cathode.

Tungsten rhenium A metal alloy with a high melting point and a high atomic number. The anode of a general purpose x-ray tube is usually made of this alloy.

U

Ulceration The process of pus formation on a free surface, such as the skin or a mucous membrane, to form an ulcer.

Umbra See *Primary radiation.*

Uncontrolled area Area such as a nearby hallway or corridor that is frequented by the general public.

Undifferentiated cells Immature or nonspecialized cells.

Unit A fixed amount of some property or characteristic (e.g., distance-meter, time-second, energy-joule) used as a measure for which other amounts of that property or characteristic can be described.

United Nations Scientific Committee on the Effects of Atomic Radiation (UNSCEAR) A group that plays a prominent role in the formulation of radiation protection guidelines. This group evaluates human and environmental ionizing radiation exposure from a variety of sources and research conclusions to derive radiation risk assessments for radiation-induced cancer and for genetic (hereditary) effects.

Unmodified scattering See *Coherent scattering.*

Unnecessary exposure Any radiation exposure that does not benefit a person in terms of diagnostic information obtained for the clinical management of medical needs or any radiation exposure that does not enhance the quality of the study.

Unnecessary radiologic procedure Radiologic examination for which there is no sufficient justification to subject a patient to the minimal risk of the absorbed radiation dose resulting from the procedure.

Uracil (U) A pyrimidine base found only in RNA. It replaces thymine (T) as the nitrogenous base in ribonucleic acid.

US Code of Federal Regulations Document prepared and distributed by the US Office of the Federal Register that contains the rules and regulations of the Nuclear Regulatory Commission (NRC) and the radiation protection standards governing occupational radiation exposure.

Use factor (U) For primary radiation, the use factor represents the portion of beam-on time that the x-ray beam is directed at a primary barrier during the week. Also known as *beam direction factor.*

Useful beam See *Primary radiation.*

V

Variable rectangular collimator A box-shaped device containing the radiographic beam-defining system; the device is most often used to define the size and shape of the radiographic beam.

Vasculitis An inflammation of the blood vessels. It causes changes in the walls of blood vessels, including thickening, weakening, narrowing, and scarring. These changes restrict blood flow, resulting in organ and tissue damage.

Verbal messages Spoken words.

Vesicle Small cavities or sacs containing liquid.

Volt (V) SI unit of electrical potential and potential difference.

Voltage Electrical potential at a point or position relative to ground potential.

Voluntary motion Motion controlled by will (i.e., skeletal muscle).

W

Wavelength Distance between two consecutive crests or troughs in a wave (given in meters).

Wave-particle duality Electromagnetic radiation can travel and interact with matter in the form of a wave or a particle. For this reason, x-rays may be described as both waves and particles.

Window level Sets the midpoint of the range of densities visible on a digital image.

Workload (W) Essentially the radiation output weighted time that the unit is actually delivering radiation during the week. It is specified either in units of milliampere-seconds (mAs) per week or milliampere-minutes (mA-min) per week.

World Health Organization The authority that directs and coordinates for health within the United Nations system.

X

X-ray beam limitation device A device that limits the parameters of the useful beam to a designated size and shape before it enters the area of clinical interest.

X-rays (x-ray photons) Electromagnetic radiation that emerges from the anode of an x-ray tube after bombardment by high-speed electrons in a highly evacuated glass tube or from an atom that has experienced a photoelectric interaction.

INDEX

Page numbers followed by "*f*" indicate figures, "*t*" indicate tables, and "*b*" indicate boxes.

Radiation therapy
  blood cell effect during treatment, 136
  orthovoltage, skin damage caused by, 151–152
  radioisotopes used in, 301–303
Radiation warning signs, 296, 296f
Radiation weighting factor (W_R), 68, 120
Radiation workers
  change in employment by, 80–83
  dose limits for, 197–198, 197t
  early medical, carcinogenesis and, 167
  larger equivalent dose allowance for, 275
  life span shortening and, 172–173
  patient safety and, 5–6
  radiation safety and, 3–4
  responsibility for maintaining ALARA and, 6, 8b
Radiationless effect, 46
Radio waves, 17b, 18t
Radioactive contamination, 309
Radioactive decay, 19
Radioactive dispersal device, 309. see also Radiation emergencies
Radiodermatitis, 59–60, 150
Radiographic contrast, photoelectric absorption on, 48–49
Radiographic density, 49f
Radiographic equipment
  diagnostic x-ray, code of standards for, 188–189, 189b
  radiation safety features of, 202–214
    compensating filters, 211, 212f
    control panel, or console, 203
    diagnostic-type protective tube housing, 202–203, 203f
    exposure linearity, 212
    exposure reproducibility, 211–212
    filtration, 208–211
    radiographic examination table, 203
    radiographic grids, 212–214, 213f
    source-to-image receptor distance indicator, 203–204
    usage of screen-film, 212
    x-ray beam limitation devices, 204–208
Radiographic examination table, 203
Radiographic fog, 40–41, 42f, 44, 44f

Radiographic grids, 212–214, 213f
  in computed radiography, 218
Radiographic image receptor, 40
Radiographic imaging
  pediatric considerations during, 251–255
  postprocessing of, quality control program for, 243
Radioisotopes, 19–20, 300–314
  medical usage of, 301–309
    nuclear medicine, 304
    positron emission tomography and computed tomography, 304–305, 306f
    radiation therapy, 301–303
    radioactive materials, handling and disposal of, 303–304
Radiologic technologists. see Radiation workers
Radiologists. see Radiation workers
Radionuclides, 21, 21t, 24
Radiosensitivity
  apoptosis and, 132
  of cells. see Cell, radiosensitivity of
  of children, 10
  embryonic cell
    during first trimester, 174
    during second and third trimester, 174–175
Radium, natural radiation from, 21–22
Radium watch-dial painters, carcinogenesis and, 166
Radon, 21, 21t, 22f–23f
Recessive point mutations, 176
Recoil electron, 50
Record, of radiation exposures, 77–78, 78t
Recovery
  from acute radiation syndrome, 148
  after radiation damage, 150
Red blood cells. see Erythrocytes
Reference values, 12
Regulatory agencies, US, 185–187, 186t
  agreement states, 186
  Environmental Protection Agency (EPA), 186–187
  Food and Drug Administration (FDA), 187
  Nuclear Regulatory Commission (NRC), 185–186
  Occupational Safety and Health Administration (OSHA), 187

Relative biologic effectiveness, 120, 120b
Relative risk models, for cancer, 164, 165f
Rem, 62
Remote control fluoroscopic systems, 286
Repair, after radiation damage, 150
Repair enzymes, 95–96
Repeat exposures, radiographic, result from poor communication, 234–235
Repeat images
  consequences of, 244
  repeat analysis program, benefit of, 244–245, 245b
Repeat rates, in digital radiography, 215–216, 217f
Replication, 111
Reproducibility, 189b, 211–212
Reproductive cells, 101, 111b, 137–138
Reproductive death, as cellular effect of irradiation, 131
Reproductive system, radiation effects on, 152–153, 152f
Restitution, 127–128, 127f
Rhodium filter, 268, 269f
Ribonucleic acid (RNA), 97
  messenger, 99, 100f
  ribosomal, 100
  structure of, 99–102, 100f
  transfer, 99–100
Ribosomal RNA (rRNA), 100
Ribosomes, 99–100, 100f, 106
Risk, 8–9
  concern about, 245
  dose limits and
    embryo-fetus vulnerability, 193
    occupational, 193
    revised concepts of, 193
  occupational, 193
Risk estimates, for cancer, 164–165
  absolute risk and relative risk models for, 164, 164f–165f
  epidemiologic studies for, 164–165
  models for extrapolation of cancer risk from high-dose to low-dose data, 165, 165f
Risk models
  for predicting cancer risk, 161–162, 162f
  for predicting leukemia and breast cancer, 162
  selection of, rationale for, 162